# Biennial Review of Infertility

Douglas T. Carrell • Catherine Racowsky
Peter N. Schlegel • Bradley J. Van Voorhis
Editors

# Biennial Review of Infertility

## Volume 1

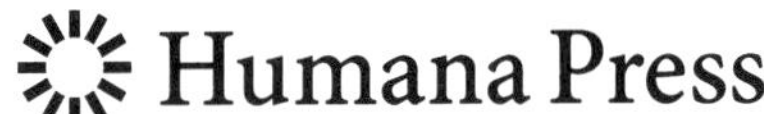

*Editors*
Douglas T. Carrell
University of Utah School of Medicine
IVF and Andrology Laboratories
675 S. Arapeen Dr.
Salt Lake City, UT 84108
Suite 205,
USA

Catherine Racowsky
Harvard Medical School
Brigham & Women's Hospital
Dept. Obstetrics & Gynecology
75 Francis St.
Boston, MA 02115
USA

Peter N. Schlegel
New York Presbyterian Hospital
Weill Cornell Medical Center
Department of Urology
525 East 68th St. Starr 900
New York, NY 10021
USA

Bradley J. Van Voorhis
University of Iowa
Carver College of Medicine
Dept. Obstetrics & Gynecology
200 Hawkins Drive
Iowa City, IA 52242
USA

ISBN: 978-1-60327-391-6 e-ISBN: 978-1-60327-392-3
DOI: 10.1007/978-1-60327-392-3
Springer Dordrecht Heidelberg London New York

Library of Congress Control Number: PCN applied for



Printed on acid-free paper

Springer is part of Springer Science+Business Media (www.springer.com)

*We dedicate this initial volume of Biennial Review of Infertility to William Harvey, Min Cheuh Chang, Robert Edwards, Patrick Steptoe, Howard and Georgeanna Jones, and the many other pioneering clinicians and scientists on whose foundation we continue to build improved care for the infertile couple.*

# Preface

Infertility is a common and profound medical disease. The speed at which our understanding of reproductive medicine grows and new technologies emerge is accelerating and daunting. The objective of this book is to present important and cutting edge topics relevant to infertility in a single volume accessible and applicable to all medical specialties involved in the care of infertile couples. We have strived to select respected, evidence-based experts as authors to present each topic in a clear manner that will benefit both clinicians and scientists.

The nature of science is that hypotheses are tested by experiment, theories are proposed, and validation studies are undertaken. Especially in medical science, study design is often, by necessity, suboptimal and the flow of resulting data may be confusing and conflicting. Therapies may be undertaken without validation, and essential science is delayed by the desire to treat the patient and stay at the cutting edge of the industry. These issues are not unexpected, but may cause confusion and ultimately are not helpful for the infertile couple. Therefore, we have specifically focused each chapter on evidence-based medicine. Despite this strong focus, limitations of our published literature exist. Where such limitations exist, we have endeavored to provide a balanced view of existing information that is clinically relevant for the evolving areas of our specialty. Additionally, we have introduced a section highlighting emerging controversies in the field of reproductive medicine in which contrasting points of view are presented. It is our hope that this section will stimulate further studies to improve understanding of the topics presented.

During clinical evaluation and therapy, an infertile couple will likely interact with a variety of health care professionals, including gynecologists, reproductive endocrinologists, urologists, andrologists, embryologists, laboratory technicians, nurses, and therapists. Indeed, appropriate patient care rests on effective communication and collaboration among such a team of experts. It has been our pleasure, as co-editors of this book, to work together as a diverse group of specialists to bring together the topics discussed herein. Our aim is that this book can act as a biennial tool to provide an ongoing appraisal of current knowledge, and to foster communication and collaboration among all those working to help couples resolve their infertility.

Salt Lake City, UT, USA — Douglas T. Carrell
Boston, MA, USA — Catherine Racowsky
New York, NY, USA — Peter N. Schlegel
Iowa City, IA, USA — Bradley J. Van Voorhis

# Contents

# Contributors

**David F. Albertini, PhD**
Department of Molecular and Integrative Physiology, Center for Reproductive Sciences, Kansas University Medical Center, Kansas City, KS, USA

**Amr A. Azim, MD, MSc, DSc, FACOG**
Department of Obstetrics and Gynecology, The Center for Reproductive Medicine & Infertility Associates, Weill-Cornell Medical College, New York, NY, USA

**Victor E. Beshay, MD**
Department of Obstetrics and Gynecology, University of Texas at Southwestern Medical Center, Dallas, TX, USA

**John J. Bromfield, PhD**
Department of Molecular and Integrative Physiology, Center for Reproductive Sciences, Kansas University Medical Center, Kansas City, KS, USA

**Bruce R. Carr, MD**
Department of Obstetrics and Gynecology, University of Texas at Southwestern Medical Center, Dallas, TX, USA

**Sandra Carson, MD**
Division of Reproductive Endocrinology and Infertility, Women and Infants Hospital, Warren Alpert Medical School of Brown University, Providence, RI, USA

**S. Temel Ceyhan, MD**
Department of Obstetrics and Gynecology, Brigham and Women's Hospital, Harvard Medical School, Boston, MA, USA

**Catherine M. H. Combelles, PhD**
Biology Department, Middlebury College, Middlebury, VT, USA

**Victoria K. Cortessis, PhD**
Department of Preventative Medicine and Norris Comprehensive Cancer Center, Keck School of Medicine, University of Southern California, Los Angeles, CA, USA

**John M. Csokmay, MD**
National Institute of Child Health and Human Development, National Institutes of Health, Bethesda, MD, USA

**Owen K. Davis, MD, FACOG**
Department of Obstetrics and Gynecology, The Center for Reproductive Medicine & Infertility Associates, Weill-Cornell Medical College, New York, NY, USA

**Alan H. DeCherney, MD**
National Institute of Child Health and Human Development, National Institutes of Health, Bethesda, MD, USA

**Anuja Dokras, MD, PhD**
Department of Obstetrics and Gynecology, University of Pennsylvania, Philadelphia, PA, USA

**Harry Fisch, MD**
Department of Urology, Columbia University Medical Center, New York, NY, USA

**Victor Y. Fujimoto, MD**
Department of Obstetrics, Gynecology, and Reproductive Sciences, University of California at San Francisco School of Medicine, San Francisco, CA, USA

**Jan Gerris, MD, PhD**
Center for Reproductive Medicine, Women's Clinic, Ghent University Hospital, Ghent, Belgium

**Linda C. Giudice, MD, PhD, MSc**
Department of Obstetrics, Gynecology, and Reproductive Sciences, University of California at San Francisco School of Medicine, San Francisco, CA, USA

**Alan H. Handyside, PhD**
The London Bridge Fertility, Gynaecology and Genetics Centre, and Bridge Genoma, London, UK

**Katharine V. Jackson, MD**
Department of Obstetrics and Gynecology, Brigham and Women's Hospital, Harvard Medical School, Boston, MA, USA

**Katie L. Jones, BS**
Department of Molecular and Integrative Physiology, Center for Reproductive Sciences, Kansas University Medical Center, Kansas City, KS, USA

**Stephan Krotz, MD**
Division of Reproductive Endocrinology and Infertility, Women and Infants Hospital, Warren Alpert Medical School of Brown University, Providence, RI, USA

**Anver Kuliev, MD, PhD**
Reproductive Genetics Institute, Chicago, IL, USA

**Dolores J. Lamb, PhD**
Scott Department of Urology and Department of Molecular and Cellular Biology, Baylor College of Medicine, Houston, TX, USA

**Joel L. Marmar, MD**
Department of Urology, UMDNJ, Robert Wood Johnson School of Medicine, Camden, NJ, USA

**Sebastiaan Mastenbroek, MSc**
Center for Reproductive Medicine, University of Amsterdam, Meibergdreef, Amsterdam, The Netherlands

**Tetsunori Mukaida, PhD**
HART Clinic, Ohtemachi, Naka-ku, Hiroshima, Japan

**Kutluk Oktay, MD**
Institute for Fertility Preservation, Center for Human Reproduction, NY, and Department of Obstetrics & Gynecology, New York Medical College-Westchester Medical Center, Valhalla, NY

**Ozgur Oktem, MD**
Institute for Fertility Preservation, Center for Human Reproduction, NY, and Department of Obstetrics & Gynecology, New York Medical College-Westchester Medical Center, Valhalla, NY

**Satin S. Patel, MD**
Department of Obstetrics and Gynecology, University of Texas at Southwestern Medical Center, Dallas, TX, USA

**Samantha M. Pfeifer, MD**
Department of Obstetrics and Gynecology, University of Pennsylvania Medical Center, Philadelphia, PA, USA

**Catherine Racowsky, PhD**
Department of Obstetrics and Gynecology, Brigham and Women's Hospital, Harvard Medical School, Boston, MA, USA

**Vanessa Y. Rawe, PhD**
Center of Studies in Gynecology and Reproduction (CEGyR), Buenos Aires, Argentina

**Sjoerd Repping, PhD**
Center for Reproductive Medicine, University of Amsterdam, Meibergdreef, Amsterdam, The Netherlands

**Glenn L. Schattman, MD**
Department of Reproductive Medicine, Weill Medical College of Cornell University, New York, NY, USA

**Peter N. Schlegel, MD, PhD**
Department of Urology, Weill Cornell Medical College, New York, NY, USA

**Petra De Sutter, PhD**
Center for Reproductive Medicine, University Hospital, Ghent, Belgium

**Mounia Tannour-Louet, PhD**
Scott Department of Urology, Baylor College of Medicine, Houston, TX, USA

**Alan R. Thornhill, PhD**
The London Bridge Fertility, Gynaecology and Genetics Centre, and Bridge Genoma, London, UK

**Fulco Van der Veen, MD, PhD**
Center for Reproductive Medicine, University of Amsterdam, Meibergdreef, Amsterdam, The Netherlands

**Yury Verlinsky, PhD**
Reproductive Genetics Institute, Chicago, IL, USA

**Matthew Wosnitzer, MD**
Department of Urology, Columbia University Medical Center, New York, NY, USA

# Section I
# Female Infertility

# Environmental Factors Affecting Female Infertility

Victor Y. Fujimoto and Linda C. Giudice

**Abstract** There is increasing concern about the effects of environmental contaminants on reproductive health. While there are limited clinical data regarding most chemical exposures and human reproduction, studies in laboratory animal models and wildlife underscore the vulnerability of the reproductive system to many environmental insults at different times of development and across the life cycle. Here, we review data implicating select environmental contaminants in compromised reproductive capacity in animals. We also review epidemiologic data in humans that suggest roles for environmental contaminants in reproductive dysfunction and infertility.

**Keywords** Environmental contaminants • Reproduction • Organic and inorganic exposures • Embryo toxicity • Oocyte toxicity

## 1 Introduction

The emerging research area of environmental and reproductive health is gaining increasing attention in the scientific and medical communities, as well as patient advocacy groups, as there is an escalation of studies citing the adverse effects of environmental exposures on human and mammalian reproduction (1–4). Several environmental chemicals that display endocrine-disrupting potential have been shown to demonstrate alterations in hormone signaling and effects on reproductive tract development and function in vivo and in vitro (5). Many environmental chemicals are inadvertantly introduced into the human system by normal daily living activities through food, water, air, personal care products, toys, infant teethers, dental sealants, and the like. For example, patients who consume higher amounts of seafood are at increased risk for the bioaccumulation of methyl mercury and polychlorinated biphenyls (PCBs) (6, 7). These and other chemicals discussed in this chapter are ubiquitous in the environment and are present in fish, wildlife, human adipose tissue, blood, and breast milk. One clear example of reproductive toxicity involves mercury. Administration of methyl mercury adversely affects the embryo viability in pregnant mice with a subsequent reduction in litter sizes (8). There are other examples of compromised embryonic development and blastocyst formation in animal models where oocytes and embryos are exposed in vitro to concentrations of PCBs, dichlorodiphenyltrichloroethane (DDT), hexachlorocyclohexane (HCH), and methoxychlor (MXC) (9–11).

While there are many classes of environmental contaminants, here we focus on the effects of smoking, pesticides, heavy metals, and a variety of other chemicals on mammalian gametogenesis and embryogenesis, as well as human clinical/epidemiologic reproductive outcomes. Where possible, we also discuss biologic mechanisms regulating these effects. There is a broad body of literature detailing environmental contamination and reproduction in avian and amphibian models, which is not included in this chapter but is available for review (12–14). Fecundity and early embryo risk are discussed; however, issues around pregnancy and birth outcome risks are not included in this chapter, as they have been comprehensively reviewed (15). In addition, the scope of effects from environmental exposures in

V.Y. Fujimoto (✉) and L.C. Giudice
Department of Obstetrics, Gynecology, and Reproductive Sciences, University of California at San Francisco, San Francisco, CA, 94115, USA
e-mail: fujimotov@obgyn.ucsf.edu

D.T. Carrell et al. (eds.), *Biennial Review of Infertility*, DOI: 10.1007/978-1-60327-392-3_1

female reproductive health and disease, i.e., endocrine disruption, gynecologic disorders, and pregnancy outcomes, is substantial and have been the subject of several recent comprehensive reviews (1–3). All the sections included here were developed through the specific environmental exposure of interest and include exposures during different developmental/adult life stages with the following categories of exposure: (1) cigarette smoking and polycyclic aromatic hydrocarbons; (2) agricultural and residential pesticides; (3) inorganic heavy metals; (4) bisphenol A; (5) polychlorinated and polybrominated biphenyl compounds; (6) DDT and DDE; and (7) dioxins. The final section discusses our current understanding of the role of the aryl hydrocarbon receptor (AhR) as a mediator of halogenated aromatic hydrocarbon contaminant effects in mammalian reproduction.

## 2 Cigarette Smoking and Polycyclic Aromatic Hydrocarbons

One in three adults smokes cigarettes (16). The demographic distribution of cigarette smokers varies widely, with the highest percentage of cigarette smokers in Europe and Asia. The environmental contaminants identified in cigarette smoke number approximately 4,000 chemical compounds (17). Cigarette smoking has long been known to induce changes in reproductive function, with effects on both oocytes and embryos. While there are behavioral changes in women that occur once they identify themselves to be pregnant, including cessation of smoking, many women remain relatively unaware of the negative impact that cigarette smoking can have on their and their offspring's reproductive health. Several epidemiologic studies and reviews have demonstrated a clear association between smoking and reduced fecundity (18–20). The time to pregnancy (TTP) is consistently delayed in smokers compared to nonsmokers (21). The American Society of Reproductive Medicine has produced a patient fact sheet on smoking and infertility and practice guidelines with a position statement on smoking and reduced fecundity, discouraging smoking in women who are considering pregnancy or attempting to conceive (22). Several systematic reviews and meta-analyses of the literature on smoking and infertility have been published, which provide a consistent negative association between female cigarette smoking exposure and fertility potential (22–24). Ex-smokers appear to have a similar fecundity rate, compared to nonsmokers, suggesting that active exposure to chemicals in cigarette smoke during the follicular phase and/or luteal phase of the menstrual cycle inhibits normal reproductive processes (19). Further evidence of the negative association of cigarette smoking by females on reproductive results comes from in vitro fertilization (IVF) data (25–29). Zenzes et al. found an increased proportion of diploid oocytes recovered during IVF and a decreased proportion of mature oocytes with cigarette smoking (29, 30). There may also be contributing endometrial dysfunction as demonstrated by Soares et al., who showed that lower pregnancy rates were associated with heavy cigarette smoking in an oocyte donation–recipient model (31). A recent study found that women exposed to secondary cigarette smoke also have lower IVF pregnancy outcomes, similar to women who smoke cigarettes directly (32). A comprehensive review of the effects of smoking on human gametes and embryos has recently been published (33).

There is also evidence that women who smoke cigarettes have an increased risk of spontaneous miscarriage (23, 34, 35). However, other studies have not clearly demonstrated an association between cigarette-smoking and risk of spontaneous abortion (36–40). In addition to the risk of spontaneous miscarriage, multiple studies have demonstrated an increased risk of ectopic pregnancy associated with active cigarette smoking (41–44). Mechanistically, tubal motility and ciliary function have been implicated as targets of cigarette contaminant exposures (45–49).

Cumulative evidence suggests mechanisms underlying adverse actions of the chemicals in cigarette smoke on ovarian, tubal, and endometrial function. One of the challenges in understanding the biologic mechanism of cigarette smoking on reproductive processes is the large number of chemicals found therein. While many of the chemicals have been poorly studied, one constituent of cigarette smoke that has been well studied is cotinine, a stable metabolite of nicotine. Cotinine levels in humans correlate strongly with tobacco consumption (50). Both cotinine and cadmium levels have been detected in human follicular fluid (FF), with higher levels in smokers than in nonsmokers (51–53). Additionally, other toxins known to exist in cigarette smoke include the class of compounds known as polycyclic aromatic hydrocarbons (PAHs) (54). PAH compounds of interest include 9,10-dimethylbenzanthracene (DMBA), 3-methylcholanthrene (3-MC), and benzo[*a*]pyrene (BaP) (see Fig. 1). BaP exposure reduces litter size and decreased survival of fetal pups in a dose-dependent fashion (55, 56). PAH compounds affect granulosa cell function and have been indirectly associated with the development of a variety of ovarian tumors (57–59). BaP levels and DNA adduct formation have been detected in luteinized granulosa cells recovered from IVF FF and correlate with cotinine levels, suggesting an increased risk in granulosa cell DNA damage with cigarette smoking (60). Various polymorphisms in metabolic genes, including CYP1A1 and GSTT1, have been associated with differences in fetal birth weight restriction associated with cigarette smoking (60).

The most profound effect of PAHs via cigarette smoking on female reproduction may be the decline in ovarian reserve associated with its exposure. This observation is consistent with the association of cigarette smoking with an earlier age at menopause (61–63). Sharara et al. described diminished ovarian reserves in women who smoke cigarettes on the basis of abnormal clomiphene challenge testing (64). Several studies have confirmed an association between cigarette smoking and elevated basal follicle-stimulating hormone (FSH) levels independent of age (65–67). DMBA, 3-MC, and BaP were all found to be ovotoxic, resulting in significant destruction of primordial and primary follicles in mice and rats (68–71). Mechanistically, there is evidence that PAH-induced reduction of primordial follicles operates via the AhR-regulated Bax expression (72, 73). That said, it is not yet clear whether ovarian antral follicle pools are diminished in humans in response to cigarette smoking when adjusted for maternal age (67, 74). Ovarian response, defined by the numbers of mature oocytes retrieved, appears to be less in cigarette smokers than nonsmokers, although age-adjusted correlations were not performed (26). Collectively, the

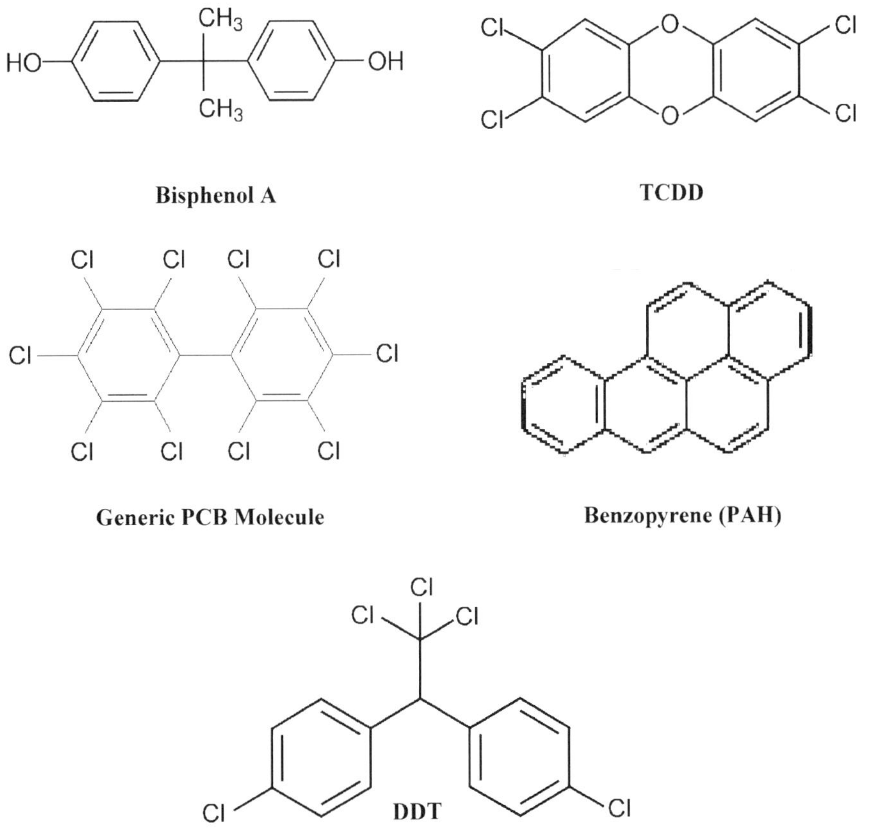

HO — CH3 — CH3 — OH

**Bisphenol A**

Cl Cl O O Cl Cl

**TCDD**

Cl Cl Cl Cl Cl Cl Cl Cl Cl Cl

**Generic PCB Molecule**

**Benzopyrene (PAH)**

Cl Cl Cl Cl Cl

**DDT**

**Fig. 1** Organic chemicals ubiquitous in the environment and responsible for reproductive effects

evidence in the literature points toward a negative impact of cigarette smoking on ovarian aging processes.

The Barker hypothesis proposes that in utero fetal exposures to nutritional (and by extrapolation, environmental) contaminants can manifest in adult life as clinical disease or altered state of health (75–77). This hypothesis with regard to environmental contaminants is supported by the recent study by Jurisicova et al., in which a decrease in the fetal ovarian follicle pool exposed to PAHs during gestation was observed and demonstrated to be via activation of the cellular apoptotic pathway mediated by the AhR (78). Furthermore, xenotransplanted human ovaries responded to PAHs similarly (78). These observations are consistent with the reduced fecundity seen in women exposed in utero to maternal cigarette smoking (79).

## 3 Agricultural and Residential Pesticide Exposures

Considerable attention has been given to the possibility that heavy pesticide exposure may cause increased reproductive difficulties. Numerous studies have addressed a possible relationship between agricultural and household pesticide use and the risk of spontaneous abortion. Although the data to date are inconclusive with regard to an association of pesticide exposures and increased risk of spontaneous abortion (80–89), a study by Greenlee et al. suggests an association between direct mixing and application of pesticides by reproductive-aged women and their likelihood of infertility within two years of direct contact with pesticides (90).

Biologic evidence has been provided implicating pesticides in affecting early embryogenesis in a study where six herbicides (atrazine, dicamba, metolachlor, 2,4-dichlorophenoxyacetic acid (2,4-D), pendimethalin, and mecoprop), three insecticides (chlorpyrifos, terbufos, and permethrin), and two fungicides (chlorothalonil and mancozeb) in combination or sometimes individually adversely affected the development of murine blastocyst embryos (91). In the early 1990s, studies demonstrated that carbendazim, the active metabolite of benomyl, a systemic benzimidazole fungicide that was banned in the United States in 2002, had direct effects on the meiotic spindle assembly of the murine oocyte. Perreault et al. found an increase in preimplantation and postimplantation pregnancy losses after acute carbendazim exposure in female hamsters during the proestrus period (92). As a result of further investigation into the etiology of this infertility causation, Zuelke and Perreault subsequently demonstrated that carbendazim induced meiotic arrest within the oocytes (93). Jeffay et al. further elucidated the carbendazim effect by inducing an arrest of preimplantation development of murine embryos to the blastocyst stage with acute carbendazim exposure in the female hamster during the proestrus–estrus transition (94). Can and Albertini were able to interrupt the meiotic spindle assembly of murine oocytes using a benzimidazole derivative, methyl 2-benzimidazolecarbamate, lending further evidence to its mechanism of action (95). While benomyl was banned from use in California in 2002, there is evidence of the persistence of carbendazim in human FF in women undergoing IVF (Fujimoto, unpublished data).

In 1993, a case–control study assessing a cluster of Down syndrome infants with an incidence of 27% in a small Hungarian village suggested trichlorfon insecticide exposure as the etiology (96). Apparently, a high consumption of fish contaminated with trichlorfon around the time of conception was associated with high meiotic II error rates, increased miscarriage, and Down syndrome offspring in exposed individuals. Yin et al. subsequently confirmed in mouse in vitro matured oocytes that trichlorfon adversely affects normal spindle formation during meiosis (97). Recent evidence suggests that pesticides can influence aromatase activity in the human choriocarcinoma JEG-3 cell line (98). These examples illustrate the potential sensitivity of the mammalian oocyte, surrounding cumulus cells, and the early embryo to pesticide exposures and lend biologic plausibility to adverse effects on human gametes and embryos.

## 4 Inorganic Heavy Metal Exposures

There are only a few studies on the effects of toxic heavy metals (arsenic (As), cadmium (Cd), lead (Pb), and mercury (Hg)) on mammalian reproduction. Several animal and human studies have linked Hg exposure to reproductive toxicity. Hg has been shown to be embryotoxic in animal studies (8, 99). In addition, it has been linked to an increased risk of spontaneous abortion and birth defects (100). Some studies of male infertility have demonstrated the potential effects of Hg on human seminiferous epithelium in the testis, but the data are controversial (101). Relatively few studies on Hg and female infertility have been published. Rowland et al. found decreased fertility among female dental assistants exposed to Hg vapor (102). In another study in Hong Kong, infertile Asian couples undergoing IVF were found to have significantly higher blood Hg concentrations than the control group and these higher concentrations were associated with higher seafood consumption (103).

There are several environmental sources of Hg, but the aquatic food chain is an important source of bioaccumulation. Seafood intake has been shown to contribute to the bodily accumulation of Hg, and Hg consumption is considered a health risk. The Environmental Protection Agency and the National Research Council recommend blood Hg levels <5.0 μg/L or hair level <1.0 μg/g (104). Populations that have a high intake of fish are at particular risk of Hg exposure, including the Nunavik Inuit communities residing in Northern Quebec and residents of the Faroe Islands and New Zealand, which has raised concerns over childhood neurodevelopmental delay in those populations (105–108). A San Francisco-based study found that patients with diets high in commercial fish consumption had blood Hg levels that far exceeded these recommended levels (7). Recently published data of the National Health and Nutrition Examination Surveys (NHANES) reveal that Asians and Pacific Islanders have significantly higher Hg than other ethnicities surveyed (109, 110), indicating that they are potentially at greater risk to the reproductive toxic effects of methyl Hg.

In addition to Hg in fish, there are high levels of Cd in cigarette smoke and Pb, Hg, and As contamination of herbal products from Asia (111–114). A specific example of herbal product contamination is ginseng extracts, of which 80% were found to have detectable levels of various pesticides and benzene derivatives (111). A case of Pb poisoning has recently been reported as a direct result of herbal product consumption during infertility treatment (115). It is currently not clear whether detectable exposures of toxic metals such as As, Pb, Hg, and Cd have deleterious effects on human reproduction. These heavy metals have all been detected in human FF (116–118). A recent IVF-based study assessing Cd, Pb, and Hg levels found a negative association between lead levels and fertilization outcomes but no effects were seen with Hg or Cd (116). There is evidence that both As and Cd adversely affect murine blastocyst development with increased apoptotic changes possibly via oxidative stress mechanisms (119–123). It should be noted, however, that further studies are needed to clarify the roles of various heavy metals in female reproduction.

## 5 Bisphenol A Exposure

Bisphenol A (BPA) is gaining considerable attention as an environmental chemical that may have adverse effects on human health and disease. The chemical name of bisphenol A is 2,2-bis(4-hydroxyphenyl) propane (see Fig. 1) (124). BPA is produced in large quantities (more than £6 billion per year) for incorporation into various resins and plastics (e.g., polycarbonate) (124). The exposure to BPA is ubiquitous, penetrating many aspects of daily living primarily through dietary consumption. A consensus statement was issued in 2007 by the Chapel Hill Bisphenol A expert panel on the relationship between BPA and human health effects (124). BPA has been shown to have endocrine-disrupting effects through steroid receptor binding. BPA binds with weak affinity to the nuclear estrogen receptor, although recent evidence suggests it may act to induce physiologic responses through cell membrane estrogen receptors in low picogram per milliliter concentrations (125). In humans, serum BPA levels have been measured within the nanogram per milliliter range (126, 127). Urinary concentrations of BPA have been measured in the microgram per liter range (128, 129). There is currently a debate as to whether the low exposure levels of BPA in humans have significant reproductive biologic effects (125, 130, 131).

The adverse female reproductive effects of BPA exposure have been described primarily on meiotic aberrations in the oocyte. Studies are based for the most part on mammalian models with little clinical evidence thus far available. There are currently four studies that detail our current understanding of BPA effects on oocyte nuclear health. In 2000, Takai et al. published their work on the effects of BPA on early embryo development (132). Two-cell mouse embryos were cultured with BPA with or without tamoxifen, a selective estrogen receptor modulator, and evaluated for blastocyst advancement. At 100 μM concentration of BPA, decreased blastocyst formation was observed and negation of the effect in the presence of tamoxifen, suggesting an estrogen receptor–mediated effect. At nanomolar concentrations of BPA, the opposite effect was seen with increased murine blastocyst formation.

Several studies have demonstrated that BPA interferes with microtubule assembly in the cultured Chinese hamster lung V79 cell line (133, 134). A direct link between BPA and murine aneuploidy was first reported by Hunt and colleagues (135). In this landmark study published in 2003, a dramatic increase from 1–2% to 40% was observed in chromosomal alignment defects in the first meiotic spindle. Furthermore, a high rate of aneuploidy (hyperploidy) was also observed in these animals. This increase was ultimately traced and attributed to the leaching of BPA from water bottles and damaged cages in which the female mice were housed during the final stages of oocyte maturation. Thus, in adult female mice completing their estrus cycles, an association between BPA exposure and meotic spindle abnormalities in their oocytes was demonstrated.

Further study of the effects of BPA on meiotic cell cycle progression was reported by Can et al. in 2005 (136) who found that mouse cumulus–oocyte complexes exposed to BPA exhibited a dose-dependent delay in the transition of oocytes from metaphase I to metaphase II. Fluorescent-labeling of oocytes with $\alpha$ + ß-tubulin and pericentrin, together with confocal imaging of the in vitro matured oocytes exposed to BPA, revealed disturbed microtubular spindle structure and pericentriolar compaction and dispersion, compared to control oocytes. In addition, the absence of chromosomes in the first polar body was commonly seen in the BPA-treated oocytes. The doses of BPA required to disrupt the meiotic spindle assembly in oocytes are lower than those required to disrupt the mitotic spindle assembly of Chinese hamster V79 cells (133, 134, 136). Can and Semiz previously demonstrated that diethylstilbestrol, a synthetic estrogen, also disrupted the progression of metaphase I oocytes to metaphase II, with fragmentation and loosening of the meiotic spindle assembly (137). BPA also induces apoptosis in murine ovarian granulosa cells. In addition, the alkylphenol, *p*-tert-octylphenol, which has endocrine-disrupting properties via the estrogen receptor, reduces bovine oocyte nuclear maturation, thereby preventing meiotic progression (138).

Perhaps the most intriguing study thus far with respect to the role BPA on oocyte integrity was published in 2007 by Susiarjo et al., in which murine fetal oocytes exposed to BPA during gestation were similarly found to have abnormal pachytene associations and abnormalities in synaptonemal complex structure, compared to unexposed murine fetal oocytes, as determined by MLH1 and SCP3 immunostaining (139). Similar to PAHs from cigarette smoking, this observation lends further support to the Barker hypothesis that in utero exposures may influence future reproductive outcomes. These data would suggest that there may be a transgenerational impact of BPA exposure in utero. Furthermore, when oocytes of 4–5 week-old pups exposed to BPA were analyzed, there was a higher rate of aneuploidy; specifically, about 40% of all oocytes were aneuploid, compared to an unexposed rate of 1.8% (139). The proposed mechanism for the effect of BPA on altering the synaptonemal complex of murine fetal oocytes, offered by these investigators, involves the estrogen receptor ß as a potential site of interaction with BPA, or at least a final common pathway for disruption. This is based on a similar meiotic phenotype in prophase fetal oocytes of ßERKO–/– mice with similar rates of synaptonemal aberrations (57%), compared to those of the BPA-exposed female murine fetus (52%).

While these murine studies collectively provide substantial evidence towards a BPA-induced effect on oogenesis and increased meiotic errors at various stages of oocyte nuclear maturation, there is little evidence to support this concept in humans. The only published clinical study comes from Japan, in which 45 patients with a history of three or more first trimester miscarriages without uterine anomaly or blood karyotype abnormality (study group) and 32 healthy non-pregnant women without prior pregnancy loss (control group) underwent serum BPA testing (140). Mean serum BPA levels were higher in the study group compared to the control group (2.59 vs. 0.77 ng/mL, $P = 0.024$), showing that serum BPA is associated with recurrent miscarriage (140). However, the limitations of this study include the short half-life of BPA that can result in substantial variability of BPA measurements, the lack of timing of BPA measurements within relevant biologic timeframes (such as during the lutenizing hormone (LH) surge when BPA exposure is most likely to affect the meiotic transition from metaphase I to metaphase II), the statistical methodology used, and the different demographics utilized for recruitment of patients and control subjects. Thus, it is currently not known to what extent BPA exposures affect human oocyte health, despite compelling murine studies. Clearly, well-designed studies are needed to establish with confidence an association of BPA exposure with aneuploidy risk and reduced reproductive potential in women.

## 6 Polychlorinated and Polybrominated Biphenyl Compound Exposures

This category of environmental toxins represents a broad family of various industrial contaminants that include PCB compounds, polychlorinated dibenzo-*p*-dioxins (PCDDs), and polychlorinated dibenzofurans (PCDFs). These chemicals are ubiquitous and persistent in the environment because of their chemical stability, lipophilic character, and low water solubility (141). Although banned from production in most countries in the 1970s, PCBs have received increasing attention as environmental contaminants of relevance to reproductive outcomes. The food chain is the primary source of human contamination with 209 congeners of these halogenated aromatic hydrocarbon compounds (see Fig. 1) (142). Because of their lipophilic nature, bioaccumulation occurs within an organism, which is magnified in each predator. PCB congeners are classified by the United States Environmental Protection Agency as probable human carcinogens of medium carcinogenic hazard. The first report of PCBs causing reproductive harm came from a study based in the Wassen Sea, Netherlands, in which a decline in the seal population was traced to reduced litters because of PCB and DDE contamination (143). Human consumption of sport-caught fish provides high exposure to PCB congeners (144, 145) and results in measurable levels of PCBs in serum and urine (146–149). Maternal serum PCB concentrations have been documented during critical windows of development including the periconception interval and early pregnancy (150). PCB levels are detectable within the human FF (151–155). A study originating from the New York Angler Cohort in the Great Lakes area demonstrated an association between maternal fish consumption and reduced fecundability (156). However, other studies have not revealed associations between maternal fish consumption and time-to-pregnancy (TTP) outcomes in areas with high PCB exposures (144, 157, 158). Given the well-documented contamination of the Great Lakes ecosystem by PCBs, dioxins, heavy metals, and pesticides, it has been hypothesized that the observations made about maternal fish consumption and increased TTP may be causally related to exposures to these various toxins (159).

Cohort studies assessing the risk of spontaneous miscarriage have found no associations with PCB exposures (160–162), and there are no studies addressing PCB exposures and reproductive outcomes within an infertile population. PCBs have also been implicated as a cause of fetal growth restriction identified with maternal contaminated fish consumption (163, 164). Beyond these limited studies focusing on fecundity and maternal fish consumption, no other evidence exists in epidemiologic studies to support the effect of contaminated fish consumption and poor reproductive potential.

Polybrominated biphenyl compounds (PBBs) are structurally similar to PCBs, except for a bromine substitution. In 1973, PBBs entered the human food chain in the United States via meat and dairy products inadvertently contaminated with PBBs (165). By recruiting exposed women identified through a registry, there was no increased risk of spontaneous abortions in women with PBB levels above 6.5 ppb, compared to women below the limit of detection (166). Associations between PBBs and infertility await further investigation.

Several studies in mammalian models demonstrate effects of PCBs on ovarian function, oogenesis, and embryogenesis. Some studies have demonstrated a disruption of both estrus and menstrual cycles (167–170). Kholkute et al. demonstrated that several PCB mixtures negatively affect the fertilizability of murine oocytes (171–173). Pocar et al. demonstrated disruption of bovine oocyte maturation with PCB exposures as low as 0.01 mg/mL and impaired fertilization and increased polyspermy at 0.001 mg/mL (174). The PCB, 3,3′,4,4′-tetrachlorobiphenyl, was also found to decrease fertilization potential in murine oocytes when female mice were fed a diet containing the PCB, tetrachloro-biphenyl (TCB), within two weeks of pairing (175). Pocar et al. also showed a dose-dependent effect on reduced bovine blastocyst formation from PCB exposures (174). Effects of organochlorine compounds on in vitro porcine oocyte maturation, fertilization, and early embryonic development (10) reveal that when cumulus oocyte complexes (COCs) are isolated, matured, fertilized, and cultured in the presence of various concentrations of an organochlorine mixture that includes the PCBs, Aroclor 1260, Aroclor 1254, PCB 126, and 3,3′, 4,4′-tetrachlorobiphenyl among other non-PCB compounds, there is marked functional disruption. These include dose-dependently reduced cumulus expansion and decreased blastocyst formation (10). A 20% reduction in blastocyst formation was also noted in female rabbits given the PCB, Aroclor 1260, three times a week at 4 mg/kg body weight dosage (176). Low concentrations (1 pg/mL range) of Aroclor 1254 disturbed bovine oocyte fertilization with increased polyspermy and reduced blastocyst formation (174). In the in vitro matured bovine oocyte model, subsequent blastocyst formation was reduced using PCB 126 in exposures ranging from 1 to 100 pg/mL (11). Thus, there is clear evidence in various mammalian models that oocyte competence and early embryo development can be compromised by exposure to PCBs.

While the mechanisms responsible for these observed effects of PCBs on early embryo development are unknown, there is evidence that PCBs have proinflammatory properties that increase oxidative stress via the AhR (177–180). There is evidence that PCB-like compounds act via the AhR, a ligand-activated transcription factor, to affect murine ovarian weight and ovarian cyclicity (181, 182). However, Schmidt et al. identified AhR –/– mice to be fertile without compromised reproduction, raising the question of whether PCB effects on reproduction are mediated via other mechanisms (183). Further evidence against a role for the AhR being involved in the embryotoxic effect of PCBs is provided by Kietz and Fischer, who demonstrated changes in rabbit blastocyst gene expression changes independent of AhR expression after exposure to PCBs (184).

## 7 DDT and DDE Exposures

1,1,1-Trichloro-2,2-bis(*p*-chlorophenyl)ethane (DDT) is an insecticide that is metabolized to 1,1-dichloro-2,2-bis(*p*-chlorophenyl)ethylene (DDE) – a persistent organochlorine pollutant (see Fig. 1) (185). Although banned in the United States in 1972, the scope and persistence of these compounds in our environment are underscored by the finding that DDT and DDE comprise 84% of the analyzed pesticide concentrations in the surface sediment layer (70 cm) of San Francisco Bay (186). This buildup clearly represents the legacy left behind by the substantial utilization of DDT from the mid-1940s through the mid-1970s as an agricultural pesticide in California. Similar to PCB exposures, DDT and DDE were present in the serum and urine of pregnant women from the San Francisco Bay area participating in the Child Health and Development Study of California (146–149, 187). Also similar to PCBs, DDT and DDE are lipophilic, slowly metabolized chemicals that accumulate in human adipose tissue (188). The persistent nature of DDE in humans is demonstrated by studies that show similar levels of DDE compared to those conducted 30 years earlier (189, 190). In a study based in Ontario, Canada, approximately 50% of IVF patients had detectable levels of DDE in serum and FF with mean levels considerably higher than any PCBs (155). In the San Francisco Bay area population, all IVF patients tested had detectable levels of FF DDE (Fujimoto, unpublished data).

DDE exposure is associated with an increased risk of spontaneous abortion (189, 191, 192). Korrick et al. found a positive association between serum DDE levels and spontaneous abortion in this case–control study, but this study was limited by the variable time frame of blood collection from the index pregnancy outcome (189). Sera from pregnant women in the Collaborative Perinatal Project from 1959 to 1965 were tested for DDE and related to prior spontaneous miscarriage history, adjusted for age, race, and smoking, with DDE levels ranging from 0 to 60 mg/L (191). An increased serum DDE level was positively associated with a fetal loss history but was limited also by the retrospective history of pregnancy loss (191). Venners et al. published a prospective study in a Chinese population of reproductive-aged, newly married women (192). Daily urine samples were collected and measured for DDT and human chorionic gonadotropin (hCG) levels, which revealed an exposure–response association between preconception DDT levels and subsequent early pregnancy losses (192). However, DDE and TTP studies have not consistently revealed differences in fecundity as a result of DDE exposures (193, 194). By Pearson correlation analysis, Younglai et al. demonstrated a negative association between serum and FF levels of DDE and IVF fertilization, but no effect was found on pregnancy outcomes (155). In a small cohort, higher serum DDE levels in women undergoing IVF were associated with reduced pregnancy rates (but not significant likely due to a lack of power) (195). An interesting study published in 2003 demonstrated reduced fecundability in daughters of mothers who were exposed during pregnancy to high levels of DDT and DDE between 1960 and 1963, suggesting an in utero effect of this endocrine disruptor on the fetal reproductive axis, similar to BPA (196).

A biologic mechanism for the effects of DDT and its metabolite, DDE, on reproductive potential remains elusive. However, studies on the effects of DDE on granulosa cells suggest endocrine-disrupting properties. DDE decreases steroidogenesis in luteinized granulosa cells but increases VEGF and IGF-1 expression in the ovarian follicle (197–200). Incubation of murine embryos with low doses of DDT reduces the growth of early stage embryos and subsequent blastocyst development, with increased apoptosis (201). A similar observation was made in bovine embryos exposed to DDT, with a reduction in blastocyst formation (9). This effect of DDT on murine blastocyst development was reversed by the addition of an estrogen receptor antagonist (202). However, a subsequent study did not reveal any effect on implantation rates or number of pups per dam after incubation of murine embryos with DDT (203). It is possible that the negative effects of DDT and DDE on early embryogenesis may be acting via oxidative stress pathways (204, 205).

## 8 Dioxin Exposures

Dioxins represent a class of organic chemicals that are structurally related to PCBs (see Fig. 1). Similar to PAHs and PCBs, dioxins are believed to activate AhR ligands with downstream gene activation and expression (206). The clinical evidence for dioxin exposure and reproductive health comes mainly from the Seveso Women's Health Study, which studied an Italian village population north of Milan exposed to high levels of 2,3,7,8-tetrachlorodibenzo-*p*-dioxin (TCDD) from a chemical plant explosion that released ~30 kg of TCDD into the atmosphere in 1976 (207). The measurable serum levels of TCDD in Seveso residents ranged from 2.5 to 56,000 ppt, with a background nonexposed level of 20 ppt (208). Unintended human exposures to TCDD generally occur via consumption of contaminated food products and air inhalation around industrial waste processing plants. TCDD has been classified as a human carcinogen by the International Agency for Research on Cancer and displays endocrine-disrupting properties (209, 210).

The clinical relevance of dioxin exposures to human reproduction is still unknown. A case–cohort study of Seveso women exposed to high levels of TCDD found a nonsignificant association with surgically diagnosed endometriosis (211). Furthermore, there is evidence in the nonhuman primate model which indicates that chronic exposure to TCDD increases the risk of endometriosis, with severity of disease that is dose dependent (212, 213). However, the association between TCDD exposure and clinically diagnosed endometriosis remains controversial in humans (214–219). Nonetheless, functional AhR receptors that are dioxin responsive are expressed in human endometrial stromal cells and endometriosis implants (220). There are no studies currently in the clinical literature that directly address the role of dioxins in human reproductive potential, and although TCDD is present in human FF (221), there are no data on direct effects of TCDD on oocyte development and function.

There are several studies, however, worthy of mention within the TCDD mammalian reproduction literature. For example, TCDD can alter murine estrous cyclicity and ovulatory events (222, 223), and TCDD administered to pairing female hamsters lengthens the time to first litter in a dose-dependent fashion (224). TCDD exposure increases the cavitation rates of murine preimplantation embryos, with accelerated differentiation (225). There is also evidence that TCDD exposure during preimplantation development alters gene expression of murine blastocysts and the methylation status of the murine imprinted genes H19 and Igf2 (226, 227). Also, when murine embryos are incubated with TCDD in concentrations found in human FF (1–5 pM range) they responded with stage-specific effects of lower eight-cell development but accelerated blastocyst development within surviving embryos (221). Murine maternal exposure of environmentally relevant doses of TCDD during the periconception period does not affect ovulation, fertilization efficiency, or embryo survival, but rather results in disrupted nuclear and cytoplasmic profiles of preblastocyst embryos (228).

Early fetal loss has been demonstrated with maternal TCDD exposure in several different mammalian models, including the primate, possibly owing to effects on uterine decidualization (229, 230). There is also evidence that TCDD acts as an endocrine disruptor to reduce estrogen biosynthesis within the ovarian follicle via actions on 17,20 lyase activity of the P450c17 enzyme complex (231). TCDD may influence ovarian reserve via the AhR receptor activation pathway, similar to PAHs (232, 233). Collectively, these studies suggest that dioxins may have direct effects on oocyte and early embryo development as well as endometrial differentiation.

## 9 Aryl Hydrocarbon Receptor in Reproduction

As has been mentioned earlier in the sections on cigarette smoking and PAHs, PCBs, and dioxins, AhR-mediated pathways appear to be important in cell signaling with these lipophilic organic chemicals (halogenated aromatic hydrocarbons) which are considered important activating ligands that bind to AhR intracellularly (234). This complex disassociates within the cell nucleus and dimerizes with AhR nuclear translocator (ARNT) to transform into a highly active transcriptional factor that regulates the transcription of cytochrome P450A1 (CYP1A1), a gene that encodes one of several xenobiotic-metabolizing enzymes (234, 235). TCDD, PAHs, and PCBs bind to AhR influencing various downstream events that effect detoxification of these lipophilic chemicals, induction of cellular apoptosis, and antagonism of normal endocrine responses (235, 236). The role of AhR in reproduction is supported by differences in fecundity between low- and high-affinity AhR (237). Bovine oocytes and surrounding cumulus cells both express AhR and ARNT (238). The use of AhR antagonists has demonstrated decreased levels of CYP1A1 in cumulus oocyte complexes with a reduced ability of bovine oocytes to undergo complete in vitro nuclear maturation (238). As discussed previously, contradictory evidence in the murine AhR knockout model exists that argues against a significant role for AhR in mammalian fertility, as the AhR−/AhR− female mouse is fertile (183). Thus, the role of AhR in fertility remains controversial, and further studies are needed to clarify the roles of halogenated aromatic hydrocarbons as ligands within the AhR-mediated pathways in reproduction.

## 10 Clinical Applications Summary

Evidence has been steadily accumulating regarding the effects of environmental contaminant exposures on mammalian and other animal reproductive systems. However, there remains controversy on the impact of environmental exposures on human reproduction. Large, prospective, epidemiologic-based studies are needed to address potentially subtle effects of various environmental contaminants on reproductive health. While cigarette smoking and its component chemicals as summarized in this chapter have substantial clinical and scientific data to support their effects on reducing the quality and quantity of oocytes, cigarette smoke is still unique as an environmental exposure as measured by the magnitude of research available that addresses its negative impact on human reproduction. PCBs, BPA, heavy metals, pesticides including DDT and dioxins are candidates as reproductive toxicants, with proposed biologic mechanisms for reproductive disruption, although they fall short in terms of clinical validation of their effects in the human population (see Table 1). Clearly, a concerted effort by the scientific and clinical communities must be made to further address and determine whether these chemicals adversely affect clinical reproductive outcomes before clinical recommendations can be made to limit exposures. However, before the results of these decade (or more)-long studies are conducted and the data analyzed, biologic plausibility recommends the limitation of exposures in accordance with the "precautionary principle." This principle states that if an action or policy might cause severe or irreversible harm to the public, precautionary measures shall be taken even if causal link has not been proven (239).

**Table 1** Reproductive compromise associated with various environmental contaminants

| | Smoking PAHs | Pesticides | Heavy metals | Bisphenol A | PCBs | DDT and DDE | Dioxins |
|---|---|---|---|---|---|---|---|
| Clinical – fecundity | +++ | ++ | NA | + | ++ | + | NA |
| Clinical spontaneous miscarriage | ++ | + | + | + | | + | NA |
| Clinical – fertility treatment outcomes | +++ | NA | + | NA | NA | NA | NA |
| Mammalian – litter sizes | ++ | ++ | | ++ | ++ | + | ++ |
| Mammalian – fertilization outcomes | NA | ++ | + | +++ | +++ | | |
| Mammalian – embryogenesis | +++ | ++ | + | +++ | +++ | ++ | ++ |

No association; +, weak association; ++, moderate association; +++, strong association; *NA* no literature available to derive a conclusion

## References


1. Caserta D, Maranghi L, Mantovani A, Marci R, Maranghi F, Moscarini M. Impact of Endocrine Disruptor Chemicals in Gynaecology. Hum Reprod Update 2008;14:59–72.
2. Fenton SE. Endocrine-Disrupting Compounds and Mammary Gland Development: Early Exposure and Later Life Consequences. Endocrinology 2006;147:s18–24.
3. McLachlan JA. Environmental Signaling: What Embryos and Evolution Teach Us About Endocrine Disrupting Chemicals. Endocr Rev 2001;22:319–41.
4. Woodruff TJ, Carlson A, Schwartz JM, Giudice LC. Proceedings of the Summit on Environmental Challenges to Reproductive Health and Fertility: Executive Summary. Fertility and Sterility 2008;89:281–300.
5. Sanderson JT. The Steroid Hormone Biosynthesis Pathway as a Target for Endocrine-Disrupting Chemicals. Toxicol Sci 2006;94:3–21.
6. Arisawa K, Matsumura T, Tohyama C, et al. Fish Intake, Plasma Omega-3 Polyunsaturated Fatty Acids, and Polychlorinated Dibenzo-p-dioxins/Polychlorinated Dibenzofurans and Co-Planar Polychlorinated Biphenyls in the Blood of the Japanese Population. Int Arch Occup Environ Health 2003;76:205–15.
7. Hightower JM, Moore D. Mercury Levels In High-End Consumers of Fish. Environ Health Perspect 2003;111:604–8.
8. Ornaghi F, Ferrini S, Prati M, Giavini E. The Protective Effects of N-Acetyl-L-Cysteine Against Methyl Mercury Embryotoxicity In Mice. Fundam Appl Toxicol 1993;20: 437–45.
9. Alm H, Torner H, Tiemann U, Kanitz W. Influence of Organochlorine Pesticides on Maturation and Postfertilization Development of Bovine Oocytes In Vitro. Reprod Toxicol 1998;12:559–63.
10. Campagna C, Sirard M-A, Ayotte P, Bailey JL. Impaired Maturation, Fertilization, and Embryonic Development of Porcine Oocytes Following Exposure to an Environmentally Relevant Organochlorine Mixture. Biol Reprod 2001;65: 554–60.
11. Krogenaes AK, Nafstad I, Skåre JU, Farstad W, Hafne AL. In Vitro Reproductive Toxicity of Polychlorinated Biphenyl Congeners 153 and 126. Reprod Toxicol 1998; 12:575–80.
12. De Luca-Abbott SB, Wong BS, Peakall DB, et al. Review of Effects of Water Pollution on the Breeding Success of Waterbirds, with Particular Reference to Ardeids in Hong Kong. Ecotoxicol Environ Saf 2001;10:327–49.
13. Guillette LJ, Jr, Edwards TM. Environmental Influences on Fertility: Can We Learn Lessons from Studies of Wildlife? Fertil Steril 2008;89:e21–e4.
14. Guillette LJJ, Moore BC. Environmental Contaminants, Fertility, and Multioocytic Follicles: A Lesson from Wildlife? Semin Reprod Med 2006;24:134–41.
15. Windham G, Fenster L. Environmental Contaminants and Pregnancy Outcomes. Fertil Steril 2008;89:e111–e6.
16. Gajalakshmi GK, Jha P, Ranson K, Nguyen S. Global patterns of smoking, and smoking-attributable mortality. In P Jha & F Chalouka (eds.), Tobacco Control in Developing Countries. Oxford: Oxford Medical Publications 2000:11–40.
17. Brunnemann KD, Hoffmann D. Analytical Studies on Tobacco-Specific N-Nitrosamines in Tobacco and Tobacco Smoke. Crit Rev Toxicol 1991;21:235–40.
18. Bolumar F, Olsen J, Rebagliato M, et al. Body Mass Index and Delayed Conception: A European Multicenter Study on Infertility and Subfecundity. Am J Epidemiol 2000;151: 1072–9.
19. Curtis KM, Savitz DA, Arbuckle TE. Effects of Cigarette Smoking, Caffeine Consumption, and Alcohol Intake on Fecundability. Am J Epidemiol 1997;146:32–41.
20. Hull MGR, North K, Taylor H, Farrow A, Ford WC. Delayed Conception and Active and Passive Smoking. Fertil Steril 2000;74:725–33.
21. Spinelli A, Figa-Talamanca I, Osborn J. Time to Pregnancy and Occupation In A Group of Italian Women. Int J Epidemiol 1997;26:601–9.
22. The Practice Committee of the American Society of Reproductive Medicine. Smoking and infertility. Fertil Steril 2006;86:S172–S7.

23. Augood C, Duckitt K, Templeton AA. Smoking and Female Infertility: A Systematic Review and Meta-Analysis. Hum Reprod 1998;13:1532–9.
24. Klonoff-Cohen H. Female and Male Lifestyle Habits and IVF: What Is Known and Unknown. Hum Reprod Update 2005;11:180–204.
25. El-Nemr A, Al-Shawaf T, Sabatini L, Wilson C, Lower AM, Grudzinskas JG. Effect of Smoking on Ovarian Reserve and Ovarian Stimulation In In Vitro Fertilization and Embryo Transfer. Hum Reprod 1998;13:2192–8.
26. Freour T, Masson D, Mirallie S, et al. Active Smoking Compromises IVF Outcome and Affects Ovarian Reserve. Reprod Biomed Online 2008;16:96–102.
27. Hughes EG, Brennan BG. Does Cigarette Smoking Impair Natural or Assisted Fecundity? Fertil Steril 1996;66: 679–89.
28. Lintsen AME, Pasker-de Jong PCM, de Boer EJ, et al. Effects of Subfertility Cause, Smoking and Body Weight on the Success Rate of IVF. Hum Reprod 2005;20:1867–75.
29. Zenzes MT, Reed TE, Casper RF. Effects of Cigarette Smoking and Age on the Maturation of Human Oocytes. Hum Reprod 1997;12:1736–41.
30. Zenzes MT, Wang P, Casper RF. Cigarette Smoking May Affect Meiotic Maturation of Human Oocytes. Hum Reprod 1995;10:3213–7.
31. Soares SR, Simon C, Remohi J, Pellicer A. Cigarette Smoking Affects Uterine Receptiveness. Hum Reprod 2007; 22:543–7.
32. Neal MS, Hughes EG, Holloway AC, Foster WG. Sidestream Smoking Is Equally As Damaging As Mainstream Smoking on IVF Outcomes. Hum Reprod 2005;20:2531–5.
33. Zenzes MT. Smoking and Reproduction: Gene Damage to Human Gametes and Embryos. Hum Reprod Update 2000;6:122–31.
34. Ness RB, Grisso JA, Hirschinger N, et al. Cocaine and Tobacco Use and the Risk of Spontaneous Abortion. N Engl J Med 1999;340:333–9.
35. Winter E, Wang J, Davies MJ, Norman R. Early Pregnancy Loss Following Assisted Reproductive Technology Treatment. Hum Reprod 2002;17:3220–3.
36. Chatenoud L, Parazzini F, Di Cintio E, et al. Paternal and Maternal Smoking Habits before Conception and During the First Trimester: Relation to Spontaneous Abortion. Ann Epidemiol 1998;8:520–6.
37. Maconochie N, Doyle P, Prior S, Simmons R. Risk Factors for First Trimester Miscarriage–Results from a UK-Population-Based Case-Control Study. BJOG: Int J Obstet Gynaecol 2007;114:170–86.
38. Nielsen A, Hannibal CG, Lindekilde BE, et al. Maternal Smoking Predicts the Risk of Spontaneous Abortion. Acta Obstetricia et Gynecologica Scandinavica 2006;85: 1057–65.
39. Rasch V. Cigarette, Alcohol, and Caffeine Consumption: Risk Factors for Spontaneous Abortion. Acta Obstetricia et Gynecologica Scandinavica 2003;82:182–8.
40. Windham GC, Swan SH, Fenster L. Parental Cigarette Smoking and the Risk of Spontaneous Abortion. Am J Epidemiol 1992;135:1394–403.
41. Coste J, Bouyer J, Ughetto S, et al. Ectopic Pregnancy Is Again on the Increase. Recent Trends in the Incidence of Ectopic Pregnancies in France (1992–2002). Hum Reprod 2004;19:2014–8.
42. Coste J, Job-Spira N, Fernandez H. Increased Risk of Ectopic Pregnancy with Maternal Cigarette Smoking. Am J Public Health 1991;81:199–201.
43. Coste J, Job-Spira N, Fernandez H, Papiemik E, Spira A. Risk Factors for Ectopic Pregnancy: A Case-Control Study in France, with Special Focus on Infectious Factors. Am J Epidemiol 1991;133:839–49.
44. Karaer A, Avsar FA, Batioglu S. Risk Factors for Ectopic Pregnancy: A Case-Control Study. Aust N Z J Obstet Gynaecol 2006;46:521–7.
45. Knoll M, Shaoulian R, Magers T, Talbot P. Ciliary Beat Frequency of Hamster oviducts Is Decreased in vitro by Exposure to Solutions of Mainstream and Sidestream Cigarette Smoke. Biol Reprod 1995;53:29–37.
46. Knoll M, Talbot P. Cigarette Smoke Inhibits Oocyte Cumulus Complex Pick-Up by the Oviduct In Vitro Independent of Ciliary Beat Frequency. Reprod Toxicol 1998;12:57–68.
47. Riveles K, Iv M, Arey J, Talbot P. Pyridines in Cigarette Smoke Inhibit Hamster Oviductal Functioning in Picomolar Doses. Reprod Toxicol 2003;17:191–202.
48. Riveles K, Roza R, Arey J, Talbot P. Pyrazine Derivatives in Cigarette Smoke Inhibit Hamster Oviductal Functioning. Reprod Biol Endocrinol 2004;2:23.
49. Riveles K, Roza R, Talbot P. Phenols, Quinolines, Indoles, Benzene, and 2-Cyclopenten-1-ones are Oviductal Toxicants in Cigarette Smoke. Toxicol Sci 2005;86:141–51.
50. Benowitz NL, Kuyt F, Jacob P, Jones RT. Cotinine Disposition and Effects. Clin Pharmacol Ther 1983;34: 604–11.
51. Weiss T, Eckert A. Cotinine Levels in Follicular Fluid and Serum of IVF Patients: Effect on Granulosa-Luteal Cell Function In Vitro. Hum Reprod 1989;4:482–5.
52. Zenzes MT, Krishnan S, Krishnan B, Zhang H, Casper RF. Cadmium Accumulation in Follicular Fluid of Women in In Vitro Fertilization-Embryo Transfer Is Higher In Smokers. Fertil Steril 1995;64:599–603.
53. Zenzes MT, Reed TE, Wang P, Klein J. Cotinine, A Major Metabolite of Nicotine, Is Detectable in Follicular Fluids of Passive Smokers in In Vitro Fertilization Therapy. Fertil Steril 1996;66:614–9.
54. Bartsch H, Nair U, Risch A, Rojas M, Wikman H, Alexandrov K. Genetic Polymorphism of CYP Genes, Alone or in Combination, as a Risk Modifier of Tobacco-related Cancers. Cancer Epidemiol Biomarkers Prev 2000;9: 3–28.
55. Archibong AE, Inyang F, Ramesh A, et al. Alteration of Pregnancy Related Hormones and Fetal Survival in F-344 Rats Exposed by Inhalation to Benzo(a)pyrene. Reprod Toxicol 2002;16:801–8.
56. Kristensen P, Eilertsen E, Einarsdóttir E, Haugen A, Skaug V, Ovrebø S. Fertility in Mice After Prenatal Exposure to Benzo[a]pyrene and Inorganic Lead. Environ Health Perspect 1995;103:588–90.
57. Buters J, Quintanilla-Martinez L, Schober W, et al. CYP1B1 Determines Susceptibility to Low Doses of 7,12-Dimethylbenz [a]anthracene-Induced Ovarian Cancers in Mice: Correlation of CYP1B1-Mediated DNA Adducts with Carcinogenicity. Carcinogenesis 2003;24:327–34.
58. Goodman MT, McDuffie K, Kolonel LN, et al. Case-Control Study of Ovarian Cancer and Polymorphisms in Genes Involved in Catecholestrogen Formation and Metabolism. Cancer Epidemiol Biomarkers Prev 2001;10:209–16.

59. Vidal JD, VandeVoort CA, Marcus CB, Lazarewicz NR, Conley AJ. In Vitro Exposure to Environmental Tobacco Smoke Induces CYP1B1 Expression in Human Luteinized Granulosa Cells. Reprod Toxicol 2006;22:731–7.
60. Wang X, Zuckerman B, Pearson C, et al. Maternal Cigarette Smoking, Metabolic Gene Polymorphism, and Infant Birth Weight. JAMA 2002;287:195–202.
61. Harlow BL, Signorello LB. Factors Associated with Early Menopause. Maturitas 2000;35:3–9.
62. Kinney A, Kline J, Levin B. Alcohol, Caffeine and Smoking in Relation to Age at Menopause. Maturitas 2006;54: 27–38.
63. Mikkelsen T, Graff-Iversen S, Sundby J, Bjertness E. Early Menopause, Association with Tobacco Smoking, Coffee Consumption and Other Lifestyle Factors: A Cross-Sectional Study. BMC Public Health 2007;7:149.
64. Sharara FI, Beatse SN, Leonardi MR, Navot D, Scott RTJ. Cigarette Smoking Accelerates the Development of Diminished Ovarian Reserve As Evidenced by the Clomiphene Citrate Challenge Test. Fertil Steril 1994;62:257–62.
65. Backer LC, Rubin CS, Marcus M, Kieszak SM, Schober SE. Serum Follicle-Stimulating Hormone and Luteinizing Hormone Levels in Women Aged 35–60 in the U.S. Population: The Third National Health and Nutrition Examination Survey (NHANES III, 1988–1994). Menopause 1999;6(1):29–35.
66. Cramer DW, Barbieri RL, Fraer AR, Harlow BL. Determinants of Early Follicular Phase Gonadotrophin and Estradiol Concentrations in Women of Late Reproductive Age. Hum Reprod 2002;17:221–7.
67. Kinney A, Kline J, Kelly A, Reuss ML, Levin B. Smoking, Alcohol and Caffeine in Relation to Ovarian Age During the Reproductive Years. Hum Reprod 2007;22:1175–85.
68. Hoyer PB, Sipes IG. Assessment of Follicle Destruction in Chemical-Induced Ovarian Toxicity. Annu Rev Pharmacol Toxicol 1996;36:307–31.
69. Mattison DR. Difference in Sensitivity of Rat and Mouse Primordial Oocytes to Destruction by Polycyclic Aromatic Hydrocarbons. Chemico-Biological Interactions 1979;28: 133–7.
70. Mattison DR. Morphology of Oocyte and Follicle Destruction by Polycyclic Aromatic Hydrocarbons in Mice. Toxicol Appl Pharmacol 1980;53:249–59.
71. Mattison DR, Shiromizu K, Nightingale MS. Oocyte Destruction by Polycyclic Aromatic Hydrocarbons. Am J Ind Med 1983;4:191–202.
72. Matikainen T, Perez GI, Jurisicova A, et al. Aromatic Hydrocarbon Receptor-Driven Bax Gene Expression is Required for Premature Ovarian Failure Caused by Biohazardous Environmental Chemicals. Nat Genet 2001;28: 355–60.
73. Matzuk MM. Eggs in the Balance. Nat Genet 2001;28: 300–1.
74. Nardo LG, Christodoulou D, Gould D, Roberts SA, Fitzgerald CT, Laing I. Anti-Mullerian Hormone Levels and Antral Follicle Count in Women Enrolled in In Vitro Fertilization Cycles: Relationship to Lifestyle Factors, Chronological Age and Reproductive History. Gynecol Endocrinol 2007;23:486–93.
75. Barker DJ, Clark PM. Fetal Undernutrition and Disease in Later Life. Rev Reprod 1997;2:105–12.
76. Barker DJP. Maternal Nutrition, Fetal Nutrition, and Disease in Later Life. Nutrition 1997;13:807–13.
77. Osmond C, Barker DJ. Fetal, Infant, and Childhood Growth are Predictors of Coronary Heart Disease, Diabetes, and Hypertension in Adult Men and Women. Environ Health Perspect 2000;108:545–53.
78. Jurisicova A, Taniuchi A, Li H, et al. Maternal Exposure to Polycyclic Aromatic Hydrocarbons Diminishes Murine Ovarian Reserve Via Induction of Harakiri. J Clin Invest 2007;117:3971–8.
79. Weinberg CR, Wilcox AJ, Baird DD. Reduced Fecundability in Women with Prenatal Exposure to Cigarette Smoking. Am J Epidemiol 1989;129:1072–8.
80. Arbuckle TE, Lin Z, Mery LS. An Exploratory Analysis of the Effect of Pesticide Exposure on the Risk of Spontaneous Abortion in An Ontario Farm Population. Environ Health Perspect 2001;109:851–7.
81. Bell EM, Hertz-Picciotto I, Beaumont JJ. A Case-Control Study of Pesticides and Fetal Death Due to Congenital Anomalies. Epidemiology 2001;12:148–56.
82. Goulet L, Thériault G. Stillbirth and Chemical Exposure of Pregnant Workers. Scand J Work Environ Health 1991;17: 25–31.
83. Hemminki K, Niemi ML, Saloniemi I, Vainio H, Hemminki E. Spontaneous Abortions by Occupation and Social Class in Finland. Int J Epidemiol 1980;9:149–53.
84. Pastore LM, Hertz-Picciotto I, Beaumont JJ. Risk of Stillbirth from Occupational and Residential Exposures. Occup Environ Med 1997;54:511–8.
85. Restrepo M, Muñoz N, Day NE, Parra JE, de Romero L, Nguyen-Dinh X. Prevalence of Adverse Reproductive Outcomes in a Population Occupationally Exposed to Pesticides in Colombia. Scand J Work Environ Health 1990;16:232–8.
86. Taha TE, Gray RH. Agricultural Pesticide Exposure and Perinatal Mortality in Central Sudan. Bull World Health Organ 1993;71:317–21.
87. Thomas DC, Petitti DB, Goldhaber M, Swan SH, Rappaport EB, Hertz-Picciotto I. Reproductive Outcomes in Relation to Malathion Spraying in the San Francisco Bay Area, 1981–1982. Epidemiology 1992;3(1):32–9.
88. Willis WO, de Peyster A, Molgaard CA, Walker C, MacKendrick T. Pregnancy Outcome Among Women Exposed to Pesticides Through Work Or Residence in an Agricultural Area. J Occup Med 1993;35:943–9.
89. Zhu JL, Hjollund NH, Andersen AM, Olsen J. Occupational Exposure to Pesticides and Pregnancy Outcomes in Gardeners and Farmers: A Study Within the Danish National Birth Cohort. J Occup Environ Med 2006;48:347–52.
90. Greenlee AR, Arbuckle TE, Chyou PH. Risk Factors for Female Infertility in An Agricultural Region. Epidemiology 2003;14:429–36.
91. Greenlee AR, Ellis TM, Berg RL. Low-Dose Agrochemicals and Lawn-Care Pesticides Induce Developmental Toxicity in Murine Preimplantation Embryos. Environ Health Perspect 2004;112:703–9.
92. Perreault SD, Jeffay SC, Poss P, Laskey JW. Use of the Fungicide Carbendazim as a Model Compound to Determine the Impact of Acute Chemical Exposure During Oocyte Maturation and Fertilization on Pregnancy Outcome in the Hamster. Toxicol Appl Pharmacol 1992;114:225–31.
93. Zuelke KA, Perreault SD. Carbendazim (MBC) Disrupts Oocyte Spindle FUnction and Induces Aneuploidy in Hamsters Exposed During Fertilization (Meiosis II). Mol Reprod Dev 1995;42:200–9.

94. Jeffay SC, Libbus BL, Barbee RR, Perreault SD. Acute Exposure of Female Hamsters to Carbendazim (MBC) During Meiosis Results in Aneuploid Oocytes with Subsequent Arrest of Embryonic Cleavage and Implantation. Reprod Toxicol 1996;10:183–9.
95. Can A, Albertini DF. Stage Specific Effects of Carbendazim (MBC) on Meiotic Cell Cycle Progression in Mouse Oocytes. Mol Reprod Dev 1997;46:351–62.
96. Czeizel AE, Elek C, Gundy S, et al. Environmental Trichlorfon and Cluster of Congenital Abnormalities. The Lancet 1993;341:539–42.
97. Yin H, Cukurcam S, Betzendahl I, Adler ID, Eichenlaub-Ritter U. Trichlorfon Exposure, Spindle Aberrations and Nondisjunction in Mammalian Oocytes. Chromosoma 1998;107:514–22.
98. Laville N, Balaguer P, Brion F, et al. Modulation of Aromatase Activity and mRNA by Various Selected Pesticides in the Human Choriocarcinoma JEG-3 cell line. Toxicology 2006;228:98–108.
99. Fuyata ea. Embryotoxic Effects of Methylmercuric Chloride Administered to Mice and Rats During Organogenesisis. Teratology 1978;18:353–66.
100. Sharara F, Seifer D, Flaws J. Environmental Toxicants and Female Reproduction. Fertil Steril 1998;70:613–22.
101. Skakkebaek N, Giwercman A, de Kretser D. Pathogenesis and Management of Male Infertility. The Lancet 1994;343: 1473–79.
102. Rowland A, Baird D, Weinberg C, Shore D, Shy C, Wilcox A. The Effect of Occupational Exposure to Mercury Vapour on the Fertility of Female Dental Assistants. Occup Environ Med 1994;51:28–34.
103. Choy C, Lam C, Cheung L, Briton-Jone C, Cheung L, Haines C. Infertility, Blood Mercury Concentrations and Dietary Seafood Consumption: A Case-Control Study. Br J Obstet Gynecol 2002;109:1121–25.
104. Mahaffey KR. Recent Advances in Recognition of Low-Level Methylmercury Poisoning. Curr Opin Neurol 2000;13:699–707.
105. Crump KS, Kjellström T, Shipp AM, Silvers A, Stewart A. Influence of Prenatal Mercury Exposure Upon Scholastic and Psychological Test Performance: Benchmark Analysis of a New Zealand Cohort. Risk Analysis 1998;18: 701–13.
106. Grandjean P, Weihe P, Burse VW, et al. Neurobehavioral Deficits Associated with PCB in 7-Year-Old Children Prenatally Exposed to Seafood Neurotoxicants. Neurotoxicol Teratol 2001;23:305–17.
107. Grandjean P, Weihe P, White RF, et al. Cognitive Deficit in 7-Year-Old Children with Prenatal Exposure to Methylmercury. Neurotoxicol Teratol 1997;19:417–28.
108. Muckle G, Ayotte P, Dewailly E, Jacobson SW, Jacobson JL. Determinants of Polychlorinated Biphenyls and Methylmercury Exposure in Inuit Women of Childbearing Age. Environ Health Perspect 2001;109:957–63.
109. Hightower JM, O'Hare A, Hernandez GT. Blood Mercury Reporting in NHANES: Identifying Asian, Pacific Islander, Native American, and Multiracial Groups. Environ Health Perspect 2006;114:173–5.
110. Mahaffey K, Clickner R, Bodurow C. Blood Organic Mercury and Dietary Mercury Intake: National Health and Nutrition Examination Survey, 1999 and 2000. Environ Health Perspect 2004;112:562–70.
111. Durgnat JM, Heuser J, Andrey D, Perrin C. Quality and Safety Assessment of Ginseng Extracts by Determination of the Contents of Pesticides and Metals. Food Addit Contam 2005;22:1224–30.
112. Ernst E. Toxic Heavy Metals and Undeclared Drugs in Asian Herbal Medicines. Trends Pharmacol Sci 2002;23: 136–9.
113. Garvey GJ, Hahn G, Lee RV, Harbison RD. Heavy Metal Hazards of Asian TRaditional Remedies. Int J Environ Health Res 2001;11:63–71.
114. Saper RB, Kales SN, Paquin J, et al. Heavy Metal Content of Ayurvedic Herbal Medicine Products. JAMA 2004;292: 2868–73.
115. Geraldine M, Herman DS, Venkatesh T. Lead Poisoning as a Result of Infertility TReatment Using Herbal Remedies. Arch Gynecol Obstet 2007;275:279–81.
116. Al-Saleh I, Coskun S, Mashhour A, et al. Exposure to Heavy Metals (Lead, Cadmium and Mercury) and Its Effect on the Outcome of In-Vitro Fertilization Treatment. Int J Hyg Environ Health 2007;211:560–79.
117. Silberstein T, Saphier O, Paz-Tal O, Gonzalez L, Keefe DL, Trimarchi JR. Trace Element Concentrations in Follicular Fluid of Small Follicles Differ from Those in Blood Serum, and may represent long-term exposure. Fertil Steril 2008; April 17 [Epub ahead of print].
118. Zenzes MT, Krishnan S, Krishnan B, Zhang H, Casper RF. Cadmium Accumulation in Follicular Fluid of Women in In Vitro Fertilization-Embryo Transfer Is Higher In Smokers. Fertil Steril 1995;64:599–603.
119. De SK, Paria BC, Dey SK, Andrews GK. Stage-Specific Effects of Cadmium on Preimplantation Embryo Development and Implantation in the Mouse. Toxicology 1993;80: 13–25.
120. Fernandez EL, Gustafson A-L, Andersson M, Hellman B, Dencker L. Cadmium-Induced Changes in Apoptotic Gene Expression Levels and DNA Damage in Mouse Embryos Are Blocked by Zinc. Toxicol Sci 2003;76:162–70.
121. Liu L, Trimarchi JR, Navarro P, Blasco MA, Keefe DL. Oxidative Stress Contributes to Arsenic-induced Telomere Attrition, Chromosome Instability, and Apoptosis. J Biol Chem 2003;278:31998–2004.
122. Navarro PAAS, Liu L, Keefe DL. In Vivo Effects of Arsenite on Meiosis, Preimplantation Development, and Apoptosis in the Mouse. Biol Reprod 2004;70:980–5.
123. Paksy K, Forgács Z, Gáti I. In VitroComparative Effect of Cd2+, Ni2+, and Co2+ on Mouse Postblastocyst Development. Env Res 1999;80:340–7.
124. vom Saal FS, Akingbemi BT, Belcher SM, et al. Chapel Hill Bisphenol A Expert Panel Consensus Statement: Integration of Mechanisms, Effects in Animals and Potential to Impact Human Health at Current Levels of Exposure. Reprod Toxicol 2007;24:131–8.
125. Welshons WV, Nagel SC, vom Saal FS. Large Effects from Small Exposures. III. Endocrine Mechanisms Mediating Effects of Bisphenol A at Levels of Human Exposure. Endocrinology 2006;147:s56–69.
126. Ikezuki Y, Tsutsumi O, Takai Y, Kamei Y, Taketani Y. Determination of Bisphenol A Concentrations in Human

Biological Fluids Reveals Significant Early Prenatal Exposure. Hum Reprod 2002;17:2839–41.
127. Takeuchi T, Tsutsumi O. Serum Bisphenol A Concentrations Showed Gender Differences, Possibly Linked to Androgen Levels. Biochemical and Biophysical Research Communications 2002;291:76–8.
128. Calafat AM, Kuklenyik Z, Reidy JA, Caudill SP, Ekong J, Needham LL. Urinary Concentrations of Bisphenol A and 4-Nonylphenol in a Human Reference Population. Environ Health Perspect 2005;113:391–5.
129. Calafat AM, Ye X, Wong LY, Reidy JA, Needham LL. Exposure of the U.S. Population to Bisphenol A and 4-Tertiary-Octylphenol: 2003–2004. Environ Health Perspect 2008;116:39–44.
130. Goodman JE, McConnell EE, Sipes IG, et al. An Updated Weight of the Evidence Evaluation of Reproductive and Developmental Effects of Low Doses of Bisphenol A. Crit Rev Toxicol 2006;36:387–457.
131. vom Saal FS, Welshons WV. Large Effects from Small Exposures. II. The Importance of Positive Controls in Low-Dose Research on Bisphenol A. Environ Res 2006; 100:50–76.
132. Takai Y, Tsutsumi O, Ikezuki Y, et al. Estrogen Receptor-Mediated Effects of a Xenoestrogen, Bisphenol A, on Preimplantation Mouse Embryos. Biochem Biophys Res Commn 2000;270:918–21.
133. Nakagomi M, Suzuki E, Usumi K, et al. Effects of Endocrine Disrupting Chemicals on the Microtubule Network In Chinese Hamster V79 Cells in Culture and in Sertoli cells in Rats. Teratog Carcinog Mutagen 2001; 21:453–62.
134. Pfeiffer E, Rosenberg B, Deuschel S, Metzler M. Interference with Microtubules and Induction of Micronuclei In Vitro By Various Bisphenols. Mutat Res 1997;390:21–31.
135. Hunt PA, Koehler KE, Susiarjo M, et al. Bisphenol A Exposure Causes Meiotic Aneuploidy in the Female Mouse. Curr Biol 2003;13:546–53.
136. Can A, Semiz O, Cinar O. Bisphenol-A Induces Cell Cycle Delay and Alters Centrosome and Spindle Microtubular Organization in Oocytes During Meiosis. Mol Hum Reprod 2005;11:389–96.
137. Can A, Semiz O. Diethylstilbestrol (DES)-Induced Cell Cycle Delay and Meiotic Spindle Disruption in Mouse Oocytes During In-Vitro Maturation. Mol Hum Reprod 2000;6:154–62.
138. Pocar P, Augustin R, Gandolfi F, Fischer B. Toxic Effects of In Vitro Exposure to p-tert-Octylphenol on Bovine Oocyte Maturation and Developmental Competence. Biol Reprod 2003;69:462–8.
139. Susiarjo M, Hassold TJ, Freeman E, Hunt PA. Bisphenol A Exposure In Utero Disrupts Early Oogenesis in the Mouse. PLoS Genetics 2007;3:e5.
140. Sugiura-Ogasawara M, Ozaki Y, Sonta S-i, Makino T, Suzumori K. Exposure to Bisphenol A Is Associated with Recurrent Miscarriage. Hum Reprod 2005;20:2325–9.
141. Safe SH. Polychlorinated Biphenyls (PCBs): Environmental Impact, Biochemical and Toxic Responses, and Implications for Risk Assessment. Crit Rev Toxicol 1994;24:87–149.
142. McFarland VA, Clarke JU. Environmental Occurrence, Abundance, and Potential Toxicity of Polychlorinated Biphenyl Congeners: Considerations for a Congener-Specific Analysis. Environ Health Perspect 1989;81:225–39.
143. Reijnders PJH. Reproductive Failure in Common Seals Feeding on Fish From Polluted Coastal Waters. Nature 1986;324:456–7.
144. Buck GM, Sever LE, Mendola P, Zielezny M, Vena JE. Consumption of Contaminated Sport Fish from Lake Ontario and Time-to-Pregnancy: New York State Angler Cohort. Am J Epidemiol 1997;146:949–54.
145. Harris SA, Jones JL. Fish Consumption and PCB-Associated Health Risks in Recreational Fishermen on the James River, Virginia. Environ Res 2008;107:254–63.
146. Anderson HA, Falk C, Hanrahan L, et al. Profiles of Great Lakes Critical Pollutants: A Sentinel Analysis of Human Blood and Urine. The Great Lakes Consortium. Environ Health Perspect 1998;106:279–89.
147. Kearney JP, Cole DC, Ferron LA, Weber J-P. Blood PCB,p,p'-DDE, and Mirex Levels in Great Lakes Fish and Waterfowl Consumers in Two Ontario Communities. Environ Res 1999;80:S138–S49.
148. Kosatsky T, Przybysz R, Shatenstein B, Weber J-P, Armstrong B. Fish Consumption and Contaminant Exposure among Montreal-Area Sportfishers: Pilot Study. Environ Res 1999;80:S150–8.
149. Turyk M, Anderson HA, Hanrahan LP, et al. Relationship of Serum Levels of Individual PCB, Dioxin, and Furan Congeners and DDE with Great Lakes Sport-Caught Fish Consumption. Environ Res 2006;100:173–83.
150. Bloom MS, Buck Louis GM, Schisterman EF, Liu A, Kostyniak PJ. Maternal Serum Polychlorinated Biphenyl Concentrations Across Critical Windows of Human Development. Environ Health Perspect 2007;115:1320–4.
151. De Felip E, Domenico Ad, Miniero R, Silvestroni L. Polychlorobiphenyls and Other Organochlorine Compounds in Human Follicular Fluid. Chemosphere 2004;54:1445–9.
152. Jarrell JF, Villeneuve D, Franklin C, et al. Contamination of Human Ovarian Follicular Fluid and Serum by Chlorinated Organic Compounds in Three Canadian Cities. CMAJ 1993;148(8):1321–7.
153. Pauwels A, Covaci A, Delbeke L, Punjabi U, Schepens PJC. The Relation Between Levels of Selected PCB Congeners in Human Serum and FOllicular Fluid. Chemosphere 1999;39:2433–41.
154. Trapp M, Baukloh V, Bohnet HG, Heeschen W. Pollutants in Human Follicular Fluid. Fertil Steril 1984;42:146–8.
155. Younglai EV, Foster WG, Hughes EG, Trim K, Jarrell JF. Levels of Environmental Contaminants in Human Follicular Fluid, Serum, and Seminal Plasma of Couples Undergoing In Vitro Fertilization. Arch Environ Contam Toxicol 2002;43:121–6.
156. Buck GM, Vena JE, Schisterman EF, et al. Parental Consumption of Contaminated Sport Fish from Lake Ontario and Predicted Fecundability. Epidemiology 2000;11:388–93.
157. Axmon A, Rylander L, Strömberg U, Hagmar L. Female Fertility in Relation to the Consumption of Fish Contaminated with Persistent Organochlorine Compounds. Scand J Work Environ Health 2002;28:124–32.

158. Buck GM, Mendola P, Vena JE, et al. Paternal Lake Ontario Fish Consumption and Risk of Conception Delay, New York State Angler Cohort. Environ Res 1999;80:S13–8.
159. Cordle F, Locke R, Springer J. Risk Assessment in a Federal Regulatory Agency: An Assessment of Risk Associated with the Human Consumption of Some Species of Fish Contaminated with Polychlorinated Biphenyls (PCBs). Environ Health Perspect 1982;45:171–82.
160. Dar E, Kanarek MS, Anderson HA, Sonzogni WC. Fish Consumption and Reproductive Outcomes in Green Bay, Wisconsin. Environ Res 1992;59:189–201.
161. Mendola P, Buck GM, Vena JE, Zielezny M, Sever LE. Consumption of PCB-Contaminated Sport Fish and Risk of Spontaneous Fetal Death. Environ Health Perspect 1995;103(5):498–502.
162. Sugiura-Ogasawara M, Ozaki Y, Sonta S-i, Makino T, Suzumori K. PCBs, Hexachlorobenzene and DDE are Not Associated with Recurrent Miscarriage. Am J Reprod Immunol 2003;50:485–9.
163. Buck G, Tee G, Fitzgerald E, et al. Maternal Fish Consumption and Infant Birth Size and Gestation: New York State Angler Cohort Study. Environ Health 2003;2:7.
164. Rylander L, Strömberg U, Hagmar L. Dietary Intake of Fish Contaminated with Persistent Organochlorine Compounds in Relation to Low Birthweight. Scand J Work Environ Health 1996;22:260–6.
165. Fries GF. The PBB Episode in Michigan: an Overall Appraisal. Crit Rev Toxicol 1985;16:105–56.
166. Small CM, Cheslack-Postava K, Terrell M, et al. Risk of Spontaneous Abortion Among Women Exposed to Polybrominated Biphenyls. Environ Res 2007;105:247–55.
167. Barsotti DA, Marlar RJ, Allen JR. Reproductive Dysfunction in Rhesus Monkeys Exposed to Low Levels of Polychlorinated Biphenyls (Aoroclor 1248). Food Cosmet Toxicol 1976;14: 99–103.
168. Brezner E, Terkel J, Perry AS. The Effect of Aroclor 1254 (PCB) on the Physiology of Reproduction in the Female Rat-I. Comp Biochem Physiol C 1984;77:65–70.
169. Jonsson HTJ, Keil JE, Gaddy RG, Loadholt CB, Hennigar GR, Walker EMJ. Prolonged Ingestion of Commercial DDT and PCB; Effects on Progesterone Levels and Reproduction in the Mature Female Rat. Arch Environ Contam Toxicol 1975;3:479–90.
170. Müller WF, Hobson W, Fuller GB, Knauf W, Coulston F, Korte F. Endocrine Effects of Chlorinated Hydrocarbons in Rhesus Monkeys. Ecotoxicol Environ Saf 1978;2:161–72.
171. Kholkute SD, Dukelow WR. Effects of Polychlorinated Biphenyl (PCB) Mixtures on In Vitro Fertilization in the Mouse. Bull Environ Contam Toxicol 1997;59:531–6.
172. Kholkute SD, Rodriguez J, Dukelow WR. Reproductive Toxicity of Aroclor-1254: Effects on Oocyte, Spermatozoa, In Vitro Fertilization, and Embryo Development in the Mouse. Reprod Toxicol 1994;8:487–93.
173. Kholkute SD, Rodriguez J, Dukelow WR. Effects of Polychlorinated Biphenyls (PCBs) on In Vitro Fertilization in the Mouse. Reprod Toxicol 1994;8:69–73.
174. Pocar P, Perazzoli F, Luciano AM, Gandolfi F. In Vitro reproductive Toxicity of Polychlorinated Biphenyls: Effects on Oocyte Maturation and Developmental Competence in Cattle. Mol Reprod Dev 2001;58:411–6.
175. Huang A, Lin S, Inglis R, Powell D, Chou K. Pre- and Postnatal Exposure to 3,3′,4,4′-Tetrachlorobiphenyl: II. Effects on the Reproductive Capacity and Fertilizing Ability of Eggs in Female Mice. Arch Environ Contam Toxicol 1998;34:209–14.
176. Seiler P, Fischer B, Lindenau A, Beier HM. Fertilization and Early Embryology: Effects of Persistent Chlorinated Hydrocarbons on Fertility and Embryonic Development in the Rabbit. Hum Reprod 1994;9:1920–6.
177. Hennig B, Meerarani P, Slim R, et al. Proinflammatory Properties of Coplanar PCBs: In Vitro and in Vivo Evidence. Toxicol Appl Pharmacol 2002;181:174–83.
178. Lehmann DW, Levine JF, Law JM. Polychlorinated Biphenyl Exposure Causes Gonadal Atrophy and Oxidative Stress in Corbicula fluminea Clams. Toxicol Pathol 2007;35:356–65.
179. Murugesan P, Muthusamy T, Balasubramanian K, Arunakaran J. Studies on the Protective Role of Vitamin C and E Against Polychlorinated Biphenyl (Aroclor 1254): Induced Oxidative Damage in Leydig Cells. Free Radic Res 2005;39:1259–72.
180. Slim R, Toborek M, Robertson LW, Lehmler HJ, Hennig B. Cellular Glutathione Status Modulates Polychlorinated Biphenyl-Induced Stress Response and Apoptosis in Vascular Endothelial Cells. Toxicol Appl Pharmacol 2000;166:36–42.
181. Gao X, Son D-S, Terranova PF, Rozman KK. Toxic Equivalency Factors of Polychlorinated Dibenzo-p-dioxins in an Ovulation Model: Validation of the Toxic Equivalency Concept for One Aspect of Endocrine Disruption. Toxicol Appl Pharmacol 1999;157:107–16.
182. Son D-S, Ushinohama K, Gao X, et al. 2,3,7,8-Tetrachlorodibenzo-p-dioxin (TCDD) Blocks Ovulation By a Direct Action on the Ovary Without Alteration of Ovarian Steroidogenesis: LAck of A Direct Effect on Ovarian Granulosa and Thecal-Interstitial Cell Steroidogenesis In Vitro. Reprod Toxicol 1999;13:521–30.
183. Schmidt JV, Su GH-T, Reddy JK, Simon MC, Bradfield CA. Characterization of a Murine Ahr Null Allele: Involvement of the Ah Receptor in Hepatic Growth and Development. Proc Nat Acad Sci 1996;93:6731–6.
184. Kietz S, Fischer B. Polychlorinated Biphenyls Affect Gene Expression in the Rabbit Preimplantation Embryo. Mol Reprod Dev 2003;64:251–60.
185. Kutz FW, Wood PH, Bottimore DP. Organochlorine Pesticides and Polychlorinated Biphenyls in Human Adipose Tissue. Rev Environ Contam Toxicol 1991;120:1–82.
186. Venkatesan MI, de Leon RP, van Geen A, Luoma SN. Chlorinated Hydrocarbon Pesticides and Poychlorinated Biphenyls in Sediment Cores from San Francisco Bay. Mar Chem 1999;64:85–97.
187. James RA, Hertz-Picciotto I, Willman E, Keller JA, Charles MJ. Determinants of Serum Polychlorinated Biphenyls and Organochlorine Pesticides Measured in Women from the Child Health and Development Study Cohort, 1963–1967. Environ Health Perspect 2002;110:617–24.
188. Murphy R, Harvey C. Residues and Metabolites of Selected Persistent Halogenated Hydrocarbons in BLood Specimens from a General Population Survey. Environ Health Perspect 1985;60:115–20.

189. Korrick SA, Chen C, Damokosh AI, et al. Association of DDT with Spontaneous Abortion: A Case-Control Study. Ann Epidemiol 2001;11:491–6.
190. O'Leary JA, Davies JE, Feldman M. Spontaneous Abortion and Human Pesticide Residues of DDT and DDE. Am J Obstet Gynecol 1970;108:1291–2.
191. Longnecker MP, Klebanoff MA, Dunson DB, et al. Maternal Serum Level of the DDT Metabolite DDE in Relation to Fetal Loss in Previous Pregnancies. Environ Res 2005;97:127–33.
192. Venners SA, Korrick S, Xu X, et al. Preconception Serum DDT and Pregnancy Loss: A Prospective Study Using a Biomarker of Pregnancy. Am J Epidemiol 2005;162: 709–16.
193. Cocco P, Fadda D, Ibba A, et al. Reproductive outcomes in DDT applicators. Environ Res 2005;98:120–6.
194. Law DCG, Klebanoff MA, Brock JW, Dunson DB, Longnecker MP. Maternal Serum Levels of Polychlorinated Biphenyls and 1,1-Dichloro-2,2-bis(p-chlorophenyl)ethylene (DDE) and Time to Pregnancy. Am J Epidemiol 2005;162:523–32.
195. Weiss JM, Bauer O, Blüthgen A, et al. Distribution of Persistent Organochlorine Contaminants in Infertile Patients from Tanzania and Germany. J Assist Reprod Genet 2006;23:393–9.
196. Cohn BA, Cirillo PM, Wolff MS, et al. DDT and DDE Exposure in Mothers and Time to Pregnancy in Daughters. The Lancet 2003;361:2205–6.
197. Chedrese JP, Falter F. The Diverse Mechanism of Action of Dichlorodiphenyldichloroethylene (DDE) and Methoxychlor in Ovarian Cells In Vitro. Reprod Toxicol 2001; 15:693–8.
198. Crellin NK, Kang HG, Swan CL, Chedrese PJ. Inhibition of Basal and Stimulated Progesterone Synthesis By Dichlorodiphenyldichloroethylene and Methoxychlor in a Stable Pig Granulosa Cell Line. Reproduction 2001;121: 485–92.
199. Crellin NK, Rodway MR, Swan CL, Gillio-Meina C, Chedrese PJ. Dichlorodiphenyldichloroethylene Potentiates the Effect of Protein Kinase A Pathway Activators on Progesterone Synthesis in Cultured Porcine Granulosa Cells. Biol Reprod 1999;61:1099–103.
200. Holloway AC, Petrik JJ, Younglai EV. Influence of Dichlorodiphenylchloroethylene on Vascular Endothelial Growth Factor and Insulin-Like Growth Factor in Human and Rat Ovarian Cells. Reprod Toxicol 2007;24:359–64.
201. Greenlee AR, Quail CA, Berg RL. Developmental Alterations in Murine Embryos Exposed In Vitro to An Estrogenic Pesticide, o,p'-DDT. Reprod Toxicol 1999; 13:555–65.
202. Greenlee AR, Quail CA, Berg RL. The Antiestrogen ICI 182,780 Abolishes Developmental Injury for Murine Embryos Exposed In Vitro to o,p'-DDT. Reprod Toxicol 2000;14:225–34.
203. Greenlee AR, Ellis TM, Berg RL, Mercieca MD. Pregnancy Outcomes for Mouse Preimplantation Embryos Exposed In vitro to the Estrogenic Pesticide o,p'-DDT. Reprod Toxicol 2005;20:229–38.
204. Dowling V, Hoarau PC, Romeo M, et al. Protein Carbonylation and Heat Shock Response in *Ruditapes decussatus* Following p,p'-dichlorodiphenyldichloroethylene (DDE) Exposure: A Proteomic Approach Reveals that DDE Causes Oxidative Stress. Aquatic Toxicology 2006; 77:11–8.
205. Pérez-Maldonado IN, Athanasiadou M, Yáñez L, González-Amaro R, Bergman A, Díaz-Barriga F. DDE-Induced Apoptosis in Children Exposed to the DDT Metabolite. Sci Total Environ 2006;370:343–51.
206. Bock KW, Köhle C. Ah Receptor: Dioxin-Mediated Toxic Responses as Hints to Deregulated Physiologic Functions. Biochem Pharmacol 2006;72:393–404.
207. Needham LL, Gerthoux PM, Patterson DGJ, et al. Serum Dioxin Levels in Seveso, Italy, Population in 1976. Teratog Carcinog Mutagen 1997;17:225–40.
208. Eskenazi B, Mocarelli P, Warner M, et al. Relationship of Serum TCDD Concentrations and Age At Exposure of Female Residents of Seveso, Italy. Environ Health Perspect 2004;112:22–7.
209. Heiden TCK, Struble CA, Rise ML, Hessner MJ, Hutz RJ, CarvanIiiMJ. Molecular Targets of 2,3,7,8-Tetrachlorodibenzo-p-dioxin (TCDD) Within the Zebrafish Ovary: Insights into TCDD-Induced Endocrine Disruption and Reproductive Toxicity. Reprod Toxicol 2008;25:47–57.
210. IARC. Polychlorinated Dibenzo-para-dioxins and Polychlorinated Dibenzofurans. IARC Monogr Eval Carcinog Risks Hum 1997:69.
211. Eskenazi B, Mocarelli P, Warner M, et al. Seveso Women's Health Study: A Study of the Effects of 2,3,7,8-Tetrachlorodibenzo- p-dioxin on Reproductive Health. Chemosphere 2000;40: 1247–53.
212. Rier SE, Martin DC, Bowman RE, Dmowski WP, Becker JL. Endometriosis in Rhesus Monkeys (Macaca mulatta) Following Chronic Exposure to 2,3,7,8-Tetrachlorodibenzo-p-dioxin. Fundam Appl Toxicol 1993;21:433–41.
213. Yang JZ, Agarwal SK, Foster WG. Subchronic Exposure to 2,3,7,8-Tetrachlorodibenzo-p-dioxin Modulates the Pathophysiology of Endometriosis in the Cynomolgus Monkey. Toxicol Sci 2000;56:374–81.
214. Foster WG. Endocrine Toxicants Including 2,3,7,8-Terachlorodibenzo-p-Dioxin (TCDD) and Dioxin-like Chemicals and Endometriosis: Is There A Link? J Toxicol Environ Health B 2008;11:177–87.
215. Heilier J-F, Nackers F, Verougstraete V, Tonglet R, Lison D, Donnez J. Increased Dioxin-Like Compounds in the Serum of Women with Peritoneal Endometriosis and Deep Endometriotic (Adenomyotic) Nodules. Fertil Steril 2005;84:305–12.
216. Koninckx PR, Braet P, Kennedy SH, Barlow DH. Dioxin Pollution and Endometriosis in Belgium. Hum Reprod 1994;9:1001–2.
217. Mayani A, Barel S, Soback S, Almagor M. Dioxin Concentrations in Women with Endometriosis. Hum Reprod 1997;12:373–5.
218. Pauwels A, Schepens PJC, D'Hooghe T, et al. The Risk of Endometriosis and Exposure to Dioxins and Polychlorinated Biphenyls: A Case-Control Study of Infertile Women. Hum Reprod 2001;16:2050–5.
219. Rier SPD, Foster WGPD. Environmental Dioxins and Endometriosis. Sem Reprod Med 2003;21:145–54.
220. Zhao D, Pritts EA, Chao VA, Savouret J-F, Taylor RN. Dioxin Stimulates RANTES Expression in An In-Vitro Model of Endometriosis. Mol Hum Reprod 2002;8: 849–54.

221. Tsutsumi O, Uechi H, Sone H, et al. Presence of Dioxins in Human Follicular Fluid: Their Possible Stage-Specific Action on the Development of Preimplantation Mouse Embryos. Biochem Biophys Res Commn 1998;250: 498–501.
222. Giavini E, Prati M, Vismara C. Embryotoxic Effects of 2,3,7,8 Tetrachlorodibenzo-p-dioxin Administered to Female Rats Before Mating. Environ Res 1983;31:105–10.
223. Li XL, Johnson DC, Rozman KK. Reproductive Effects of 2,3,7,8-Tetrachlorodibenzo-p-dioxin (TCDD) in Female Rats: Ovulation, Hormonal Regulation, and Possible Mechanism(s). Toxicol Appl Pharmacol 1995;133:321–7.
224. Yellon SM, Singh D, Garrett TM, Fagoaga OR, Nehlsen-Cannarella SL. Reproductive, Neuroendocrine, and Immune Consequences of Acute Exposure to 2,3,7, 8-Tetrachlorodibenzo-p-Dioxin in the Siberian Hamster. Biol Reprod 2000;63:538–43.
225. Blankenship AL, Suffia MC, Matsumura F, Walsh KJ, Wiley LM. 2,3,7,8-Tetrachlorodibenzo-p-dioxin (TCDD) Accelerates Differentiation of Murine Preimplantation Embryos In Vitro. Reprod Toxicol 1993;7:255–61.
226. Wu Q, Ohsako S, Baba T, Miyamoto K, Tohyama C. Effects of 2,3,7,8-Tetrachlorodibenzo-p-dioxin (TCDD) on Preimplantation Mouse Embryos. Toxicology 2002; 174:119–29.
227. Wu Q, Ohsako S, Ishimura R, Suzuki JS, Tohyama C. Exposure of Mouse Preimplantation Embryos to 2,3,7, 8-Tetrachlorodibenzo-p-dioxin (TCDD) Alters the Methylation Status of Imprinted Genes H19 and Igf2. Biol Reprod 2004;70:1790–7.
228. Hutt K, Shi Z, Albertini D, Petroff B. The Environmental Toxicant 2,3,7,8-tetrachlorodibenzo-p-dioxin Disrupts Morphogenesis of the Rat Pre-implantation Embryo. BMC Dev Biol 2008;8:1.
229. Guo Y, Hendrickx AG, Overstreet JW, et al. Endocrine Biomarkers of Early Fetal Loss in Cynomolgus Macaques (*Macaca fascicularis*) Following Exposure to Dioxin. Biol Reprod 1999;60:707–13.
230. Li B, Liu HY, Dai LJ, Lu JC, Yang ZM, Huang L. The Early Embryo Loss Caused by 2,3,7,8-Tetrachlorodibenzo-p-dioxin May Be Related to the Accumulation of this Compound in the Uterus. Reprod Toxicol 2006;21:301–6.
231. Moran FM, VandeVoort CA, Overstreet JW, Lasley BL, Conley AJ. Molecular Target of Endocrine Disruption in Human Luteinizing Granulosa Cells by 2,3,7,8-Tetrachlorodibenzo-p-dioxin: Inhibition of Estradiol Secretion Due to Decreased 17Alpha-hydroxylase/17,20-Lyase Cytochrome P450 Expression. Endocrinology 2003;144:467–73.
232. Abbott BD, Schmid JE, Pitt JA, et al. Adverse Reproductive Outcomes in the Transgenic Ah Receptor-Deficient Mouse. Toxicol Appl Pharmacol 1999;155:62–70.
233. Benedict JC, Lin T-M, Loeffler IK, Peterson RE, Flaws JA. Physiological Role of the Aryl Hydrocarbon Receptor in Mouse Ovary Development. Toxicol Sci 2000;56:382–8.
234. Kishi R, Sata F, Yoshioka E, et al. Exploiting Gene-Environment Interaction to Detect Adverse Health Effects of Environmental Chemicals on the Next Generation. Basic Clin Pharmacol Toxicol 2008;102:191–203.
235. Pocar P, Fischer B, Klonisch T, Hombach-Klonisch S. Molecular Interactions of the Aryl Hydrocarbon Receptor and Its Biological and Toxicological Relevance for Reproduction. Reproduction 2005;129:379–89.
236. Pocar P, Nestler D, Risch M, Fischer B. Apoptosis in Bovine Cumulus-Oocyte Complexes After Exposure to Polychlorinated Biphenyl Mixtures During In Vitro Maturation. Reproduction 2005;130:857–68.
237. Nebert DW, Brown DD, Towne DW, Eisen HJ. Association of fertility, fitness and longevity with the murine Ah locus among (C57BL/6N) (C3H/HeN) recombinant inbred lines. Biol Reprod 1984;30:363–73.
238. Pocar P, Augustin R, Fischer B. Constitutive Expression of CYP1A1 in Bovine Cumulus Oocyte-Complexes in Vitro: Mechanisms and Biological Implications. Endocrinology 2004;145:1594–601.
239. Raffensperger C, Tickner J, Schettler T, Jordan A. And Can Mean Saying “Yes” to Innovation. Nature 1999;401: 207–8.

# Metformin for the Treatment of Polycystic Ovary Syndrome (PCOS)

Satin S. Patel, Victor E. Beshay, and Bruce R. Carr

**Abstract** Because of the high prevalence of insulin resistance, there is a growing interest in the application of insulin sensitizing agents in patients with polycystic ovary syndrome (PCOS). Metformin is the most widely prescribed insulin sensitizing agent in patients with PCOS. In this chapter, we address the importance of lifestyle modification as the initial intervention in patients with PCOS. Furthermore, we discuss the efficacy of metformin compared to low-dose estrogen/progestin oral contraceptives in restoring menstrual cyclicity, reducing androgen excess, and protecting against uterine malignancies. Additionally, the role of metformin in PCOS patients with infertility is addressed.

**Keywords** Metformin • Polycystic ovary syndrome • PCOS • Hyperinsulinemia • Anovulation • Androgen

## 1 Introduction

Polycystic ovary syndrome (PCOS) is the most common endocrinopathy in women, affecting 5–10% of all females of reproductive age (1–5). According to the Rotterdam criteria, PCOS is characterized by increased ovarian androgen production, menstrual cycle irregularity, and polycystic morphology on ovarian ultrasound (6). PCOS comprises a spectrum of metabolic abnormalities encompassing hirsutism, acne, and often infertility (7). Additionally, since many PCOS patients are anovulatory, owing to unopposed estrogen secretion, they are at a significantly higher risk for endometrial hyperplasia and subsequently frank carcinoma (8, 9). More recent studies have highlighted the link between PCOS and metabolic syndrome, a condition marked by hyperlipidemia and insulin resistance (10, 11). Hence, early diagnosis of PCOS, along with vigilant long-term screening for signs of diabetes and cardiovascular diseases is imperative.

Although the pathophysiology of PCOS still remains largely uncharacterized, insulin resistance and compensatory hyperinsulinemia appear to be a prominent feature of this phenotype (10, 12). Several studies have demonstrated a causative association between hyperandrogenemia and underlying hyperinsulinemia (10, 12–15). Elevated insulin levels have been shown to increase serum androgen levels both directly, via effects on the ovary and adrenal, as well as via lutenizing hormone (LH) secretion by the pituitary (16–19). Furthermore, studies in the theca cell model have delineated that insulin normally functions to exert an inhibitory effect on 17-$\alpha$ hydroxylase (CYP17), thereby inhibiting androgen production. *In vitro* studies using theca cells from PCOS patients have demonstrated exaggerated androgen synthesis (20, 21). Moreover, hyperinsulinemia has been shown to inhibit hepatic synthesis of sex hormone binding globulin (SHBG), in turn increasing the bioavailability of free androgens (13, 22). This resulting hyperinsulinemic androgen excess state in PCOS patients is believed to be the underlying cause of anovulatory infertility as well as the worrisome metabolic sequelae associated with PCOS.

Therefore, targeting insulin resistance has been the key focus in the PCOS realm of pharmacologic development. The application of several insulin sensitizing agents, many of which have exhibited promise in Type

S.S. Patel, V.E. Beshay, and B.R. Carr (✉)
University of Texas at Southwestern Medical Center, Department of OB/GYN, Division of Reproductive Endocrinology & Infertility, 5323 Harry Hines Blvd., Dallas, TX, 75390-9032, USA
e-mail: Bruce.carr@utsouthwestern.edu

D.T. Carrell et al. (eds.), *Biennial Review of Infertility,* DOI: 10.1007/978-1-60327-392-3_2

II diabetes, has been studied in the PCOS population. Metformin, an oral biguanide, is the most widely used insulin sensitizing agent in the United States (23–29). Moreover, it is the recommended first-line treatment in newly diagnosed patients with type II diabetes mellitus (30). By enhancing the binding of insulin to the insulin receptor, thereby stimulating postreceptor action, metformin is believed to enhance insulin signaling (31). Metformin exerts its metabolic effects by decreasing lipolysis, hepatic gluconeogenesis, and intestinal glucose absorption, thereby reducing the requirement for insulin secretion (29, 32–34). Additionally, metformin has been shown to act directly on the theca cell, reducing CYP17 expression and subsequently depressing theca cell androstenedione production (35, 36).

The steadily increasing prevalence of obesity and diabetes in developing countries has led to an increased awareness of diabetes prevention. Oral glucose tolerance testing is being increasingly implemented in selected patients in efforts to diagnose "prediabetic" high-risk patients. Understandably, patients suffering from PCOS comprise a large fraction of this population. Although our success with diagnosing patients with glucose intolerance has been favorable, directing the subsequent long-term management of these patients is a subject of much controversy. Most clinicians unanimously agree that weight reduction should be of paramount concern (37). A recent meta-analysis revealed that metformin does not result in weight loss among overweight and obese patients with PCOS (27). Hence initial interventions should focus primarily on routine exercise along with lifestyle and dietary modification. The place of insulin sensitizing agents in these patients is a question that remains unanswered at this time.

## 2 Metformin in the Prevention of Diabetes

Recent studies have taken an interest in the potential role of metformin in the prophylaxis against insulin resistance and, ultimately, the development of diabetes. In a randomized controlled trial, the NIH Diabetes Prevention Project compared the benefit from metformin therapy to lifestyle intervention in patients exhibiting glucose intolerance (38). Treatment arms consisted of weight loss via dietary modification and exercise in comparison to metformin monotherapy. With a mean follow-up of 2.8 years, the incidence of diabetes was reduced by 58% with lifestyle intervention and 31% with metformin, as compared to placebo (38). This finding underscores that even in patients who are at high risk for developing diabetes, lifestyle intervention is superior to pharmacologic prophylaxis with metformin (38).

As in the case with diabetes prevention, insulin sensitizing agents have similarly met marginal success in the prevention of cardiovascular disease. In fact, some agents have surprisingly been found to exacerbate preexisting cardiac disease. Nissen (2007) demonstrated a 43% increase in risk of myocardial infarction among patients taking rosiglitazone (39). This resulted in a black box warning by the FDA, advising against the use of rosiglitazone in patients at high risk for cardiovascular disease. Therefore, the use of insulin sensitizing agents, particularly of the thiazolidinedione class, should be minimized in patients with known cardiovascular disease.

## 3 Metformin in the Treatment of Menstrual Irregularities

Owing to the interdependence of hyperinsulinemia and androgen excess in PCOS patients, the effectiveness of metformin in ameliorating aberrations of an androgen excess state has also been studied. Oligomenorrhea is one of the most common complaints amongst PCOS patients. Fleming (2002) reported that 30% of oligomenorrheic PCOS patients achieve restoration of a normal ovarian rhythm after 16 weeks of metformin therapy (40).

However, it is important to note that in comparison to metformin, combined estrogen–progestin oral contraceptives as well as cyclic progestin therapy have been found to yield superior results in terms of restoration of menstrual cyclicity. Furthermore, oral contraceptive pill (OCP) treatment also reduces symptoms of androgen excess and menorrhagia, which often improves anemia (41). Since patients with oligomenorrhea are at risk for endometrial hyperplasia and potentially invasive carcinoma, protection of the endometrium is of crucial concern. PCOS patients who are on OCPs have a lower incidence of endometrial hyperplasia, a known precursor to endometrial carcinoma (42, 43). Similarly, a significantly reduced risk of ovarian cancer has been demonstrated among OCP users (42). Additionally, the use of hormonal agents also offers the added benefit of contraceptive protection in selected patients. Therefore, if metformin is used in the treatment of PCOS patients, it may be advisable to add OCPs to better prevent endometrial hyperplasia. However, at this time, there are only a few short-term studies investigating the combination of metformin and OCPs.

## 4 Metformin in the Treatment of Hyperandrogenism

The phenotypic manifestations of PCOS, hirsutism, acne, and alopecia, are usually the driving force for patients to seek medical attention. Given the association between androgen excess and insulin resistance, many studies have investigated the effect of metformin monotherapy on these symptoms. Unfortunately, studies thus far have failed to show a significant improvement with metformin monotherapy (44). In contrast, OCPs have been shown to significantly reduce hirsutism, acne, and alopecia (41). The Endocrine Society Clinical Practice Guidelines (2008) advises against using metformin to treat hirsutism in premenopausal women; estrogen/progestin OCPs are the recommended first-line treatment (45). Additionally, OCPS have also been shown to be superior with respect to menstrual cycle restoration and protection of the endometrium against hyperplasia and malignancy (41).

Owing to the heterogeneity of PCOS, the treatment approach should be guided by the specific metabolic disturbances at hand. In the patient with frank diabetes, metformin therapy should be the first line of treatment. Nondiabetic, normoinsulinemic PCOS patients with complaints of clinical manifestations of androgen excess should be treated with a trial of OCPs without metformin. If PCOS patients display evidence of glucose intolerance without a diagnosis of overt diabetes, lifestyle and dietary modification should be recommended as the initial intervention. In selected patients who fail conservative management, metformin therapy may be instituted.

Small studies have found that older, higher dose OCPs may increase the risk of insulin resistance and lipid abnormalities in PCOS patients (46). However, no long-term placebo-controlled study has demonstrated that current low-dose OCPs increase the risk of diabetes, hyperlipidemia, or cardiovascular disease in both patients with or without PCOS (47, 48).

## 5 Metformin for the PCOS Patient with Infertility

PCOS is the most common cause of infertility among reproductive-aged women. Most cases of infertility in this population are believed to arise from ovulatory dysfunction. In fact, PCOS accounts for nearly 75% of all cases of anovulatory infertility in women seeking fertility treatment. Additionally, even after attaining successful conception, women with PCOS remain at a threefold increased risk for pregnancy loss, implicating additional factors in the multifaceted etiology of PCOS-related reproductive dysfunction.

PCOS is a complex and heterogeneous disorder characterized by dysfunctional ovarian steroidogenesis. Cultured theca cells from PCOS patients display markedly increased androgen secretion, likely as a result of hyperinsulinemia (49–51). This hyperandrogenic milieu alters the intrafollicular microenvironment, leading to aberrant folliculogenesis. *In vitro* studies have demonstrated that developing follicles exposed to a high androgen environment are prone to result in follicular arrest at the 4–8 diameter size (52). Failure to produce a dominant follicle in turn leads to anovulation. Hence the underlying insulin resistance, hyperandrogenemia and the resulting aberrant follicular growth, is thought to result in the common PCOS phenotype of oligoovulation, androgen excess, and anovulatory infertility (53).

Fortunately, many treatment options are available to infertile couples suffering from PCOS. Since the majority of these patients are anovulatory, initial efforts are geared towards restoring ovulation. Clomiphene citrate (CC) is typically the first-line pharmacologic agent recommended. CC successfully restores ovulation in 70–85% of women (54). This allows for a 50% pregnancy rate within three consecutive cycles of CC among anovulatory PCOS patients. Some authors have reported a cumulative pregnancy rate exceeding 90% in PCOS patients using CC for at least six cycles (55).

Since CC is an antiestrogen, it functions by dampening the negative feedback of estrogen on the anterior pituitary, leading to a net increase in gonadotropin (follicle-stimulating hormone (FSH) and luteinizing hormone (LH) production). Note, however, that there are several limitations of CC therapy. CC is known to exert an antiestrogenic effect on the cervical mucus and endometrial lining (56, 57). Additionally, CC use increases the patient's risk of twin gestation, with an absolute risk of roughly 4–10% (58, 59).

In cases where ovulation using CC fails to occur, stimulation of the PCOS ovary may be attempted using exogenous gonadotropins. Currently, recombinant FSH preparations are the most widely used form of gonadotropin ovulation induction. Of note, PCOS patients undergoing ovulation induction with gonadotropins require close surveillance, since they are at elevated risk for ovarian hyperstimulation syndrome (60). In a patient in whom CC or gonadotropin therapy fails, *in vitro* fertilization may be necessary. Newer advanced reproductive techniques, such as *in vitro* maturation, appear to minimize the patient's risk for ovarian hyperstimulation syndrome (61, 62). However, pregnancy rates with *in vitro* maturation are low at this time and therefore this practice is currently considered experimental.

In patients with insulin resistance, improving insulin sensitivity via pharmacologic agents would logically appear to increase ovulation rates (31, 49, 50). Unlike treatment with CC or gonadotropins, metformin therapy does not appear to accelerate follicular recruitment. Instead, it is theorized to enhance the microfollicular milieu, in which a narrow range of insulin levels is thought to be critical for healthy monofollicular gonadal function (63, 64).

Studies using metformin monotherapy in infertile patients with anovulatory infertility have demonstrated an improvement in ovulatory rates (31). In a recent meta-analysis, Creanga (2008) reported a nearly threefold improvement in ovulatory rates in PCOS women undergoing metformin treatment (65). Unfortunately, this success in bolstering ovulatory rates does not appear to translate to actual improved pregnancy rates. In a prospective randomized, controlled trial of 626 infertile PCOS women, Legro (2007) reported a markedly lower live-birth rate with metformin treatment compared to those receiving CC monotherapy. The live-birth rate in the CC group was 22.5% compared to only 7.2% in the metformin group; this difference was statistically significant. Furthermore, these conclusions are in accord with the recent meta-analyses by Moll (2007) and Creanga (2008) evaluating the effectiveness of metformin in improving ovulatory and subsequently pregnancy rates (65, 66). Additionally, studies investigating the combination of CC and metformin failed to provide any added benefit over CC monotherapy (67). Moreover, supplementing CC with metformin does not lower the threshold CC dose that is necessary for ovulation (68). Hence, metformin appears to be an inferior choice in the initial management for PCOS patients with infertility. The most appropriate first-line therapy in anovulatory PCOS patients desiring conception is CC (67).

## 6 Metformin Following Conception

Whether PCOS patients should continue metformin therapy following conception is a subject of debate. The U.S. Food and Drug Administration (FDA) has classified metformin as "Pregnancy category B," indicating that safety in pregnant women has not been definitively established but no experimental animal evidence suggesting teratogenicity has been reported (69). Given that PCOS patients are at greater risk of miscarriage in the first trimester of gestation, many practitioners opt to continue metformin use until fetal cardiac activity has been documented, while others continue treatment until the end of the first trimester (70). However, in a large prospective randomized, controlled trial, continued use of metformin in early pregnancy was not associated with a reduced miscarriage rate as compared to women not on metformin who used CC alone for ovulation induction (67).

## 7 Precautions with Metformin

All women undergoing metformin therapy should be counseled on the risk of adverse events associated with this medication (71). The most worrisome of these side effects is lactic acidosis (71, 72). Although the actual incidence is rare (1:33,000), those that are affected face a grim prognosis, with mortality rates approaching 50% (73–75). Moreover, symptoms of lactic acidosis are often subtle and nonspecific. Affected patients may present with generalized fatigue, abdominal pain, and myalgia. In more pronounced cases, symptoms may progress to respiratory depression. Suspected cases should be attended to promptly with particular attention to correcting abnormalities in serum electrolytes, ketones, glucose, pH, and lactate levels (76). Cases with marked anion-gap metabolic acidosis may benefit from prompt hemodialysis (77, 78).

Fortunately, the enforcement of preventative measures has helped reduce the incidence of lactic acidosis. Such measures include the discontinuation of metformin 24–48 h prior to any planned surgery or imaging study requiring the use of intravenous contrast. Additionally, even mild renal impairment is a contraindication to metformin use (79).

More commonly, patients undergoing metformin treatment have gastrointestinal complaints (32). In fact, up to 30% of patients taking metformin report suffering from nausea, vomiting, diarrhea, bloating, flatulence, or a combination of these symptoms. Metformin-induced gastrointestinal discomfort is believed to result from drug accumulation in the intestinal wall, and side effects are more prevalent at higher dosages (80, 81). For this reason, a gradual stepwise increase in metformin dosage may allow the patient to acclimate in a more comfortable fashion (29). Newer extended-release formulations may be associated with fewer side effects.

## 8 Alternatives to Metformin

The utility of other classes of oral hypoglycemic agents have also been studied in PCOS patients. Increasing attention is particularly being drawn to the thiazolidinedione (glitazones) class of drugs. These agents function by increasing insulin sensitivity, without simulating insulin secretion (82–84). As in the case with metformin, glitazones have been found to increase ovulatory rates in PCOS patients (85). However, also similarly, neither metformin nor glitazones have demonstrated a benefit on pregnancy rates or live-birth rates compared to CC monotherapy. Additionally, glitazone therapy has been demonstrated to result in weight gain, which may further exacerbate the patient's infertility and other PCOS-associated sequelae (30). Moreover, glitazones have been found to have a worrisome side effect profile, leading to the withdrawal of Troglitazone from the U.S. market by the FDA in 1999, due to numerous reports of fatal liver toxicity (86, 87). Subsequently, rosiglitazone also received a black box warning from the FDA after Nissen (2007) reported a 43% increased risk of myocardial infarction among patients taking rosiglitazone (39). Because of these findings, it follows that only a limited number of short-term studies evaluating glitazones in PCOS has been reported.

## 9 Conclusions

At this time, the only indication for metformin therapy approved by the FDA is type II diabetes (29, 81, 88). Although a large fraction of patients with PCOS display signs of impaired glucose tolerance, lifestyle intervention has been found to be more effective than metformin therapy for the prevention of diabetes (38). Furthermore, low-dose estrogen/progestin oral contraceptives have been shown to have superior results in alleviating symptoms of androgen excess, restoring menstrual cyclicity, and protecting against endometrial malignancies (41–43, 45). Although metformin appears to improve ovulatory rates in some patients, ovulation induction using clomiphene citrate results in higher live-birth rates compared to metformin therapy. Hence the evidence to date suggests that metformin therapy in patients with PCOS should be reserved for CC-resistant patients and patients with frank type II diabetes.

## References

1. Hull MG. Epidemiology of infertility and polycystic ovarian disease: endocrinological and demographic studies. Gynecol Endocrinol 1987;1:235–45.
2. Polson DW, Adams J, Wadsworth J, Franks S. Polycystic ovaries–a common finding in normal women. Lancet 1988;1: 870–2.
3. Asuncion M, Calvo RM, San Millan JL, Sancho J, Avila S, Escobar-Morreale HF. A prospective study of the prevalence of the polycystic ovary syndrome in unselected Caucasian women from Spain. J Clin Endocrinol Metab 2000;85: 2434–8.
4. Franks S. Polycystic ovary syndrome. N Engl J Med 1995; 333:853–61.
5. Lam PM, Cheung LP, Haines C. Revisit of metformin treatment in polycystic ovarian syndrome. Gynecol Endocrinol 2004;19:33–9.
6. Revised 2003 consensus on diagnostic criteria and long-term health risks related to polycystic ovary syndrome (PCOS). Hum Reprod 2004;19:41–7.
7. Ehrmann DA. Polycystic ovary syndrome. N Engl J Med 2005;352:1223–36.
8. Hardiman P, Pillay OC, Atiomo W. Polycystic ovary syndrome and endometrial carcinoma. Lancet 2003;361: 1810–2.
9. Gadducci A, Gargini A, Palla E, Fanucchi A, Genazzani AR. Polycystic ovary syndrome and gynecological cancers: is there a link? Gynecol Endocrinol 2005;20:200–8.
10. Dunaif A. Insulin resistance and the polycystic ovary syndrome: mechanism and implications for pathogenesis. Endocr Rev 1997;18:774–800.

11. Poretsky L, Cataldo NA, Rosenwaks Z, Giudice LC. The insulin-related ovarian regulatory system in health and disease. Endocr Rev 1999;20:535–82.
12. Dunaif A, Graf M. Insulin administration alters gonadal steroid metabolism independent of changes in gonadotropin secretion in insulin-resistant women with the polycystic ovary syndrome. J Clin Invest 1989;83:23–9.
13. Nestler JE, Powers LP, Matt DW, Steingold KA, Plymate SR, Rittmaster RS, et al. A direct effect of hyperinsulinemia on serum sex hormone-binding globulin levels in obese women with the polycystic ovary syndrome. J Clin Endocrinol Metab 1991;72:83–9.
14. Richardson MR. Current perspectives in polycystic ovary syndrome. Am Fam Physician 2003;68:697–704.
15. Barbieri RL, Smith S, Ryan KJ. The role of hyperinsulinemia in the pathogenesis of ovarian hyperandrogenism. Fertil Steril 1988;50:197–212.
16. Nahum R, Thong KJ, Hillier SG. Metabolic regulation of androgen production by human thecal cells in vitro. Hum Reprod 1995;10:75–81.
17. Prelevic GM, Wurzburger MI, Balint-Peric L. LH pulsatility and response to a single s.c. injection of buserelin in polycystic ovary syndrome. Gynecol Endocrinol 1990;4:1–13.
18. Bergh C, Carlsson B, Olsson JH, Selleskog U, Hillensjo T. Regulation of androgen production in cultured human thecal cells by insulin-like growth factor I and insulin. Fertil Steril 1993;59:323–31.
19. Willis D, Franks S. Insulin action in human granulosa cells from normal and polycystic ovaries is mediated by the insulin receptor and not the type-I insulin-like growth factor receptor. J Clin Endocrinol Metab 1995;80:3788–90.
20. Escobar-Morreale HF, Luque-Ramirez M, San Millan JL. The molecular-genetic basis of functional hyperandrogenism and the polycystic ovary syndrome. Endocr Rev 2005;26:251–82.
21. Nelson VL, Qin KN, Rosenfield RL, Wood JR, Penning TM, Legro RS, et al. The biochemical basis for increased testosterone production in theca cells propagated from patients with polycystic ovary syndrome. J Clin Endocrinol Metab 2001;86:5925–33.
22. Azziz R. Androgen excess is the key element in polycystic ovary syndrome. Fertil Steril 2003;80:252–4.
23. Ibanez L, Valls C, Ferrer A, Ong K, Dunger DB, De Zegher F. Additive effects of insulin-sensitizing and anti-androgen treatment in young, nonobese women with hyperinsulinism, hyperandrogenism, dyslipidemia, and anovulation. J Clin Endocrinol Metab 2002;87:2870–4.
24. Harborne L, Fleming R, Lyall H, Norman J, Sattar N. Descriptive review of the evidence for the use of metformin in polycystic ovary syndrome. Lancet 2003;361:1894–901.
25. Haas DA, Carr BR, Attia GR. Effects of metformin on body mass index, menstrual cyclicity, and ovulation induction in women with polycystic ovary syndrome. Fertil Steril 2003; 79:469–81.
26. Velazquez EM, Mendoza S, Hamer T, Sosa F, Glueck CJ. Metformin therapy in polycystic ovary syndrome reduces hyperinsulinemia, insulin resistance, hyperandrogenemia, and systolic blood pressure, while facilitating normal menses and pregnancy. Metabolism 1994;43:647–54.
27. Lord JM, Flight IH, Norman RJ. Metformin in polycystic ovary syndrome: systematic review and meta-analysis. BMJ 2003;327:951–3.
28. Elizur SE, Tulandi T. Drugs in infertility and fetal safety. Fertil Steril 2008;89:1595–602.
29. Ben-Haroush A, Yogev Y, Fisch B. Insulin resistance and metformin in polycystic ovary syndrome. Eur J Obstet Gynecol Reprod Biol 2004;115:125–33.
30. Ortega-Gonzalez C, Luna S, Hernandez L, Crespo G, Aguayo P, Arteaga-Troncoso G, et al. Responses of serum androgen and insulin resistance to metformin and pioglitazone in obese, insulin-resistant women with polycystic ovary syndrome. J Clin Endocrinol Metab 2005;90:1360–5.
31. Pirwany IR, Yates RW, Cameron IT, Fleming R. Effects of the insulin sensitizing drug metformin on ovarian function, follicular growth and ovulation rate in obese women with oligomenorrhoea. Hum Reprod 1999;14:2963–8.
32. Bailey CJ, Turner RC. Metformin. N Engl J Med 1996;334: 574–9.
33. Patane G, Piro S, Rabuazzo AM, Anello M, Vigneri R, Purrello F. Metformin restores insulin secretion altered by chronic exposure to free fatty acids or high glucose: a direct metformin effect on pancreatic beta-cells. Diabetes 2000; 49:735–40.
34. Kirpichnikov D, McFarlane SI, Sowers JR. Metformin: an update. Ann Intern Med 2002;137:25–33.
35. Attia GR, Rainey WE, Carr BR. Metformin directly inhibits androgen production in human thecal cells. Fertil Steril 2001;76:517–24.
36. Adashi EY, Resnick CE, D'Ercole AJ, Svoboda ME, Van Wyk JJ. Insulin-like growth factors as intraovarian regulators of granulosa cell growth and function. Endocr Rev 1985;6:400–20.
37. Kiddy DS, Hamilton-Fairley D, Bush A, Short F, Anyaoku V, Reed MJ, et al. Improvement in endocrine and ovarian function during dietary treatment of obese women with polycystic ovary syndrome. Clin Endocrinol (Oxf) 1992;36: 105–11.
38. Knowler WC, Barrett-Connor E, Fowler SE, Hamman RF, Lachin JM, Walker EA, et al. Reduction in the incidence of type 2 diabetes with lifestyle intervention or metformin. N Engl J Med 2002;346:393–403.
39. Nissen SE, Wolski K. Effect of rosiglitazone on the risk of myocardial infarction and death from cardiovascular causes. N Engl J Med 2007;356:2457–71.
40. Fleming R, Hopkinson ZE, Wallace AM, Greer IA, Sattar N. Ovarian function and metabolic factors in women with oligomenorrhea treated with metformin in a randomized double blind placebo-controlled trial. J Clin Endocrinol Metab 2002;87:569–74.
41. Costello MF, Shrestha B, Eden J, Johnson NP, Sjoblom P. Metformin versus oral contraceptive pill in polycystic ovary syndrome: a Cochrane review. Hum Reprod 2007;22: 1200–9.
42. Vessey M, Painter R. Oral contraceptive use and cancer. Findings in a large cohort study, 1968–2004. Br J Cancer 2006;95:385–9.
43. Schlesselman JJ. Risk of endometrial cancer in relation to use of combined oral contraceptives. A practitioner's guide to meta-analysis. Hum Reprod 1997;12:1851–63.
44. Cosma M, Swiglo BA, Flynn DN, Kurtz DM, Labella ML, Mullan RJ, et al. Clinical review: insulin sensitizers for the treatment of hirsutism: a systematic review and metaanalyses of randomized controlled trials. J Clin Endocrinol Metab 2008;93:1135–42.

45. Martin KA, Chang RJ, Ehrmann DA, Ibanez L, Lobo RA, Rosenfield RL, et al. Evaluation and treatment of hirsutism in premenopausal women: an endocrine society clinical practice guideline. J Clin Endocrinol Metab 2008;93:1105–20.
46. Godsland IF, Walton C, Felton C, Proudler A, Patel A, Wynn V. Insulin resistance, secretion, and metabolism in users of oral contraceptives. J Clin Endocrinol Metab 1992;74:64–70.
47. Diamanti-Kandarakis E, Baillargeon JP, Iuorno MJ, Jakubowicz DJ, Nestler JE. A modern medical quandary: polycystic ovary syndrome, insulin resistance, and oral contraceptive pills. J Clin Endocrinol Metab 2003;88:1927–32.
48. Vrbikova J, Cibula D. Combined oral contraceptives in the treatment of polycystic ovary syndrome. Hum Reprod Update 2005;11:277–91.
49. Gilling-Smith C, Willis DS, Beard RW, Franks S. Hypersecretion of androstenedione by isolated thecal cells from polycystic ovaries. J Clin Endocrinol Metab 1994;79:1158–65.
50. Gilling-Smith C, Story H, Rogers V, Franks S. Evidence for a primary abnormality of thecal cell steroidogenesis in the polycystic ovary syndrome. Clin Endocrinol (Oxf) 1997;47:93–9.
51. Wickenheisser JK, Quinn PG, Nelson VL, Legro RS, Strauss JFIII, McAllister JM. Differential activity of the cytochrome P450 17alpha-hydroxylase and steroidogenic acute regulatory protein gene promoters in normal and polycystic ovary syndrome theca cells. J Clin Endocrinol Metab 2000;85:2304–11.
52. Fujiwara T, Sidis Y, Welt C, Lambert-Messerlian G, Fox J, Taylor A, et al. Dynamics of inhibin subunit and follistatin mRNA during development of normal and polycystic ovary syndrome follicles. J Clin Endocrinol Metab 2001;86: 4206–15.
53. Laven JS, Imani B, Eijkemans MJ, Fauser BC. New approach to polycystic ovary syndrome and other forms of anovulatory infertility. Obstet Gynecol Surv 2002;57:755–67.
54. Costello MF, Eden JA. A systematic review of the reproductive system effects of metformin in patients with polycystic ovary syndrome. Fertil Steril 2003;79:1–13.
55. Macgregor AH, Johnson JE, Bunde CA. Further clinical experience with clomiphene citrate. Fertil Steril 1968;19: 616–22.
56. Randall JM, Templeton A. Cervical mucus score and in vitro sperm mucus interaction in spontaneous and clomiphene citrate cycles. Fertil Steril 1991;56:465–8.
57. Nakamura Y, Ono M, Yoshida Y, Sugino N, Ueda K, Kato H. Effects of clomiphene citrate on the endometrial thickness and echogenic pattern of the endometrium. Fertil Steril 1997;67:256–60.
58. Kousta E, White DM, Franks S. Modern use of clomiphene citrate in induction of ovulation. Hum Reprod Update 1997; 3:359–65.
59. Eijkemans MJ, Imani B, Mulders AG, Habbema JD, Fauser BC. High singleton live birth rate following classical ovulation induction in normogonadotrophic anovulatory infertility (WHO 2). Hum Reprod 2003;18:2357–62.
60. Tulandi T, McInnes RA, Arronet GH. Ovarian hyperstimulation syndrome following ovulation induction with human menopausal gonadotropin. Int J Fertil 1984;29:113–7.
61. Child TJ, Abdul-Jalil AK, Gulekli B, Tan SL. In vitro maturation and fertilization of oocytes from unstimulated normal ovaries, polycystic ovaries, and women with polycystic ovary syndrome. Fertil Steril 2001;76:936–42.
62. Chian RC, Buckett WM, Tulandi T, Tan SL. Prospective randomized study of human chorionic gonadotrophin priming before immature oocyte retrieval from unstimulated women with polycystic ovarian syndrome. Hum Reprod 2000;15: 165–70.
63. Nestler JE, Strauss JFIII. Insulin as an effector of human ovarian and adrenal steroid metabolism. Endocrinol Metab Clin North Am 1991;20:807–23.
64. Nestler JE, Jakubowicz DJ, Evans WS, Pasquali R. Effects of metformin on spontaneous and clomiphene-induced ovulation in the polycystic ovary syndrome. N Engl J Med 1998;338:1876–80.
65. Creanga AA, Bradley HM, McCormick C, Witkop CT. Use of metformin in polycystic ovary syndrome: a meta-analysis. Obstet Gynecol 2008;111:959–68.
66. Moll E, van der Veen F, van Wely M. The role of metformin in polycystic ovary syndrome: a systematic review. Hum Reprod Update 2007;13:527–37.
67. Legro RS, Barnhart HX, Schlaff WD, Carr BR, Diamond MP, Carson SA et al. Clomiphene, metformin, or both for infertility in the polycystic ovary syndrome. N Engl J Med 2007;356:551–66.
68. Cataldo NA, Barnhart HX, Legro RS, Myers ER, Schlaff WD, Carr BR et al. Extended-release metformin does not reduce the clomiphene citrate dose required to induce ovulation in polycystic ovary syndrome. J Clin Endocrinol Metab 2008;93:3124–7.
69. Sills ES, Perloe M, Palermo GD. Correction of hyperinsulinemia in oligoovulatory women with clomiphene-resistant polycystic ovary syndrome: a review of therapeutic rationale and reproductive outcomes. Eur J Obstet Gynecol Reprod Biol 2000;91:135–41.
70. Jakubowicz DJ, Iuorno MJ, Jakubowicz S, Roberts KA, Nestler JE. Effects of metformin on early pregnancy loss in the polycystic ovary syndrome. J Clin Endocrinol Metab 2002;87:524–9.
71. Spiller HA, Sawyer TS. Toxicology of oral antidiabetic medications. Am J Health Syst Pharm 2006;63:929–38.
72. Gan SC, Barr J, Arieff AI, Pearl RG. Biguanide-associated lactic acidosis. Case report and review of the literature. Arch Intern Med 1992;152:2333–6.
73. Huckabee WE. Lactic Acidosis. Am J Cardiol 1963;12: 663–6.
74. Tucker GT, Casey C, Phillips PJ, Connor H, Ward JD, Woods HF. Metformin kinetics in healthy subjects and in patients with diabetes mellitus. Br J Clin Pharmacol 1981;12:235–46.
75. Ficicioglu C, Api M, Ozden S. The number of follicles and ovarian volume in the assessment of response to clomiphene citrate treatment in polycystic ovarian syndrome. Acta Obstet Gynecol Scand 1996;75:917–21.
76. Adrogue HJ. Metabolic acidosis: pathophysiology, diagnosis and management. J Nephrol 2006;19 Suppl 9:S62–9.
77. Heaney D, Majid A, Junor B. Bicarbonate haemodialysis as a treatment of metformin overdose. Nephrol Dial Transplant 1997;12:1046–7.
78. Luft FC. Lactic acidosis update for critical care clinicians. J Am Soc Nephrol 2001;12 Suppl 17:S15–9.
79. Snyder RW, Berns JS. Use of insulin and oral hypoglycemic medications in patients with diabetes mellitus and advanced kidney disease. Semin Dial 2004;17:365–70.
80. DeFronzo RA, Goodman AM. Efficacy of metformin in patients with non-insulin-dependent diabetes mellitus. The Multicenter Metformin Study Group. N Engl J Med 1995; 333:541–9.

81. Garber AJ, Duncan TG, Goodman AM, Mills DJ, Rohlf JL. Efficacy of metformin in type II diabetes: results of a double-blind, placebo-controlled, dose-response trial. Am J Med 1997;103:491–7.
82. Iwamoto Y, Kosaka K, Kuzuya T, Akanuma Y, Shigeta Y, Kaneko T. Effects of troglitazone: a new hypoglycemic agent in patients with NIDDM poorly controlled by diet therapy. Diabetes Care 1996;19:151–6.
83. Wojcicki J, Szwed G, Drozdowska-Ksiazek D. The antitussive and expectorant drug Duopect evaluated by the preferential test. Arch Immunol Ther Exp (Warsz) 1976;24: 549–52.
84. Yki-Jarvinen H. Thiazolidinediones. N Engl J Med 2004; 351:1106–18.
85. Mitwally MF, Kuscu NK, Yalcinkaya TM. High ovulatory rates with use of troglitazone in clomiphene-resistant women with polycystic ovary syndrome. Hum Reprod 1999;14:2700–3.
86. Baillargeon JP, Iuorno MJ, Nestler JE. Insulin sensitizers for polycystic ovary syndrome. Clin Obstet Gynecol 2003; 46:325–40.
87. Ehrmann DA, Rychlik D. Pharmacologic treatment of polycystic ovary syndrome. Semin Reprod Med 2003;21:277–83.
88. Campbell RK, White JRJr., Saulie BA. Metformin: a new oral biguanide. Clin Ther 1996;18:360–71; discussion 59.

# Minimally Invasive Approaches to Treat Symptomatic Uterine Myomas

Samantha M. Pfeifer

**Abstract** Uterine myomas are common in reproductive-aged women. Traditionally, treatment for symptomatic myomas in women wishing to preserve their ability to have children has been abdominal myomectomy. While this procedure is very successful in improving symptoms related to the myomas, it is associated with surgical morbidity, patient hospitalization, and a prolonged postoperative recovery. Newer, less invasive techniques are now available to treat symptomatic uterine myomas including laparoscopic and robotically assisted laparoscopic myomectomy, uterine artery embolizaiton, and MRI-guided ultrasound focused surgery. These techniques have the advantage of less morbidity and quick recovery. Many studies have shown promising results with regard to improvement in myoma-related symptoms. However, concerns have been raised about using these procedures for women who would like to become pregnant. Further studies are needed to evaluate the risks and benefits compared to standard treatment options.

**Keywords** Myoma • Myomectomy • Embolization • Laparoscopy • Uterus

## 1 Introduction

Uterine myomas are among the most common solid tumors of the female reproductive tract, affecting approximately 20–50% of reproductive-aged women (1, 2). Common symptoms are related to the number and size of the myomas, as well as their location in the uterus, and include pressure, discomfort, excess bleeding, urinary frequency, or retention and constipation. Myomas have also been implicated as a cause of infertility and pregnancy loss. Obstetrical outcomes with myomas include increased risk of transfusion, abruption, malpresentation, and preterm delivery (1, 2).

Surgical treatment for symptomatic myomas in those wishing to preserve fertility has traditionally involved abdominal myomectomy. The goal of abdominal myomectomy is to remove the visible and accessible myomas and then reconstruct the uterus. This procedure has been shown to improve quality of life, decrease bleeding, and reduce uterine volume (3). The procedure is safe and can be performed with minimal blood loss and complications (4). Following abdominal myomectomy, myomas can recur, leading to clinically significant symptoms in 10% by 5 years and in 27% by 10 years (5, 6). Recurrence is more common following removal of multiple myomas compared to solitary myomectomy (7). Published term pregnancy rates following myomectomy range from 40 to 50% and live birth rates as high as 70–100% (8). The drawback of abdominal myomectomy is hospital stay postoperatively (mean 2.5 days) and time to return to work (mean 44 days) (3).

Less invasive alternatives such as laparoscopic myomectomy, robotic-assisted laparoscopic myomectomy, uterine fibroid embolization, and MRI-guided focused ultrasound surgery are now available. These procedures have the advantage of quick recovery and less morbidity. Use of less invasive procedures in women desiring fertility, as well as the efficacy and advantages over myomectomy, need to be assessed.

S.M. Pfeifer
University of Pennsylvania Medical Center,
3701 Market Street, Suite 800, Philadelphia, PA
e-mail: spfeifer@obgyn.upenn.edu

D.T. Carrell et al. (eds.), *Biennial Review of Infertility,* DOI: 10.1007/978-1-60327-392-3_3

## 2 Laparoscopic Myomectomy

Laparoscopic myomectomy was first proposed in the 1970s, and advances in equipment and experience have led to significant improvements in this technique (9). A laparoscopic approach offers the advantages of shorter hospital stay, faster recovery, decreased blood loss, and reduced postoperative pain when compared to laparotomy (10, 11). The application of this technique, however, is limited by the size and number of myomas to be removed and the technical challenge of laparoscopic suturing. The goal of laparoscopic myomectomy is to achieve closure of the uterus that is comparable to, or superior to, abdominal myomectomy. It is one of the more challenging laparoscopic procedures and requires a skilled surgeon.

Laparoscopic myomectomy is well suited to patients with a few fibroids of medium size (approximately 5 cm) in the subserosal or intramural location. These limitations are primarily due to time and technical difficulties relating to suturing and removal of the myomas by morcellation. In a review of a series of laparoscopic myomectomy, the mean myoma size was 4 to 7 cm and number removed 1–3 (12). In a randomized, controlled study of 40 women, comparing myomectomy through laparoscopy to laparotomy, the mean number of myomas was 2.5 and 2.3, respectively, and the mean diameter for each group was <5 cm (range 3–6 cm) (10). In another randomized, controlled study of 131 patients for laparoscopic versus abdominal myomectomy, the myoma size was ≥5 cm for each group and the number of myomas removed was <4 (11). Removal of large myomas by laparoscopy has been described. One case study described 51 patients who underwent laparoscopic myomectomy with removal of at least one myoma >9 cm (13). Removal of submucosal myomas poses the additional challenge of closing the endometrial cavity. In a case series of 34 women who underwent laparoscopic myomectomy for myomas penetrating the uterine cavity, the mean diameter of the myomas removed was 6.7 cm (range 4–15 cm) (14). In the 23 patients wishing to conceive postoperatively, 21 had a normal uterine cavity as demonstrated by hysteroscopy.

The technique for laparoscopic myomectomy should mirror that for abdominal myomectomy. Laparoscopic port placement is important to facilitate enucleation of the myomas and repair of the defect. Placing two ports on the primary surgeon's side of the table, one in the lower quadrant and the other lateral to the umbilical port, is recommended (9). Dilute pitressin may be injected into the uterus for hemostasis, although in some cases adequate hemostasis can be achieved using electrocautery or harmonic scalpel. A transverse incision over the myoma is recommended with laparoscopic myomectomy, in contrast to what is typically done at laparotomy, to facilitate suturing the defect given the ergonomics and limited instrument motion with laparoscopy (9). Closure of the defect is the most technically challenging aspect of laparoscopic myomectomy. Principles of closing the defect laparoscopically should be the same as in laparotomy with the goals of hemostasis and, when indicated, future pregnancy in mind. A multilayered closure is preferred. This can be done with either interrupted or running stitches. A self-righting needle driver facilitates suturing.

Removal of the myomas is typically done by morcellation, though colpotomy has been described. Morcellation can be time consuming, especially with large or numerous myomas. Morcellation of the myoma in situ has recently been described as a way to decrease operative time during laparoscopic myomectomy (15). It is important to remove all fragments of myoma following morcellation because of the risk of developing parasitic myomas. Multiple peritoneal parasitic myomas have been described months to years after myomectomy and morcellation located in previous laparoscopic port sites, in the pelvis near the uterus and ovaries, and in paracolic gutters (16–18).

Laparoscopic myomectomy has been shown to be an effective and safe alternative to abdominal myomectomy in selected patient populations. Randomized, controlled studies comparing the two techniques have used strict inclusion criteria such as limiting size and number of myomas to be removed (10, 11, 19). These studies have shown shorter hospitalization and less postoperative pain with laparoscopic myomectomy. Blood loss and operative time in all studies was similar, but laparoscopic myomectomy time was longer when more myomas were removed. Pregnancy rates for laparoscopic versus abdominal myomectomy were not significantly different: 54 vs. 56% (11).

Short-term outcomes following laparoscopic myomectomy have been evaluated in several large case studies. A retrospective study of 332 laparoscopic myomectomies evaluated outcomes relative to experience and technique (20). The majority of cases (209) were performed from 1998 to 2003, in the era of electromechanic morcellation and vasoconstrictive agents. The majority of patients (47%) had more than one myoma removed with a mean number of 2.2 and a maximum number of 8. Average size of myomas was 6 cm with a range of 1–20 cm. With experience and improved technology, the length of time of the procedure decreased and the mean dimension of the largest myoma increased from 5 to 7 cm. Conversion rate to laparotomy in this study was 1.5% and was due to anesthetic problems in three patients and to the size and limited mobility of the myoma in a narrow space in the other two.

In another retrospective study of 407 laparoscopic myomectomies, conversion rate to laparotomy was 2.9%, and the risk increased with size, number, location in the anterior uterus, and presence of adenomyosis (21). In a case series of 386 patients undergoing laparoscopic myomectomy, intraoperative complication rate was 3.3%, including bleeding requiring autologous transfusion in 2.7% (22). Postoperative complication rate was low, with three patients requiring blood transfusion and two requiring a second laparoscopy.

Recurrence of myomas following laparoscopic myomectomy appears to be similar to that in abdominal myomectomy, although with laparoscopy, fewer fibroids are generally removed. In one study, 81 patients were randomized to laparoscopic or abdominal myomectomy and were assessed for myomas recurrence postoperatively by ultrasound (19). The groups were similar in number of myomas per patient and presenting symptoms. Recurrence of myoma >1 cm by ultrasound at 40 months was 27% in the laparoscopic group and 23% in the abdominal group, which are not significantly different. In one multicenter retrospective study, 512 women underwent laparoscopic myomectomy (23). Recurrence was assessed by appearance of myomas on ultrasound. The cumulative recurrence was 12% at 1 year, 53% at 5 years, and 84% at 8 years. The cumulative probability of reoperation for recurrent myomas was 6.7% at 5 years and 16% at 8 years. Risk factors for recurrence were preoperative number of myomas, preoperative uterine size, and delivery after myomectomy. These compare with abdominal myomectomy where the 5-year recurrence by ultrasound is 51–63% (24, 25).

There are no prospective randomized, controlled studies comparing the rate of adhesion formation after laparoscopic compared to abdominal myomectomy. Adhesion rate following abdominal myomectomy has been reported to be 80–100% (26–28), with the highest rate of bowel and adnexal adhesions seen with a posterior incision on the uterus (26). Several case series have evaluated adhesion formation following laparoscopic myomectomy by second-look laparoscopy. These studies have, in general, shown adhesion formation to be lower than described with abdominal myomectomy. However, it is difficult to compare the results, as the indications for abdominal myomectomy and laparoscopic myomectomy are different and more complex procedures are usually performed by laparotomy. Early case studies utilizing second-look laparoscopy after laparoscopic myomectomy showed postmyomectomy adhesions in 29–36% of patients (29, 30). Risk of adhesions was increased with use of suture to close the uterine defect and with posterior uterine incision primarily involving the rectosigmoid. A prospective observational study involved second-look laparoscopy in 372 patients following laparoscopic myomectomy from 2000 to 2005 (31). Adhesion barriers (fibrin gel, fibrin sheath, Seprafilm™, Interceed™) were used in 84% of patients, and in the remaining 16% no adhesion-preventing agent was used. Use of an adhesion barrier was at the discretion of the surgeon. At second-look laparoscopy, adhesions were seen at the site of the uterine wound in 38% of patients and were more common on the posterior wall (69%). The size and number of myomas removed correlated with increased risk of adhesion formation.

Prospective randomized studies have shown that adhesion barriers are associated with a decrease in adhesion following laparoscopic myomectomy. One study evaluated the use of oxidized regenerated cellulose and found significantly fewer adhesions in the treatment compared to control group (40 vs. 88%) (32). Hyaluronic acid gel is easier to use than oxidized cellulose at the time of laparoscopy, as has been evaluated in two prospective randomized studies (33, 34). In one study of 36 patients evaluated at second-look laparoscopy, the rate of adhesion formation was significantly lower with the hyaluronic acid gel than without it (28 vs. 78%) (33). However, in this study there were significantly more adhesions with serosal closure with interrupted "figure 8" stitches compared to subserosal closure, emphasizing the importance of the surgical technique. In the other study of 52 patients randomized to receive hyaluronic acid or no treatment at the time of laparoscopic myomectomy, there was no difference in the incidence of adhesions between the two groups, but the severity of adhesions was less in the group treated with the adhesion barrier (34).

Pregnancy rates following laparoscopic myomectomy are comparable to those seen after abdominal myomectomy (9). One randomized, controlled trial evaluated pregnancy outcome in 115 patients undergoing laparoscopic or abdominal myomectomy (10). Pregnancy rates in the laparoscopic compared to the abdominal groups were similar (54 and 56%, respectively), as were the cumulative pregnancy rates and abortion rates. A recent randomized, controlled study evaluated the reproductive outcomes with laparoscopic versus minilaparotomic myomectomy (35). A total of 136 patients completed the study. The characteristics of each group were similar. Cumulative pregnancy rates were not statistically different between laparoscopic versus minilaparotomy groups (53 vs. 38%, $p = 0.9$), nor were live birth and abortion rates.

Concern has been raised regarding the risk of uterine rupture at the myomectomy incision during pregnancy following laparoscopic myomectomy. There have been several case reports describing uterine rupture, and all have occurred during the third trimester of pregnancy (28–36 weeks gestation) (9, 21, 36). However, not all reports have specified the location of the rupture, nor how the previous defect at myomectomy was repaired. In the largest series of 100 deliveries following laparoscopic myomectomy, there was one uterine rupture that occurred at the prior myomectomy scar. The patient had a laparoscopic myomectomy previously repaired by a single-layer closure, and at second-look laparoscopy was found to have a fistula in the myomectomy scar which was repaired again with a single-layer closure. During the subsequent pregnancy, she had spontaneous uterine rupture at the myomectomy scar during the third trimester, not associated with labor. It appears that the risk of uterine rupture with laparoscopic myomectomy is very low when the uterine defect is repaired adequately.

Laparoscopic myomectomy has been used for many years to treat symptomatic uterine myomas in those wishing to preserve their uterus. As technology has improved, more complex myomectomies involving large myomas and those located in submucosal locations are being performed laparoscopically. This is considered one of the most challenging laparoscopic procedures, mostly due to the skill required to close the uterine defects. In the hands of an experienced and skilled surgeon, outcomes appear comparable to those with laparotomy with the advantage of quicker recovery. Subsequent pregnancy carries a low risk of uterine rupture if the uterine defect is closed adequately.

## 3 Robotic-Assisted Laparoscopic Myomectomy

The use of robotic technology in gynecologic surgery has increased since the late 1990s. In April 2005, the Food and Drug Administration (FDA) approved the da Vinci surgical system for gynecologic applications. The da Vinci system is comprised of three components: (1) the surgeon console housing the stereoscopic viewer and instrument controls; (2) the InSite vision system (Intuitive Surgical, Sunnyvale, CA) providing three-dimensional stereoscopic imaging through a 12-mm endoscope; (3) three or four robotic arms able to hold a vast array of laparoscopic instruments. These instruments possess seven degrees of freedom which replicate the full range of motion of the surgeon's hands, overcoming the limited mobility seen in conventional laparoscopy. Advantages of the robotic approach over traditional laparoscopic surgery include improved dexterity and precision with laparoscopic instruments, three-dimensional imaging, and scaling of the surgeon's movements to negate tremor (37). The improved dexterity is a particular benefit with respect to suturing and may offer an advantage over laparoscopic myomectomy where one of the limitations is the inability to perform layered closure of deep intramural or transmural defects. This may not pose a problem for hemostasis, but may potentially lead to compromise in uterine integrity during a subsequent pregnancy. The advantages of the robotic approach must be weighed against the disadvantages of lack of tactile sensation, bulkiness of the system, and cost.

There have been a few published studies of robotic-assisted laparoscopic myomectomy. The first series in 2004 described the experience with 35 patients (38). The mean number of myomas removed was 1.6 (range 1–5), and the mean diameter was 8 cm. A subsequent retrospective case–control study of 58 patients compared the outcome of robotic-assisted laparoscopic myomectomy with laparotomy (39). The patients did not differ in age, body-mass index, or mean myoma weight. The robotic-assisted group compared to the laparotomy group had significantly fewer complications, less blood loss with the procedure, and shorter length of stay (1.5 vs. 3.6 days). Operative times as well as professional and hospital charges were statistically higher for the robotic group.

Another retrospective matched-control study compared robotic-assisted myomectomy with standard laparoscopic myomectomy (40). Fifteen patients who underwent robotic-assisted myomectomy were compared to 35 matched controls who were treated by standard laparoscopic myomectomy. The groups were matched for age, body mass index, and prior abdominopelvic surgery, as well as the size, number, and location of myomas. The robotic group had significantly longer mean operative time compared to the standard group (234 vs. 203 min, $p = 0.03$), while blood loss and hospital stay were comparable. Further studies are needed to determine which patients would benefit from this technology and what the long-term advantages are with respect to reproductive outcome.

## 4 Uterine Artery Embolization for Myomas

Uterine artery embolization (UAE) or uterine fibroid embolization (UFE) was first described in 1995 as a treatment for symptomatic myomas (41). The procedure involves percutaneous cannulation of the femoral artery and embolization of the uterine artery and its branches directly feeding the myomas by injecting substances (gelatin sponges, polyvinyl alcohol particles, or tris-acryl gelatin microspheres) until occlusion or slow flow is documented. Radiation exposure is relatively low, approximately 15 rads (42). One-day hospital admission is required for pain management.

This procedure was initially not recommended for women who desired future childbearing, owing to potential risks to pregnancy associated with uterine artery occlusion. Initial studies, therefore, focused on successful resolution of symptoms related to myomas. Short-term follow-up from embolization at 3 months in 555 women revealed improvement in menorrhagia in 83% of women, dysmenorrhea in 77%, and urinary frequency in 86% (43). A study of 400 women who were followed for an average of 16.7 months after embolization for fibroids showed that menstrual bleeding and pain were improved in 84 and 79%, respectively (44). A retrospective study comparing 51 women post UAE and 38 women post myomectomy for 3–5 years showed that the overall symptoms were improved with UAE and myomectomy (92 and 90%, respectively) (45). However, embolization patients were more likely to have subsequent invasive procedures for myomas compared to myomectomy patients (29 vs. 3%, $p = .004$) Following UAE, approximately 10% of women experienced postembolization syndrome characterized by abdominal pain, nausea, vomiting, fever, malaise, and leukocytosis.

Concerns regarding the use of this technique in women who desire future childbearing include risk of ovarian failure, risk of hysterectomy, and potential risks to the fetus due to residual myomas and as a result of uterine artery occlusion.

Amenorrhea has been described in women following UAE. The reason is felt to be migration of the occluding material with resulting occlusion of the ovarian vessels. In women <40 years of age the rate of amenorrhea following UAE was 3% (95%CI 1–7%) compared to 41% in women $^{3}$50 years of age (95%CI 26–58) (43). Ovarian function was assessed in a randomized controlled study comparing UAE to myomectomy in 63 women with an average age of 32 years (46). Three women (10%) demonstrated FSH values >20 mIU/mL post embolization compared to none in the myomectomy group. A subsequent randomized controlled study of UAE versus myomectomy showed FSH > 10 IU/L in 13.8% of UAE patients and in 3.2% of myomectomy patients ($p < .05$) (47).

Another concern with UAE for those wishing to preserve fertility is insufficient fibroid reduction. Since fibroids have been shown to increase risk of abruption, malpresentation, hemorrhage, and preterm labor, residual large myomas following UAE may result in complications during subsequent pregnancy. The mean percent volume reduction of myomas with UAE has been shown to be 44% at 3 months and 58% at 12 months follow-up (48). When comparing myomectomy and UAE in a randomized controlled study, ultrasound monitoring at 6 month intervals post procedure revealed absence of significant pathology in 43% of patients who had UAE and in 82% of those who underwent myomectomy ($p < .01$) (46).

Although the use of UAE for women with reproductive plans is controversial, pregnancies after UAE have been reported, and one prospective randomized, controlled study evaluating UAE and myomectomy in women with at least one fibroid >4 cm but not exceeding 12 cm has been published (47). One hundred twenty-one women were randomized to UAE or myomectomy and the reproductive outcome was compared: pregnancy rate (50 vs. 78%), delivery rate (19 vs. 48%), and abortion rate (64 vs. 23%). The authors conclude that although UAE is as safe and effective as myomectomy, myomectomy has a greater chance of success in women who plan to get pregnant after the procedure. However, longer term follow-up in these patients is necessary. A retrospective case series reported on 56 completed pregnancies following UAE for symptomatic myomas (49). Term delivery rate was 82%.

Pregnancy complications were assessed and compared to rates from the general obstetric population reported from the literature. The rate of preterm delivery (18.2%) and postpartum hemorrhage (18.2%) were increased compared to the general population. Rate of miscarriage was not increased. Cesarean section rate was 72.7%, and of those 54% were elective, the main indication being uterine myoma in 70%. Another retrospective case study compared 53 pregnancies following UAE to 139 pregnancies after myomectomy (50). Pregnancies following UAE had a higher rate of preterm delivery (odds ratio 6.2; 95%CI 1.4, 27.7) and malpresentation (odds ratio 4.3, 95% CI 1.0, 20.5) compared to pregnancies following laparoscopic myomectomy.

UAE has been shown to be effective in the treatment of myomas with improvement in symptoms. Until more studies have evaluated the effect in subsequent pregnancies, use of UAE in women who desire future childbearing should be done with caution. This technique may have value in treating women who have recurrence of myomas following myomectomy and in whom the risks associated with repeat myomectomy are significant. Women with solitary myomas who desire fertility would probably benefit from surgical excision of the myoma.

## 5 MRI-Guided Focused Ultrasound Surgery

MRI-guided system for the localization and treatment of uterine myomas with focused ultrasound therapy was approved for use by the FDA in 2004. This technique directs high-intensity ultrasound waves into a focal volume of a myoma. The ultrasound energy creates sufficient heat at the focal point so that protein denaturation, irreversible cell damage, and coagulative necrosis occur. Concurrent MRI allows precise tissue targeting and monitoring of therapy by assessing the temperature of the treated area. Since specific myomata are targeted for treatment, some may go untreated owing to time or technical limitations, adding a potential variable in treatment outcome. The procedure is performed on an outpatient basis, and patients may return to normal activity in one day.

Treatment outcomes at 6 and 12 months were reported for 109 women who underwent MRI-guided focused ultrasound surgery (51, 52). Reduction in uterine volume was modest: 13.5% at 6 months and 9.4% at 12 months. Symptoms were improved in 71% of women at 6 months but only 51% at 12 months. Improvement in symptoms correlates with thoroughness of treatment (53). This procedure is currently not recommended for women who desire childbearing. However, an uneventful pregnancy has been reported following focused ultrasound surgery for a single, large anterior myoma (54). Long-term studies are needed to evaluate the efficacy of this procedure as well as its use for women desiring pregnancy.

## 6 Conclusions

Minimally invasive alternatives to abdominal myomectomy are available. All the techniques have the benefit of less pain and shorter duration of recovery. In women desiring fertility, laparoscopic myomectomy appears to be safe in the hands of a skilled surgeon. However, the applicability of this technique is limited by the size and number of myomas. UAE and MRI-focused ultrasound surgery are less invasive procedures, but experience in women who wish to conceive is limited. Prospective studies are needed to determine the long-term efficacy and ideal patient populations for these procedures.

## References

1. Buttram VC, Reiter RC. Uterine leiomyomate: etiology, symptomatology, and management. Fertil Steril 1981;36:433–5.

2. Day Baird D, Dunson DB, Hill MC, Cousins D, Schectman JM. High cumulative incidence of uterine leiomyoma in black and white women: ultrasound evidence. Am J Obstet Gynecol 2003;188:100–7.
3. Goodwin SC, Bradley LD, Lipman JC, et al. Uterine artery embolization versus myomectomy: a multiceter comparative study. Fertil Steril 2006;85:14–21.
4. Sawin SW, Pilevsky ND, Berlin JA, Barnhart KT. Comparability of perioperative morbidity between abdominal myomectomy and hysterectomy for women with uterine leiomyomas. Am J Obstet Gynecol 2000;183:1448–55.
5. Fauconnier A, Chapron C, Babaki-Fard K, Dubuisson JB. Recurrence of leiomyomata after myomectomy. Hum Reprod Update 2000;6:595–602.
6. Candiani GB, Fedele L, Parazzini F, Villa L. Risk of recurrence after myomectomy. Br J Obstet Gynecol 1991;98: 385–9.
7. Malone LJ. Moymectomy: recurrence after removal of solitary and multiple myomas. Obstet gynecol 1969;43:200–3.
8. Practice Committee of the American Society for Reproductive Medicine. Myomas and reproductive function. Fertil Steril 2006;86:S194–9.
9. Hurst BS, Matthews ML, Marshburn PB. Laparoscopic myomectomy for symptomatic uterine myomas. Fertil Steril 2005;83:1–23.
10. Mais V, Ajossa S, Gueriero S, et al. Laparoscopic versus abdominal myomectomy: a prospective, randomized trial to evaluate benefits in early outcome. Am J Obstet Gynecol 1996;174:654–8.
11. Seracchioli R, Rossi S, Govoni F, et al. Fertility and obstetric outcome after laparoscopic myomectomy of large myomata: a randomized comparison with abdominal myomectomy. Hum Reprod 2000;15:2663–8.
12. Dubuisson JB, Fauconnier A, Babaki-Fard K, Chapron C. Laparoscopic myomectomy: a current view. Hum Reprod Update 2000;6:588–94.
13. Sinha K, Hedge A, Warty N, Patil N. Laparoscopic excision of very large myomas. J Am Assoc Gynecol Laparosc 2003; 10:461–8.
14. Seracchioli R, Colombo FM, Bagnoli A, et al. Laparoscopic myomectomy for fibroids penetrating the uterine cavity: is it a safe procedure? Br J Obstet Gynaecol 2003;110:236–40.
15. Torng P, Hwang J, Huang S, et al. Effect of simultaneous morcellation in situ on operative time during laparoscopic myomectomy. Hum Reprod 2008;23(10):2220–6.
16. Paul PG, Koshy AK. Multiple peritoneal parasitic myomas after laparoscopic myomectomy and morcellation. Fertil Steril 2006;85:492–3.
17. Kumar S, Sharma JB, Verma D, et al.. Disseminated peritoneal leiomyomatosis: an unusual complication of laparoscopic myomectomy. Arch Gynecol Obstet 2008;278:93–5.
18. Moon HS, Koo JS, Park SH, et al. Parasitic leiomyoma in the abdominal wall after laparoscopic myomectomy. Fertil Steril 2008;90(4):1201.e1–2.
19. Rossetti A, Sizzi O, Soranna L, et al. Long-term results of laparoscopic myomectomy: recurrence rate in comparison with abdominal myomectomy. Hum Reprod 2001;16: 770–4.
20. Rossetti A, Sizzi O, Chiarotti F, Florio G. Developments in techniques for laparoscopic myomectomy. J Soc Laparoendos Surg 2007;11:34–40.
21. Dubuisson JB, Fauconnier A, Deffarges JV, et al.. Pregnancy outcome and deliveries following laparoscopic myomectomy. Hum Reprod 2000;15:869–73.
22. Landi S, Zaccoletti R, Ferrari L, Minelli L. Laparoscopic myomectomy: technique, complications, and ultrasound scan evaluations. J Am Assoc Gynecol Laparosc 2001;8: 231–40.
23. Yoo EH, Lee PI, Huh CY, et al.. Predictors of leiomyoma recurrence after laparoscopic myomectomy. J Minim Invas Gynecol 2007;14:690–7.
24. Fedele L, Parazzuni F, Luchini L, et al. Recurrence of fibroids after myomectomy: a transvaginal ultrasonographic study. Hum Reprod 1995;10:1795–6.
25. Hanafi M. Predictors of leiomyoma recurrence after myomectomy. Obstet Gynecol 2005;105:877–81.
26. Tulandi T, Murray C, Guralnick M. Adhesion formation and reproductive outcome after myomectomy and second-look laparoscopy. Obstet Gynecol 1993;82:213–5.
27. The Myomectomy Adhesion Multicenter Study Group. An expanded polytetrafluotoethylene barrier (Gore-tex Surgical Membrane) reduces post-myomectomy adhesion formation. Fertil Steril 1995;63:491–3.
28. Ugur M, Turan C, Mungan T, et al. Laparoscopy for adhesion prevention folloiwng myomectomy. Int J Gynecol Obstet 1996;53:145–9.
29. Takeuchi H, Kitade M, Kikuchi I, et al. Influencing factors of adhesion development and the efficacy of adhesion-preventing agents in patients undergoing laparoscopic myomectomy as evaluated by a second-look laparoscopy. Fertil Steril 2008;89: 1247–53.
30. Dubuisson JB, Fauconnier A, Chapron C, Kreiker G, Norgaard C. Second look after laparoscopic myomectomy. Hum Reprod 1998;13:2102–6.
31. Takeuchi H, Kitade M, Kikuchi I, et al. Influencing factors of adhesion development and the efficacy of adhesion-preventing agents in patients undergoing laparoscopic myomectomy as evaluated by a second-look laparoscopy. Fertil Steril 2008;89:1247–53.
32. Mais V, Ajossa S, Piras B, et al. Prevention of de-novo adhesion formation after laparoscopic myomectomy: a randomized trial to evaluate the effectiveness of an oxidized regenerated cellulose absorbable barrier. Hum Reprod 1995;10:3133–5.
33. Pellicano M, Bramante S, Cirillo D, et al. Effectiveness of autocrosslinked hyaluronic acid gel after laparoscopic myomectomy in infertile patients: a prospective, randomized, controlled study. Fertil Steril 2003;80:441–4.
34. Mais V, Bracco GL, Litta P, Gargiulo T, Melis GB. Reduction of postoperative adhesions with an auto-crosslinked hyaluronan gel in gynaecological laparoscopic surgery: a blinded, controlled, randomized, multicentre study. Hum Reprod 2006;21:1248–54.
35. Palomba S, Zupi E, Falbo A, et al. A multicenter randomized, controlled study comparing laparoscopic versus minilaparotomic myomectomy: reproductive outcomes. Fertil Steril 2007;88:933–41.
36. Seinera P, Farina C, Todros T. Laparoscopic myomectomy and subsequent pregnancy: results in 54 patients. Hum Reprod 2000;15:1993–6.
37. Advincula AP, Song A. The role of robotic surgery in gynecology. Curr Opin Obstet Gynecol 2007;19:331–6.

38. Advincula AP, Song A, Burke W, Reynolds RK. Preliminary experience with robot-assisted laparoscopic myomectomy. J Am Assoc Gynecol Laparosc 2004;11:511–18.
39. Advincula AP, Xu X, Goudeau S, Ransom SB. Robot-assisted laparoscopic myomectomy versus abdominal myomectomy: a comparison of short-term surgical outcomes and immediate costs. J Minim Invas Gynecol 2007;14:698–705.
40. Nezhat C, Lavie O, Hsu S, et al. Robotic-assisted laparoscopic myomectomy compared with standard laparoscopic myomectomy- a retrospective matched control study. Fertil Steril 2008 March 28 [Epub ahead of print]
41. Ravina JH, Ciraru-Vigneron N, Bouret JM, et al. Arterial embolisation to treat uterine myomata. Lancet 1995;346:671–2.
42. Parker WH. Uterine myomas: management. Fertil Steril 2007;88:255–71.
43. Pron G, Bennett J, Common A, et al. The Ontario uterine fibroid embolization trial. Part 2. Uterine fibroid reduction and symptom relief after uterine artery embolization for fibroids. Fertil Steril 2003;79:120–7.
44. Walker WJ, Pelage JP. Uterine artery embolisation for symptomatic fibroids: clinical results in 400 women with imaging follow up. Br J Obstet Gynaecol 2002;109:1262–72.
45. Broder MS, Goodwin S, Chen Get al. comparison of long-term outcomes of myomectomy and uterine artery embolization. Obstet gynecol 2002;100:864–8.
46. Mara M, Fucikova Z, Maskova J, Kuzel D, Haakova L. Uterine fibroid embolization versus myomectomy in women wishing to preserve fertility: preliminary results of a randomized controlled trial. Eur J Obstet Gynecol Reprod Biol 2006;126:226–33.
47. Mara M, Maskova J, Fucikova Z, et al. Midterm clinical and first reproductive results of a randomized controlled trial comparing uterine fibroid embolization and myomectomy. Cardiovasc Interv Radiol 2008;31:73–85.
48. Spies JB, Bruno J, Czeyda-Pommersheim F, et al. Long-term outcome of uterine artery embolization for leiomyomata. Obstet Gynecol 2005;106:933–9.
49. WalkerWJ, McDowell SJ. Pregnancy after uterine artery embolization for lieomyomata: a series of 56 completed pregnancies. Am J Obstet Gynecol 2006;195:1266–71.
50. Goldberg J, Pereira L, Berghella V, et al. Pregnancy outcomes after treatment for fibromyomata: uterine artery embolization versus laparoscopic myomectomy. Am J Obstet Gynecol 2004;191:18–21.
51. Hindley J, Gedrovc WM, Regan L, et al. MRI guidance of focused ultrasound therapy of uterine fibroids; early results. Am J Roentgenol 2004;183:1713–9.
52. Stewart EA, Rabinovici J, Tempany CM, et al. Clinical outcomes of focused ultrasound surgery for the treatment of uterine fibroids. Fertil Steril 2006;85:22–9.
53. Stewart E, Gostout M, Rabinovici J, et al. Sustained relief of leiomyoma symptoms by using focused ultrasound surgery. Obstet Gynecol 2007;110:279–87.
54. Morita Y, Ito N, Ohashi H. Pregnancy following MR-guided focused ultrasound surgery for a uterine fibroid. Int J Gynecol and Obstet 2007;99:56–68.

# Poor Response to Controlled Ovarian Hyperstimulation

Amr A. Azim and Owen K. Davis

**Abstract** Poor response to controlled ovarian hyperstimulation is associated with low estradiol and follicular response to gonadotropins, reduced number of retrieved oocytes and available embryos for transfer and unsatisfactory IVF outcomes. The prevalent opinion is that it represents an early stage of ovarian senescence. Poor responders are difficult to identify prior to gonadotropin stimulation and are generally resistant to a multitude of intervention strategies.

The aim of this chapter is to present the physiological basis for low response and to analyze the literature regarding identification and management of poor responders.

**Keywords** Poor responders • Ovarianreserve • Controlled ovarian hyperstimulation • Genetics of poor response • Gonadotropin releasing hormone agonists and antagonists • Gonadotropins • Clomiphene • Letrozole • Growth hormone

## 1 Introduction

Of the major challenges facing an ART (assisted reproductive technology) program, the accurate identification and efficient management of poor responders (1) remains one of the most enigmatic. The goal of controlled ovarian hyperstimulation (COH) is multifollicular recruitment with retrieval of multiple oocytes in an effort to compensate for the "inefficiencies" of the embryology laboratory and the poor predictive value of current criteria for embryo selection (2). Poor response to ovarian stimulation generally connotes a quantitative reduction of follicular response and thus the number of oocytes retrieved after COH. On the other hand, ovarian reserve is defined as the numerical and qualitative endowment of germ cells remaining in the ovary. Although tests for ovarian reserve have reasonable capacity to predict poor response to ovarian stimulation (3), the exact relationship between these tests remains to be defined. Diminished ovarian reserve and poor response to COH appear to be part of a continuum of the reproductive aging process, as considerable evidence indicates that they predict an increased propensity for an early and accelerated development of the menopausal transition (4–6). The incidence of poor response to ovarian stimulation has been estimated to be between 9 and 26% (7). In the US, diminished ovarian reserve was the sole diagnostic category in 8.2% of ART cycles (8). In addition to the variability of demographic characteristics between centers, this wide range in the incidence of poor response can in part be explained by the lack of a uniform definition for poor responders (9). The aim of this chapter is to review the literature on poor response to ovarian stimulation and discuss the rationale and outcomes of various strategies developed to optimize outcomes.

## 2 Definition of Poor Response to COH

Garcia et al. (10) defined poor response as a peak estradiol ($E_2$) < 300 pg/mL after human menopausal gonadotropin (hMG) stimulation. Since then, the defining criteria for poor response have evolved to include the number of large follicles, number of oocytes retrieved, peak $E_2$ level, mean daily and total gonadotropin doses, length of gonadotropin stimulation,

A.A. Azim and O.K. Davis (✉)
The Center for Reproductive Medicine & Infertility, Weill-Cornell Medical College, 1305 York Avenue, 7th floor, New York, NY, 10021, USA
e-mail: okdavis@med.cornell.edu

D.T. Carrell et al. (eds.), *Biennial Review of Infertility,* DOI: 10.1007/978-1-60327-392-3_4

low antral follicle count (AFC), elevated basal serum FSH and/or FSH/LH ratio, age and combinations of these criteria (9) (Table 1). Due to these variations in both the definition and end points, different intervention strategies are not readily comparable. There has been a tendency to designate the number of follicles or oocytes as the defining criterion in recent publications. Some studies also require the use of an aggressive starting dose (300–450 U) of gonadotropins, a high total dose (>3,000 U) or median dose (total units/days of stimulation of ≥300 U) before classifying a patient as a poor responder (18), to avoid the possibility of decreased sensitivity to FSH, e.g., due to FSH receptor (FSHR) polymorphism (vide infra). If a poor response is unexpectedly encountered at a "standard" dose of gonadotropins, consideration should be given to cancelling oocyte retrieval and initiating another cycle with a maximal starting dose of gonadotropins to avoid ascertainment bias (24). Moreover, "overzealous" oocyte retrieval in poor responders may artificially inflate the total number of oocytes obtained at the expense of increasing the number and proportion of immature oocytes. The issue is further complicated in that all poor responders are not equivalent in terms of prognosis. Young poor responders manifest significantly better outcomes

**Table 1** Definition of poor response to controlled ovarian hyperstimulation

| Study | Criteria for poor response | Protocol in first cycle | *N* (%) | Outcome on subsequent cycles |
|---|---|---|---|---|
| Saldeen et al. (11) | ≤5 follicles at retrieval | OC-long GnRHa-rFSH | 290 (17) | N/A |
| Frankfurter et al. (12) | Peak E < 1,000 pg/mL & <5 oocytes retrieved | GnRHa or ant | 12 (?) | MPA + ant suppression before antagonist protocol. PR 21% |
| Baka et al. (13) | ≤3oocytes retrieved or $E_2$ < 500 pg/mL | Long GnRHa | 96(?) | Short GnRHa PR 12.5%/cycle |
| Pennarubia et al. (14) | Cycle cancellation due to poor follicular response | Long GnRHa | 129 (?) | Increased gonadotropin dose. PR/cycle 13% |
| Malmusi et al. (15) | No response when ≥300 IU FSH for ≥15 days or <5 oocytes retrieved | Long GnRHa ICSI | 60 (?) | FSH 450–600 U/day Flare; 3.5 ± 1.4 oocytes Ant; 2.5 ± 1.2 oocytes |
| Marci et al. (16) | $E_2$ < 600 pg/ml on hCG & <3 oocytes retrieved | Long GnRHa- rFSH 225 U/day | 60 (?) | FSH 375 U/day ongoing PR GnRHa; 0 Ant 13.3% |
| Klinkert et al. (17) | Expected; AFC <5 Actual; <4 oocytes or cancellation (<3 follicles) | Long GnRHa rFSH 150–300 U | 52 (10) | N/A |
| Klinkert et al. (18) | <4 oocytes retrieved or cycle cancellation (<3 follicles). Starting dose 150–225 U | Long GnRHa | 225 (12–16) | Increased gonadotropin dose. Cumulative (three cycles) ongoing pregnancy; 37–47% (unexpected poor responders; <41, normal FSH), 16–19% (expected poor responders) |
| Hellberg et al. (19) | True poor responder 1–2oocytes retrieved Intermediate 3–4 oocytes | Long GnRHa | 1699 (?) | Second cycle;delivery 9.5% (true)-16.5% (intermediate) third cycle; delivery 7.3% |
| Morgia et al. (20) | ≤3 follicles | ? | 129 (?) | ICSI in all cycles flare-FSH 600 U; 6.9% natural cycle; 6.1% (PR/cycle) |
| Khalaf et al. (21) | $E_2$ < 100 pg/mL on day 6 | Long GnRHa rFSH increased to 450 U | 193(?) | N/A |
| Akman et al. (22) | Two cancelled IVF for FSH > 15 mIU/mL, $E_2$ on hCG < 500 pg/mL or <4 oocytes retrieved | Long GnRHa ICSI-AH | 48 (?) | FSH 300 U + hMG300 U/day flare; 16.7% Ant; 12.5% (ongoing pregnancy/cycle) |
| Garcia-Velasco et al. (23) | <3 follicles ≥18 mm | Long GnRHa-FSH225- 150 + hMG75 U/day | 70 (?) | FSH 375 + hMG 225 U//day GnRHa stop; 17.6% nonstop 14.9% PR/cycle |

*GnRHa* gonadotropin releasing hormone agonist; *Ant* antagonist; *PR* pregnancy rate; *rFSH* recombinant follicle stimulating hormone; (? ) not specified

than older poor responders despite similar numbers of retrieved oocytes (11, 25, 26). It is plausible that the definition should vary depending on the treatment plan. One study suggested critical oocyte threshold below which the clinical pregnancy rate was significantly diminished, specifically five, six or eight oocytes for patients treated with ICSI, IVF, and TESE/ICSI, respectively (27). In addition to agreeing on uniform criteria for defining a poor response, the reproductive medicine community should define what constitutes a clinically meaningful increase in the number of retrieved oocytes after any proposed intervention. One paper (28) proposed that an increase by two oocytes (with a standard deviation of 2.5) would be the cutoff for a minimally important difference (MID). In addition to low peak $E_2$, low number of oocytes retrieved, low conception rates and increased abortion rate, IVF cycles in poor responders can be associated with low AFC (17), high FSH/LH ratio (29), discrepancy in antral follicle sizes, the presence of large follicles/cysts before gonadotropin stimulation (30), premature LH surge possibly due to lowered circulating gonadotrophin surge-attenuating factor (GnSAF) bioactivity (31), elevated serum progesterone prior to hCG administration (32), drop of $E_2$ levels during stimulation (33) and a long stimulation cycle (17).

## 3 Risk Factors for Poor Response to COH

### 3.1 *Genetic Risk Factors*

Accumulating evidence in the literature implicates chromosomal (numerical or structural) aberrations as well as mutations or variability in specific genes in reproductive aging, the earliest manifestation of which is poor response to COH (34–36). Due to the complexity of regulation of oogenesis and folliculogenesis, it is highly unlikely that a single gene or a small number of genes is in control of the response to COH (37). The aim of identifying these key genes (e.g., FSH receptor genotyping) is to predict response to COH in the individual patient, select the most appropriate gonadotropin dose and counsel patients about their prognosis for IVF (For reviews see ref. 38, 39). Research on genetic influences on response to COH is still in a nascent stage and the relationship of the most promising candidate genes to clinical outcomes are not uniformly accepted (40). The aim here is to present the evidence for such genetic variation and poor response to COH. Mutations with severe impairment of fertility will not be discussed. (Table 2, Fig. 1). There is also ongoing research linking antimullerian hormone (AMH) and its type II receptor (AMHRII) polymorphism with age at menopause (55). The most promising of these markers is FSHR polymorphism; sparse data exist for the other markers. So far there are no prospective studies investigating the predictability of poor response to COH in the treatment naïve patients, especially considering variability in the prevalence of these genetic differences among different population groups. More importantly there are no randomized clinical trials to indicate an improvement in pregnancy and spontaneous abortion rates employing any of the available strategies in poor responders predicted by these tests. Data so far imply that these genetic differences have a modest ability to identify poor responders to COH and that multiple genetic and environmental factors control the response to ovarian stimulation.

### 3.2 *Acquired Risk Factors*

A number of risk factors have been discussed in the literature in relation to poor response to COH. Pelvic infection as evident by pelvic adhesions, extensive tubal damage or Chlamydia IgG antibodies is associated with poor ovarian response (56). Ovarian endometriomas are associated with a small numbers of retrieved oocytes (57) and their resection can be associated with further reduction in oocyte yield (58). Ovarian response is also impaired after laparoscopic ovarian cystectomy for nonendometriotic cysts (59). Women who have undergone bilateral ovarian drilling can be at risk for poor response to ovarian stimulation (60). Exposure to chemotherapy for malignancies or autoimmune diseases, or prior to hematopoietic stem cell transplantation is associated with a marked reduction in ovarian reserve and poor response to ovarian stimulation (61, 62). Additionally, smoking is associated with reduced response to COH (63).

**Table 2** Genetic variation linked to poor response to controlled ovarian hyperstimulation

| Gene | Locus | Genetic variation | Phenotype | Clinical effects | Ref |
|---|---|---|---|---|---|
| FSHR | 2p21-p16 Exon 10 | Two SNPs *919A→G;* T307A (extracellular domain) and *2039A→G*; N680S (intracellular domain) | The$^{307}$-Asn$^{680}$ or Ala$^{307}$-Ser$^{680}$ (allelic frequency variable in different population) | Ser$^{680}$/Ser$^{680}$ (Compared to Asn$^{680}$ /Asn$^{680}$) is associated with; Higher concentration of basal FSH levels. Higher AFC. Longer menstrual cycles due to longer period needed for in vivo maturation. Lower follicle production, oocyte yield and low $E_2$ in COH. Require higher FSH dose to achieve similar $E_2$ on hCG day. Interact with other loci predicting poor response (ERα, ERβ). Probably can detect <40% of poor responders | (37, 40–48) |
| ERα | 6q24-27 Intron 1 | Two SNPs *Pvu*II (P); *938C→T* and *Bst*UI (B) | No aa difference in ERα | PP (compared to pp and Pp) is associated with; Significantly less oocytes or mature oocytes retrieved. Significantly *higher* peek $E_2$ Significantly lower pregnancy rate. Probably cannot discriminate between poor and normal responders B allele was not informative | (39, 49, 50) |
| ERβ | Exon 8, Exon 5 | Two SNPs *Alu*I (A); 39A→G and *Rsa*I (R) | aa change in DNA binding domain | Maybe associated with ovulatory dysfunction. No evidence of separate effect on COH. May interact with other polymorphisms | (37, 51) |
| CYP19A1 | 15q21.1-q21.3 Exon 10 | 1672C→T | | No evidence of independent effect on COH. May interact with other genes | (37) |
| FMR1 FMR2 | Xq27.3 Exon 1 Xq28 | $(CGG)_{55-200}$ Premutation 0.04% microdel | Decreased absent FMRP1 | Increased risk (15–20%) for premature ovarian failure and early menopause (5 years) especially with paternal inheritance ± intention tremors & ataxia, behavioral and cognitive symptoms. Elevated basal serum FSH Response to COH not reported | (52–54) |

*SNP* single nucleotide polymorphism, aa; amino acid; *ER* estrogen receptor; *FSHR* FSH receptor; *Microdel* microdeletion; *FMRP* fragile X protein; *COH* controlled ovarian hyperstimulation

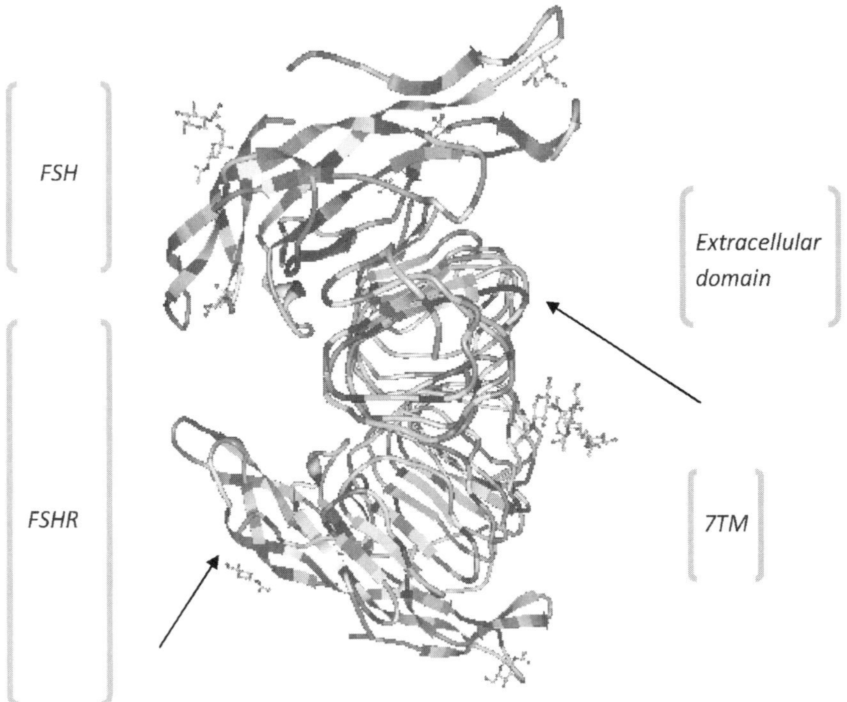


**Fig. 1** Crystal structure of human follicle stimulating hormone complexed with its Receptor. Protein data bank PDB code: 1XWD. Each color represents a separate amino acid. Arrow in the extracellular domain indicates the site of 307 Thr→Ala. Arrow in the intracellular domain indicates the site of 680 Asn→Ser. 7TM; transmembrane domain. Accessed at the web at www.pdb.org/pdb/explore/images.do?structureId=1XWD

## 4 Ovarian Reserve Testing

Ovarian reserve (OR) is usually defined as the number and quality of oocytes left in the ovaries and correlates with fertility potential in the female (64). Methods of screening for low ovarian reserve will be summarized.

### 4.1 Clinical

#### 4.1.1 Age

"Advanced" age appears to be the most important determinant of the number and quality of oocytes remaining in the ovary. Poor response to COH is an early manifestation of reproductive aging (4–6). The largest report of the effect of age on fertility (6.4 million pregnancies between 1990 and 2000) depicts a marked reduction in the incidence of pregnancy and a sharp increase in reproductive loss with increasing chronological age. These trends become evident at and above age 30 (65). In ART, birth rates drop from 20% of started cycles for ages 38–40 to 11% at ages 41–42 and 4% in women older than 42 years (8). Chronological age alone, however, is not an accurate reflection of reproductive performance. Marked variability in OR is seen if age is the only factor considered. Age will not identify younger women with poor reserve and older women with good reserve (11, 18, 64–66). This limits accurate counseling, individualization of treatment protocols and prediction of occurrence of pregnancy and live birth. Because of poor performance as a screening test women should not be denied treatment based solely on a single elevated value of basal serum FSH (67, 68). Finally, an elevated FSH level is a risk factor for first trimester spontaneous abortion (69, 70).

#### 4.1.2 History of Poor Response to COH

The magnitude of ovarian response in prior IVF cycles has been used to predict response in subsequent cycles (Table 3). Some studies found that prior cycle cancellation due to poor response is a better negative predictor

**Table 3** Prediction of poor response to controlled ovarian hyperstimulation after prior poor response

| Study | *N* | Mean age (year) | Inclusion criteria | Protocol in first cycle | Recurrence of poor response |
|---|---|---|---|---|---|
| Baka et al. (13) | 96 | 36 | ≤3 oocytes retrieved or $E_2$ < 500 pg/mL | Long GnRHa | three oocytes 58.3%, two 34.4%, one oocyte 7.3% of cycles. PR/cycle 12.5%, no pregnancy if one oocyte retrieved |
| Pennarubia et al. (14) | 129 | 36 | Cycle cancellation due to poor follicular response | Long GnRHa | Increased gonadotropin dose. PR/cycle 13% |
| Veleva et al. (71) | 80 | 34 | ≤3 oocytes retrieved in ≥1 cycle three IVF cycles Starting dose in first cycle 150–300 U | Long GnRHa | 2.5% LR in all three cycles. Increase in FSH dose resulted in a higher number of oocytes in women with an initial LR (from 2.1 ± 0.9 to 6.7 ± 2.7) but the PR/cycle remained low |
| Klinkert et al. (18) | 225 | 35–41 | <4 oocytes retrieved or cycle cancellation (<3 follicles). Starting dose 150–225 U | Long GnRHa | 64% (expected), 31% (unexpected) had good response in later cycles. Cumulative (three cycles) ongoing PR; 37–47% (unexpected poor responders; <41, normal FSH), 16–19% (expected poor responders) |
| Hellberg et al. (19) | 1,699 | | True poor responder 1–2 oocytes retrieved intermediate 3–4 oocytes | Long GnRHa | Second cycle; delivery 9.5% (true) – 16.5% (intermediate). Third cycle; delivery 7.3% irrespective of number retrieved |

*GnRHa* gonadotropin releasing hormone agonist; *PR* pregnancy rate; *rFSH* recombinant follicle stimulating hormone; *LR* low response; *NR* normal response; *U* unitv

for subsequent pregnancy rates than age (71) or basal serum FSH (14). Others have disputed the predictive value of history of prior poor response especially in young poor responders and those with normal FSH levels (14, 26).

## 4.2 Biochemical Methods

### 4.2.1 Basal Serum FSH

In 1975, Sherman and Korenman reported that women experiencing normal ovulatory cycles nonetheless exhibit subtle elevation in FSH levels starting around their mid thirties (72). The earliest description of the relationship between IVF pregnancy rates and basal FSH levels was published by Mausher and Rosenwaks in 1988 (73). Cutoffs for normal basal serum FSH should be defined by each center (11–15 mIU/mL). The serum FSH exhibits significant intercycle variability; women with FSH <15 mIU/ml display minimal intercycle variability (2.6) while those with FSH >15 mIU/mL exhibit marked variability (7.4). High intercycle variability appears to correlate with diminished ovarian reserve. The highest FSH value appears to be the most predictive (74–76). Obtaining a history of FSH levels confers important prognostic information. Oocyte yields were lower in patients with a history of elevated basal FSH across all age groups. Over the age of 40 years, both implantation and clinical pregnancy rates were lower in these patients, with no significant decrement observed in patients under the age of 40 years. In one study, no pregnancies were observed in patients with a history of three or more elevated FSH levels, regardless of age (77). Evidence in the literature indicates that older women (>40 years) with normal FSH respond differently to COH when compared with younger women presenting with high FSH >15 mIU/mL (26). Younger women with high FSH produce fewer oocytes and have higher cycle cancellation rates but experience lower aneuploidy rates and higher implantation and ongoing pregnancy rates when compared to their older counterparts (26, 78), although their aneuploidy rates are higher than young women with normal basal FSH concentration. To date, at least 37 studies examined the performance of basal FSH as a screening test for OR. Systematic review of these studies (3) indicated that FSH has a modest ability to identify poor responders. If a "very high" cutoff value of FSH is chosen (20–25 mIU/mL), which applies only to a minority of the infertility population, the probability of poor response is around 70%. Moreover, for the same reason, FSH had a poor ability to predict a low pregnancy rate of <5%. Because of poor performance as a screening test women should not be denied treatment based solely on a single elevated value of basal serum FSH (68). Finally, an elevated FSH level is a risk factor for first trimester spontaneous abortion (69).

### 4.2.2 Basal Serum $E_2$

Combining the day 3 basal $E_2$ with the FSH level improves the prediction of a poor response to COH. In one study, no pregnancy occurred when $E_2$ exceeded 75 pg/mL with a significant reduction in the number of oocytes retrieved once the $E_2$ levels exceed 60 pg/mL (70). Analysis of ten published studies indicates, however, that basal serum $E_2$ has a low predictive value for poor ovarian response and a very poor ability to predict the nonoccurrence of pregnancy after IVF (26).

### 4.2.3 Inhibin B

Inhibin B is a heterodimeric glycoprotein member of the TGFb superfamily, and is secreted by granulosa cells, principally in preantral follicles. In the largest study to date, a day 3 serum inhibin B of <45 ng/mL correlated with reduced response to COH and diminished pregnancy rates (79). In a systematic review of nine published studies on inhibin B, the accuracy in the prediction of poor response and nonpregnancy is only modest and at a very low threshold level. Inhibin B appears to be inferior to most of the other tests used to screen for diminished ovarian reserve. If a low threshold (45 ng/mL) is chosen as a cutoff, the test would detect approximately 50% of poor responders. Moreover this low threshold is encountered in a small proportion of women seeking IVF (26). There is a renewed interest in the change of serum inhibin B (Δ inhibin B) in response to dynamic testing for OR (vide infra).

### 4.2.4 Antimullerian Hormone (AMH)

AMH is a homodimeric glycoprotein member of the TGFb superfamily. AMH is produced exclusively by the gonads. It is produced by granulosa cells in the developing pool of follicles to the early antral stage (3–8 mm), independent of FSH stimulation. It is not expressed by primordial follicles, late antral/preovulatory follicles, atretic follicles or corpora lutea (80). An ultrasensitive sandwich ELISA assay (sensitivity < 0.1 ng/mL) is now available for AMH but no assay of international standard is yet available. A major practical advantage to AMH measurement is minimal intracycle (81) and intercycle (82) variability in the follicular phase of cycling women even after oral or vaginal sex steroid administration (83) and prolonged GnRH agonist suppression (84). Its measurement is not affected by the early recruitment of large follicles that often takes place in the preceding luteal phase of poor responders (85). After the commencement of gonadotropin stimulation, the levels progressively drop due to loss of expression by the predominant late antral follicles in the ovary (86). These data indicate that AMH is an FSH- and cycle-independent, marker for OR. DeVet et al. in 2002 (87) reported on the correlation of AMH and reproductive aging. In the setting of IVF, AMH was shown to correlate more strongly with AFC than any of the other markers for OR (88, 89), response to COH or number of oocytes retrieved (Table 4). An association of basal AMH (92, 95) or AMH levels on the day of hCG (96) with oocyte or embryo quality has been suggested but this is not uniformly accepted (97). In summary, AMH appears to be a good and convenient single marker for predicting response to COH and a modest predictor for the occurrence or failure of pregnancy in IVF cycles.

## 4.3 Dynamic Testing

### 4.3.1 Clomiphene Citrate Challenge Test (CCCT)

The potential utility of this test for the assessment of OR was initially reported in 1987 (98). The CCCT entails measurement of FSH on day 3 and then on day 10 of the cycle after administration of 100 mg daily of clomiphene citrate (day 5–9). Interpretation is based on the day 10 or sum of day 3 and day 10 values (91). In one study, if the sum of the two FSH values exceeded 22 mIU/mL, a poor response was correctly predicted in 89% of cases. A value >22 mIU/mL value was, however, present in only 16% of their population. If a lower cut-off is chosen, the ability to detect poor responders

**Table 4** Prediction of poor response to controlled ovarian hyperstimulation by AMH

| Study | *N* | Mean age(year) | Mean or cutoff for AMH level (ng/mL) | Retrieved oocytes (mean) | Comments |
|---|---|---|---|---|---|
| Nelson (90) | LR 53 | 37 | 0.6 for LR, 0.3 for no response. | 0–2 | AMH strongly correlates with oocyte yield & better predictor of live birth while FSH is a better predictor of poor response |
| | NR 250 | 34 | 1.4 for NR | 8.5 | |
| Kwee et al. (91) | LR 29 | 35 | 1.48 | 3 | Number of follicles increase by 2.5/1 ng/mL increase in AMH. PPV 67%. Comparable to other tests for prediction of poor response |
| | NR 81 | 33 | 3.5 | 14.9 (ongoing PR 10 vs. 24%) | |
| Lekamge et al. (92) | LR 54 | 36.6 | ≤2 | 5 (2.1 embryos) | Low AMH was excellent predictor (83%) for low oocytes yield and modest predictor (64%) for pregnancy (projected cumulative PR/cycle 28 vs. 74%) |
| | NR 72 (both had FSH<10 mIU/mL) | 34.3 | >2 | 11.9 (6.4 embryos) | |
| Tremellen et al. (93) | LR 20 | 38 | 0.83 | 2.4 | Prediction of poor response; PPV 67%, NPV 92% for AMH |
| | NR 55 | 32 | 2.4 Cut-off 1.1 | 15.1 | |
| Muttukrishna et al. (94) | LR 17 | ? | Cut-off for poor response 0.2 | 0 in poor responders (cycle cancelled) | Basal AMH was the best predictor of number of oocytes retrieved. AMH <0.2 predicts 78% of poor responders |
| | NR 52 | | | | |
| Van Rooij et al. (89) | LR 35 | 33.8 | 0.2 | 2 | Excellent correlation with AFC and oocytes retrieved. AMH < 0.1 predicts 77% poor responders |
| | NR 84 | 36.8 | 1.4 | 9 | |

*N* number of poor and normal responders (given separately); *rFSH* recombinant follicle stimulating hormone; *LR* low response; *NR* normal response; PPV and positive predictive values; *NPV* negative predictive value; *PR* pregnancy rate per started cycle. Wide variations exist between commercial assays (92)

markedly decreases (99). Analysis of 12 published studies utilizing the CCCT revealed that the test is inferior to basal FSH and AFC in prediction of poor response to COH and prediction of no pregnancy after IVF (3).

### 4.3.2 Exogenous FSH Ovarian Reserve Test (EFORT)

Fanchin (100) reported the use of EFORT for evaluation of ovarian reserve and prediction of response to COH. On cycle day 3, baseline FSH and $E_2$ were measured followed by injection of 300 IU rFSH. $E_2$ was remeasured on cycle day 4. Both FSH and $\Delta E_2$ were ascertained. More recently, there was a renewed interest in including basal serum inhibin B and Δ inhibin B in interpreting the outcome of this test (84, 98). The cut-off for $\Delta E_2$ is generally set at 30 pg/mL (94, 98, 99) and that of Δ inhibin B at 40 pg/mL. Studies were not consistent regarding the predictive value of $\Delta E_2$ (40–79%). On the other hand, Δinhibin B was found to predict the strongest association with response to COH (98, 99) compared to all other OR tests, including AMH. The test is less practical than other predictors for OR and IVF outcomes and more research is required to determine its true validity before widespread application.

### 4.3.3 Gonadotropin Stimulating Hormone Agonist Stimulation Test (GAST)

Muasher et al. (101) used the GAST to evaluate response to COH. In this test, a GnRHa is administered on cycle day 2 after measuring serum FSH and $E_2$. $E_2$ is then remeasured on day 3. The test is considered abnormal if either FSH is abnormal or $\Delta E_2 < 20–50$ pg/mL (102). The ability of this test to correctly identify poor responders is not higher than other OR tests. The test is also a poor predictor of pregnancy (103).

## 4.4 Biophysical Methods

### 4.4.1 Antral Follicle Count

Reuss et al. (104) demonstrated that transvaginal ultrasonographic assessment of the number of antral follicles >2 mm in the ovaries correlates negatively with age. Thereafter, multiple studies evaluated the validity of the number of follicles ≤10 mm in the early follicular phase in predicting response to COH and pregnancy in IVF cycles. The threshold value for low AFC has varied between 2 and 9 follicles in different studies (3, 105). AFC can be equally well assessed by 2D (7.5 mHz vaginal probe) or 3D ultrasound (106). There is evidence to indicate that the AFC shows minimal intercycle variability (±4 follicles), when compared to FSH and ovarian volume, and that the observed variability is operator dependent (107). Recently, it was shown that the AFC strongly correlates with and has similar predictive value to serum AMH measurement (88, 91, 94). Another use of AFC is to adjust the gonadotropin starting dose in IVF cycles. Popovic-Todorovic et al. in a prospective randomized study (108) showed that, compared to a standard dose, the use of a "normogram" including the AFC to individualize the starting FSH dose improves ovarian response and pregnancy rates. A meta-analysis of 11 randomized trials including about 1,400 patients also indicated that the AFC can be an important determinant of the starting FSH dose in IVF cycles (109). We commonly adjust the starting gonadotropin dose based on AFC. In the largest study to date (372 cycles), a cut-off of <3 follicles was significantly associated with reduced numbers of oocytes retrieved. The number of retrieved oocytes could potentially be predicted from the regression equation "retrieved oocytes = 0.8AFC + 2" (110). A meta-analysis of 17 studies however, indicated that the AFC has a modest capacity to detect low response to COH and is unable to detect the occurrence of no pregnancy (3, 105).

### 4.4.2 Ovarian Volume (OVVOL)

Decrease in the mean ovarian volume with age was first documented in 1987 (111). Ovarian volume is usually measured using the ellipsoid formula ($D_1 \times D_2 \times D_3 \times 0.53$) and the mean of the two ovarian volumes is considered. The largest study on OVVOL and its relation to IVF outcomes (267 patients) indicated that mean ovarian volume >2–3 mL correlates with AFC, number of oocytes retrieved and occurrence of pregnancy (112). A meta-analysis of nine published reports indicated that OVVOL measurement has a minimal ability to predict failure to conceive after IVF. The test also has a limited value to detect poor responders as a very low threshold (close to zero) would have to be employed. In both cases the AFC was a better test than OVVOL for predicting IVF outcomes (105).

#### 4.4.3 Ovarian Blood Flow

Ovarian stromal flow has been suggested as an OR test. A stromal flow index <11 was associated with increased age, fewer retrieved oocytes and nonpregnancy after IVF (108, 113). The sensitivity and specificity at this cutoff were 30 and 96%, respectively. Studies so far do not permit accurate analysis of the performance of this test. Recent reports implicating genes related to vascular insufficiency and earlier menopause (Factor V Leiden and apolipoprotein E-2) (114) may render this test attractive for further investigation.

### *4.5 Direct Assessement of OR; Ovarian Biopsy*

Follicular studies utilizing autopsy (115) and surgical (116) specimens have determined that the number of germ cells in human ovaries declines from birth through menopause. Ovarian biopsy has been suggested as a test of OR (117). Clearly, its utility is negated by invasiveness, risk and the potential for topographical variation in follicle density. Its sole benefit resides in estimating the quality of ovarian strips destined for cryopreservation prior to gonadotoxic treatment in cancer patients (118).

### *4.6 Concluding Remark on OR Testing*

All available OR tests have, at best, a modest ability to predict either poor response to COH or the occurrence of pregnancy following IVF. Data so far do not allow any single test or combination of tests to be an absolute deterrent from pursuing at least one cycle of COH before exclusion from autologous treatment. Response to ovarian stimulation and the production of good quality oocytes/embryos are of greater predictive value (1). Age remains a critical predictor of OR and IVF outcomes, taking into consideration quantity as well as quality of oocytes remaining in the ovary (1, 26, 119)

## 5 Physiological Basis for Intervention in Poor Responders

Based on our current understanding of the basic science and clinical endocrinology of the ovarian cycle and the pharmacology of COH, interventions to improve the response to COH can be summarized in the following general categories.

### *5.1 Enhanced Secretion of Endogenous Gonadotropins*

In 1983, Wide and Hobson reported that FSH from postmenopausal women is more active than FSH from premenopausal women (120). Since then, marked heterogeneity of the FSH molecule has been recognized and is due to variations in carbohydrate moieties, especially sialic acid. The sialic acid residues of the terminal oligosaccharide chain determine the rate of metabolic clearance and biological activity. Less acidic isoforms (lower sialic acid content) are cleared more rapidly and have higher bioactivity (receptor binding) than the more acidic isoforms (121). Isoform expression is variable, depending on the stage of the menstrual cycle (less sialylated FSH isoforms are preferentially secreted during the periovulatory period). Estradiol increases the secretion of less acidic isoforms. There is also a role for GnRH in the modulation of FSH heterogeneity (121). Moreover, variation in FSH structure is seen when comparing natural, urinary and recombinant products. The biological effects of these observations have been partially elucidated. Less acidic isoforms are more potent in stimulating aromatase, while more acidic isoforms induce higher $\alpha$-inhibin m-RNA production. There is some evidence implicating an rFSH effect on antral follicles reflecting "overexposure" to gonadotropins, when compared with pituitary FSH (slower preantral growth rate, smaller end size and theca cell hypertrophy). Intact follicle cultures also suggest that variation in FSH isoforms may impact oocyte maturity (122). Although no firm evidence from clinical trials or meta-analyses is available to establish the superiority of one gonadotropin preparation (2) or an improved response to COH with regimens that induce the release of endogenous gonadotropins, these remain a theoretical basis for intervention in poor responders. As with FSH, heterogeneity of LH has been also reported. Basic isoforms with shorter half life and higher biopotency predominate in young "estrogen rich" women and in the follicular phase and midcycle while acidic long acting forms predominate in older women (123).

## 5.2 Increase the Sensitivity of FSHR to its Ligand; Role of Sex Steroids

Human and primate studies have demonstrated an important role for sex steroids in FSHR expression. So far, there is no conclusive evidence that estrogens have an obligatory role in folliculogenesis in primates and humans (124). There is evidence of an indirect effect for estradiol on enhancing FSHR stimulation. The human FSHR gene has an imperfect, 5¢ half consensus estrogen receptor response element (ERE). Estrogen by itself has no effect on the distribution or number of FSHRs as it does not affect the levels of FSHR-mRNA or affinity of FSH binding to granulosa cells, but it does increase the aromatase expression (125). Estrogen synergizes with FSH and cAMP to increase the number of FSH receptors. This appears to be mediated via the proliferative action of estrogen on granulosa cells, rather than through a direct effect on transcription (126). The role of androgens appears to be different. Testosterone and dihydrotestosterone increase FSHR mRNA in bovine and primate granulosa cells in primary follicles (125, 127). Moreover, there is evidence that androgens promote growth and reduce apoptosis of follicles ≤1 mm in primate ovaries (128). Androgen effects may be mediated through an increased synthesis of IGF-I (129).

## 5.3 Increase Stimulation of the FSHR by Increased Exogenous Gonadotropin Dosage

Regimens tailored to improve the follicular response in COH often employ higher doses of gonadotropins to increase FSH levels above the thresholds for the less sensitive follicles. Some poor responders appear to be less responsive to FSH either due to reduced expression of FSHR (130) or to variation in the internal structure of the receptor (see section on genetic risk factors).

## 5.4 Improve Antral Follicle Maturation; Role of LH

Recent work in humans and primates appears to challenge the importance of LH as established by "the two gonadotropin-two cell hypothesis" a key concept in steroidogenesis initially proposed in 1941 (131). As the follicles acquire LH receptors, they progress from FSH-dependent growth to LH-responsive maturation. LH has a facilitatory, not an obligatory, role in follicle maturation by increasing androgen substrate and estradiol production and possibly by improving oocyte competence (132, 133). Further studies led to the development of the "LH-threshold" and "ceiling" concepts. The threshold level of LH for beneficial effects is low, probably not exceeding 1 mIU/mL. LH should be below a ceiling value to avoid potentially deleterious effects on folliculogenesis. No such level has been strictly defined (134). Clinical studies, however, do not support the concept that LH supplementation improves response to COH in normogonadotropic women undergoing assisted reproduction cycles (135). Improved response to COH has been suggested in a subset of patients including those with profound LH suppression and poor responders (131, 132).

## 5.5 Luteal Phase Synchronization

Heterogeneity in the size of antral follicles and their sensitivity to FSH in the luteal phase of the menstrual cycle is well documented in the human ovary (136–138). The FSH rise during the luteal-follicular transition may account for this heterogeneity, by accelerating the growth of the more sensitive follicles (139). This incoordinate growth may ultimately lead to fewer follicles reaching a stage of final maturation. Consequently, fewer oocytes are retrieved after COH. This could be one contributing factor in the apparently lower pregnancy rates in antagonist cycles compared to long GnRH agonist cycles (140). Integral to the events that take place proximate to the luteal-follicular shift is the stimulus for luteolysis in human and nonhuman primates. Studies with GnRH antagonists indicate that withdrawal of the luteal phase LH stimulus for 3 days is required for irreversible degeneration of the corpus luteum (141, 142) and allowing for the first wave of follicular recruitment to progress. The use of a GnRH antagonist to affect luteolysis and menstruation to accelerate the initiation of COH (143) and the use of estradiol to synchronize follicular recruitment in the luteal phase of the preceding menstrual cycle were reported (144). Estrogen itself does not appear to enhance follicular growth, at least in primate ovaries (145). The feasibility of synchronization of early antral follicle growth in the luteal phase prior to COH in antagonist cycles was investigated in a series of studies by Fanchin et al. (146–149). Luteal estradiol administration did not delay the onset of menstruation but slightly prolonged the follicular phase of the stimulation cycle (147, 148). $E_2$ adminstration resulted in higher basal estradiol levels and lower basal FSH and inhibin levels before the initiation of gonadotropins, reducing the value of these levels as OR markers in the cycle of treatment (146, 147). This team also noticed a significant reduction in the diameter and size discrepancy of antral follicles when compared to controls. Moreover, there was a significant increase in the number of follicles ≥16 mm on the day of hCG, the number of oocytes retrieved and a nonsignificant trend towards increased pregnancy rates (146–148). The same group reported on the use of a GnRH antagonist in the luteal phase in order to synchronize antral follicles. The use of the antagonist was associated with lower basal serum FSH, $E_2$ and inhibin B as well as a significant reduction in the discrepancy in antral follicle size (149). These studies furnish the physiological basis for luteal synchronization of antral follicles in antagonist cycles. Our group and others have described a modified protocol for the synchronization of antral follicles in poor responders (150).

### 5.6 *Reduced Suppression of the Pituitary*

Animal and human data suggest that it may be desirable to reduce the GnRHa dose and duration of injections in down-regulated agonist cycles. GnRH type I and II molecules as well as their mutual GnRHR type I receptor protein are expressed in the human ovary in preovulatory follicles and corpora lutea (78, 151). GnRH can inhibit FSH-stimulated steroid hormone production by granulosa cells (152), induce granulosa cell apoptosis and may affect implantation (153, 154). These effects are exerted at concentrations much lower than those used in clinical practice. Excessive suppression of the pituitary gland is associated with the need for higher doses of gonadotropins and a reduced IVF success rate in low responders. The avoidance of early suppression of the pituitary gland is an additional rationale for using GnRH antagonists in poor responders.

## 6 Effectiveness of Therapeutic Interventions to Improve Ovarian Response and IVF Outcomes in Low Responders

Numerous studies have been published with the goal of improving IVF outcomes in this challenging patient population. Although multiple interventions are usually incorporated, we will attempt to evaluate the evidence for or against the clinical application of each strategy separately. In most studies a treatment-independent improvement in ovarian response cannot be excluded, in large measure due to the retrospective nature of the overwhelming majority of these publications. “Improvement,” in other words, can stem from intercycle variability or the phenomenon of regression to the mean.

### 6.1 *COH Initiation in a Cycle with Normal OR Markers*

Patients with abnormal OR markers (specifically high basal serum FSH) are commonly serially monitored for a cycle with normal FSH levels prior to initiation of COH in the hope of obtaining a better follicular response. Although a common clinical practice, there is little evidence to support its efficacy. Intercycle variability in basal FSH levels was shown to predict poor response to COH, especially for levels >15 mIU/mL (75, 76). The few studies that investigated this approach (Table 5) were retrospective and included a small number of patients. Initiating COH in cycles with normal serum FSH levels appears to be associated with a large (40%) drop-out rate due to self exclusion from treatment and about 60% of those who came back are expected to have a second value that is abnormal (158). The validity of these studies is affected by the exclusion

**Table 5** Initiation of COH in a cycle with normal basal FSH in women with history of high FSH

| Study | *N* | Mean age (year) | Mean serum FSH (mIU/mL) | Inclusion criteria of study group | Retrieved oocytes (mean) | Comments |
|---|---|---|---|---|---|---|
| Abdalla et al. (155) | High FSH 39 cycles | 39.1 | 13.9 | One cycle FSH >10 & one cycle <10, ≤12 months apart *IVF irrespective of FSH levels* | 4.5 (LB 12.8%) | Repeated testing has no value. Subsequent cycle should be offered irrespective of FSH |
| | Normal FSH 39 cycles | 39.2 | 7.3 | | 4.2 (LB 5.1%) | |
| Roberts et al. (77) | History of high FSH | | 7.5 | *History of FSH ≥ 20 IVF only if repeat FSH<20 & $E_2$< 75 pg/mL (both RIA)* | | History of high FSH predicts lower yield in cycles with normal FSH and in patients <40 year; no reduction in PR >40 year; low PR |
| | 30 | <35 | | | 8.4 (33.3%) | |
| | 56 | 35–40 | | | 7 (35.7%) | |
| | 94 | >40 | | | 5.2 (9.6%) | |
| | No history | | 8.3 | | | |
| | 550 | <35 | | | 11.6 (51.5) | |
| | 651 | 35–40 | | | 9.7 (43.3%) | |
| | 547 | >40 | | | 7.7 (26.2%) | |
| Lass et al. (156) | History of high FSH | | | ≥38 Year and/or history of poor response, FSH >12. *IVF if repeat <12* | | Repeat FSH is abnormal in about 60% of samples If repeat <12; >40 year 43% cancellation <40 year 13% cancellation |
| | 30 | 39.2 | 9.3 | | 6.4 (LB 14.6%) | |
| | No history | | | | | |
| | 63 | 37.4 | 7.7 | | 8.6 (LB 12.7%) | |
| Martin et al. (157) | FSH >20 53 cycles | 33.8 | ? | *IVF irrespective of FSH levels in the immediate preceding cycle* | 5.3 (0) | Repeat testing is very predictive of IVF outcomes. IVF only if FSH <20 Discourage IVF if ≥2 abnormal tests |
| | FSH <20 + history of one >20 54 cycles | 33.1 | ? | | 7.4 (5.6%) | |
| | FSH <20 + history of two or more >20 11 cycles | 33.5 | ? | | 6 (0) | |
| | FSH <20 1,750 cycles | 32.4 | ? | | 8.9 (16.5%) | |
| Scott et al. (75) | Highest FSH ? | ? | 19.2 | Three attempts within 2 years 81 patients-281 cycle (RIA) *IVF irrespective of FSH levels* | 2.1 | Intercycle variability cannot be used to select optimal cycle for stimulation. Large variability is associated with poor response |
| | Lowest FSH ? | 35.6 in all cycles? | 9.1 | | 2.6 | |

*N* number of patients unless indicated; *RIA* radioimmunoassay; *PR* pregnancy rate per started cycle. Numbers in parenthesis are PR unless indicated, *LB* live birth. Assays use chemelumiscent method unless indicated; ? not specified

of patients with a poorer prognosis. Moreover, the cut-off used for postponing IVF may have a profound effect on the evaluation of the efficacy of this practice. There is evidence to indicate that the highest value is more predictive than the current value for serum FSH (159). Finally, the argument that in cycles with high FSH, prognosis is poor because the patient is already maximally stimulated by her pituitary FSH secretion (and will not respond to exogenous FSH) may not always be true because of the differences in isoform bioactivity between endogenous and exogenous FSH. A history of ≥2 elevations in serum FSH can predict IVF outcomes in cycles with normal FSH levels. Younger women (<38 years) with moderate elevations of FSH (≤15 mIU/mL, within the upper limit of variability of the FSH assay) can attempt ovarian stimulation without delay.

## *6.2 Increasing the Daily Dose of Gonadotropins*

Proactively, increasing the initial gonadotropin dose in poor responders or reactively, during the course of COH for an unexpected poor response, is a common practice in reproductive medicine. On the other hand, a high starting dose of gonadotropins(≥300 U/day), is generally required to ascertain the diagnosis of poor response (24) and to avoid the possibility of reduced FSHR sensitivity due to polymorphism (37, 41–48). In a randomized clinical trial, Kilnkert et al. (13) showed that the expected poor response based on basal AFC <5 is not rectified by increasing the starting FSH dose from 150 to 300 U/day. The median number of retrieved oocytes was three in both groups. There was no significant difference in the ongoing pregnancy rate (8% in the 150 U vs. 4% in the 300 U group). Several studies investigated the effect of a higher starting gonadotropin dose in expected poor responders or increasing the dose in response to low follicular or estradiol response in the first few days of stimulation (28, 160–168). The dose was increased to 300–450 U/day. No significant increase in the number of oocytes or pregnancy rates was detected. Several randomized clinical trials investigated dose increases in normal responders (100–150 × 200–250 U). A higher starting dose increased the number of oocytes and reduced the cancellation rate but did not improve the pregnancy rate. The increased oocyte yield was mainly observed in younger patients (169). One "statistical" explanation to any observed increase in oocyte yield after gonadotropin dose increase is the phenomenon of regression to the mean. Rombauts (169) analyzed outcomes of suboptimal responders from the Monash IVF database and found a significant increase in the number of retrieved oocytes whether the starting dose was increased to 300 or maintained at 225 U in their subsequent cycles. The number of oocytes also significantly dropped in high responders although their starting dose remained at 225 U in both cycles. There is no specific biological explanation as to why women with poor ovarian reserve or a history of poor response are resistant to increased doses of gonadotropins. Experimental evidence indicates that the FSHR undergoes desensitization after prolonged exposure to its ligand (170). Moreover, exposure to higher FSH doses early in the follicular phase may not circumvent the early follicular recruitment that takes place in the previous luteal phase. Possible deleterious effects of higher doses of FSH on oocyte quality have recently been suggested. Animal data indicate that excessive exposure to gonadotropins can induce chromosomal abnormalities in murine oocytes (171, 172). The results of a recent randomized clinical trial detected a higher proportion of aneuploid embryos with conventional stimulation than with "milder" stimulation regimens (173). It is possible that these effects are exaggerated in poor responders and ultimately limit the pregnancy rate even if the number of oocytes is increased.

## *6.3 Reduction or Cessation of GnRH Agonist*

Several studies have demonstrated that the pituitary gland can be desensitized using half the standard dose of GnRH agonist. Moreover, once desensitization is achieved, LH remains suppressed for 15–22 days even if the agonist is discontinued. Half the regular daily subcutaneous dose, starting before or on the day of gonadotropin initiation, or half the depot intramuscular dose is associated with a similar steroid hormone pattern, duration of desensitization and recovery, less profound suppression of serum LH and a similar incidence of premature LH surges (174–180). These randomized trials, however, did not find a significant increase in the number of retrieved oocytes or clinical pregnancy rates except when half-dose depot or reduced daily dose were compared to full-dose depot formulations. Further reduction in agonist dose (25–33 mg of triptorelin) has also been investigated in women with serum FSH >10 mIU/mL with no significant difference in retrieved oocytes or pregnancy rate (181). Retrospective studies in poor responders indicated that reduced daily GnRH agonist dose was associated with lower cycle cancellation, higher numbers of oocytes and embryos and a trend towards a higher pregnancy rate (182–187) Controlled studies on the "stop" protocol are presented in Table 6. In summary, it appears reasonable to use a lower dose or a stop regimen if an agonist protocol is employed but low dose agonist or stop protocols do not appear to clearly improve outcomes in poor responders.

## 6.4 Microdose/Flare GnRH Agonist Protocols

After the initial reports of the use of GnRHa microdose/flare regimens for COH (191–198), several studies adapting this protocol for poor responders appeared in the literature (199–204). Pretreatment with a low dose oral contraceptive pill (OCs) or progestins is employed to prevent corpus luteum rescue and is followed on cycle day 1 or 2 by the administration of minidose GnRHa e.g., 80 μg/day leuprolide acetate in one or two divided doses, until the day before hCG administration. The flare effect continues for the first 3 days and downregulation is achieved in 4 days. Gonadotropins are initiated on cycle day 3–5 at a dose of 300–600 U/day. A modification of this regimen is the short or flare protocol. A full dose of GnRHa is started on the first or second day of the cycle and maintained or reduced after a few days until the day of hCG, while gonadotropins are started 1–3 days after the agonist. The use of short protocols is associated with an increased risk for premature elevation of LH, serum androgens and progesterone, especially in poor responders. This might reduce oocyte yield and increase spontaneous abortion rates (198, 199, 204). Although gonadotropins are commonly administered in a fixed high dose fashion, Cedrin-Durnerin and colleagues demonstrated that a step-down regimen is not detrimental and is associated with reduced cancellation rates and cost containment (205). We generally administer hCG on flare protocols once two follicles attain a diameter of 16–17 mm. Retrospective studies appraising the microdose protocol in poor responders have yielded contradicting results. Scott and Navot demonstrated that a short protocol enhanced follicular response in 34 patients who demonstrated poor response after luteal agonist administration (200). In a similar design (patient as own control), Surrey et al. (202) detected an improvement of response in 34 patients with a history of poor response on a long protocol, when stimulated using microdose of leuprolide acetate. There were no significant differences in premature LH surges, serum progesterone on the day of hCG or the number of retrieved oocytes and number of ongoing pregnancies although there was a significant reduction in cycle cancellations (21 vs. 65%) in the microdose group. Leondires and colleagues (203) detected no significant differences between low responders stimulated with microdose agonist and age-matched controls stimulated with a long protocol. In fact, cycle cancellation was actually more common in the microdose group (22.5 vs. 8.2%). Schoolcraft et al. (201) compared the response of a cohort of 32 patients who were previously cancelled due to poor response on a standard long agonist protocol with their response in subsequent cycles utilizing a microdose protocol, additionally incorporating adjuvant growth hormone. An ongoing pregnancy rate of 43.8% of started cycles was described with a cancellation rate of 12.5%. Karacan et al. retrospectively compared outcomes in 111 poor responders and 33 good responders who did not conceive, both after long protocol stimulation. Forty percent of poor responders were cancelled and a mean of 7.1 oocytes per patient were obtained. The clinical pregnancy rate per initiated cycle was 9.9% and live birth 2.5%. In this study, the live birth rate was not improved in poor responders (or normal responders) who failed luteal GnRHa (206). Spandorfer et al. in a noncontrolled study (207), analyzed the largest experience from a single center with a flare protocol (1 mg of leuprolide reduced by day 5–0.5 mg/day). Of 450 cycles, the cancellation rate was 24% with a 14% delivery rate per initiated cycle. The magnitude of the estradiol flare correlated with a lower risk for cycle cancellation. Antagonist protocols have also been compared to the flare approach. Fasouliotis et al. (207) reported results of 53 patients who failed to conceive on a microdose protocol and were subsequently stimulated using a GnRH antagonist. There were no significant differences in IVF outcomes except for a notable increase in

**Table 6** Gonadotropin releasing hormone agonist stop protocol for poor responders to COH

| Study | *N* | Mean age (year) | Definition of poor response and inclusion criteria | Protocol | Retrieved oocytes (mean) | Comments |
|---|---|---|---|---|---|---|
| Dirnfeld et al. (188) (RCT) | GnRHa Stop 40 cycles | 33.4 | $E_2$ < 500 pg/mL, ≤4 mature oocytes) FSH 9–12 mIU/mL and age <42 years | buserelin 1 mg/day or treptorelin 0.1 mg/day Stop; CD3 Gn 225–375 U | 6.5 (7.5%) | Higher cancellation rate in stop protocol (22.5 vs. 5%, one LH surge) No difference in other outcomes. Higher oocyte yield in women with history of high FSH |
| | Long GnRH 38 cycles | 35.5 | | | 7.7 (7.9%) | |
| Garcia- Velasco et al. (23) (RCT) | GnRHa stop 34 cycles | 34.4 | Cycle cancellation; <3 follicles ≥18 mm FSH < 12 mIU/mL | Leuprolide 1 mg/day | 8.7 (17.6%) | More oocytes retrieved. No difference in cancellation rate (5.9 vs. 2.8%) and pregnancy rates |
| | long GnRH 36 cycles | 34 | | Stop; menses Gn 300 U | 6.2 (13.9%) | |
| Schachter et al. (189) (case-control) | GnRHa stop 36 cycles | 34.7 | ≤5 oocytes or poor quality embryos | Nafarelin 600 µg/day | 5.9 (0) | No significant increase in oocyte yield. Better cleavage and embryo morphology |
| | Long GnRH 36 cycles | 34.7 | | Stop; CD8 Gn | 7.2 (20%) | |
| Arslan et al. (190) | GnRHa stop 245 cycles | 37.1 | FSH>10 mIU/mL, $E_2$ >90 pg/mL, age > 37 years, $E_2$ < 900 pg/mL, <5 mature oocytes, cancellation <4 dominant follicles after 6 days of stimulation | Leuprolide 0.5 mg/day stop; menses Leuprolide 40 µg/12 h Flexible Gn 450 U | 9.5 (35% per transfer) | Significantly higher delivery rate per transfer (27, 12, 20%). No difference in other outcomes |
| | OC-Microflare 85 cycles | 37.9 | | | 6.9 (21% per transfer) | |
| | OC-Antagonist 138 cycles | 35.4 | | | 7.8 (28% per transfer) | |

*N* number of patients or cycles; *PR* pregnancy rate per started cycle; *CD* cycle day, Numbers in parenthesis are PR unless indicated; *LB* live birth; *Gn* gonadotropin dose in units/day; *RCT* randomized clinical trial

the ongoing pregnancy rate (23.9 vs. 7.3%). Finally, Mohamed and colleagues (208) compared outcomes in 77 patients stimulated with a flare and 57 patients with an antagonist protocol. Both groups had previously failed long down regulation regimens. Stimulation was prolonged in the flare group and the cancellation rate was reduced (0 vs. 7%). There were no significant differences in other outcomes. A number of studies suffer from significant methodological flaws that are prevalent in intervention trials in reproductive medicine (209, 210). In some, the reader is cautioned that the unrealistic outcomes following intervention cast doubt on the accuracy of the definition of poor response. RCTs using short protocols in poor responders are presented in Table 7. Meta-analysis of studies comparing short GnRHa and standard antagonist protocols (215, 216) favors the short protocol with respect to the number of retrieved oocytes (weighted mean difference 0.48, 95% confidence interval 0.08–0.87). One of these studies reported a significantly higher pregnancy rate with an antagonist as compared to a short agonist approach. Low dose long GnRHa was superior to the short protocol in the two randomized studies published to date. In summary, any clear superiority of flare protocols is not supported by current evidence.

## 6.5 GnRH Antagonist Protocols

Following experience in a primate model (217), several studies in the 1990s have established the optimal dose GnRH antagonist in ovarian stimulation. A meta-analysis of randomized clinical trials (RCT) comparing antagonist to long agonist protocols indicated that the antagonist protocol required a shorter duration of gonadotropin administration but was associated with a lower pregnancy rate (OR 0.84, 95% CI 0.72–0.97) in mostly normal responders undergoing ART (140). Craft and colleagues suggested that GnRH antagonists offer a viable option for ovarian stimulation in low responders (218). In antagonist protocols, gonadotropins are started on cycle day 2, and the antagonist is started on either a fixed cycle day; 2 (early), 6–8 (delayed) or once the lead follicle reaches 12–14 mm or $E_2$ reaches 250–400 pg/mL (flexible). So far there appears to be no clear advantage to any of these approaches, although there was a trend towards higher pregnancy rates in delayed fixed regimens (219). These strategies were not investigated in poor responders. Arslan et al. retrospectively compared GnRH agonist (245 patients), microflare (85 patients) and antagonist protocols (138 patients). Only the delivery rate per transfer was significantly different between the three groups: 27, 12 and 20%, respectively (220). RCTs comparing GnRH antagonists with long protocols are presented in Table 8. One advantage of antagonists is the ability to add other adjuvant ovarian stimulants that have the potential for improving response. Regimens utilizing CC, aromatase inhibitors or modified natural cycles in combination with an antagonist protocol are discussed elsewhere in this chapter. It appears from the limited data available (215, 216, Tables 7 and 8) that the antagonist protocol tends to result in a higher oocyte yield and pregnancy rate than long and short agonist protocols (though differences were not significant).

## 6.6 Luteal Phase Synchronization

This protocol is designed to target the lack of synchronization of the basal follicular cohort prior to initiation of ovarian stimulation (223). An antagonist, estradiol or both are administered in the latter part of the luteal phase for follicular synchronization. The antagonist also induces luteolysis. Stimulation is started on cycle day 2, typically with high dose gonadotropins, and the antagonist is reintroduced once the lead follicle reaches 12–14 mm, $E_2$ reaches 250–400 pg/mL or on cycle day 6–8. The protocol used at the Cornell IVF program is presented in Fig. 2 (223). Others have employed estradiol only or antagonist only for luteal synchronization (Table 9). Estradiol pretreatment was compared to no pretreatment in normal responders stimulated using gonadotropins and GnRH antagonists. No significant difference was detected in the number or quality of oocytes retrieved and other IVF outcomes (228). In poor responders, however, there was a general trend towards reduced cycle cancellation and increased number of retrieved oocytes.

## 6.7 Oral Contraceptive Pills (OCs)

Check and Chase in 1984 used estrogen rebound therapy to induce ovulation in women with hypergonadotropic amenorrhea (229). Pretreatment suppression was

**Table 7** Microdose/flare gonadotropin releasing hormone agonist in poor responders: RCTs

| Study | Number of cycles | Mean age (year) | Definition of poor response and inclusion criteria | Protocol | Retrieved oocytes (mean) | Comments |
|---|---|---|---|---|---|---|
| *Short vs. long agonist* | | | | | | |
| Sbracia et al. (211) | GnRHa Flare 110 cycles | 41.6 | Age > 40 years (FSH ≤ 10 mIU/mL) | OCs-buserelin 0.4 mg/day starting CD1 or luteal buserelin 0.4 mg till hCG. Gn starting CD3, FSH 300 U | 4.5 (clinical PR/ cycle 10.9%) | Long protocol is superior to flare protocol in oocyte yield and pregnancy rates. No difference in cycle cancellation (4 vs. 4) |
| | GnRH agonist 110 cycles (ICSI in all cycles) | 42.4 | | | 8.4 (clinical PR/ cycle 22.7%) | |
| Weissman et al. (212) | GnRHa Flare 29 cycles | 39.2 | <5 oocytes or <3 follicles > 16 mm or $E_2$ < 500 pg/mL. (FSH < 20 mIU/mL) | OCs-triptorelin 0.5 mg/day starting CD2 for 4 days then 0.1 mg/day or triptorelin 0.1 mg/day till downregulation then 1/2 dose till hCG Gn starting CD3, FSH 375 U × 3days then hMG 375 U till hCG | 3.1 (clinical PR/ cycle 3.4%) | Modified long protocol is superior to flare protocol in oocyte yield and pregnancy rates. No difference in cycle cancellation (2 vs. 1) |
| | GnRH agonist 31 cycles (uterine ET or ZIFT) | 38.5 | | | 4.4 (clinical PR/ cycle 22.6%) | |
| *Short vs. antagonist* | | | | | | |
| Akman et al. (22) | GnRHa microdose 24 cycles | 38 | ≥2 failed cycles due to FSH >15 mIU/mL, $E_2$ on hCG day <500 pg/mL or mature oocytes <4 | OCs then leuprolide 40 µg/day starting CD2 or cetrorelix 0.25 mg/day when follicles ≥14 mm. Starting Gn FSH 300 + hMG 300 U | 5.5 (ongoing PR/ trans 21.05%) | No significant difference in cancellation rate (21 and 25%), the number of mature oocytes retrieved, clinical and ongoing pregnancy rates |
| | GnRH antagonist 24 cycles (ICSI in all cycles) | 38.5 | | | 4.5 (ongoing PR/ trans 16.6%) | |
| Schmidt et al. (213) | GnRHa microdose 24 cycles | ? | Peak $E_2$ ≤ 850 pg/mL or ≤4 follicles >15 mm on hCG day in prior cycles with starting dose of 300 U per day | OCs- leuprolide 40 µg/12 h starting 3 days after last pill or ganirelex 0.25 mg/day when follicles ≥12 mm or $E_2$ ≥ 250 pg/mL. Starting Gn FSH 300 + hMG 150 U | Nine (clinical PR/ trans 36.4%) | No significant difference in cancellation rate (50 and 42%), the number of oocytes retrieved and clinical pregnancy rates |
| | GnRH antagonist 24 cycles | ? | | | 8.9 (clinical PR/ trans 38.5%) | |
| Malmusi et al. (15) | GnRHa flare 30 cycles | 36.6 | No follicular response or <5 oocytes after stimulation starting Gn dose of 300 U | Treptorelin 0.1 mg/day starting CD 1 or ganirelex 0.25 mg/day when follicles ≥14 mm. Starting Gn FSH 450 U. Dose increase to 600 U after 6 days if no response | 3.5 (clinical PR/ cycle 20%) | Significant increase in oocytes and mature oocytes retrieved and fertilization rate. Trend towards higher pregnancy rate |
| | GnRH antagonist 25 cycles (ICSI in all cycles) | 36.2 | | | 2.5 (clinical PR/ cycle 12%) | |

| | | | | | | |
|---|---|---|---|---|---|---|
| De Placido et al. (214) | GnRHa flare 67 cycles | 37.3 | Age ≥ 37, basal FSH ≥ 9 mIU/mL or cycle cancellation due to <3 follicles ≥18 mm with FSH < 12 mIU/mL | Treptorelin 0.1 mg/day on CD 2 or cetrorelix 0.125 mg/day when follicles ≥14 mm for 2 days then 0.25 mg/day. Starting Gn FSH 300 U. recLH 150 U added in both groups at follicles 14 mm | 6.5 (clinical PR/cycle 21.2%) | More mature oocytes were retrieved in antagonist group (4.6 vs. 5.7). No difference in all other outcomes |
| | GnRH antagonist 66 cycles (ICSI in all cycles) | 37.2 | | | 6.8 (clinical PR/cycle 25.4%) | |
| Lainas et al. (215) | GnRHa flare 90 cycles | 39.3 | ≥1 failed IVFcycle with ≤5 oocytes, basal FSH ≥ 9 mIU/mL | Treptorelin 0.05 mg/day on CD 2 or ganirelix 0.25 mg/day when follicles ≥14 mm or LH ≥ 10 mIU/mL. Starting Gn FSH 400 U. (all treatment included day of hCG) | Three (ongoing PR/cycle 4.4%) | Higher pregnancy rates. No difference in all other outcomes. |
| | GnRH antagonist 180 cycles (ICSI in all cycles) | 38.4 | | | Three (clinical PR/cycle 12.2%) | |
| Short vs. natural cycle | | | | | | |
| Morgia et al. (20) | GnRHa flare 101 cycles | 37.3 | Age ≤ 43, cancellation due to ≤3 follicles in prior cycles | Buserelin 0.1 mg/day on CD 1 or Natural cycle. Starting Gn FSH 600 U on CD 3 in microdose group | 2.1 (clinical PR/cycle 6.9%) | Higher implantation rate in natural cycles (14.9 vs. 5.5). No difference in other outcomes (oocytes obtained 77.2% vs. 82.2% in microdose cycles) |
| | Natural cycle 114 cycles (ICSI in all cycles) | 37.2 | | | 0.8 (clinical PR/cycle 6.1%) | |

*ICSI* intracytoplasmic sperm injection; *ZIFT* zygote intrafallopian transfer; *ET* embryo transfer; *GnRHa* gonadotropin releasing hormone agonist; *PR* pregnancy rate per started cycle; *CD* cycle day; *Gn* gonadotropin dose in units/day; *RCT published* randomized clinical trial; *recLH* recombinant leutinizing hormone; ? not specified

**Table 8** Gonadotropin releasing hormone antagonist vs. luteal agonist in poor responders: RCTs

| Study | Number of cycles | Mean age (year) | Definition of poor response and inclusion criteria | Protocol | Retrieved oocytes (mean) | Comments |
|---|---|---|---|---|---|---|
| Tazegül et al. (221) | GnRHa antagonist 44 cycles | 38.3 | <4 mature oocytes in prior stimulation cycles and $E_2$ on hCG day <500 pg/mL | OCs in all cycles Antagonist 0.25 mg/day when lead follicle ≥14 mm or luteal lueoprolide 1 mg/day reduced to 0.5 mg with stimulation Gn starting CD2, FSH 300 U | 5.44 (clinical PR/cycle 22.7%) | Shorter stimulation in antagonist. No difference in other outcomes. No difference in cycle cancellation (9 vs. 6.6%) |
| | Long GnRH agonist 45 cycles (all ICSI) | 37.9 | | | 5.47 (clinical PR/cycle 24.4%) | |
| Cheung et al. (222) | GnRHa antagonist 33 cycles | 36 | <3 follicles or FSH > 10 mIU/mL | OCs in all cycles cetrorelix 0.25 mg/day starting CD 6 or luteal buserelin 0.6 mg till hCG. Gn starting CD2, FSH 300 U | 5.9 (clinical PR/cycle 16.1%) | Shorter stimulation and more embryos in antagonist. No difference in other outcomes. No difference in cycle cancellation (38.7 vs. 34.4%) |
| | Long GnRH agonist 33 cycles | 36.3 | | | 5.6 (clinical PR/cycle 9.4%) | |
| Marci et al. (16) | GnRHa antagonist 30 cycles | 38.8 | <3 follicles and $E_2$ on hCG day <600 pg/mL with prior long protocol | OCs in all cycles cetrorelix 0.25 mg/day when two lead follicles 14 mm or luteal agonist 3.75 mg. Gn starting CD2, FSH 375 U | 5.6 (ongoing PR/cycle 13.3%) | Shorter stimulation and more oocytes in antagonist. No difference in other outcomes. No difference in cycle cancellation (3.3 vs. 13.3%) |
| | Long GnRH agonist 30 cycles | 39 | | | 4.3 (ongoing PR/cycle 0) | |

*ICSI* intracytoplasmic sperm injection; *GnRHa* gonadotropin releasing hormone agonist; *PR* pregnancy rate per started cycle; *CD* cycle day; *Gn* gonadotropin dose in units/day; *RCT published* randomized clinical trial. OR for clinical pregnancy 1.78 (Cheung (222)) and 2.8 (Marci (16))

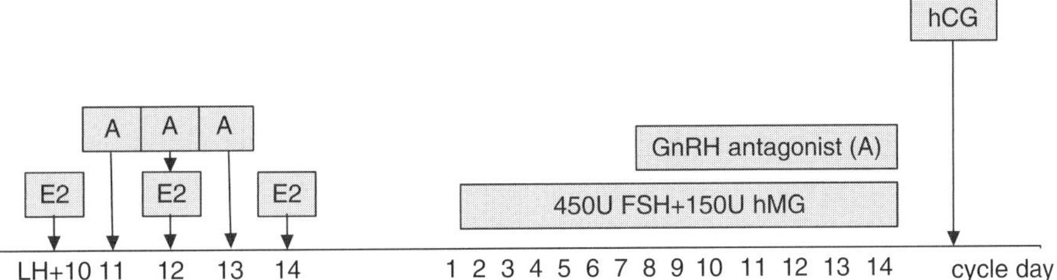


**Fig. 2** Luteal phase synchronization before ovarian stimulation (OD protocol). $E_2$; micronized estradiol transdermal patches 2 mg. LH+; days after lutinizing hormone surge.Estradiol patches are started ten days after LH surge and replaced every other day. The last patch is not removed till it falls on its own. A; 0.25 mg ganirelex or cetrorelix. The antagonist is started in the day following the first patch and for three successive days. Gonadotropin stimulation is started the second day of menestration

associated with a rebound increase in FSH levels (223) and occasional pregnancy. Lindheim and colleagues reported a trend towards higher pregnancy rates and lower cancellation rates in women pretreated with OCs compared to COH without pretreatment (190). In normal responders, there is no conclusive evidence of improved outcome in women pretreated with OCs (230). Collateral benefits have been cited for the use of OCs including ease of scheduling, prevention of an LH surge, reduction of hypoestrogenic side effects, prevention of ovarian cysts in the early follicular phase and possible improved outcomes in a subset of normal and hyper-responders (231). Our concern here is to evaluate their effect, in conjunction with "poor responder protocols," on IVF success (Table 10). Kovacs et al. retrospectively compared suppression using OCs or a GnRH agonist prior to COH and detected no improvement in the OC group (233). Al-Mizayen compared pretreatment suppression using a gestogen or OCs prior to microflare agonist administration in poor responders. No differences in IVF outcomes were observed (220). Arslan et al. (2005) compared OCs to no OCs prior to microdose agonist use in poor responders. There was a small but significant increase in the number of retrieved oocytes but no difference in pregnancy rates (234). Finally, Shapiro compared the effects of OC pretreatment prior to an antagonist protocol in a mixed population of poor and normal responders. The pregnancy rate per started cycle was 33.1 in the OCs group and 33.7% in the no-OCs group (235). It appears from this data that OCs do not hold significant promise to improve response to COH. Indeed, they may increase the gonadotropin dose requirement, at least when used as an adjuvant to microflare or antagonist protocols, owing to their profound suppression of the hypothalamo-pituitary-gonadal axis and possibly decreasing serum androgen levels (236–238). Moreover, there has been some recent concern regarding the profound suppression of LH activity, and possibly increased pregnancy loss after IVF (239). Although this question is still open for debate (135), it suggests some caution in consideration of OCs prior to COH in poor responders.

## 6.8 LH Supplementation

The introduction of recombinant LH (rLH) in addition to available preparations with LH activity (hMG and low dose hCG) have led to investigation of the relative importance of LH in COH (131–133, 239, 240). One possible role for rLH is in normal responders who demonstrate an initial hypo-response to COH on FSH alone as opposed to true poor responders. In normal responders stimulated following depot agonist and exhibiting initial low response, De Placido et al. demonstrated, in two randomized clinical trials, that LH (241) or hMG (242) supplementation is superior to FSH step-up in terms of the number of retrieved oocytes and pregnancy rates. Likewise, Ferraretti demonstrated that LH supplementation is superior to FSH step up and hMG regarding pregnancy and delivery rates (243). Hence, it is important to differentiate between poor responders with diminished ovarian reserve and normal responders experiencing excessive LH suppression following down-regulation. In true poor responders, LH supplementation has been described in a number of regimens, such as rLH 75–150 U starting on cycle day 6–8 (Table 11), hMG 75–150 U/day (242) or a low dose hCG of 50–225 U/day (239, 246). There is no apparent advantage for one type of gonadotropin over the other. Gomez demonstrated in a

**Table 9** Luteal phase synchronization in poor responders

| Study | Number of cycles | Mean age (year) | Definition of poor response and inclusion criteria | Protocol | Retrieved oocytes (mean) | Comments |
|---|---|---|---|---|---|---|
| Estradiol and luteal antagonist | | | | | | |
| Dragisic et al. (150) (Cross- over case- control study) | Luteal agonist + $E_2$ 66 cycles | 41.6 | <5 oocytes, FSH > 12 mIU/mL or $E_2$ on hCG day <500 pg/mL | Strting day LH+ 10; $E_2$ patch 0.1 mg every other day ×3 (keep last one), ganirelex 0.25 mg × 3 the second day of the patch. Gn CD2 ≥ FSH 150 + hMG 150 U. Ganirelex on follicle ≥13 mm, $E_2$ ≥ 300 pg/mL or day 7. or Antagonist, microdose or long agonist protocol | 8.3 (clinical PR/cycle 30.3%) | No significant improvement in number of oocytes or embryos transferred. Less cycle cancellation (13.6 vs. 33.3%) |
| | Other protocols 66 cycles | 42.4 | | | 6.4 (clinical PR/cycle 7.4%) | |
| Luteal antagonist | | | | | | |
| Humaidan et al. (224) (Cross- over case- control study) | Luteal antagonist 24 cycles | 33.4 | <5 oocytes, Gn dose >2,000 U in prior long agonist cycles, age <40 years | Cetrorelix 3 mg day 23 Cetrorelix 0.25 mg/day when follicles ≥14 mm. Starting CD2, Gn ≥ 300 U × 8 days then individualized | 4.3 (clinical PR/cycle 27.7%) | Significant increase in the number of oocytes and good quality embryos. Live birth per cycle in pretreatment group 19.2% |
| | GnRH antagonist 24 cycles | ? | | | 2.4 (ongoing PR/cycle 0) | |
| Fridén et al. (225) (Cross- over case- control study) | Luteal antagonist 30 cycles | 36.5 | <5 oocytes in prior agonist cycles | Cetrorelix 3 mg day 23 Cetrorelix 0.25 mg/day when follicles ≥14 mm. Starting Gn CD2 FSH + hMG dose individualized | 4.2 (clinical PR/cycle 14%) | Possible improved outcome |
| | Long agonist 30 cycles | ? | | | ? clinical PR/cycle 0 | |
| Luteal estradiol | | | | | | |
| Frattarelli et al. (226) (Cross- over case- control study) | Luteal $E_2$ pretreatment 60 cycles | 37.9 | History of poor response on antagonist or microdose agonist protocols. Same patient was stimulated using the same protocol after $E_2$ pretreatment | Oral $E_2$ 2 mg × 2/day (day 21 to day 3), microdose leoprolide or flexible antagonist protocol or Microdose leuprolide or flexible antagonist Starting Gn FSH 375–450 U/day on CD2 + hCG 10–50 U/d | 11.8 (clinical PR/cycle 38.3%)) | More retrieved oocytes and embryos >7 cells. No significant difference in pregnancy rates |
| | No pretreatment 60 cycles | 37.7 | | | 9.5 (clinical PR/cycle 0) | |
| Hill et al. (227) (matched case- control study) | Luteal $E_2$ pretreatment 57 cycles | 36.6 | ≤5 oocytes, poor quality or cancellation on antagonist or microdose agonist protocols. Matched 1:4 controls, using the same protocol | Oral $E_2$ 2 m × 2/day (day 21 to day3), microdose leoprolide or flexible antagonist protocol or Microdose leuprolide or flexible antagonist Starting Gn FSH 375–450 U/day on CD3 + hCG 10–50 U/d | 11.2 (clinical PR/cycle 38.6%) | No significant difference in retrieved oocytes, embryos >7 cells and pregnancy rates |
| | No pretreatment 228 cycles | 36.6 | | | 10.8 (clinical PR/cycle 36.4%) | |

*GnRHa* gonadotropin releasing hormone agonist; *PR* pregnancy rate per started cycle; *CD* cycle day; *Gn* gonadotropin dose; ? not specified

**Table 10** Oral contraceptive pill pretreatment in poor responders

| Study | Number of cycles | Mean age (year) | Definition of poor response and inclusion criteria | Protocol | Retrieved oocytes (mean) | Comments |
|---|---|---|---|---|---|---|
| Duvan et al. (231) (case- control study) | OC-Microdose agonist 26 cycles | 36.3 | <4 mature follicles, maximal $E_2$ <500 pg/ml, prior cancellation of flare cycle, FSH >10 pg/ml or age > 39 | 21 days of OCs (150 mcg desogestrel, 20 mcg ethinyl estradiol), 2 days later leuprolide 40 μg/12 h or Microdose leuprolide Gn start 2 days after agonist | 6.1 (clinical PR/cycle 15%) | Significant icrease in Gn dose and length of stimulation. No difference in other outcomes |
| | Microdose agonist 27 cycles | 36.5 | | | 6.1 (clinical PR/cycle 14%) | |
| Bendikson et al. (232) (case- control study) | OC- antagonist 146 cycles | 38.4 | FSH >10 mIU/mL, <4 oocytes or age > 40 years | OCs (desogen or orthonovum 1/35) × 15–30 days. Antagonist 0.25 mg when lead follicle 14 mm | 7.2 (clinical PR/cycle 10.6%) | Higher Gn dose in OC group. No difference in other outcomes |
| | antagonist 48 cycles | 37.7 | | | 7.3 (ongoing PR/cycle 14.6%) | |

*GnRHa* gonadotropin releasing hormone agonist; *PR* pregnancy rate per started cycle; *CD* cycle day, Gn gonadotropin dose

**Table 11** Luteinizing hormone supplementation during ovarian stimulation in poor responders: RCTs

| Study | Number of cycles | Mean age (year) | Definition of poor response and inclusion criteria | Protocol | Retrieved oocytes (mean) | Comments |
|---|---|---|---|---|---|---|
| Barrene-txea et al. (244) | rLH 42 cycles | 42.1 | FSH ≥ 10 pg/ml or age ≥ 40. Only first IVF cycle included (MEAN FSH 13.9 & 13.2 mIU/mL) | Leuprolide flare 0.5 mg CD2 + rFSH 375 U CD2 + rLH 150 U & drop rFSH to 300 U CD7 or leuprolide flare 0.5 mg CD2 + rFSH 375 U CD2. Drop rFSH to 300 U CD7 | 5.4 (clinical PR/cycle 23.8%) | No significant difference in all outcomes. (pregnancy loss 30 vs. 22.2%) |
| | No LH 42 cycles (ICSI all) | 41.8 | | | 5.7 (clinical PR/cycle 21.4%) | |
| Fábre- gues et al. (245) | rLH 60 cycles | 38.4 | Age > 35 years. Only first IVF cycle included. | Long treptorelin+ rFSH 450 U + rLH 150 U CD6 or Long treptorelin + rFSH 450 U. (drop rFSH to 300 U next day in both groups) | 6.3 (clinical PR/cycle 40%) | Significantly more oocytes and embryos in non-LH group. No difference in other outcomes (pregnancy loss 13 vs. 16%) |
| | No LH60 cycles (ICSI all) | 38.2 | | | 7.9 (ongoing PR/cycle 42%) | |
| De- Placido et al. (213) | Antagonist + rLH 66 cycles | 37.2 | Age ≥ 37 years or FSH ≥9 pg/ml. Only first IVF cycle included | cetrorelix 0.125 × 2 day @ 14 mm then 0.25 mg/day or Treptorelin 0.1 mg/day on CD 2 Gn rFSH 300 U CD2 + rLH 150 U @14 mm | 6.8 (clinical PR/cycle 25.4%) | Significantly more *mature* oocytes in antagonist group. No difference in other outcomes (Pregnancy loss 10 vs. 25%) |
| | Flare + rLH 67 cycles (ICSI all) | 37.3 | | | 6.5 (ongoing PR/cycle 21.2%) | |

*rLH* recombinant luteinizing hormone; *PR* pregnancy rate; *CD* cycle day; *ICSI* intracytoplasmic sperm injection; *RCT* randomized clinical trial

randomized trial that 75 U of rLH is as effective as 75 U of hMG in promoting follicular recruitment in women 38 years or older (247). A meta-analysis of 14 randomized clinical trials including 2,612 women suggested that LH supplementation was not associated with a significant improvement in the occurrence of clinical or ongoing pregnancy rates (240). Although the authors detected an improved pregnancy rate in "poor responders" supplemented with LH, their conclusion was based on data including normogonadotropic women with an initial low response in addition to actual poor responders. When studies of women at high risk for poor response to COH are analyzed (Table 11), it appears that LH supplementation is not associated with any clear advantage as an adjuvant to currently employed FSH-based COH regimens. Some have suggested that older women may benefit from LH supplementation during COH (248). The results of the largest randomized study to date, however, did not demonstrate that LH improves IVF outcome in women older than 38 (249). Finally, the results of randomized trials and multiple meta-analyses comparing recombinant and urinary preparations of FSH have failed to demonstrate any superiority of one preparation over the other (2).

## 6.9 Clomiphene Citrate (CC) – Gonadotropins

This protocol exploits the CC-induced increase in endogenous gonadotropin secretion, while minimizing pituitary suppression through the use of an antagonist. In one such protocol, CC 100 mg/day is orally administered on cycle days 2–6, with gonadotropins starting on cycle day 2 and addition of an antagonist by cycle day 6–8. HCG is administered when the lead follicles reach 18 mm or more. The addition of CC to an antagonist protocol is associated with higher intrafollicular levels of LH when compared to gonadotropin-only cycles, which can therefore lead to lower fertilization rates and increased embryonic loss (250). It has been suggested that a higher dose of the antagonist e.g., cetrorelix 3 mg followed by 0.25 mg daily doses after 3 days if required may be preferred to daily antagonist administration (251). It was further shown, in one randomized clinical trial, that overlapping the administration of gonadotropins in a CC-based protocol (starting two days after CC initiation) was associated with a higher incidence of premature LH surges (28.5 vs. 11.1%) but with lower cycle cancellation due to poor follicular development (7 vs. 22%) and higher numbers of mature oocytes and pregnancy rates (250). This further underscores the fact that daily antagonist administration is not always sufficient to suppress an LH surge. Weigert compared an OCs-CC 100 mg/day-rFSH 225 U-rLH 75 U regimen with a long agonist-rFSH 150 U/day regimen in an unselected IVF population (252). The number of oocytes retrieved in the agonist protocol was significantly higher (8.7 vs. 7.7) with no significant difference in pregnancy rate per initiated cycle (35.1 vs. 29.3%, respectively). Studies utilizing CC protocols in poor responders are outlined in Table 12. It appears that CC with gonadotropins may be a promising protocol with the potential to improve the response to stimulation.

## 6.10 Aromatase Inhibitors (AI)

After initial primate work examining the effects of aromatase inhibitors on folliculogenesis (256, 257); their potential application for ovarian stimulation in humans was recognized by Metwally and Casper in 2000 (for review see ref 258). These authors were also the first to suggest that AI might improve the response of poor responders (259). Aromatase inhibitors stimulate ovulation/augment follicular growth by releasing the hypothalamus from the negative feed-back effects of estradiol (central mechanism) and/or via the accumulation of intrafollicular androgen substrate, which may increase the expression of FSHR (peripheral mechanism) (258) and *possibly* other intraovarian factors (e.g., gonadotropin surge attenuating factor) (260). It is this peripheral mechanism that may hold promise for an improved ovarian response. Lossl et al. (261) and Garcia-Velasco et al. (262) demonstrated in randomized clinical trials that letrozole stimulation is associated with higher levels of testosterone and androstenedione in follicular fluid and that it is associated with improved follicular recruitment. For ovarian stimulation, an AI (frequently letrozole) is administered orally at a daily dose of 2.5–5 mg on cycle days 2–6. Gonadotropins are introduced on cycle days 4 or 5. An LH surge is prevented with an antagonist and ovulation is triggered once the lead follicle reaches 18 mm in mean diameter. In the general IVF population, the use of letrozole is associated with higher follicular

**Table 12** Comiphene citrate-gonadotropin-antagonist protocol in poor responders

| Study | Number of cycles | Mean agwe (year) | Definition of poor response and inclusion criteria | Protocol | Retrieved oocytes (mean) | Comments |
|---|---|---|---|---|---|---|
| D'Amato et al. (253) (RCT) | CC-rFSH-delayed antagonist 85 cycles | 34 | <4 mature oocytes in prior two long agonist stimulation cycles or prior cycle cancellation after a mean FSH dose of 4,750U (FSH 13.7 vs. 11.8) | CC 100 mg/day + rFSH 300 U CD2-6. Cetrorelix 0.25 mg/day when lead follicle ≥16 mm or $E_2$ > 100 pg/mL or luteal lueoprolide single dose. Gn flexible starting dose after desensitization | 5.6 (Clinical PR/cycle 22.2%) | Significantly higher Gn dose in CC group, more oocytes and good quality embryos, lower cancellation (4.7 vs. 33%). No difference in PR, IR |
| | Long GnRH agonist 60 cycles | 33 | | | 3.4 (Clinical PR/cycle 15.3%) | |
| Nikoletos et al. (254) (Case-control study) | CC-hMG-antagonist 15 cycles | 30.7 | ? (ICSI all) | CC 100 mg/day CD 2–8 + hMG 225 U CD6. Cetrorelix 0.25 mg/day CD6 or Depot treptorelin + flexible hMG dose | Three (clinical PR/cycle 14.3%) | Significantly less gonadotropin dose and days of stimulation. No differences in other outcomes |
| | Long GnRH agonist 21 cycles | 30.7 | | | Three (clinical PR/cycle 9.5%) | |
| Craft et al. (218) (Case-control study) | CC-hMG-antagonist 24 cycles | 36.2 | Failed prior agonist cycles or >FSH 600 U per oocyte (IVF or GIFT) | CC 100 mg/day CD 2–5 + flexible dose hMG CD5. Cetrorelix 0.25 mg/day CD6 or @ 14 mm follicle or agonist + Flexible hMG dose | 6.4 (PR/cycle 23.5%) | Significantly lower cancellation (29.2 vs. 56.5%). No significant difference s in other outcomes |
| | hMG + agonist 23 cycles | 36.2 | | | 4.7 (PR/cycle 10%) | |
| Benadiva et al. (255) (Case-control study) | CC-hMG-antagonist 93 cycles | 36.2 | Failed prior gonadotropin ± agonist cycles | CC 100 mg/day CD 2–6 + hMG CD5. or Flexible hMG dose ± agonist | 5.8 (Delivery/cycle 17.2%) | Significantly less Gn & oocytes in CC group. No difference in the number of embryos, lower cancellation (24 vs. 34%) and higher PR |
| | hMG ± agonist 182 cycles | 36.2 | | | 8.7 (delivery/cycle 0) | |

*ICSI* intracytoplasmic sperm injection; *GnRH* gonadotropin releasing hormone; *PR* pregnancy rate per started cycle; *IR* implantation rate; *CD* cycle day; *Gn* gonadotropin dose in units/day; *RCT published* randomized clinical trial; ? not specified

androgens but no change in serum androgens, midfollicular elevation of LH levels, significantly lower peak estradiol levels, thicker endometrium and a possible increase in the number of retrieved oocytes (263). Even more than with the CC protocol, the risk of premature LH surges appears to be increased in AI protocols (264) and they additionally tend to occur at lower estradiol levels (260). Optimal antagonist administration in these cycles has not yet been accurately defined. Cetrorelix 0.25 mg daily initiated at 14 mm follicle size, is only partially successful in preventing an LH surge (incidence 19.4% with the antagonist and 43.4% without the antagonist) indicating that higher doses and/or earlier administration may be needed (264). Aged ovaries are more prone to the deleterious effects of this protocol with respect to premature LH surges (260). In poor responders, randomized trials (Table 12) have suggested that letrozole might have the potential to improve response to COH. More experience will be required to establish the benefit of AI in poor responders (Table 13).

## 6.11 Androgens (A)

The published literature regarding the role of androgens (A) in folliculogenesis is conflicting. The androgen receptor (AR) is expressed in preantral and early antral follicles in murine, nonhuman primate and human ovaries. In human follicles this expression starts in transitional follicles possibly prior to that of FSHR and AMH receptor II (267). While some data indicate that A are atretogenic to granulosa cells in preantral follicles of A treated hypophysectomized rats (268, 269), others have suggested that A stimulate isolated murine follicles (270, 271). Nonhuman primate studies predominantly suggest that A stimulate folliculogenesis in adult ovaries of (127–129, 272). Other studies, however, failed to demonstrate an enhanced FSH/LH stimulated estradiol production after exogenous A treatment in rhesus monkeys (273). Additionally, insulin growth factor I stimulation did not increase estrogen secretion (274). In humans, a hyperandrogenic ovarian milieu as in polycystic ovary syndrome and congenital adrenal hyperplasia is associated with multicystic ovaries (275). High intrafollicular A is associated with increased granulosa cell production of AMH (276). Finally, low baseline A levels were associated with lower numbers of retrieved oocytes after COH (236–238). Data on A pretreatment is still preliminary. The optimal timing, duration and specific agents as well as resulting blood levels and adverse effects are yet to be identified. It is also not clear whether pharmacologic manipulation should target intraovarian (AI or hCG) or systemic (testosterone or dehydroepiandrosterone) androgen levels. Studies on testosterone pretreatment are presented in Table 14. Treatments appear to be generally well tolerated but results are somewhat contradictory. Casson et al. reported an improved ovarian response to ovarian stimulation in five poor responders after treatment with dehydroepiandrosterone (DHEA), 80 mg/day for 2 months (279). A recent retrospective study compared ovarian response in 190 women supplemented with 75 mg/day of DHEA for a mean of 3.8 months and 101 women who did not receive DHEA, prior to COH (280). Both groups were classified as having diminished ovarian reserve (FSH >12 mIU/mL) or "ovarian aging" (>95% confidence interval for mean FSH for age). Both groups were stimulated with a flare protocol and a starting gonadotropin dose of 450–600 U. Significantly fewer oocytes were retrieved in the DHEA group (3.9 vs. 5.8 oocytes) but the clinical pregnancy rate was higher (28.1 vs. 10.9). Interestingly, serum DHEA levels were in the low normal range in the study group. Mild cosmetic side effects were reported. RCTs will be required to validate the potential use of DHEA as an adjuvant to ovarian stimulation.

## 6.12 Natural Cycles and Minimal Stimulation

"Natural cycle" protocols (NC) entail one of three regimens; "pure" natural cycles (no medications except for hCG), modified natural cycles (75–150 U of hMG + antagonist once a dominant follicle of 12–14 mm diameter is reached) and minimal stimulation (75–150 U of gonadotropins starting cycle day 3–5 with an addition of an antagonist once a dominant follicle develops) (281). For oocyte maturation, the hCG trigger is administered at a mean follicular diameter of 16–18 mm. Oocyte retrieval is undertaken 32–36 following hCG injection. In vitro maturation can be employed to increase the yield of MII oocytes. Though not uniformly accepted, there is some evidence that follicular flushing in NC-IVF increases oocyte recovery from 47 to 85% and that oocytes recovered after

**Table 13** Aromatase inhibitor-gonadotropin-antagonist protocols in poor responders: RCTs

| Study | Number of cycles | Mean age (year) | Definition of poor response and inclusion criteria | Protocol | Retrieved oocytes (mean) | Comments |
|---|---|---|---|---|---|---|
| School-craft (265) (RCT) | Let-rFSH-antagonist 179 cycles | 38 | Age > 41 years, FSH>10 mIU/mL, <6 antral follicles, prior cycle cancellation, prior poor response ($E_2$ < 500 pg/mL or<6 oocytes) | Let 2.5 mg/day CD3–7. Antagonist 0.25 mg/day when lead follicle ≥14 mm or Lueoprolide 40 µg/12 h. Gn starting dose FSH 300 U + hMG150 U CD2 | 12 (ongoing PR/cycle 37%) | Significantly higher ongoing PR. No significant differences in other outcomes. Cancellation 9 vs.4.3% |
| | OC-Flare agonist 355 cycles | 38 | | | 13 (ongoing PR/cycle 52%) | |
| Garcia- Velasco et al. (262) (RCT) | Let-Gn-antagonist 71 cycles | 36.5 | Cancelled long agonist cycle due to <6 follicles or $E_2 \leq 500$ pg/mL | Let 2.5 mg/day CD 2–6. or No letr. Gn starting dose FSH 225 U + hMG150 U CD2 Ganirelex 0.25 mg/day when lead follicle ≥14 mm | 6.1 (Clinical PR/cycle 22.4%) | No difference in the number of MII. Higher IR in let group. No difference in other outcomes. Cancell ation for poor response 15.5 vs. 19.7% |
| | Gn-antagonist 76 cycles | 37.4 | | | 4.3 (Clinical PR/cycle 15.2%) | |
| Goswami et al. (266) (RCT) | Let-FSH-13 cycles | 38.5 | >35 years *and* failed prior 1–3 agonist cycles due to poor response | Let 2.5 mg/day CD 3–7 + FSH 75 U CD3 and 8 or Leuprolide 0.5 mg starting dose FSH 300 U | 1.6 (PR/cycle 23%) | Significantly lower total Gn (150 vs. 2,900 U). No significant difference in other outcomes.Cancellation 7.7 vs. 4% |
| | Long agonist 25 cycles | 39.1 | | | 2.1 (PR/cycle 24%) | |

*OC* oral contraceptive pills; *Let* letrozole; *GnRH* gonadotropin releasing hormone; *PR* pregnancy rate per started cycle; *IR* implantation rate; *MII* mature oocytes; *CD* cycle day; *Gn* gonadotropin dose in units/day; *RCT published* randomized clinical trial

**Table 14** Androgen supplementation in poor responders

| Study | Number of cycles | Mean age (year) | Definition of poor response and inclusion criteria | Protocol | Retrieved oocytes (mean) | Comments |
|---|---|---|---|---|---|---|
| Balasch (277) (pro-spective self controlled) | T-long agonist 25 cycles | 38 | Age 31–39 years, FSH < 10 mIU/mL, Two cancelled long agonist cycles due to poor response | T patch 20 µg/Kg/day × 5 days before Gn. Leuprolide 0.5 mg/day reduced to 0.25 mg with stimulation. Gn FSH 300 U + hMG 300 U (third) or Two long lueoprolide cycles. Gn starting dose FSH 300 U + hMG300 U (second) or FSH 450, 300, 150 days 3, 4, 5 (first cycle) | 5.8 (clinical PR/cycle 24%) | Higher AFC, 80% retrieval and transfer, reduction of Gn dose in T cycle. |
| | Two long agonist 25 cycles × 2 | 38 | | | 0 (clinical PR/cycle 0%) | Cancellation 20 vs. 100% |
| Massin et al. (278) (RCT) | T-long agonist 27 cycles | 36.9 | Poor response due to <6 oocytes or $E_2 \leq 1{,}200$ pg/mL and diminished ovarian reserve; FSH > 12 mIU/mL, $E_2 > 70$ pg/mL, inhibin <45 pg/mL and age < 42 years | T gel 10 mg/day 15–20 days during pituitary desensitization. or Placebo gel + Long agonist | 5.3 (clinical PR/cycle 16.7%) | No effect on AFC & AMH. |
| | Placebo- long agonist 26 cycles | 37.3 | | | 5.0 (clinical PR/cycle 4%) | |

*OC* oral contraceptive pills; *Let* letrozole; *GnRH* gonadotropin releasing hormone; *PR* pregnancy rate per started cycle; *IR* implantation rate; *MII* mature oocytes; *CD* cycle day; *Gn* gonadotropin dose in units/day; *RCT published* randomized clinical trial

flushing are of better morphology and may produce higher quality embryos than those floating in the liquor folliculi (282). NCs are associated with a low risk for multiple pregnancies, lower per-cycle cost and potentially less discomfort. Minimal stimulation also theoretically avoids the putative deleterious effects of high doses of gonadotropins on the meiotic competence of oocytes and subsequent embryonic development (171–173, 283). NC might theoretically be associated with higher implantation rates than stimulated cycles. The main disadvantages are high cycle cancellation rate due to premature ovulation, unsuccessful oocyte recovery and fertilization failure. Intrauterine insemination can be performed in appropriate patients if premature ovulation occurs. A review of 1,800 NC in 20 studies indicated that approximately 30% of the cycles were cancelled, primarily due to an LH surge. Embryo transfer was performed in 45.5% of started cycles resulting in an ongoing pregnancy rate 7.2% per initiated cycle and 15.8% of transfers. A cumulative ongoing pregnancy rate after up to nine modified NC (mean four cycles) in 268 patients was 44.4% (7.9% per started cycle, 20.7% per embryo transfer). Pregnancy rates did not decline in high order cycle numbers (284). Results of studies utilizing NC in poor responders are summarized in Table 15. A true comparison with ovarian stimulation will require randomized studies. In a cost-effectiveness analysis, Ubaldi et al. reported that if the pregnancy rate remains constant across four NC-IVF, it is possible to achieve a cumulative pregnancy rate of 40 vs. 8% from one stimulated cycle in poor responders while spending equal monetary units in both scenarios (293). Another application of the NC is NC-IUI (intrauterine insemination). The Lister group analyzed outcomes of 1,759 IUI cycles. In this report, women older than 37 years with tubal patency and no significant male factor achieved significantly higher live birth rates after NC-IUI (133 cycles) than following gonadotropin (426) or clomiphene (140) cycles (7.5 vs. 3.5 vs. 2.1%, respectively) (294). Outcomes of NC-IUI, in appropriately selected patients, appeared to be comparable to NC-IVF (Table 15).

## 6.13 Glucocorticoids

In 1956, Greenblat, used cortisone alone for the treatment of infertility (295). Since then, glucocorticoids have been used in conjunction with ovarian stimulation mainly to inhibit adrenal androgen production. In human preovulatory follicles, there is a sharp increase in the free cortisol concentrations compared to the serum (296, 297) probably due to activation of ovarian 11b hydroxysteroid dehydrogenase type I, thus increasing the conversion of cortisone to cortisol.

Glucocorticoids were shown to exert the following biological effects on the follicular system prior to ovulation:

1. Decreased granulosa cell apoptosis through increased expression of Bcl-2 and decreased expression of p53, and enhanced integrity of gap junctions through an increase in connexin 43 and cadherins as well as cell cytoskeleton (298, 299) and possibly decreased oocyte apoptosis.
2. Enhanced gonadotropin/c-AMP induced steroidogenesis (299).
3. Possible increase in serum growth hormone and production of IGF-I that partially mediates FSH effects (300).
4. Anti-inflammatory effects in the periovulatory period (298).
5. Possible positive effect on oocyte maturation and implantation. Keay reported higher cortisol/cortisone ratios in follicular fluid from conception cycles in women undergoing follicular puncture in unstimulated (301) and stimulated cycles (302). Glucocorticoids may interact with zona proteins.

Three studies investigated the effect of glucorticoids on response to COH in a general IVF population (Table 16). Although results are conflicting and require confirmation in well designed trials, the reduced cycle cancellation and low incidence of poor response was encouraging.

Although glucocorticoids were used in women with autoimmune premature ovarian failure with variable success, these data cannot be extrapolated to indicate their effects on response to COH.

## 6.14 Growth Hormone (GH) and Growth Hormone Releasing Factor (GHRH)

Evidence from murine and human follicular systems indicates that GH may exert direct and indirect (through IGF-I) effects on in vivo follicular maturation. GH, IGFs and their receptors and binding proteins are present in the human ovary (305, 306). While IGF-I is

**Table 15** Natural cycle/minimal stimulation in poor responders

| Study | Number of cycles | Mean age (year) | Definition of poor response and inclusion criteria | Cycles with transfer% | IR% | PR% |
|---|---|---|---|---|---|---|
| Controlled studies | | | | | | |
| Morgia et al. (20) (RCT) | Natural cycle 114 cycles | 37.2 | Age ≤ 43, cancellation due to ≤3 follicles in prior cycles | 41.2 | 14.9 | Clinical PR/cycle 6.1 |
| | Agonist flare 101 cycles buserelin 0.1 mg/day CD 1. Gn FSH 600 U on CD 3 | 37.3 | | 68.3 hCG at ≥16 mm follicles, retrieval at 36 h ICSI in all cycles | 5.5 $p < 0.05$ | Clinical PR/cycle 6.9 No pregnancies after three cycles |
| Elizur et al. (285) (Case control study) | Modified NC 52 cycles antagonist 0.25 mg + hMG 150–225 @ 13 mm | 39 | ≤4 oocytes or $E_2$ < 100 pg/mL on hCG | 67.4 | 10 | Clinical PR/cycle 9.5 |
| | Antagonist 200 cycles FSH ≥ 225 U/day CD2. Antagonist 0.25 mg @13 mm | 38.4 | | 83 | 6.8 | Clinical PR/cycle 8.5 |
| | Long agonist 288 cycles treptorelin depot FSH ≥ 225 U/day | 38.1 | | 81.6 | 7.4 | Clinical PR/cycle 8.6 |
| Feldman et al. (286) (Case- control study) | Natural cycle 44 cycles | 37 | Age < 40, ≤3follicles or cancellation in prior long agonist cycles | 41 | 20 | Delivery/cycle 4.5 |
| | Stimulated 55 cycles leuprolide 1 mg/day reduced to 0.5. Gn300–600 U | 36.7 | | ? hCG at ≥18 mm follicles, retrieval at 36 h | ? | PR 0 |
| Bassil et al. (287) | Natural cycle 16 cycles | 36.6 | Cancellation or poor response (one follicle) in two cycles | 37.5 Urine LH/6 h at 17 mm, hCG at ≥18 mm, retrieval at 35 h (33 h after surge) | 50 | Clinical PR/cycle 18.8 |
| | Stimulated cycles 25 cycles | 36.6 | | 20 | 0 | Clinical PR/cycle 0 |
| Lindheim et al. (288) (Case- control study) | Natural cycle 30 cycles | 37 | Age < 40, ≤3follicles or cancellation in prior long agonist cycles | 76.7 | 33 | PR/retrieval 16.6 |
| | Long agonist 27 cycles Leuprolide 1 mg/day reduced to 0.5. Gn300–600 U | 36.7 | | 77.8 hCG at ≥18 mm follicles, retrieval at 36 h | 7 $p < 0.01$ | PR/retrieval 7.4 |
| Case series | | | | | | |
| Check et al. (289) | Natural Cycle 92 cycles E$E_2$ 20 µg/day pretreatment for high FSH | 35.1–36.4 | Age ≤ 39 FSH >12 mIU/mL, antral follicle count ≤3, ≤3 mature oocytes Antagonist 0.25 mg + 75 U FSH if LH doubled. hCG at ≥17 mm follicles, retrieval at 33 h (30 h after surge) | 20.6 | 21.1 | clinical PR/cycle 4.3 |
| | Modified NC 116 cycles 75 U/day at 10 mm | | | 50.9 | 28.8 | clinical PR/cycle 14.7 |
| | Minimal stimulation 188 cycles 75 U/day CD2 | | | 27.1 | 29.4 | Clinical PR/cycle 8 |
| Papaleo et al. (290) | Modified NC 26 cycles antagonist 0.25 mg/day at 13 mm | 40.2 | FSH > 10 mIU/mL, low antral follicle count | 57.7 hCG at ≥16 mm follicles, retrieval (FF) at 36 h. ICSI in all cycles | 20 | Clinical PR/cycle 11.5 |

(continued)

**Table 15** (continued)

| Study | Number of cycles | Mean age (year) | Definition of poor response and inclusion criteria | Cycles with transfer% | IR% | PR% |
|---|---|---|---|---|---|---|
| Branco et al. (291) | Modified NC 158 cycles cetrorelix at 13 mm + hMG 150 U | 36.9 | Age < 38 FSH > 10 mIU/mL, $E_2$ > 60 pg/mL, and/or inhibin B <45 pg/mL, or <5 follicles on mean daily Gn 250U | 42.4 hCG at ≥16 mm follicles, retrieval at 36 h | 28.3 | Clinical PR/cycle 12 cumulative clinical PR (3 cycles) 35.2 |
| Koli-bianakis et al. (292) | Modified NC 78 cycles ganirelex 0.25 mg + FSH 100 U at 14 mm | 38.4 | FSH >12 mIU/mL, and ≤5 oocytes on mean startin Gn 466 U (median FSH in prior cycles 21.9) | 24.4 hCG at ≥16 mm follicles, retrieval at 32 h (double lumen), ICSI considered in all patients | 0 | Clinical PR/cycle 0 |
| Ubaldi et al. (293) | Modified NC 258 cycles ganirelex 0.25 mg + FSH 75-100 U at 14–15 mm | ? | Cancellation or ≤2 oocytes in ≥2cycles of ovarian stimulation | 51.5 hCG at ≥16 mm follicles, retrieval at 35 h, ICSI all cycles for male factor | 27.4 | Clinical PR/cycle 13.5 |

*NC* natural cycle; *GnRH* gonadotropin releasing hormone; *PR* pregnancy rate per started cycle; *IR* implantation rate; *CD* cycle day; *Gn* gonadotropin dose in units/day; *RCT published* randomized clinical trial; *FF* follicular flushing; *ICSI* intracytoplasmic sperm injection. All differences are not significant unless indicated; ? not specified

**Table 16** Glucocorticoid supplementation during COH

| Study | Number of cycles | Mean age (year) | Inclusion criteria | Protocol | Retrieved oocytes (mean) | Comments |
|---|---|---|---|---|---|---|
| Ubaldi (302) (RCT) | Predni- solone 20 mg/day 159 cycles<br>None 156 cycles | 33.1<br>32.7 | Age < 39, normal day 3 hormone levels, no history of poor response, no contraindications to steroids | Prednisolone 10 mg twice a day on first day of stimulation. Long buserelin protocol. FSH 200–225 U starting dose. ICSI in all cycles | 11.9 (clinical PR/cycle 46.5%)<br>12 (clinical PR/cycle 46.1%) | No significant differ-ences between groups. No side effects |
| Keay et al. (303) (RCT) | Dexa- methasone 1 mg/day 145 cycles<br>Placebo 145 cycles | 32.5<br>32.2 | Age < 40 No contraindications | Dexamethasone 1 mg or placebo at 11 pm. Long buserelin protocol. FSH or hMG 150–300 U starting dose | 11 (Clinical PR/cycle 26.9%)<br>10 (Clinical PR/cycle 17.2%) | Cancellation due to poor response 2.8 vs. 12.4%. No significant difference in other outcomes |
| Kemeter et al. (304) (RCT) | Predni-Solone 7.5 mg/day 73 cycles<br>None agonist 73 cycles | 34.4<br>34.2 | All except if hormonal abnormalities or other medications | Clomiphene 100 mg/day and/or gonadotropins 150 U/day | 4.6 (clinical PR/cycle 11%)<br>3.8 (Clinical PR/cycle 8.2%) | Significantly higher pregnancy rate |

*PR* pregnancy rate per started cycle; *RCT published* randomized clinical trial

**Table 17** Growth hormone and growth hormone releasing hormone supplementation in poor responders during COH: RCTs

| Study | Number of cycles | Inclusion criteria | Protocol | Comments |
|---|---|---|---|---|
| Kucuk et al. (314) | GH 31 cycles<br>None 30 cycles | Mean age 35.8 and 35.2 years. Poor response to high dose Gn? | GH 12 IU/day SC in all agonist days. Long treptorelin protocol. Gn 450 U. ICSI all cycles | Significantly more oocytes in GH group (6.5 vs. 3.2 and embryos) Cancellation 0 vs. 16.7%. No significant difference in PR (32.3 vs. 16.7%) and IR (11.7 vs.31.5%) |
| Tesarik et al. (311) | GH 50 cycles<br>Placebo 50 cycles | 41–44 (mean 42.3 and 42.2 years) (ICSI all cycles) | GH 8 IU/day SC from day 7 of gonadotrophin administration till the day following hCG. Long treptorelin protocol. Gn FSH 450 U + hMG 150 U | No difference in retrieved oocytes (5.8 vs. 5.6). Higher clinical PR (26 vs. 6%), IR (6.2 vs. 1.7%) & delivery rate (22 vs. 4%) |
| Howles et al. (315) | GRF 96 cycles<br>Placebo agonist 100 cycles | Age 18–40 ≥2 cycles with ≤3 follicles >16 mm on hCG day or cancellation, or >41 ampoules of Gn in a short protocol or 47 ampoules in long protocol | GRF 500 μg SC twice daily till day of hCG or 14 days. Long buserelin or treptorelin protocol. Gn 300 U | Increase GH and IGF-I. No significant difference in other outcomes |
| Suikkari et al. (316) | GH 16 cycles<br>Placebo six cycles | Age 25–40 ≥2 cycles ≤2 oocytes or ≥48 ampoules hMG consumed | GH 4 or 12 U/day SC starting day 3 leuprolide flare 0.75 mg in the morning in spontaneous cycles. Gn 300 U | No significant differences |
| Dor et al. (317) | GH 7 cycles<br>Placebo seven cycles | Age 30–45 $E_2$ < 500 pg/ml on day of hCG, <3 oocytes | GH 18 IU/day SC on days 2, 4, 6, and 8 of stimulation. Short GnRHa/hMG protocol | No significant differences (retrieved oocytes 2.2 vs. 1.9) |
| Bergh et al. (318) | GH 9 cycles<br>Placebo nine cycles | Age 25–38 ≥2 failed cycles with <5 oocytes | Long buserelin protocol. GH 0.1 IU/kg/day SC or placebo after downregulation starting 7 days before stimulation. FSH and/or hMG 150–300 U starting dose | No significant differences between groups except fertilization rate and IGF-I in FF |
| Zhuang et al. (319) | GH 12 cycles<br>Placebo 15 cycles | Mean age 33.2 and 32.3 years. Prior poor response? | GH 12 IU/day IM on alternate days. Long buserelin protocol | Significantly higher pregnancy rate |
| Hughes et al. (320) | GH ? cycles<br>Placebo ? cycles | Poor responders to high dose hMG? | GH 12 IU/day. Long buserelin /hMG. | No significant differences |
| Owen et al. (321) | GH 13 cycles<br>Placebo 12 cycles | Age 25–38 >1 cycles with <6 oocytes and <3 embryos (18 PCO patients!) | GH 24 IU IM or placebo, days 1, 3, 5, 7, 9, and 11 of hMG treatment, during long GnRHa protocol | Significant increase in the number of oocytes |

*GH* growth hormone; *GRF* growth hormone releasing factor; *GnRH* gonadotropin releasing hormone; *PR* pregnancy rate per started cycle; *IR* implantation rate; *CD* cycle day; *Gn* gonadotropin dose in units/day; *RCT published* randomized clinical trial; *ICSI* intracytoplasmic sperm injection; *SC* subcutaneous; ? not specified

required for fertility (at least in some species) GH appears to be facilitatory. GH actions may include early follicular recruitment, late follicular development, oocyte maturation and steroidogenesis (307, 308 for reviews). Although GH may enhance responsiveness to gonadotropins, this appears to be restricted to women with relative GH deficiency (309), hypoestrogenic women on GnRH agonist (310) or lower GH concentration in women with advanced reproductive age (311). Hypergonadotropic women are nonresponsive to the enhancing effect of GH (312). Some reports of GH cotreatment indicate an improved response to COH and higher pregnancy rates (200). A meta-analysis of nine randomized clinical trials (3 in 91 normal responders and 6 in 302 poor responders) indicated that there is no evidence that GH improves live birth or other secondary outcomes in either IVF population. However when one study utilizing GH releasing factor (GRF) was excluded from analysis an improvement in live birth rate of borderline significance was detected (313). The optimal method (early vs. late administration) and dose (4–12 IU) of GH is yet to be defined. RCT utilizing GH or GRF in poor responders are presented in Table 17. In studies showing improvement in pregnancy rates, the number of retrieved oocytes was not uniformly increased by GH cotreatment indicating that an effect on oocyte quality or an endometrial effect may be responsible for these outcomes. Cotreatment with GH could be promising if large studies confirm its efficacy and define patient characteristics that might benefit from it.

## 7 Clinical Application Summary

Patients with diminished ovarian reserve and ovarian hypo-responsiveness to pharmacologic stimulation remain one of the thorniest challenges in the practice of ART. Documentation of prior poor response and/or the presence of positive clinical markers for diminished ovarian reserve mandate careful consideration of available stimulation strategies. Chronologic age is of paramount importance, as younger women with a poor response still manifest implantation rates roughly commensurate with their age. It is therefore reasonable to consider the option of oocyte donation sooner in the care of the reproductively "older" patient, although some of these women may also achieve successful pregnancies with autologous oocytes. At Cornell, we have had extensive experience utilizing luteal "estrogen priming," either estradiol alone or in combination with a GnRH-antagonist, and have additionally enjoyed some degree of success with agonist "flare" protocols. Most importantly, the choice of protocol should be tailored to the individual patient, taking into account her previous clinical experience in addition to biological markers including basal FSH with estradiol and antral follicle counts.

## References


1. Kligman I, Rosenwaks Z. Differentiating clinical profiles: predicting good responders, poor responders, and hyper-responders. Fertil Steril 2001, 76(6):1185–90 (Level III).
2. Macklon N, Stouffer R, Giudice L, Fauser B. The Science behind 25 years of ovarian stimulation for in vitro Fertilization. Endo Rev 2006, 27(2):170–207 (Level III).
3. Broekmans F, Kwee J, Hendriks D, Mol B, Lambalk C. A systematic review of tests predicting ovarian reserve and IVF outcome. Hum Reprod Update 2006, 12:685–718 (Level III).
4. Lawson R, El-Toukh Y T, Kassab A, et al. Poor response to ovulation induction is a stronger predictor of early menopause than elevated basal FSH: a life table analysis. Hum Reprod 2003, 18(3):527–33 (Level II-2).
5. de Boer E, Tonkelaar I, te Velde E, Burger C, van Leeuwen FE. Increased risk of early menopausal transition and natural menopause after poor response at first IVF treatment. Hum Reprod 2003, 18(7):1544–52 (Level II-2).
6. de Boer E, Tonkelaar I, te Velde E, Burger C, Klip H, van Leeuwen F. A low number of retrieved oocytes at in vitro fertilization treatment is predictive of early menopause. Fertil Steril 2002, 77(5):978–85 (Level II-2).
7. Keay S, Liversedge N, Mathur R, Jenkins J. Assisted conception following poor ovarian response to gonadotrophin stimulation. B J Obstet Gynaecol 1997, 104:521–7 (Level III).
8. Center for Disease Control and Prevention. 2005 ART report. Accessed at http://www.cdc.gov/ART/ART2005/section2b.htm#f19 on December 30, 2007 (Level III).
9. Surrey E, Schoolcraft W. Evaluating strategies for improving ovarian response of the poor responder undergoing assisted reproductive techniques. Fertil Steril 2000, 73(4):667–76 (Level III).
10. Garcia J, Jones G S, Acosta A A, Wright G. Human menopausal gonadotropin/human chorionic gonadotropin follicular maturation for oocyte aspiration: phase II, 1981. Fertil Steril 1983, 39:174–9.
11. Saldeen P, Llen K, Sundstrom P. The probability of successful IVF outcome after poor ovarian response. Acta Obstet Gynecol 2007; 86:457–61 (Level II-3).
12. Frankfurter D, Dayal M, Dubey A, Peak D, Gindoff P. Novel follicular-phase gonadotropin-releasinghormone antagonist stimulation protocol for in vitro fertilization in the poor responder. Fertil Steril 2007, 88(5):1442–5 (Level II-3).
13. Baka S, Makrakis E, Tzanakaki D, et al. Cancellation of a first cycle is not predictive of a subsequent failure. Ann N Y Acad Sci 2006, 1092:418–25 (Level II-3).

14. Pennarubia J, Fabregues F, Manau D, et al. Previous cycle cancellation due to poor follicular development as a predictor of ovarian response in cycles stimulated with gonadotrophin-releasing hormone agonist-gonadotrophin treatment. Hum Reprod 2005, 20(3):622–8 (Level II-2).
15. Malmusi S, La Marca A, Giulini S, et al. Comparison of a gonadotropin-releasing hormone (GnRH) antagonist and GnRH agonist flare-up regimen in poor responders undergoing ovarian stimulation. Fertil Steril 2005, 84(2):402–6 (Level I).
16. Marci R, Oaserta D, Dolo V, Tatone C, Pavan A, Moscarini M. GnRH antagonist in IVF poor-responder patients: results of a randomized trial. Reprod Biomed Online 2005, 11(2):189–93 (Level I).
17. Klinkert E, Broekmans F, Looman C, Habbema J, te Velde E. Expected poor responders on the basis of an antral follicle count do not benefit from a higher starting dose of gonadotrophins in IVF treatment: a randomized controlled trial. Hum Reprod 2005, 20(3):611–15 (Level I).
18. Klinkert E, Broekmans F, Looman C, te Velde E. A poor response in the first in vitro fertilization cycle is not necessarily related to a poor prognosis in subsequent cycles. Fertil Steril 2004, 81(5):1247–53 (Level II-2).
19. Hellberg D, Waldenstrom U, Nilsson S. Defining a poor responder in in vitro fertilization. Fertil Steril 2004, 82(2):488–90 (Level II-3).
20. Morgia F, Sbracia M, Schimberni M, et al. A controlled trial of natural cycle versus microdose gonadotropin-releasing hormone analog flare cycles in poor responders undergoing in vitro fertilization. Fertil Steril 2004, 81(6):1542–7 (Level I).
21. Khalaf Y, El-Toukhy T, Taylor A, Braude P. Increasing the gonadotrophin dose in the course of an in vitro fertilization cycle does not rectify an initial poor response. Eur J Obstet Gynecol 2002, 103:146–9 (Level II-2).
22. Akman M, Halit E, Tosun S, Bayazit N, Esra A, Behceci M. Comparison of agonist-flare-up protocol and antagonistic multidose protocol in ovarian stimulation in poor responders: results of a prospective randomized trial. Hum Reprod 2001, 16(5):868–70 (Level I).
23. Garcia-Velasco J, Isaza V, Requena A, et al. High doses of gonadotrophins combined with stop versus non-stop protocol of GnRH analogue administration in low responder IVF patients: a prospective, randomized, controlled trial. Hum Reprod 2000, 15(11):2292–6 (Level I).
24. Kailasam C, Keay S D, Wilson P, Ford W C, Jenkins J M. Defining poor ovarian response during IVF cycles, in women aged <40 years, and its relationship with treatment outcome. Hum Reprod 2004, 19(7):1544–7 (Level III).
25. DeSutter P, Dhont M. Poor response after hormonal stimulation for in vitro fertilization is not related to ovarian aging. Fertil Steril 2003, 79(6):1294–8 (Level II-2).
26. van Rooij I, Bancsi L, Broekmans F, Looman C, Habbema J, te Velde E. Women older than 40 years of age and those with elevated follicle-stimulating hormone levels differ in poor response rate and embryo quality in in vitro fertilization. Fertil Steril 2003, 79(3):482–8 (Level II-3).
27. Sallam H N, Ezzeldin F, Agameya A F, Rahman A F, El-Garem Y. Defining poor responders in assisted reproduction. Int J Fertil Womens Med 2005, 50(3):115–20 (Level II-3).
28. Sunkara S K, Coomarasamy A, Khalaf Y, Braude P. A three arm randomised controlled trial comparing Gonadotrophin Releasing Hormone (GnRH) agonist long regimen versus GnRH agonist short regimen versus GnRH antagonist regimen in women with a history of poor ovarian response undergoing in vitro fertilisation (IVF) treatment: Poor responders intervention trial (PRINT). Reprod Health. 2007, 4(1):12. Accessed at http://www.reproductive-health-journal.com/content/4/1/12 on 2/17/2008 (Level III).
29. Ho J, Guu H, Yi Y, Chen M, Ho E. The serum follicle-stimulating hormone-to-luteinizing hormone ratio at the start of stimulation with gonadotropins after pituitary down-regulation is inversely correlated with a mature oocyte yield and can predict "low responders." Fertil Steril 2005, 83(4):883–8.
30. Fanchin R, Schonäuer L M, Cunha-Filho J S, Méndez Lozano D H, Frydman R. Coordination of antral follicle growth: basis for innovative concepts of controlled ovarian hyperstimulation. Semin Reprod Med 2005, 23(4):354–62 (Level III).
31. Martinez F, Barri P, Coroleu B, et al. Women with poor response to IVF have lowered circulating gonadotrophin surge-attenuating factor (GnSAF) bioactivity during spontaneous and stimulated cycles. Hum Reprod 2002, 17(3):634–40 (Level II-3).
32. Younis J S, Matilsky M, Radin O, Ben-Ami M. increased progesterone/estradiol ratio in the late follicular phase could be related to low ovarian reserve in in vitro fertilization-embryo transfer cycles with a long gonadotropin-releasing hormone agonist. Fertil Steril 2001, 76(2):294–9 (Level II-3).
33. Fisher S, Grin A, Paltoo A, Shapiro H M. Falling estradiol levels as a result of intentional reduction in gonadotrophin dose are not associated with poor IVF outcomes, whereas spontaneously falling estradiol levels result in low clinical pregnancy rates. Hum Reprod 2005, 20(1):84–8 (Level II-2).
34. Goswami D, Conway G. Premature ovarian failure. Hum Reprod Update 2005, 11(4):391–410 (Level III).
35. Broekmans F, Knauff E, te Velde E, Macklon N, Fauser B. Female reproductive ageing: current knowledge and future trends. Trends Endocrinol Metab 2007, 18(2):58–65 (Level III).
36. Toniolo D, Rizzolio F. X chromosome and ovarian failure. Semin Reprod Med 2007, 25(4):264–71 (Level III).
37. de Castro F, Morón F J, Montoro L, et al. Human controlled ovarian hyperstimulation outcome is a polygenic trait. Pharmacogenetics 2004, 14(5):285–93.
38. Gerb R, Behre H, Simoni M. Pharmacogenetics in ovarian stimulation – current concepts and future options. Reprod Biomed Online 2005, 11(5): 589–600 (Level III).
39. Hirschhorn J N, Daly M J Genome-wide association studies for common diseases and complex traits. Nat Rev Genet 2005, 6:95–108 (Level III).
40. Klinkert E, te Velde E, Weima S, van Zandvoort P, Hanssen R, Nilsson P, de Jong F, Looman C, Broekmans F. FSH receptor genotype is; associated with pregnancy but not with ovarian response in IVF. Reprod Biomed Online 2006, 13(5):687–95 (Level II-3).
41. Perez Mayorga M, Gromoll J, Behre HM, Gassner C, Nieschlag E, Simoni M. Ovarian response to follicle-stimulating hormone (FSH) stimulation depends on the FSH receptor genotype. J Clin Endocrinol Metab 2000, 85(9):3365–9 (Level II-3).
42. de Koning C, Benjamins T, Harms P, et al. The distribution of FSH receptor isoforms is related to basal FSH levels in subfertile women with normal menstrual cycles. Hum Reprod 2006, 21(2):443–6 (Level II-2).
43. Falconer H, Andersson E, Aansen A, Fried G. Follicle-stimulating hormone receptor polymorphisms in a population

of infertile women. Acta Obstet Gynecol Scand 2005, 84:806–11. (Level II-2)

44. Behre H, Greb R, Mempel A, et al. Significance of a common single nucleotide polymorphism in exon 10 of the follicle-stimulating hormone (FSH) receptor gene for the ovarian response to FSH: a pharmacogenetic approach to controlled ovarian hyperstimulation. Pharmacogenet Genomics 2005, 15:451–6 (Level I).
45. Jun J, Yoon J, Ku S, et al. Follicle-stimulating hormone receptor gene polymorphism and ovarian responses to controlled ovarian hyperstimulation for IVF-ET. J Hum Genet 2006, 51:665–70 (Level II-3).
46. Loutradis D, Patsoula E, Minas V, et al. FSH receptor gene polymorphisms have a role for different ovarian response to stimulation in patients entering IVF/ICSI-ET programs. J Assist Reprod Genetics 2006, 23(4):177–84 (Level-3).
47. Sudo S, Kudo M, Wada S, Sato O, Hsueh A J, Fujimoto S. Genetic and functional analyses of polymorphisms in the human FSH receptor gene. Mol Hum Reprod 2002, 8(10):893–9 (Level-2).
48. de Castro F, Ruiz R, Montoro L, et al. Role of follicle-stimulating hormone receptor Ser680Asn polymorphism in the efficacy of follicle-stimulating hormone. Fertil Steril 2003, 80(3):571–6 (Level II-3).
49. Georgiou I, Konstantelli M, Syrrou M, Messinis I, Lolis D. Oestrogen receptor gene polymorphisms and ovarian stimulation for in-vitro fertilization. Hum Reprod 1997, 12(7):1430–3 (Level II-2).
50. Sundarrajan C, Liao W, Roy A C, Ng S C. Association of oestrogen receptor gene polymorphisms with outcome of ovarian stimulation in patients undergoing IVF. Mol Hum Reprod 1999, 5(9):797–02 (Level II-2).
51. Sundarrajan C, Liao W X, Roy A C, Ng S C. Association between estrogen receptor-beta gene polymorphisms and ovulatory dysfunctions in patients with menstrual disorders. J Clin Endocrinol Metab 2001, 86(1):135–9 (Level II-2).
52. Allen E, Sullivan A, Marcus M, et al. Examination of reproductive aging milestones among women who carry the FMR1 premutation. Hum Reprod 2007, 22(8):2142–52 (Level III).
53. Wittenberger M, Hagerman R, Sherman S, et al. The FMR1 premutation and reproduction, Fertil Steril 2007, 87(3):456–65 (Level III).
54. Murray A, Webb J, Dennis N, Conway G, Morton N. Microdeletions in FMR2 may be a significant cause of premature ovarian failure. J Med Genet 1999, 36:767–70 (Level II-3).
55. Kevenaar M, Themmen A, Rivadeneira F, et al. A polymorphism in the AMH type II receptor gene is associated with age at menopause in interaction with parity. Hum Reprod 2007, 22(9):2382–8 (Level II-2).
56. Keay S, Barlow R, Eley A, Masson G, Anthony F, Jenkins J. The relation between immunoglobulin G antibodies to Chlamydia trachomatis and poor ovarian response to gonadotropin stimulation before in vitro fertilization. Fertil Steril 1998, 70(2):214–8 (Level III).
57. Suzuki T, Izumi S, Matsubayashi H, Awaji H, Yoshikata K, Makino T. Impact of ovarian endometrioma on oocytes and pregnancy outcome in in vitro fertilization. Fertil Steril 2005, 83(4):908–13 (Level II-2).
58. Esinler I, Bozdag G, Aybar F, Bayar, Yarali H. Outcome of in vitro fertilization/intracytoplasmic sperm injection after laparoscopic cystectomy for endometriomas. Fertil Steril 2006, 85(6):1730–5 (Level II-2).
59. Somigliana E, Ragni G, Infantino M, Benedetti F, Arnoldi M, Crosignani P G. Does laparoscopic removal of nonendometriotic benign ovarian cysts affect ovarian reserve? Acta Obstet Gynecol Scand 2006, 85(1):74–7 (Level II-2).
60. Kandil M, Selim M. Hormonal and sonographic assessment of ovarian reserve before and after laparoscopic ovarian drilling in polycystic ovary syndrome. BJOG 2005, 112(10):1427–30 (Level II-2).
61. Ginsburg E,Yanushpolsky E, Jackson K. In vitro fertilization for cancer patients and survivors. Fertil Steril 2001, 75(10):705–10 (Level III).
62. Anderson R, Themmen A, Al-Qahtani A, Groome N, Cameron D. The effects of chemotherapy and long-term gonadotrophin suppression on the ovarian reserve in premenopausal women with breast cancer. Hum Reprod 2006, 21(10):2583–92 (Level III).
63. El-Nemr A, Al-Shawaf T, Sabatini L, Wilson C, Lower A M, Grudzinskas J G. Effect of smoking on ovarian reserve and ovarian stimulation in in-vitro fertilization and embryo transfer. Hum Reprod 1998, 13(8):2192–8 (Level II-2).
64. Te Velde E, Pearson P. The variability of female reproductive ageing. Hum Reprod Update 2002, 8(2):141–54 (Level III).
65. Ventura S, Abma J, Mosher W, Henshaw S. Estimated pregnancy rates for the United states, 1990–2000: an update. National vital statistics report 52 no 23, Hyattsville, Maryland. CDC, 2004 (Level III).
66. El-Toukhy T, Khalaf Y, Hart R, Taylor A, Braude P. Young age does not protect against the adverse effects of reduced ovarian reserve – an eight year study. Hum Reprod 2002, 17(6):1519–24 (Level III).
67. van Rooij IA, de Jong E, Broekmans FJ, Looman CW, Habbema JD, te Velde ER. High follicle-stimulating hormone levels should not necessarily lead to the exclusion of subfertile patients from treatment. Fertil Steril 2004, 81(6): 1478–85 (Level III).
68. Lambalk C. Value of elevated basal follicle-stimulating hormone levels and the differential diagnosis during the diagnostic subfertility work-up. Fertil Steril 2003, 79(3): 489–90 (Level III).
69. Levi A, Raynault M, Bergh P, Drews M, Miller B, Scott R, Jr. Reproductive outcome in patients with diminished ovarian reserve. Fertil Steril 2001, 76(4):666–9 (Level III).
70. Licciardi F, Liu H, Rosenwaks Z. Day 3 estradiol serum concentrations as prognosticators of ovarian stimulation response and pregnancy outcome in patients undergoing in vitro fertilization. Fertil Steril 1995, 64(5):991–4 (Level III).
71. Veleva Z, Järvelä I, Nuojua-Huttunen S, Martikainen H, Tapanainen J. An initial low response predicts poor outcome in in vitro fertilization/intracytoplasmic sperm injection despite improved ovarian response in consecutive cycles. Fertil Steril 2005, 83(5):1384–90 (Level II-2).
72. Sherman B M, Korenman S G. Hormonal characteristics of the human menstrual cycle throughout reproductive life. J Clin Invest 1975, 55(4):699–706 (Level III).
73. Muasher S J, Oehninger S, Simonetti S, et al. The value of basal and/or stimulated serum gonadotropin levels in

prediction of stimulation response and in vitro fertilization outcome. Fertil Steril 1988, 50(2):298–307 (Level III).

74. Djerassi A, Coutifaris C, West V A, Asa S L, et al. Gonadotroph adenoma in a premenopausal woman secreting follicle-stimulating hormone and causing ovarian hyperstimulation. J Clin Endocrinol Metab 1995, 80:591–4 (Level III).
75. Scott R T Jr, Hofmann G E, Oehninger S, Muasher S J. Intercycle variability of day 3 follicle-stimulating hormone levels and its effect on stimulation quality in in vitro fertilization. Fertil Steril 1990, 54(2):297– 302 (Level II-2).
76. Kwee J, Schats R, McDonnell J, Lambalk C B, Schoemaker J. Intercycle variability of ovarian reserve tests: results of a prospective randomized study. Hum Reprod 2004, 19(3):590–5 (Level I).
77. Roberts J E, Spandorfer S, Fasouliotis S J, Kashyap S, Rosenwaks Z. Taking a basal follicle-stimulating hormone history is essential before initiating in vitro fertilization. Fertil Steril 2005, 83(1):37–41 (Level II-3).
78. Choi J H, Gilks C B, Auersperg N, Leung P C. Immunolocalization of gonadotropin-releasing hormone (GnRH)-I, GnRH-II, and type I GnRH receptor during follicular development in the human ovary. J Clin Endocrinol Metab 2006, 91(11):4562–70.
79. Seifer D, Lambert-Messerlian G, Hogan J, Gardiner A, Blazar A, Berk C. Day 3 serum inhibin-B is predictive of assisted reproductive technologies outcome. Fertil Steril 1997, 67(1):110–4 (Level III).
80. Visser J, de Jong F, Laven J, Themmen A. Anti-Mullerian hormone: a new marker for ovarian function. Reproduction 2006, 131:1–9 (Level III).
81. Hehenkamp W, Looman C, Themmen A, de Jong F, Te Velde E, Broekmans F. Anti-Mullerian hormone levels in the spontaneous menstrual cycle do not show substantial fluctuation. J Clin Endocrinol Metab 2006, 91(10):4057–63 (Level III).
82. Fanchin R, Taieb J, Lozano D H, Ducot B, Frydman R, Bouyer J. High reproducibility of serum anti-Mullerian hormone measurements suggests a multi-staged follicular secretion and strengthens its role in the assessment of ovarian follicular status. Hum Reprod 2005, 20(4):923–7 (Level II-3).
83. Streuli I, Fraisse T, Pillet C, Ibecheole V, Bischof P, de Ziegler D. Serum antimüllerian hormone levels remain stable throughout the menstrual cycle and after oral or vaginal administration of synthetic sex steroids. Fertil Steril 2007. Accessed on the web at www.fertster.org on 1/20/2007 (Level I).
84. Mohamed K, Davies W, Lashen H. Antimüllerian hormone and pituitary gland activity after prolonged down-regulation with goserelin acetate. Fertil Steril 2006, 85(5):1515–17 (Level III).
85. Fanchin R, Louafi N, Mendez Lozano D, Frydman N, Frydman R, Taieb J. Per-follicle measurements indicate that anti-Mullerian hormone secretion is modulated by the extent of follicular development and luteinization and may reflect qualitatively the ovarian follicular status. Fertil Steril 2005, 84(1):167–73 (Level II-2).
86. Fanchin R, Schonäuer L M, Righini C, Frydman N, Frydman R, Taieb J. Serum anti-Müllerian hormone dynamics during controlled ovarian hyperstimulation. Hum Reprod 2003, 18(2):328–32 (Level III).
87. de Vet A, Laven JS, de Jong FH, Themmen AP, Fauser BC. Antimüllerian hormone serum levels: a putative marker for ovarian aging. Fertil Steril 2002, 77(2):357–62 (Level II-2).
88. Fanchin R, Schonäuer LM, Righini C, Guibourdenche J, Frydman R, Taieb J. Serum anti-Müllerian hormone is more strongly related to ovarian follicular status than serum inhibin B, estradiol, FSH and LH on day 3. Hum Reprod 2003, 18(2):323–7 (Level II-3).
89. van Rooij I, Broekmans F, te Velde E, et al. Serum anti-Müllerian hormone levels: a novel measure of ovarian reserve. Hum Reprod 2002, 17(12):3065–71 (Level II-2).
90. Nelson SM, Yates RW, Fleming R. Serum anti-Müllerian hormone and FSH: prediction of live birth and extremes of response in stimulated cycles – implications for individualization of therapy. Hum Reprod 2007, 22(9):2414–21 (Level II-3).
91. Kwee J, Schats R, McDonnell J, Themmen A, de Jong F, Lambalk C. Evaluation of anti-Mullerian hormone as a test for the prediction of ovarian reserve. Fertil Steril 2007. Accessed on the web at www.fertsteril.org on 1/20/2008 (Level I).
92. Lekamge DN, Barry M, Kolo M, Lane M, Gilchrist RB, Tremellen KP. Anti-Müllerian hormone as a predictor of IVF outcome. Reprod Biomed Online 2007, 14(5):602–10 (Level II-2).
93. Tremellen KP, Kolo M, Gilmore A, Lekamge DN. Anti-mullerian hormone as a marker of ovarian reserve. Aust N Z J Obstet Gynaecol 2005, 45(1):20–4 (Level II-2).
94. Muttukrishna S, McGarrigle H, Wakim R, Khadum I, Ranieri DM, Serhal P. Antral follicle count, anti-mullerian hormone and inhibin B: predictors of ovarian response in assisted reproductive technology? BJOG 2005, 112(10):1384–90 (Level II-3).
95. Ebner T, Sommergruber M, Moser M, Shebl O, Schreier-Lechner E, Tews G. Basal level antimullerian hormone is associated with oocyte quality in stimulated cycles. Hum Reprod 2006, 21:2022–6.
96. Silberstein T, MacLaughlin DT, Shai I, Trimarchi JR, Lambert-Messerlian G, Seifer DB. mullerian inhibitory substance levels at the time of hCG administration in IVF cycles predict both ovarian reserve and embryo morphology. Hum Reprod 2006, 21:159–63.
97. Smeenk JM, Sweep FC, Zielhuis GA, Kremer JA, Thomas CM, Braat DD. Antimullerian hormone predicts ovarian responsiveness, but not embryo quality or pregnancy, after in vitro fertilization or intracyoplasmic sperm injection. Fertil Steril 2007, 87:223–6.
98. Navot D, Rosenwaks Z, Margalioth EJ. Prognostic assessment of female fecundity. Lancet 1987, 2(8560):645–7 (Level II-3).
99. Kwee J, Elting MW, Schats R, Bezemer PD, Lambalk CB, Schoemaker J. Comparison of endocrine tests with respect to their predictive value on the outcome of ovarian hyperstimulation in IVF treatment: results of a prospective randomized study. Hum Reprod 2003, 18(7):1422–7 (Level I).
100. Fanchin R, de Ziegler D, Olivennes F, Taieb J, Dzik A, Frydman R. Exogenous follicle stimulating hormone ovarian reserve test (EFORT): a simple and reliable screening test for detecting "poor responders" in in-vitro fertilization. Hum Reprod 1994, 9(9):1607–11 (Level III).

101. Muasher SJ, Oehninger S, Simonetti S, et al. The value of basal and/or stimulated serum gonadotropin levels in prediction of stimulation response and in vitro fertilization outcome. Fertil Steril 1988, 50(2):298–307 (Level III).
102. Ranieri DM, Phophong P, Khadum I, Meo F, Davis C, Serhal P. Simultaneous evaluation of basal FSH and oestradiol response to GnRH analogue (F-G-test) allows effective drug regimen selection for IVF. Hum Reprod 2001, 16(4):673–5 (Level II-3).
103. Hendriks DJ, Broekmans FJ, Bancsi LF, Looman CW, de Jong FH, te Velde ER. Single and repeated GnRH agonist stimulation tests compared with basal markers of ovarian reserve in the prediction of outcome in IVF. J Assist Reprod Genet 2005, 22(2):65–73 (Level II-2).
104. Reuss ML, Kline J, Santos R, Levin B, and Timor-Tritsch I. Age and the ovarian follicle pool assessed with transvaginal ultrasonography. Am J Obstet Gynecol 1996, 174:624–7 (Level III).
105. Hendriks DJ, Kwee J, Mol BW, te Velde ER, Broekmans FJ. Ultrasonography as a tool for the prediction of outcome in IVF patients: a comparative meta-analysis of ovarian volume and antral follicle count. Fertil Steril 2007, 87(4):764–75 (Level II-3).
106. Jayaprakasan K, Hilwah N, Kendall NR, et al. Does 3D ultrasound offer any advantage in the pretreatment assessment of ovarian reserve and prediction of outcome after assisted reproduction treatment? Hum Reprod 2007, 22(7):1932–41 (Level II-2).
107. Jayaprakasan K, Campbell B, Hopkisson J, Clewes J, Johnson I, Raine-Fenning N. Establishing the intercycle variability of three-dimensional ultrasonographic predictors of ovarian reserve. Fertil Steril. 2008. Assessed online at fertsteril.org (Level III).
108. Popovic-Todorovic B, Loft A, Bredkjaeer HE, Bangsbøll S, Nielsen IK, Andersen AN. A prospective randomized clinical trial comparing an individual dose of recombinant FSH based on predictive factors versus a "standard" dose of 150 IU/day in "standard" patients undergoing IVF/ICSI treatment. Hum Reprod 2003, 18(11):2275–82 (Level I).
109. Howles CM, Saunders H, Alam V, Engrand P. The FSH Treatment Guidelines Clinical Panel. Predictive factors and a corresponding treatment algorithm for controlled ovarian stimulation in patients treated with recombinant human follicle stimulating hormone (follitropin alfa) during assisted reproduction technology (ART) procedures. An analysis of 1378 patients. Curr Med Res Opin 2006, 22(5):907–18 (Level III).
110. Hsieh YY, Chang CC, Tsai HD. Antral follicle counting in predicting the retrieved oocyte number after ovarian hyperstimulation. J Assist Reprod Genet 2001, 18(6): 320–4 (Level II-2).
111. Andolf E, Jörgensen C, Svalenius E, Sundén B. Ultrasound measurement of the ovarian volume. Acta Obstet Gynecol Scand 1987, 66(5):387–9 (Level II-3).
112. Frattarelli JL, Levi AJ, Miller BT, Segars JH. Prognostic use of mean ovarian volume in in vitro fertilization cycles: a prospective assessment. Fertil Steril 2004, 82(4):811–5 (Level II-3).
113. Kupesic S, Kurjak A, Bjelos D, Vujisic S. Three-dimensional ultrasonographic ovarian measurements and in vitro fertilization outcome are related to age. Fertil Steril 2003, 79(1):190–7 (Level II-3).
114. Tempfer CB, Riener EK, Keck C, et al. Polymorphisms associated with thrombophilia and vascular homeostasis and the timing of menarche and menopause in 728 white women. Menopause 2005, 12(3):325–30 (Level II-2).
115. Block E. Quantitative morphological investigations of the follicular system in women; variations at different ages. Acta Anat (Basel) 1952, 14(1–2):108–23 (Level II-3).
116. Baker TG. A quantitative and cytological study of germ cells in human ovaries. Proc R Soc Lond B Biol Sci 1963, 158:417–33 (Level II-3).
117. Lass A, Silye R, Abrams DCet al. Follicular density in ovarian biopsy of infertile women: a novel method to assess ovarian reserve. Hum Reprod 1997, 12(5):1028–31 (Level II-3).
118. Lass A. Assessment of ovarian reserve: is there still a role for ovarian biopsy in the light of new data? Hum Reprod 2004, 19(3):467–9 (Level III).
119. Chuang CC, Chen CD, Chao KH, Chen SU, Ho HN, Yang YS. Age is a better predictor of pregnancy potential than basal follicle-stimulating hormone levels in women undergoing in vitro fertilization. Fertil Steril 2003, 79(1):63–8 (Level II-3).
120. Wide L, Hobson BM. Qualitative difference in follicle-stimulating hormone activity in the pituitaries of young women compared to that of men and elderly women. J Clin Endocrinol Metab 1983, 56(2):371–5 (Level II-2).
121. Ulloa-Aguirre A, Midgley AR, Beitins IZ, Padmanabhan V. Follicle-stimulating isohormones: characterisation and physiological relevance. Endocr Rev 1995, 16:765–87 (Level III).
122. Nayudu PVitt U, Ulloa-Aguirre A, Barrios de Tomasi J, Pancharatna K. Intact follicle culture: what it can tell us about the roles of FSH glycoforms during follicle development. Reprod BioMed Online 2002, 5(3):240–53 (Level III).
123. Veldhuis JD, Beitins IZ, Johnson ML, Serabian MA, Dufau ML. Biologically active luteinizing hormone is secreted in episodic pulsations that vary in relation to stage of the menstrual cycle. J Clin Endocrinol Metab 1984, 58(6):1050–8 (Level II-3).
124. Palter S, Tavares A, Hourvitz A, Veldhuis J, Adashi E. Are estrogens of import to primate/human ovarian folliculogenesis? Endocrine Rev 2001, 22(3):389–424 (Level III).
125. Luo W, Wiltbank M. Distinct regulation by steroids of messenger RNAs for FSHR and CYP19A1 in bovine granulosa cells. Biol Reprod 2006, 75:217–25.
126. Findlay J, Drummond A. Regulation of the FSH receptor in the ovary. Trend Endocrinol Metab 1999, 10(5):183–8 (Level III).
127. Weil S, Vendola K, Zhou J, Bondy CA. Androgen and follicle-stimulating hormone interactions in primate ovarian follicle development. J Clin Endocrinol Metab 1999, 84(8):2951–6.
128. Vendola KA, Zhou J, Adesanya OO, Weil SJ, Bondy CA. Androgens stimulate early stages of follicular growth in the primate ovary. J Clin Invest 1998, 101(12):2622–9.
129. Vendola K, Zhou J, Wang J, Bondy CA. Androgens promote insulin-like growth factor-I and insulin-like growth factor-I receptor gene expression in the primate ovary. Hum Reprod 1999, 14(9):2328–32.

130. Cai J, Lou H, Dong M, et al. Poor ovarian response to gonadotropin stimulation is associated with low expression of follicle-stimulating hormone receptor in granulosa cells. Fertil Steril 2007, 87(6):1350–6 (Level II-2).
131. Levy DP, Navarro JM, Schattman GL, Davis OK, Rosenwaks Z. The role of LH in ovarian stimulation. Exogenous LH: let's design the future. Hum Reprod 2000, 15(11):2258–65 (Level III).
132. Balasch J, Fábregues F. Is luteinizing hormone needed for optimal ovulation induction? Curr Opin Obstet Gynecol 2002, 14(3):265–74 (Level III).
133. Filicori M, Cognigni GE, Pocognoli P, Ciampaglia W, Bernardi S. Current concepts and novel applications of LH activity in ovarian stimulation. Trends Endocrinol Metab 2003, 14(6):267–73 (Level III).
134. Shoham Z. The clinical therapeutic window for luteinizing hormone in controlled ovarian stimulation. Fertil Steril 2002, 77:1170–7 (Level III).
135. Kolibianakis EM, Zikopoulos K, Schiettecatte J, et al. Profound LH suppression after GnRH antagonist administration is associated with a significantly higher ongoing pregnancy rate in IVF. Hum Reprod 2004, 19(11):2490–6 (Level II-3).
136. McNatty KP, Hillier SG, van den Boogaard AM, Trimbos-Kemper TC, Reichert LE Jr., van Hall EV. Follicular development during the luteal phase of the human menstrual cycle. J Clin Endocrinol Metab 1983, 56(5):1022–31 (Level III).
137. Gougeon A. Regulation of ovarian follicular development in primates: facts and hypotheses. Endocr Rev 1996, 17:121–55 (Level III).
138. Mais V, Cetel NS, Muse KN, Quigley ME, Reid RL, Yen SS. Hormonal dynamics during luteal-follicular transition. J Clin Endocrinol Metab 1987, 64:1109–14 (Level III).
139. Fanchin R, Schonäuer LM, Cunha-Filho JS, Méndez Lozano DH, Frydman R. Coordination of antral follicle growth: basis for innovative concepts of controlled ovarian hyperstimulation. Semin Reprod Med 2005, 23(4):354–62 (Level III).
140. Al-Inany HG, Abou-Setta AM, Aboulghar M. Gonadotrophin-releasing hormone antagonists for assisted conception. Cochrane Database Syst Rev 2006, (3) CD001750. DOI: 10.1002/14651858.CD001750.pub2. Accessed at the web at http://mrw.interscience.wiley.com/cochrane/clsysrev/articles/CD001750/frame.html on 1, February 2008.
141. Fraser HM, Nestor JJ, Jr., Vickery BH. Suppression of luteal function by a luteinizing hormone-releasing hormone antagonist during the early luteal phase in the stumptailed macaque monkey and the effects of subsequent administration of human chorionic gonadotropin. Endocrinol 1987, 121(2):612–8.
142. Dubourdieu S, Charbonnel B, Massai MR, Marraoui J, Spitz I, Bouchard P. Suppression of corpus luteum function by the gonadotropin-releasing hormone antagonist Nal-Glu: effect of the dose and timing of human chorionic gonadotropin administration. Fertil Steril 1991, 56(3):440–5 (Level II-3).
143. Anderson RA, Kinniburgh D, Baird DT. Preliminary experience of the use of a gonadotrophin-releasing hormone antagonist in ovulation induction/in-vitro fertilization prior to cancer treatment. Hum Reprod 1999, 14(10):2665–8 (Level III).
144. de Ziegler D, Jääskeläinen AS, Brioschi PA, Fanchin R, Bulletti C. Synchronization of endogenous and exogenous FSH stimuli in controlled ovarian hyperstimulation (COH). Hum Reprod 1998, 13(3):561–4 (Level III).
145. Koering MJ, Danforth DR, Hodgen GD. Early follicle growth in the juvenile macaca monkey ovary: the effects of estrogen priming and follicle-stimulating hormone. Biol Reprod 1994, 50(3):686–94.
146. Fanchin R, Cunha-Filho JS, Schonäuer LM, Kadoch IJ, Cohen-Bacri P, Frydman R. Coordination of early antral follicles by luteal estradiol administration provides a basis for alternative controlled ovarian hyperstimulation regimens. Fertil Steril 2003, 79(2):316–21 (Level II-2).
147. Fanchin R, Cunha-Filho JS, Schonäuer LM, Righini C, de Ziegler D, Frydman R. Luteal estradiol administration strengthens the relationship between day 3 follicle-stimulating hormone and inhibin B levels and ovarian follicular status. Fertil Steril 2003, 79(3):585–9 (Level II-2).
148. Fanchin R, Salomon L, Castelo-Branco A, Olivennes F, Frydman N, Frydman R. Luteal estradiol pre-treatment coordinates follicular growth during controlled ovarian hyperstimulation with GnRH antagonists. Hum Reprod 2003, 18(12):2698–703 (Level I).
149. Fanchin R, Castelo Branco A, Kadoch IJ, et al. Premenstrual administration of gonadotropin-releasing hormone antagonist coordinates early antral follicle sizes and sets up the basis for an innovative concept of controlled ovarian hyperstimulation. Fertil Steril 2004, 81(6):1554–9 (Level II-2).
150. Dragisic KG, Davis OK, Fasouliotis SJ, Rosenwaks Z. Use of a luteal estradiol patch and a gonadotropin-releasing hormone antagonist suppression protocol before gonadotropin stimulation for in vitro fertilization in poor responders. Fertil Steril 2005, 84(4):1023–6 (Level II-3).
151. Bramley TA, Menzies GS, Baird DT. Specific binding of gonadotrophin-releasing hormone and an agonist to human corpus luteum homogenates: characterization, properties, and luteal phase levels. J Clin Endocrinol Metab 1985, 61(5):834–41.
152. Hsueh AJ, Erickson GF. Extrapituitary action of gonadotropin-releasing hormone: direct inhibition ovarian steroidogenesis. Science 1979, 204(4395):854–5.
153. Zhao S, Saito H, Wang X, Saito T, Kaneko T, Hiroi M. Effects of gonadotropin-releasing hormone agonist on the incidence of apoptosis in porcine and human granulosa cells. Gynecol Obstet Invest 2000, 49:52–6.
154. Cheng CK, Leung PC. Molecular biology of gonadotropin-releasing hormone (GnRH)-I, GnRH-II, and their receptors in humans. Endocr Rev 2005, 26(2):283–306 (Level III).
155. Abdalla H, Thum MY. Repeated testing of basal FSH levels has no predictive value for IVF outcome in women with elevated basal FSH. Hum Reprod 2006, 21(1):171–4 (Level II-2).
156. Lass A, Gerrard A, Abusheikha N, Akagbosu F, Brinsden P. IVF performance of women who have fluctuating early follicular FSH levels. J Assist Reprod Genet 2000, 17(10):566–573 (Level II-2).
157. Martin JS, Nisker JA, Tummon IS, Daniel SA, Auckland JL, Feyles V. Future in vitro fertilization pregnancy potential of women with variably elevated day 3 follicle-stimulating hormone levels. Fertil Steril 1996, 65(6):1238–40 (Level II-2).
158. Thum MY, Abdalla HI, Taylor D. Relationship between women's age and basal follicle-stimulating hormone levels with aneuploidy risk in in vitro fertilization treatment.

Fertil Steril 2007. Accessed at the web at fertilsteril.org (Level II-2).

159. Esposito MA, Coutifaris C, Barnhart KT. A moderately elevated day 3 FSH concentration has limited predictive value, especially in younger women. Hum Reprod 2002, 17(1):118–23 (Level II-3).
160. Out HJ, Braat DD, Lintsen BM, et al. Increasing the daily dose of recombinant follicle stimulating hormone (Puregon) does not compensate for the age-related decline in retrievable oocytes after ovarian stimulation. Hum Reprod 2000, 15(1):29–35 (Level I).
161. van Hooff MH, Alberda AT, Huisman GJ, Zeilmaker GH, Leerentveld RA. Doubling the human menopausal gonadotrophin dose in the course of an in-vitro fertilization treatment cycle in low responders: a randomized study. Hum Reprod 1993, 8(3):369–73 (Level I).
162. Hock DL, Louie H, Shelden RM, Ananth CV, Kemmann E. The need to step up the gonadotropin dosage in the stimulation phase of IVF treatment predicts a poor outcome. J Assist Reprod Genet 1998, 15(7):427–30 (Level II-2).
163. Karande VC, Jones GS, Veeck LL, Muasher SJ. High-dose follicle-stimulating hormone stimulation at the onset of the menstrual cycle does not improve the in vitro fertilization outcome in low-responder patients. Fertil Steril 1990, 53(3):486–9 (Level II-2).
164. Pantos C, Thornton SJ, Speirs AL, Johnston I. Increasing the human menopausal gonadotropin dose – does the response really improve? Fertil Steril 1990, 53(3):436–9 (Level II-2).
165. Land JA, Yarmolinskaya MI, Dumoulin JC, Evers JL. High-dose human menopausal gonadotropin stimulation in poor responders does not improve in vitro fertilization outcome. Fertil Steril 1996, 65(5):961–5 (Level II-3).
166. Stadtmauer L, Ditkoff EC, Session D, Kelly A. High dosages of gonadotropins are associated with poor pregnancy outcomes after in vitro fertilization-embryo transfer. Fertil Steril 1994, 61(6):1058–64 (Level II-3).
167. Lashen H, Ledger W, López Bernal A, Evans B, Barlow D. Superovulation with a high gonadotropin dose for in vitro fertilization: is it effective? J Assist Reprod Genet 1998, 15(7):438–43 (Level II-3).
168. Manzi DL, Thornton KL, Scott LB, Nulsen JC. The value of increasing the dose of human menopausal gonadotropins in women who initially demonstrate a poor response. Fertil Steril 1994, 62(2):251–6 (Level II-3).
169. Rombauts L. Is there a recommended maximum starting dose of FSH in IVF? J Assist Reprod Genet 2007, 24(8):343–9 (Level III).
170. Amsterdam A, Hanoch T, Dantes A, Tajima K, Strauss JF, Seger R. Mechanisms of gonadotropin desensitization. Mol Cell Endocrinol 2002, 187(1–2):69–74.
171. Vogel R, Spielmann H. Genotoxic and embryotoxic effects of gonadotropin-hyperstimulated ovulation of murine oocytes, preimplantation embryos, and term fetuses. Reprod Toxicol 1992, 6(4):329–33.
172. Van Blerkom J, Davis P. Differential effects of repeated ovarian stimulation on cytoplasmic and spindle organization in metaphase II mouse oocytes matured in vivo and in vitro. Hum Reprod 2001, 16(4):757–64.
173. Baart EB, Martini E, Eijkemans MJ, et al. Milder ovarian stimulation for in-vitro fertilization reduces aneuploidy in the human preimplantation embryo: a randomized controlled trial. Hum Reprod 2007, 22(4):980–8 (Level I).
174. Vauthier D, Lefebvre G. The use of gonadotropin-releasing hormone analogs for in vitro fertilization: comparison between the standard form and long-acting formulation of D-Trp-6-luteinizing hormone-releasing hormone. Fertil Steril 1989, 51(1):100–4.
175. Balasch J, Gómez F, Casamitjana R, Carmona F, Rivera F, Vanrell JA. Pituitary-ovarian suppression by the standard and half-doses of D-Trp-6-luteinizing hormone-releasing hormone depot. Hum Reprod 1992, 7(9):1230–4 (Level I).
176. Dal Prato L, Borini A, Coticchio G, Cattoli M, Flamigni C. Half-dose depot triptorelin in pituitary suppression for multiple ovarian stimulation in assisted reproduction technology: a randomized study. Hum Reprod 2004, 19(10):2200–5 (Level I).
177. Yim SF, Lok IH, Cheung LP, Briton-Jones CM, Chiu TT, Haines CJ. Dose-finding study for the use of long-acting gonadotrophin-releasing hormone analogues prior to ovarian stimulation for IVF. Hum Reprod 2001, 16(3):492–4 (Level I).
178. Takeuchi S, Minoura H, Shibahara T, Tsuiki Y, Noritaka F, Toyoda N. A prospective randomized comparison of routine buserelin acetate and a decreasing dosage of nafarelin acetate with a low-dose gonadotropin-releasing hormone agonist protocol for in vitro fertilization and intracytoplasmic sperm injection. Fertil Steril 2001, 76(3):532–7 (Level I).
179. Safdarian L, Mohammadi FS, Alleyassin A, Aghahosseini M, Meysamie A, Rahimi E. Clinical outcome with half-dose depot triptorelin is the same as reduced-dose daily buserelin in a long protocol of controlled ovarian stimulation for ICSI/embryo transfer: a randomized double-blind clinical trial (NCT00461916). Hum Reprod 2007, 22(9):2449–54 (Level I).
180. Fábregues F, Peñarrubia J, Creus M, Casamitjana R, Vanrell JA, Balasch J. Effect of halving the daily dose of triptorelin at the start of ovarian stimulation on hormone serum levels and the outcome of in vitro fertilization. Fertil Steril 2005, 83(3):785–8 (Level I).
181. Ku SY, Choi YS, Jee BC, et al. A preliminary study on reduced dose (33 or 25 microg) gonadotropin-releasing hormone agonist long protocol for multifollicular ovarian stimulation in patients with high basal serum follicle-stimulating hormone levels undergoing in vitro fertilization-embryo transfer. Gynecol Endocrinol 2005, 21(4):227–31 (Level II-2).
182. Feldberg D, Farhi J, Ashkenazi J, Dicker D, Shalev J, Ben-Rafael Z. Minidose gonadotropin-releasing hormone agonist is the treatment of choice in poor responders with high follicle-stimulating hormone levels. Fertil Steril 1994, 62(2):343–6 (Level II-2).
183. Avrech OM, Orvieto R, Pinkas H, Sapir-Rufas O, Feldberg D, Fisch B. Inclusion of standard and low-dose gonadotropin releasing hormone-analog (short protocol) in controlled ovarian hyperstimulation regimens in normogonadotropic patients aged 40–48 years who are undergoing in vitro fertilization. Gynecol Endocrinol 2004, 19(5):247–52 (Level I).
184. Pantos K, Meimeth-Damianaki T, Vaxevanoglou T, Kapetanakis E. Prospective study of a modified gonadotropin-releasing hormone agonist long protocol in an in vitro fertilization program. Fertil Steril 1994, 61(4):709–13 (Level I).

185. Simons AH, Roelofs HJ, Schmoutziguer AP, Roozenburg BJ, van't Hof-van den Brink EP, Schoonderwoerd SA. Early cessation of triptorelin in in vitro fertilization: a double-blind, randomized study. Fertil Steril 2005, 83(4):889–96 (Level I).
186. Faber BM, Mayer J, Cox B, Jones D, Toner JP, Oehninger S, Muasher SJ. Cessation of gonadotropin-releasing hormone agonist therapy combined with high-dose gonadotropin stimulation yields favorable pregnancy results in low responders. Fertil Steril 1998, 69(5):826–30 (Level III).
187. Wang PT, Lee RK, Su JT, Hou JW, Lin MH, Hu YM. Cessation of low-dose gonadotropin releasing hormone agonist therapy followed by high-dose gonadotropin stimulation yields a favorable ovarian response in poor responders. J Assist Reprod Genet 2002, 19(1):1–6 (Level III).
188. Dirnfeld M, Fruchter O, Yshai D, Lissak A, Ahdut A, Abramovici H. Cessation of gonadotropin-releasing hormone analogue (GnRH-a) upon down-regulation versus conventional long GnRH-a protocol in poor responders undergoing in vitro fertilization. Fertil Steril 1999, 72(3):406–11 (Level I).
189. Schachter M, Friedler S, Raziel A, Strassburger D, Bern O, Ron-el R. Improvement of IVF outcome in poor responders by discontinuation of GnRH analogue during the gonadotropin stimulation phase – a function of improved embryo quality. J Assist Reprod Genet 2001, 18(4):197–204 (Level II-3).
190. Lindheim SR, Barad DH, Witt B, Ditkoff E, Sauer MV. Short-term gonadotropin suppression with oral contraceptives benefits poor responders prior to controlled ovarian hyperstimulation. J Assist Reprod Genet 1996, 13(9):745–7 (Level II-2).
191. Howles CM, Macnamee MC, Edwards RG. Short term use of an LHRH agonist to treat poor responders entering an in-vitro fertilization programme. Hum Reprod 1987, 2(8):655–6 (Level III).
192. Brzyski RG, Muasher SJ, Droesch K, Simonetti S, Jones GS, Rosenwaks Z. Follicular atresia associated with concurrent initiation of gonadotropin-releasing hormone agonist and follicle-stimulating hormone for oocyte recruitment. Fertil Steril 1988, 50(6):917–21 (Level III).
193. Sharma V, Williams J, Collins W, Riddle A, Mason B, Whitehead M, The sequential use of a luteinizing hormone-releasing hormone (LH-RH) agonist and human menopausal gonadotropins to stimulate folliculogenesis in patients with resistant ovaries. J In Vitro Fert Embryo Transf 1988, 5:38–42 (Level III).
194. Pellicer A, Simón C, Miró F, Castellví RM, Ruiz A, Ruiz M, Pérez M, Bonilla-Musoles F. Ovarian response and outcome of in-vitro fertilization in patients treated with gonadotrophin-releasing hormone analogues in different phases of the menstrual cycle. Hum Reprod 1989, 4(3):285–9 (Level I).
195. Garcia JE, Padilla SL, Bayati J, Baramki TA. Follicular phase gonadotropin-releasing hormone agonist and human gonadotropins: a better alternative for ovulation induction in in vitro fertilization. Fertil Steril 1990, 53(2):302–5.
196. Navot D, Rosenwaks Z, Anderson F, Hodgen GD. Gonadotropin-releasing hormone agonist-induced ovarian hyperstimulation: low-dose side effects in women and monkeys. Fertil Steril 1991, 55:1069–75 (Level III).
197. San Roman GA, Surrey ES, Judd HL, Kerin JF. A prospective randomized comparison of luteal phase versus concurrent follicular phase initiation of gonadotropin-releasing hormone agonist for in vitro fertilization and gamete intrafallopian transfer cycles. Fertil Steril 1992, 58:744–9 (Level I).
198. Tan SL, Kingsland C, Campbell S, et al. The long protocol of administration of gonadotropin-releasing hormone agonist is superior to the short protocol for ovarian stimulation for in vitro fertilization. Fertil Steril 1992, 57(4):810–4 (Level I).
199. Sims JA, Seltman HJ, Muasher SJ. Early follicular rise of serum progesterone concentration in response to a flare-up effect of gonadotrophin-releasing hormone agonist impairs follicular recruitment for in-vitro fertilization. Hum Reprod 1994, 9(2):235–40 (Level III).
200. Scott RT, Navot D. Enhancement of ovarian responsiveness with microdoses of gonadotropin-releasing hormone agonist during ovulation induction for in vitro fertilization. Fertil Steril 1994, 61(5):880–5 (Level III).
201. Schoolcraft W, Schlenker T, Gee M, Stevens J, Wagley L. Improved controlled ovarian hyperstimulation in poor responder in vitro fertilization patients with a microdose follicle-stimulating hormone flare, growth hormone protocol. Fertil Steril 1997, 67(1):93–7 (Level III).
202. Surrey ES, Bower J, Hill DM, Ramsey J, Surrey MW. Clinical and endocrine effects of a microdose GnRH agonist flare regimen administered to poor responders who are undergoing in vitro fertilization. Fertil Steril 1998, 69:419–24 (Level III).
203. Leondires MP, Escalpes M, Segars JH, Scott RT Jr, Miller BT. Microdose follicular phase gonadotropin-releasing hormone agonist (GnRH-a) compared with luteal phase GnRH-a for ovarian stimulation at in vitro fertilization. Fertil Steril 1999, 72(6):1018–23 (Level II-2).
204. Karacan M, Erkan H, Karabulut O, Sarikami B, Camlibel T, Benhabib M. Clinical pregnancy rates in an IVF program. Use of the flare-up protocol after failure with long regimens of GnRH-a. J Reprod Med 2001, 46(5):485–9 (Level II-2).
205. Cedrin-Durnerin I, Bständig B, Hervé F, Wolf J, Uzan M, Hugues J. A comparative study of high fixed-dose and decremental-dose regimens of gonadotropins in a minidose gonadotropin-releasing hormone agonist flare protocol for poor responders. Fertil Steril 2000, 73(5):1055–6 (Level I).
206. Spandorfer S, Navarro J, Kump LM, Liu HC, Davis OK, Rosenwaks Z. "Co-Flare" stimulation in the poor responder patient: predictive value of the flare response. J Assist Reprod Genet 2001, 18(12):629–33 (Level III).
207. Fasouliotis SJ, Laufer N, Sabbagh-Ehrlich S, Lewin A, Hurwitz A, Simon A. Gonadotropin-releasing hormone (GnRH)-antagonist versus GnRH-agonist in ovarian stimulation of poor responders undergoing IVF. J Assist Reprod Genet 2003, 20(11):455–60 (Level II-3).
208. Mohamed KA, Davies WA, Lashen H. Effect of gonadotropin-releasing hormone agonist and antagonist on steroidogenesis of low responders undergoing in vitro fertilization. Gynecol Endocrinol 2006, 22(2):57–62 (Level II-2).
209. Vail A, Gardener E. Common statistical errors in the design and analysis of subfertility trials. Hum Reprod 2003, 18:1000–4 (Level III).

210. Daya S. Pitfalls in the design and analysis of efficacy trials in subfertility. Hum Reprod 2003, 18(5):1005–9 (Level III).
211. Sbracia M, Farina A, Poverini R, Morgia F, Schimberni M, Aragona C. Short versus long gonadotropin-releasing hormone analogue suppression protocols for superovulation in patients > or = 40 years old undergoing intracytoplasmic sperm injection. Fertil Steril 2005, 84(3):644–8 (Level I).
212. Weissman A, Farhi J, Royburt M, Nahum H, Glezerman M, Levran D. Prospective evaluation of two stimulation protocols for low responders who were undergoing in vitro fertilization-embryo transfer. Fertil Steril 2003, 79(4): 886–92. (Level I).
213. Schmidt DW, Bremner T, Orris JJ, Maier DB, Benadiva CA, Nulsen JC. A randomized prospective study of microdose leuprolide versus ganirelix in in vitro fertilization cycles for poor responders. Fertil Steril 2005, 83(5):1568–71. (Level I).
214. De Placido G, Mollo A, Clarizia R, Strina I, Conforti S, Alviggi C. Gonadotropin-releasing hormone (GnRH) antagonist plus recombinant luteinizing hormone vs. a standard GnRH agonist short protocol in patients at risk for poor ovarian response. Fertil Steril 2006, 85(1):247–50 (Level I).
215. Lainas TG, Sfontouris IA, Papanikolaou EG, et al. Flexible GnRH antagonist versus flare-up GnRH agonist protocol in poor responders treated by IVF: a randomized controlled trial. Hum Reprod 2008 Apr 10. Accessed at http://humrep.oxfordjournals.org/cgi/reprint/den107v1on 4/10/2008 (Level I).
216. Sunkara SK, Tuthill J, Khairy M, et al. Pituitary suppression regimens in poor responders undergoing IVF treatment: a systematic review and meta-analysis. Reprod Biomed Online 2007, 15(5):539–46 (Level III).
217. Kenigsberg D, Littman BA, Hodgen GD. Medical hypophysectomy: I. Dose-response using a gonadotropin-releasing hormone antagonist. Fertil Steril 1984, 42(1):112–5.
218. Craft I, Gorgy A, Hill J, Menon D, Podsiadly B. Will GnRH antagonists provide new hope for patients considered "difficult responders" to GnRH agonist protocols? Hum Reprod 1999, 14(12):2959–62 (Level III).
219. Al-Inany H, Aboulghar MA, Mansour RT, Serour GI. Optimizing GnRH antagonist administration: meta-analysis of fixed versus flexible protocol. Reprod Biomed Online 2005, 10(5):567–70 (Level III).
220. al-Mizyen E, Sabatini L, Lower AM, Wilson CM, al-Shawaf T, Grudzinskas JG. Does pretreatment with progestogen or oral contraceptive pills in low responders followed by the GnRHa flare protocol improve the outcome of IVF-ET? J Assist Reprod Genet 2000, 17(3):140–6 (Level II-2).
221. Tazegül A, Görkemli H, Ozdemir S, Aktan TM.Comparison of multiple dose GnRH antagonist and minidose long agonist protocols in poor responders undergoing in vitro fertilization: a randomized controlled trial. Arch Gynecol Obstet 2008, 278:467–72 (Level I).
222. Cheung LP, Lam PM, Lok IH, et al. GnRH antagonist versus long GnRH agonist protocol in poor responders undergoing IVF: a randomized controlled trial. Hum Reprod 2005, 20(3):616–21 (Level I).
223. Cédrin-Durnerin I, Bständig B, Parneix I, Bied-Damon V, Avril C, Decanter C, Hugues JN. Effects of oral contraceptive, synthetic progestogen or natural estrogen pre-treatments on the hormonal profile and the antral follicle cohort before GnRH antagonist protocol. Hum Reprod 2007, 22(1):109–16 (Level I).
224. Humaidan P, Bungum L, Bungum M, Hald F, Agerholm I, Blaabjerg J, Yding Andersen C, Lindenberg S. Reproductive outcome using a GnRH antagonist (cetrorelix) for luteolysis and follicular synchronization in poor responder IVF/ICSI patients treated with a flexible GnRH antagonist protocol. Reprod Biomed Online 2005, 11(6):679–84 (Level II-3).
225. Fridén BE, Nilsson L. Gonadotrophin-releasing hormone-antagonist luteolysis during the preceding mid-luteal phase is a feasible protocol in ovarian hyperstimulation before in vitro fertilization. Acta Obstet Gynecol Scand 2005, 84(8):812–6 (Level II-3).
226. Frattarelli JL, Hill MJ, McWilliams GD, Miller KA, Bergh PA, Scott RT Jr. A luteal estradiol protocol for expected poor-responders improves embryo number and quality. Fertil Steril 2007. Accessed at www.fertsteril.org on 15 March 2008 (Level II-3).
227. Hill MJ, McWilliams GD, Miller KA, Scott RT Jr, Frattarelli JL. A luteal estradiol protocol for anticipated poor-responder patients may improve delivery rates. Fertil Steril 2008. Accessed at www.fertsteril.org on 15 March 2008 (Level II-2).
228. Cunha Filho JS, Terres LF, Holanda F, et al. Luteal phase oestradiol administration in ovarian stimulation cycles with GnRH antagonist is comparable to the GnRH agonist (long) protocol. J Assist Reprod Genet 2007, 24(8):326–30 (Level II-2).
229. Check JH, Chase JS. Ovulation induction in hypergonadotropic amenorrhea with estrogen and human menopausal gonadotropin therapy. Fertil Steril 1984, 42(6):919–22 (Level III).
230. Griesinger G, Venetis CA, Marx T, Diedrich K, Tarlatzis BC, Kolibianakis EM. Oral contraceptive pill pretreatment in ovarian stimulation with GnRH antagonists for IVF: a systematic review and meta-analysis. Fertil Steril 2007. Accessed at www.fertsteril.org on 15 March 2008 (Level III).
231. Duvan CI, Berker B, Turhan NO, Satiroglu H. Oral contraceptive pretreatment does not improve outcome in microdose gonadotrophin-releasing hormone agonist protocol among poor responder intracytoplasmic sperm injection patients. J Assist Reprod Genet 2008, 25 (2–3):89–93 (Level II-2).
232. Bendikson K, Milki AA, Speck-Zulak A, Westphal LM. Comparison of GnRH antagonist cycles with and without oral contraceptive pretreatment in potential poor prognosis patients. Clin Exp Obstet Gynecol 2006, 33(3):145–7 (Level II-2).
233. Kovacs P, Barg PE, Witt BR. Hypothalamic-pituitary suppression with oral contraceptive pills does not improve outcome in poor responder patients undergoing in vitro fertilization-embryo transfer cycles. J Assist Reprod Genet 2001, 18(7):391–4 (Level II-2).
234. Arslan M, Bocca S, Mirkin S, Barroso G, Stadtmauer L, Oehninger S. Controlled ovarian hyperstimulation protocols for in vitro fertilization: two decades of experience after the birth of Elizabeth Carr. Fertil Steril 2005,

84(3):555–69; Erratum in: Fertil Steril 2005, 84(5):1557 (Level II-2).
235. Shapiro DB, Mitchell-Leef D, Carter M, Nagy ZP. Ganirelix acetate use in normal- and poor-prognosis patients and the impact of estradiol patterns. Fertil Steril 2005, 83(3):666–70 (Level III).
236. Frattarelli JL, Gerber MD. Basal and cycle androgen levels correlate with in vitro fertilization stimulation parameters but do not predict pregnancy outcome. Fertil Steril 2006, 86(1):51–7 (Level II-3).
237. Barbieri RL, Sluss PM, Powers RD, et al. Association of body mass index, age, and cigarette smoking with serum testosterone levels in cycling women undergoing in vitro fertilization. Fertil Steril 2005, 83(2):302–8 (Level III).
238. Frattarelli JL, Peterson EH. Effect of androgen levels on in vitro fertilization cycles. Fertil Steril 2004, 81(6):1713–4 (Level II-3).
239. Meldrum DR, Scott RT Jr, Levy MJ, Alper MM, Noyes N. Oral contraceptive pretreatment in women undergoing controlled ovarian stimulation in ganirelix acetate cycles may, for a subset of patients, be associated with low serum luteinizing hormone levels, reduced ovarian response to gonadotropins, and early pregnancy loss. Fertil Steril 2008. Accessed at www.fertsteril.org on 15 March 2008 (Level III).
240. Mochtar MH, Van der Veen, Ziech M, van Wely M. Recombinant Luteinizing Hormone (rLH) for controlled ovarian hyperstimulation in assisted reproductive cycles. Cochrane Database Syst Rev 2007, (2):CD005070 (Level III).
241. De Placido G, Alviggi C, Perino A, et al. Italian Collaborative Group on Recombinant Human Luteinizing Hormone. Recombinant human LH supplementation versus recombinant human FSH (rFSH) step-up protocol during controlled ovarian stimulation in normogonadotrophic women with initial inadequate ovarian response to rFSH. A multicentre, prospective, randomized controlled trial. Hum Reprod 2005, 20(2):390–6 (Level I).
242. De Placido G, Mollo A, Alviggi C, et al. Rescue of IVF cycles by HMG in pituitary down-regulated normogonadotrophic young women characterized by a poor initial response to recombinant FSH. Hum Reprod 2001, 16(9): 1875–9 (Level I).
243. Ferraretti AP, Gianaroli L, Magli MC, D'angelo A, Farfalli V, Montanaro N. Exogenous luteinizing hormone in controlled ovarian hyperstimulation for assisted reproduction techniques. Fertil Steril 2004, 82(6):1521–6 (Level I).
244. Barrenetxea G, Agirregoikoa JA, Jiménez MR, de Larruzea AL, Ganzabal T, Carbonero K. Ovarian response and pregnancy outcome in poor-responder women: a randomized controlled trial on the effect of luteinizing hormone supplementation on in vitro fertilization cycles. Fertil Steril 2008, 89(3):546–53 (Level I).
245. Fábregues F, Creus M, Peñarrubia J, Manau D, Vanrell JA, Balasch J. Effects of recombinant human luteinizing hormone supplementation on ovarian stimulation and the implantation rate in down-regulated women of advanced reproductive age. Fertil Steril 2006, 85(4):925–31 (Level I).
246. Van Horne AK, Bates GW Jr, Robinson RD, Arthur NJ, Propst AM. Recombinant follicle-stimulating hormone (rFSH) supplemented with low-dose human chorionic gonadotropin compared with rFSH alone for ovarian stimulation for in vitro fertilization. Fertil Steril 2007, 88(4):1010–3 (Level II-2).
247. Gómez-Palomares JL, Acevedo-Martín B, Andrés L, Ricciarelli E, Hernández ER. LH improves early follicular recruitment in women over 38 years old. Reprod Biomed Online 2005, 11(4):409–14; Erratum in: Reprod Biomed Online 2006, 12(1):132 (Level I).
248. Marrs R, Meldrum D, Muasher S, Schoolcraft W, Werlin L, Kelly E. Randomized trial to compare the effect of recombinant human FSH (follitropin alfa) with or without recombinant human LH in women undergoing assisted reproduction treatment. Reprod Biomed Online 2004, 8(2):175–82 (Level I).
249. Nyboeandersen A, Humaidan P, Fried G, et al. Nordic LH study group. Recombinant LH supplementation to recombinant FSH during the final days of controlled ovarian stimulation for in vitro fertilization. A multicentre, prospective, randomized, controlled trial. Hum Reprod 2008, 23(2):427–34 (Level I).
250. Tavaniotou A, Albano C, Van Steirteghem A, Devroey P. The impact of LH serum concentration on the clinical outcome of IVF cycles in patients receiving two regimens of clomiphene citrate/gonadotrophin/0.25 mg cetrorelix. Reprod Biomed Online 2003, 6(4):421–6 (Level I).
251. Engel JB, Olivennes F, Fanchin R, et al. Single dose application of cetrorelix in combination with clomiphene for friendly IVF: results of a feasibility study. Reprod Biomed Online 2003, 6(4):444–7 (Level I).
252. Weigert M, Krischker U, Pöhl M, Poschalko G, Kindermann C, Feichtinger W. Comparison of stimulation with clomiphene citrate in combination with recombinant follicle-stimulating hormone and recombinant luteinizing hormone to stimulation with a gonadotropin-releasing hormone agonist protocol: a prospective, randomized study. Fertil Steril 2002, 78(1):34–9 (Level I).
253. D'Amato G, Caroppo E, Pasquadibisceglie A, Carone D, Vitti A, Vizziello GM. A novel protocol of ovulation induction with delayed gonadotropin-releasing hormone antagonist administration combined with high-dose recombinant follicle-stimulating hormone and clomiphene citrate for poor responders and women over 35 years. Fertil Steril 2004, 81(6):1572–7 (Level I).
254. Nikolettos N, Al-Hasani S, Felberbaum R, et al. Gonadotropin-releasing hormone antagonist protocol: a novel method of ovarian stimulation in poor responders. Eur J Obstet Gynecol Reprod Biol 2001, 97(2):202–7 (Level II-3).
255. Benadiva CA, Davis O, Kligman I, Liu HC, Rosenwaks Z. Clomiphene citrate and hMG: an alternative stimulation protocol for selected failed in vitro fertilization patients. J Assist Reprod Genet 1995, 12(1):8–12 (Level II-3).
256. Zelinski-Wooten MB, Hess DL, Baughman WL, Molskness TA, Wolf DP, Stouffer RL. Administration of an aromatase inhibitor during the late follicular phase of gonadotropin-treated cycles in rhesus monkeys: effects on follicle development, oocyte maturation, and subsequent luteal function. J Clin Endocrinol Metab 1993, 76(4):988–95.
257. Shetty G, Krishnamurthy H, Krishnamurthy HN, Bhatnagar S, Moudgal RN. Effect of estrogen deprivation on the reproductive physiology of male and female primates. J Steroid Biochem Mol Biol 1997, 61(3–6):157–66.

258. Mitwally MF, Casper RF, Diamond MP. The role of aromatase inhibitors in ameliorating deleterious effects of ovarian stimulation on outcome of infertility treatment. Reprod Biol Endocrinol 2005, 3:54. Acessed at http://www.rbej.com/content/3/1/54 on 3/20/2008 (Level III).
259. Mitwally MF, Casper RF. Aromatase inhibition improves ovarian response to follicle-stimulating hormone in poor responders. Fertil Steril 2002, 77(4):776–80.
260. de Ziegler D, Mattenberger C, Schwarz C, Ibecheole V, Fournet N, Bianchi-Demicheli F. New tools for optimizing endometrial receptivity in controlled ovarian hyperstimulation: aromatase inhibitors and LH/(mini)hCG. Ann N Y Acad Sci 2004, 1034:262–77 (Level III).
261. Lossl K, Andersen AN, Loft A, Freiesleben NL, Bangsbøll S, Andersen CY. Androgen priming using aromatase inhibitor and hCG during early-follicular-phase GnRH antagonist down-regulation in modified antagonist protocols. Hum Reprod 2006, 21(10):2593–600 (Level I).
262. Garcia-Velasco JA, Moreno L, Pacheco A, et al. The aromatase inhibitor letrozole increases the concentration of intraovarian androgens and improves in vitro fertilization outcome in low responder patients: a pilot study. Fertil Steril 2005, 84(1):82–7 (Level I).
263. Verpoest WM, Kolibianakis E, Papanikolaou E, Smitz J, Van Steirteghem A, Devroey P. Aromatase inhibitors in ovarian stimulation for IVF/ICSI: a pilot study. Reprod Biomed Online 2006, 13(2):166–72 (Level I).
264. Lee TH, Lin YH, Seow KM, Hwang JL, Tzeng CR, Yang YS. Effectiveness of cetrorelix for the prevention of premature luteinizing hormone surge during controlled ovarian stimulation using letrozole and gonadotropins: a randomized trial. Fertil Steril 2007. Accessed at www.fertsteril.org on 15 March 2008 (Level I).
265. Schoolcraft WB, Surrey ES, Minjarez DA, Stevens JM, Gardner DK. Management of poor responders: can outcomes be improved with a novel gonadotropin-releasing hormone antagonist/letrozole protocol? Fertil Steril 2008, 89(1):151–6 (Level I).
266. Goswami SK, Das T, Chattopadhyay R, et al. A randomized single-blind controlled trial of letrozole as a low-cost IVF protocol in women with poor ovarian response: a preliminary report. Hum Reprod 2004, 19(9):2031–5 (Level I).
267. Rice S, Ojha K, Whitehead S, Mason H. Stage-specific expression of androgen receptor, follicle-stimulating hormone receptor, and anti-Müllerian hormone type II receptor in single, isolated, human preantral follicles: relevance to polycystic ovaries. J Clin Endocrinol Metab 2007, 92(3):1034–40.
268. Hillier SG, Ross GT. Effects of exogenous testosterone on ovarian weight, follicular morphology and intraovarian progesterone concentration in estrogen-primed hypophysectomized immature female rats. Biol Reprod 1979, 20(2):261–8.
269. Billing H, Furuta I, H sueh AJ. Estrogens inhibit and androgens enhance ovarian granulosa cell apoptosis. Endocrinology 1993, 133(5):2204–12.
270. Hillier SG, Groom GV, Boyns AR, Cameron EH. Development of polycystic ovaries in rats actively immunised against T-3-BSA. Nature 1974, 250(465):433–4.
271. Murray AA, Gosden RG, Allison V, Spears N. Effect of androgens on the development of mouse follicles growing in vitro. J Reprod Fertil 1998, 113(1):27–33.
272. Vendola K, Zhou J, Wang J, Famuyiwa OA, Bievre M, Bondy CA. Androgens promote oocyte insulin-like growth factor I expression and initiation of follicle development in the primate ovary. Biol Reprod 1999 ,61(2):353–7.
273. Zeleznik AJ, Little-Ihrig L, Ramasawamy S. Administration of dihydrotestosterone to rhesus monkeys inhibits gonadotropin-stimulated ovarian steroidogenesis. J Clin Endocrinol Metab 2004, 89(2):860–6.
274. Zeleznik AJ, Little-Ihrig L, Ramasawamy S. Administration of insulin-like growth factor I to rhesus monkeys does not augment gonadotropin-stimulated ovarian steroidogenesis. J Clin Endocrinol Metab 2002, 87(12):5722–9.
275. Wang JG, Lobo RA The complex relationship between hypothalamic amenorrhea and polycystic ovary syndrome. J Clin Endocrinol Metab 2008. Accessed at http://jcem.endojournals.org/cgi/rapidpdf/jc.2007–1716v1 on 3/25/2008 (Level III).
276. Andersen CY, Lossl K. Increased intrafollicular androgen levels affect human granulosa cell secretion of anti-müllerian hormone and inhibin-B. Fertil Steril 2007. Accessed atAccessed at www.fertsteril.org on 25 March 2008 (Level II-2).
277. Balasch J, Fábregues F, Peñarrubia J, et al. Pretreatment with transdermal testosterone may improve ovarian response to gonadotrophins in poor-responder IVF patients with normal basal concentrations of FSH. Hum Reprod 2006, 21(7):1884–93 (Level I).
278. Massin N, Cedrin-Durnerin I, Coussieu C, Galey-Fontaine J, Wolf JP, Hugues JN. Effects of transdermal testosterone application on the ovarian response to FSH in poor responders undergoing assisted reproduction technique – a prospective, randomized, double-blind study. Hum Reprod 2006, 21(5):1204–11 (Level I).
279. Casson PR, Lindsay MS, Pisarska MD, Carson SA, Buster JE. Dehydroepiandrosterone supplementation augments ovarian stimulation in poor responders: a case series. Hum Reprod 2000, 15(10):2129–32 (Level III).
280. Barad D, Brill H, Gleicher N. Update on the use of dehydroepiandrosterone supplementation among women with diminished ovarian function. J Assist Reprod Genet 2007, 24(12):629–34 (Level II-2).
281. Check JH. Mild ovarian stimulation. J Assist Reprod Genet 2007, 24(12):621–7 (Level III).
282. Mendez Lozano DH, Brum Scheffer J, Frydman N, Fay S, Fanchin R, Frydman R. Optimal reproductive competence of oocytes retrieved through follicular flushing in minimal stimulation IVF. Reprod Biomed Online 2008, 16(1): 119–23 (Level II-3).
283. Munne S, Magli C, Adler A, et al. Treatment-related chromosome abnormalities in human embryos. Hum Reprod 1997, 12(4):780–4 (Level II-3).
284. Pelinck MJ, Vogel NE, Arts EG, Simons AH, Heineman MJ, Hoek A. Cumulative pregnancy rates after a maximum of nine cycles of modified natural cycle IVF and analysis of patient drop-out: a cohort study. Hum Reprod 2007, 22(9):2463–70 (Level III).
285. Elizur SE, Aslan D, Shulman A, Weisz B, Bider D, Dor J. Modified natural cycle using GnRH antagonist can be an optional treatment in poor responders undergoing IVF. J Assist Reprod Genet 2005, 22(2):75–9.
286. Feldman B, Seidman DS, Levron J, Bider D, Shulman A, Shine S, Dor J. In vitro fertilization following natural

cycles in poor responders. Gynecol Endocrinol 2001, 15(5):328–34.
287. Bassil S, Godin PA, Donnez J. Outcome of in-vitro fertilization through natural cycles in poor responders. Hum Reprod 1999, 14(5):1262–5 (Level II-3).
288. Lindheim SR, Vidali A, Ditkoff E, Sauer MV, Zinger M. Poor responders to ovarian hyperstimulation may benefit from an attempt at natural-cycle oocyte retrieval. J Assist Reprod Genet 1997, 14(3):174–6 (Level II-3).
289. Check JH, Summers-Chase D, Yuan W, Horwath D, Wilson C. Effect of embryo quality on pregnancy outcome following single embryo transfer in women with a diminished *egg* reserve. Fertil Steril 2007, 87(4):749–56 (Level III).
290. Papaleo E, De Santis L, Fusi F, et al. Natural cycle as first approach in aged patients with elevated follicle-stimulating hormone undergoing intracytoplasmic sperm injection: a pilot study. Gynecol Endocrinol 2006, 22(7):351–4 (Level III).
291. Castelo Branco A, Achour-Frydman N, Kadoch J, Fanchin R, Tachdjian G, Frydman R. In vitro fertilization and embryo transfer in seminatural cycles for patients with ovarian aging. Fertil Steril 2005, 84(4):875–80 (Level III).
292. Kolibianakis E, Zikopoulos K, Camus M, Tournaye H, Van Steirteghem A, Devroey P. Modified natural cycle for IVF does not offer a realistic chance of parenthood in poor responders with high day 3 FSH levels, as a last resort prior to oocyte donation. Hum Reprod 2004, 19(11):2545–9 (Level III).
293. Ubaldi F, Rienzi L, Ferrero S, et al. Natural in vitro fertilization cycles. Ann N Y Acad Sci 2004, 1034:245–51 (Level III).
294. Kalu E, Thum MY, Abdalla H. Intrauterine insemination in natural cycle may give better results in older women. J Assist Reprod Genet 2007, 24(2–3):83–6 (Level II-2).
295. Greenblatt RB, Barfield WE, Lampros CP. Cortisone in the treatment of infertility. Fertil Steril 1956, 7(3):203–12 (Level III).
296. Andersen CY, Hornnes P. Intrafollicular concentrations of free cortisol close to follicular rupture. Hum Reprod 1994, 9(10):1944–9.
297. Harlow CR, Jenkins JM, Winston RM. Increased follicular fluid total and free cortisol levels during the luteinizing hormone surge. Fertil Steril 1997, 68(1):48–53.
298. Sasson R, Shinder V, Dantes A, Land A, Amsterdam A. Activation of multiple signal transduction pathways by glucocorticoids: protection of ovarian follicular cells against apoptosis. Biochem Biophys Res Commun 2003, 311(4):1047–56.
299. Sasson R, Amsterdam A. Stimulation of apoptosis in human granulosa cells from in vitro fertilization patients and its prevention by dexamethasone: involvement of cell contact and bcl-2 expression. J Clin Endocrinol Metab 2002, 87(7):3441–51.
300. Miell JP, Taylor AM, Jones J, et al. The effects of dexamethasone treatment on immunoreactive and bioactive insulin-like growth factors (IGFs) and IGF-binding proteins in normal male volunteers. J Endocrinol 1993, 136(3):525–33.
301. Keay SD, Harlow CR, Wood PJ, Jenkins JM, Cahill DJ. Higher cortisol:cortisone ratios in the preovulatory follicle of completely unstimulated IVF cycles indicate oocytes with increased pregnancy potential. Hum Reprod 2002, 17(9):2410–4.
302. Ubaldi F, Rienzi L, Ferrero S, Anniballo R, Iacobelli M, Cobellis L, Greco E. Low dose prednisolone administration in routine ICSI patients does not improve pregnancy and implantation rates. Hum Reprod 2002, 17(6):1544–7 (Level I).
303. Keay SD, Lenton EA, Cooke ID, Hull MG, Jenkins JM. Low-dose dexamethasone augments the ovarian response to exogenous gonadotrophins leading to a reduction in cycle cancellation rate in a standard IVF programme. Hum Reprod 2001, 16(9):1861–5 (Level I).
304. Kemeter P, Feichtinger W. Prednisolone supplementation to Clomid and/or gonadotrophin stimulation for in-vitro fertilization – a prospective randomized trial. Hum Reprod 1986, 1(7):441–4 (Level I).
305. Abir R, Garor R, Felz C, Nitke S, Krissi H, Fisch B. Growth hormone and its receptor in human ovaries from fetuses and adults. Fertil Steril 2007. Accessed at www.fertsteril.org on 25 March 2008.
306. Slot KA, Kastelijn J, Bachelot A, Kelly PA, Binart N, Teerds KJ. Reduced recruitment and survival of primordial and growing follicles in GH receptor-deficient mice. Reproduction 2006, 131(3):525–32.
307. Poretsky L, Cataldo NA, Rosenwaks Z, Giudice LC. The insulin-related ovarian regulatory system in health and disease. Endoc Rev1999, 20:535–582 (Level III).
308. Hull KL, Harvey S. Growth hormone: roles in female reproduction. J Endocrinol 2001, 168(1):1–23 (Level III).
309. Blumenfeld Z, Amit T, Barkey RJ, Lunenfeld B, Brandes JM. Synergistic effect of growth hormone and gonadotropins in achieving conception in "clonidine-negative" patients with unexplained infertility. Ann N Y Acad Sci 1991, 626:250–65 (Level I).
310. Younis JS, Simon A, Koren R, Dorembus D, Schenker JG, Laufer N. The effect of growth hormone supplementation on in vitro fertilization outcome: a prospective randomized placebo-controlled double-blind study. Fertil Steril 1992, 58(3):575–80 (Level I).
311. Tesarik J, Hazout A, Mendoza C. Improvement of delivery and live birth rates after ICSI in women aged >40 years by ovarian co-stimulation with growth hormone. Hum Reprod 2005, 20(9):2536–41.
312. Homburg R, Farhi J. Growth hormone and reproduction. Curr Opin Obstet Gynecol 1995, 7(3):220–3 (Level III).
313. Harper K, Proctor M, Hughes E. Growth hormone for in vitro fertilization. Cochrane Database Syst Rev 2003, (3):CD000099. Accessed at http://www.mrw.interscience.wiley.com/cochrane/clsysrev/articles/CD000099/frame.html on 4/10/2008 (Level III).
314. Kucuk T, Kozinoglu H, Kaba A. Growth hormone co-treatment within a GnRH agonist long protocol in patients with poor ovarian response: a prospective, randomized, clinical trial. J Assist Reprod Genet 2008. Assessed at http://www.springerlink.com/content/3j2665q7j37j2102/fulltext.pdf on 4/10/2008 (Level I).
315. Howles CM, Loumaye E, Germond M, et al. Does growth hormone-releasing factor assist follicular development in poor responder patients undergoing ovarian stimulation for in-vitro fertilization? Hum Reprod 1999, 14(8):1939–43 (Level I).
316. Suikkari A, MacLachlan V, Koistinen R, Seppälä M, Healy D. Double-blind placebo controlled study: human biosynthetic

growth hormone for assisted reproductive technology. Fertil Steril 1996, 65(4):800–5 (Level I).
317. Dor J, Seidman DS, Amudai E, Bider D, Levran D, Mashiach S. Adjuvant growth hormone therapy in poor responders to in-vitro fertilization: a prospective randomized placebo-controlled double-blind study. Hum Reprod 1995, 10(1):40–3 (Level I).
318. Bergh C, Hillensjö T, Wikland M, Nilsson L, Borg G, Hamberger L. Adjuvant growth hormone treatment during in vitro fertilization: a randomized, placebo-controlled study. Fertil Steril 1994, 62(1):113–20 (Level I).
319. Zhuang GL, Wong SX, Zhou CQ. The effect of co-administration of low dosage growth hormone and gonadotropin for ovarian hyperstimulation in vitro fertilization and embryo transfer. Chung-Hua Fu Chan Ko Tsa Chih (Chinese J Obstet Gynaecol) 1994, 29(8): 471–4.
320. Hughes SM, Huang ZH, Morris ID, Matson PL, Buck P, Lieberman BA. A double-blind cross-over controlled study to evaluate the effect of human biosynthetic growth hormone on ovarian stimulation in previous poor responders to in-vitro fertilization. Hum Reprod 1994, 9(1):13–8 (Level I).
321. Owen EJ, Shoham Z, Mason BA, Ostergaard H, Jacobs HS. Cotreatment with growth hormone, after pituitary suppression, for ovarian stimulation in in vitro fertilization: a randomized, double-blind, placebo-control trial. Fertil Steril 1991, 56(6):1104–10 (Level I).

Note: Evidence was stratified using the system developed by the U.S. Preventive Services Task Force for ranking evidence about the effectiveness of treatments or screening:

- Level I: Evidence obtained from at least one properly designed randomized controlled trial.
- Level II-1: Evidence obtained from well-designed controlled trials without randomization.
- Level II-2: Evidence obtained from well-designed cohort or case-control analytic studies, preferably from more than one center or research group.
- Level II-3: Evidence obtained from multiple time series with or without the intervention. Dramatic results in uncontrolled trials might also be regarded as this type of evidence.
- Level III: Opinions of respected authorities, based on clinical experience, descriptive studies, or reports of expert committees.

# Ectopic Pregnancy

Stephan Krotz and Sandra Carson

**Abstract** The incidence of ectopic pregnancies has risen significantly to 2% of all pregnancies. A thorough clinical evaluation for surgical and gynecologic history and social risk factors can alert the clinician to patients at risk. Patients at risk or high suspicion should be followed closely until their β-hCG exceeds the discriminatory zone at which time ultrasound and dilation and curettage can be used to diagnose the presence of an intrauterine pregnancy. Methotrexate is now the standard for the medical treatment of ectopic pregnancy. Multi-dose methotrexate is 4–5 times less likely to fail than the single-dose regimen, which is more patient-convenient. Attempts to "split the difference" have resulted in the design of hybrid protocols to allow initial treatment to begin with fewer doses and abbreviated follow-up compared to the multidose regimen. Ectopic pregnancy in sites other than the fallopian tube are becoming more frequent and can be associated with the higher incidence of traditional risk factors, greater use of in vitro fertilization and cesarean delivery. Although treatment algorithms have not yet been codified for nontubal ectopic pregnancies, systemic methotrexate, local injection or laparoscopy remain the main options and the patient's safety remains the primary consideration in choosing an option. Accepted treatment modalities, methotrexate or surgery, have comparable outcomes with regard to future fertility for women at the reproductive age.

**Keywords** Ectopic pregnancy • Tubal pregnancy • Methotrexate • Human chorionic gonadotropin

S. Krotz(✉) and S. Carson
Reproductive Endocrinology and Infertility, Women and Infants Hospital, Rhode Island, Warren Alpert Medical School of Brown University, 385 Westminster Street #3A, Providence, RI 02903, USA
e-mail: skrotz@wihri.org

## 1 Introduction

Ectopic pregnancy is the leading cause of maternal death in the first trimester (1) and contributes to 9% of all pregnancy- related deaths. The incidence of ectopic pregnancy has increased fivefold since the early 1970s and now accounts for 2% of all pregnancies (2). While increased diagnostic sensitivity may play a role, the increased incidence is generally attributed to the increase in three main factors: sexually transmitted infections (3), tubal sterilization (4) and the use of fertility drugs. While the mortality rate has decreased tenfold over this same period (1) due to earlier diagnosis (5, 6) and outpatient management with methotrexate (7), mortality still remains sixfold higher than miscarriages, live births and elective terminations (8).

## 2 Risk Factors

In the emergency room setting, up to 45% of women with an ectopic pregnancy may be sent home with an incorrect diagnosis (9) as the triad of amenorrhea followed by abdominal pain and irregular vaginal bleeding traditionally associated with ectopic pregnancy occurs in less than half of the patients affected. Identification of risk factors related to ectopic pregnancy, which occur in 55% of affected patients, will allow earlier diagnosis and reduce related morbidities. Generally, risk factors can be stratified into three categories, which include tubal and uterine factors behavioral and clinical factors that correlate well with the relative risk for an ectopic pregnancy (Table 1).

Tubal factors include all causes of tubal trauma such as previous tubal surgeries, prior ectopic pregnancies and pelvic pathology (10–12) and increase the

D.T. Carrell et al. (eds.), *Biennial Review of Infertility*, DOI: 10.1007/978-1-60327-392-3_5

**Table 1** Ectopic pregnancy risk factors relative to all pregnant patients

| | Odds ratio |
|---|---|
| **Tubal and uterine factors** | |
| Tubal pathology (45) | 3.5–25 |
| Infertility (45) | 2.5–21 |
| Previous tubal surgery (45) | 21 |
| Two prior ectopics (12) | 16 |
| Tubal sterilization (10) | 9.3 |
| Previous surgery for ectopic (45) | 8.3 |
| Intrauterine DES exposure(10) | 5.6 |
| Prior ectopic pregnancy (12) | 3.0 |
| **Behavioral fctors** | |
| Smoking ≥1 pack per day (15) | 3.9 |
| Smoking ≥½ pack per day (15) | 3.7 |
| Chlamydia (45) | 2.8–3.7 |
| Gonorrhea (45) | 2.9 |
| Ever smoking (10, 15) | 1.5–2.5 |
| Pelvic inflammatory disease (45, 10) | 1.5–2.5 |
| >1 Lifetime sexual partners (45) | 2.1 |
| Age at first intercourse <18 (45) | 1.6 |
| **Clinical factors** | |
| Age ≥40 (15) | 2.9 |
| Infertility (45) | 2.0–2.5 |
| Parity ≥4 (12) | 1.8 |
| Oral contraceptives (10) | 1.8 |
| Beta hCG 501-2000 (12) | 1.7 |
| IUD in place (10) | 1.6 |
| Primigravida (12) | 1.6 |
| Prior live births (12) | 1.4 |
| Pain at presentation (12) | 1.4 |
| Moderate to severe vaginal bleeding (12) | 1.4 |
| Age 30–39 (15) | 1.3–1.4 |

risk for ectopic pregnancy significantly. While the risk of one previous tubal pregnancy increases the risk for a future ectopic pregnancy threefold, a history of two ectopic pregnancies (Table 1) or prior tubal surgery increases the risk 8–25-fold. Additionally, uterine factors such as a previous history of intrauterine diethylstilbestrol exposure can significantly increase a patient's risk for ectopic pregnancy, presumably by interfering with the embryo's passage into the uterine cavity (10, 12). Screening all pregnant patients with risk factors for ectopic pregnancies may seem justifiable, especially when there is a 10–27% rate of recurrence (13), but is not warranted as the high false positive rates lead to unnecessary medical intervention (14).

Behavioral Risk Factors moderately increase a patient's risk for ectopic pregnancy and are predominantly related to smoking and sexually transmitted infections. The relation between smoking and ectopic pregnancy is dose-related and tobacco is thought to have a negative impact on ovulation, fertilization, embryo transport and implantation (15). For patients who smoke a half or full pack of cigarettes daily, the odds of having an ectopic pregnancy can increase 3.7–3.9-fold. A history of gonorrhea, chlamydia or pelvic inflammatory disease, all increase the risk through resulting intraluminal adhesions which interfere with embryonic transport to the uterus(10, 11). The number of lifetime sexual partners, pelvic inflammatory disease and the risk of ectopic pregnancy also positively correlate (11, 16). Patients with more than five lifetime partners have 2.8 times the risk of pelvic inflammatory disease and ten times the risk of sexually transmitted bacterial infections compared to their counterparts with a single partner (16). Patients less than 21 years of age were 5.5 times as likely to have a concurrent gonorrhea or Chlamydia infection as compared to older women when diagnosed with an ectopic pregnancy (17).

Clinical factors related to the patient's obstetrical and gynecologic history and clinical presentation increase the risk for ectopic pregnancy minimally. More recently, age has been reexamined as an independent risk factor for ectopic pregnancy. Patients who are less than 21-years old presenting to the emergency room with classic symptoms are half as likely as older patients to have an ectopic pregnancy (17), presumably from lower exposure to tubal surgery and a lower incidence in tubal damage secondary to infectious processes. In contrast, patients older than 30 have a significantly increased risk for ectopic pregnancy (15) as expected from the aforementioned exposures (12). Interestingly, advanced maternal age has also been found to be independently linked to ectopic risk although the cause is still unclear (15). Birth control pills and intrauterine devices lower the overall risk of pregnancy but, when contraception fails, both increase the risk of ectopic pregnancy (10). Presenting symptoms and signs such as abdominal or pelvic pain, moderate to severe bleeding, and beta human chorionic gonadotropin concentrations below 2,000 mIU/mL (12) increase the risk of ectopic pregnancy only minimally.

Infertility has also been shown to increase the relative risk of ectopic pregnancy at least twofold, which is most likely related to the association of pelvic infection and tubal pathology. A recent study found the risk of ectopic pregnancy in all patients undergoing ART to be 2.1% (18), which is the same as in the general population. Zygote intrafallopian transfer (ZIFT) was the only ART procedure that has definitively been shown to increase the risk of ectopic pregnancy to 3.6%. Use of donor oocytes or a surrogate gestational carrier lowers the risk to 1.4% and 0.9% respectively (18). Additionally, transfer of two or less high quality embryos during in vitro fertilization (IVF) lowers the risk of ectopic pregnancy by 30%. Therefore, the risks associated with infertility treatment most likely stem from the cause of infertility as opposed to the treatment.

Nontubal pelvic surgery and cesarean sections have all been implied but never clearly associated with ectopic pregnancies. Past IUD use and previous medical abortion or miscarriage are still disputed as risk factors (11, 12).

# 3 Diagnosis

## *3.1 Presentation*

All patients at the reproductive age who present with vaginal bleeding or abdominal pain should have the urine or serum pregnancy test performed on initial evaluation. On confirmation of pregnancy, all patients without a confirmed intrauterine pregnancy are to be evaluated for an ectopic pregnancy. The diagnosis of ectopic pregnancy is made with the combination of serum beta human chorionic gonadotropin (β-hCG) concentrations and radiologic imaging, or by surgical means when necessary. Heterotopic pregnancy is the only exception to this rule as confirmation of an intrauterine pregnancy does not rule out an ectopic pregnancy. As the risk for heterotopic pregnancies is 24 times higher when pregnancy has been achieved through ART compared to spontaneous conception, a higher index of suspicion is warranted (18, 19). The risk of heterotopic pregnancies in ART cycles, however, still remains low at 0.15%.

## *3.2 Radiologic Imaging*

Determining which management option to employ in the treatment of an ectopic pregnancy is influenced by the location. More than 95% of ectopic pregnancies are tubal, and of those 70% are ampullary. The remainder are interstitial or cornual (2%), abdominal (1.4%), ovarian (0.2–3.2%) or cervical (0.2%) (20, 21). More recently described, rare implantation sites include the abdomen and previous cesarean scars.

### 3.2.1 Pelvic Ultrasound

Ectopic pregnancy can be definitively diagnosed by an ultrasound examination only by the visualization of fetal cardiac activity in the adnexa. However, there are other findings strongly suggestive of the presence of an ectopic pregnancy. After clinical evaluation, a diagnostic sequence of the pelvic ultrasound followed by β-hCG (Fig. 1) minimizes the risk of missing ectopic and interrupting intrauterine pregnancies (22). While an intrauterine pregnancy can be identified as early as 4.5 weeks by the decidual reaction (echogenic rim in the endometrial cavity surrounding a fluid collection) (23), the most reliable and safest sign to use is the double decidual sac sign ("double ring sign") or yolk sac nearer to 5 weeks of pregnancy (24). The presence of a fetal heartbeat or pole in the uterus unquestionably confirms an intrauterine pregnancy. The most useful radiologic sign in the diagnosis of an ectopic pregnancy when no intrauterine pregnancy or extrauterine pregnancy with fetal heart tones is seen, is echogenic fluid in the pelvis, which has a 90% positive predictive value (25). The "ring of fire" sign, thought to represent blood flow around the ectopic pregnancy, should be interpreted with caution as it may represent luteal blood flow (26) in a normal pregnancy. Endometrial stripe thickness has no utility in differentiating ectopic pregnancies from symptomatic intrauterine pregnancies or spontaneous abortions (27).

A pelvic ultrasound is less useful when the serum β-hCG concentration is below the discriminatory zone. The discriminatory zone is the threshold of β-hCG values above which a normal intrauterine pregnancy is usually seen, and ranges from 1,500 to 2,000 mIU/mL, but will vary between institutions. The sensitivity of ultrasound in detecting ectopic pregnancies below 1,500 mIU/mL, between 1,500 and 2,000 mIU/mL and greater than 2,000 mIU/mL is 29, 92 and 100% respectively (28–30). Absence of an intrauterine pregnancy on ultrasound above a β-hCG level of 2,000 mIU/mL is suggestive of an abnormal or ectopic pregnancy, and dilation and curettage or manual vacuum aspiration can be performed to differentiate between the two possibilities. In patients with β-hCG values below 1,500 mIU/mL, serial β-hCG are to be drawn until the

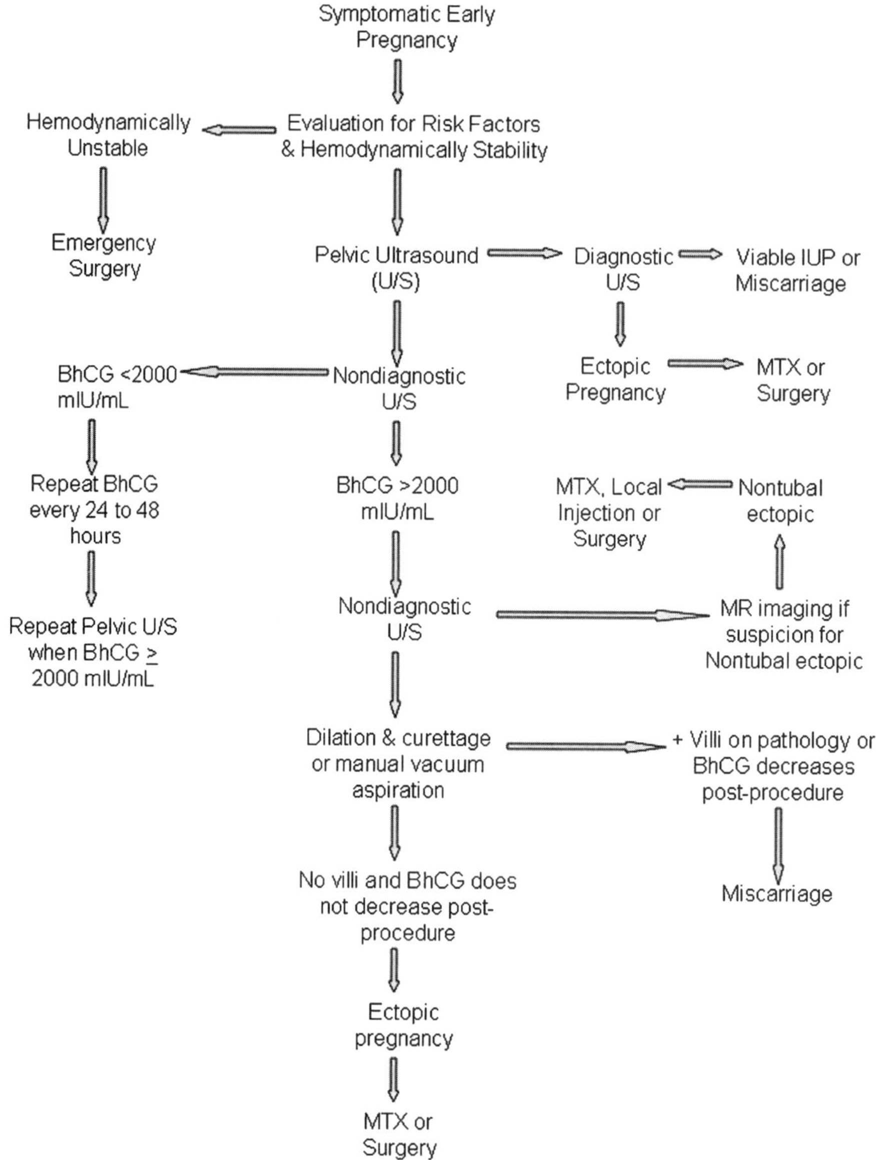


**Fig. 1** Ectopic pregnancy management algorithm

values rise above the discriminatory zone and an intrauterine pregnancy can be ruled out by ultrasound.

### 3.2.2 Magnetic Resonance Imaging

In cases in which a pelvic ultrasound does not clearly localize a pregnancy and in which a nontubal ectopic pregnancy is suspected, magnetic resonance imaging (MRI) can be very useful (31–33). Early use of MRI to differentiate cornual from tubal ectopic pregnancies may prevent catastrophic uterine rupture and hemorrhage (34).

## 3.3 Serum Tests

### 3.3.1 Beta Human Chorionic Gonadotropin

Currently, serial serum β-hCG values are the only clinically useful laboratory tests in differentiating between a normal and abnormal pregnancy. About 75–80% of patients with vaginal bleeding or abdominal pain presenting for an evaluation for ectopic pregnancy have β-hCG values below 1,500 mIU/mL. Defining the minimum expected rise and fall in serum β-hCG concentrations in patients with normal pregnancies or miscarriages can therefore alert clinicians to patients who may have an ectopic pregnancy. The minimum rise in serum β-hCG for a normal pregnancy was first described in 1981 (35) as 66% over 48 h. By 2006, this minimum rise was redefined to 35% over 48 h based on the management of more than 1,000 patients (36). Serum β-hCG concentrations decline in spontaneous abortions at a minimum of 21% in 2 days and 60% in 7 days for patients with an initial β-hCG less than 10,000 mIU/mL, and more rapidly with β-hCG concentrations higher than 10,000 mIU/mL. Any rise or decline slower than the stated thresholds suggests that an ectopic pregnancy or retained trophoblasts from a spontaneous abortion exist (37), and require dilation and curettage or manual vacuum aspiration to differentiate between the two possibilities. Up to 21% of ectopic pregnancies can "mimic" the rise and fall in serial serum β-hCG concentrations of viable intrauterine pregnancies or spontaneous abortions (36).

### 3.3.2 Progesterone

Progesterone concentrations, while traditionally used in diagnostic algorithms, only provide clinically useful values at the extremes and in certain circumstances may prove detrimental in identifying patients with ectopic pregnancies (22). A progesterone concentration less than 5 ng/mL suggests an abnormal pregnancy in 99.8% (38) of patients and no normal pregnancies have ever been documented with a value below 2.5 ng/mL. The risk of an ectopic pregnancy occurring above 25 ng/mL is only 3% but does not definitively rule one out (22).

### 3.3.3 Other Serum Markers

Many markers including glycoledin, pregnancy specific B1-glycoledin, leukemia inhibiting factor, human placental lactogen, and pregnancy-associated plasma protein A (PAPP-A) and VEGF have been evaluated in the diagnosis of ectopic pregnancy and are not clinically useful at this time (39, 40).

## *3.4 Diagnosis by Curettage*

The diagnosis of ectopic pregnancy by curettage is made by the plateau or rise of β-hCG concentrations after uterine curettage or manual vacuum aspiration. The procedure may be performed in the office and in patients in whom β-hCG values are above the discriminatory zone but have no identifiable fetal heart rate in the adnexa on imaging. Up to 38% of patients without an identifiable intrauterine pregnancy on imaging with β-hCG values above 2,000 mIU/mL may be experiencing a spontaneous abortion (41), so treating these patients empirically with methotrexate will unnecessarily subject them to the potential side-effects and risks of the medication. Curettage is considered the definitive diagnostic and treatment modality for patients in this circumstance except for those with a heterotopic pregnancy. Endometrial biopsy is an unreliable substitute for dilation and curettage or manual vacuum aspiration due to its low diagnostic sensitivity (42, 43). β-hCG concentrations are to be drawn 12–24 h after the procedure as chorionic villi cannot be identified in up to 20% of spontaneous abortion pathology specimens (44). Failure of β-hCG concentrations to decrease at the expected rate for a spontaneous abortion and lack of chorionic villi in the retrieved operative specimens is diagnostic for an ectopic pregnancy. There is no need to await histologic examination of the uterine currettings for the presence or absence of villi. Villi should be examined by a pathologist to confirm the diagnosis.

# 4 Expectant Management

Success rates reported in the literature have ranged between 48 and 100% (45), with an average reported success rate of 68% (45). At this moment, there are no standard criteria to determine who will be a candidate. According to four studies, the average range of β-hCG values for patients successfully managed, ranged between 246 and 583 mIU/mL (46). The average range of values for patients who failed expectant management fell between 470 and 2,000 mIU/mL. Currently, expectant management cannot be recommended as the standard of care.

# 5 Medical Treatment

## *5.1 Methotrexate: Who is a Candidate?*

Methotrexate, a chemotherapeutic agent (47) originally used for choriocarcinoma (48), was first used to treat an ectopic pregnancy in 1982 (49). Methotrexate targets rapidly divide cells by inhibiting dihydrofolate reductase (DHFR), which reduces folate to tetrahydrofolate, a cofactor required for DNA and RNA synthesis (50). Head-to-head comparison with laparoscopic salpingostomy has proved methotrexate equally efficacious (51). Currently methotrexate is the standard of care for patients who are hemodynamically stable, willing to comply with the treatment regimen and possess no contraindications to treatment (Table 2) (45). Prior to methotrexate administration, it is important to screen for relative and absolute contraindications by history and examination. Additionally, patients benefit by screening for any underlying medical problem with the serum tests including complete blood count, liver function tests, electrolytes and their blood type with Rh factor. A chest x-ray prior to methotrexate administration (52) is recommended in patients with a history of lung disease due to the risk of interstitial pneumonitis.

Determining which of the patients have a reasonable chance for successful outpatient management with methotrexate is as important as determining their medical eligibility. Patients with relative contraindications can still be treated with methotrexate but they possess a higher risk of rupture. Traditionally hemoperitoneum, a gestational sac size greater than 4 cm, and embryonic cardiac activity were all considered relative contraindications to methotrexate (45). However, hemoperitoneum and gestational sac size have been shown not to correlate with methotrexate success rates (53).

**Table 2** Contraindications to MTX therapy

| |
|---|
| **Absolute contraindications** |
| Intrauterine pregnancy |
| Evidence of immunodeficiency |
| Moderate to severe anemia, leukopenia or thrombocytopenia |
| Sensitivity to MTX |
| Active pulmonary disease |
| Active peptic ulcer disease |
| Clinically important hepatic dysfunction |
| Clinically important renal dysfunction |
| Breastfeeding |
| **Relative contraindications** |
| Embryonic cardiac activity detected by transvaginal ultrasonography |
| High initial hCG concentration (>5,000 mIU/mL) |
| Ectopic pregnancy greater than 4 cm on transvaginal ultrasonography |
| Refusal to accept blood transfusion |
| Inability to participate in follow-up |

Permission granted by Elsevier publishing (45)

According to one study (53), the percentage of ectopic pregnancies demonstrating embryonic cardiac activity for β-hCG values below 5,000 mIU/mL, from 5,000 to 9,999 mIU/mL, and from 10,000 to 14,999 mIU/mL was 5, 27 and 41% respectively. In general, the percentage of ectopic pregnancies with cardiac activity correlates with the serum β-hCG concentration on a continuum. Unlike serum β-hCG concentrations, however, cardiac activity cannot be measured on a continuum. Therefore, an initial β-hCG concentration is the best indicator for the success of the treatment with "single-dose" methotrexate and the chance of success correlates inversely with the β-hCG concentration (53). A recent review of patients treated with the single-dose protocol demonstrated a clinically significant decrease in success rates for patients with an initial β-hCG concentration above 5,000 mIU/mL, supporting the idea of a β-hCG threshold as a relative contraindication (54). Success rates for patients below this threshold ranged from 94–99% but in patients above 5,000 mIU/mL threshold, success rates decreased to 81–85%, and decreased even further for patients with β-hCG concentrations above 15,000 mIU/mL (53). Success for multiple dose methotrexate is not completely dependent on β-hCG concentrations and therefore it may be used at higher β-hCG concentrations.

Additional prognostic factors may be considered when deciding whether methotrexate is clinically appropriate. Clinical signs and symptoms including pelvic pain, vaginal bleeding and rate of rise in β-hCG concentrations may correspond with a higher risk of methotrexate failure (55). A rapid rise in β-hCG values of 66% over 48 h prior to methotrexate administration may place patients with a tubal pregnancy at a ninefold increased risk of rupture (56).

## 5.2 Methotrexate Dosing

The first protocols using methotrexate for ectopic pregnancy were multidose, based on the treatment for gestational trophoblastic disease and confirmed to be effective by several case series (57, 58). Starting on day 1, methotrexate (1 mg/kg intramuscularly) is given every other day alternating with days on which leucovorin rescue is given (Table 3). Leucovorin (folinic acid) is a methotrexate antagonist given to reduce the side-effects from methotrexate that may otherwise be prohibitive

**Table 3** Comparison of single-dose, multidose and two-dose methotrexate regimens

| | Single-dose (45) | Multidose (45) | Two-dose (62) |
|---|---|---|---|
| Day 0 | | | MTX 50 mg/m$^2$ IM<br>BhCG<br>CBC w/ platelets<br>Liver function tests<br>Creatinine |
| Day 1 | MTX 50 mg/m$^2$ IM<br>BhCG<br>CBC w/ platelets<br>Liver function tests<br>Creatinine | MTX 1 mg/kg IM<br>BhCG<br>CBC w/ platelets<br>Liver function tests<br>Creatinine | |
| Day 2 | | Leucovorin 0.1 mg/kg IM<br>BhCG | |
| Day 3 | | MTX 1 mg/kg IM | |
| Day 4 | BhCG | Leucovorin 0.1 mg/kg IM<br>BhCG | MTX 50 mg/m$^2$ IM<br>BhCG |
| Day 5 | | MTX 1 mg/kg IM | |
| Day 6 | | Leucovorin 0.1 mg/kg IM<br>BhCG | |
| Day 7 | BhCG<br>Evaluate for tx success<br>MTX 50 mg/m$^2$ IM[a] | MTX 1 mg/kg IM | BhCG<br>Evaluate for tx success<br>MTX 50 mg/m$^2$ IM |
| Day 8 | | Leucovorin 0.1 mg/kg IM<br>BhCG | |
| Day 11 | | | BhCG<br>MTX 50 mg/m$^2$ IM[a] |
| Day 14 | | | BhCG[b]<br>CBC w/ platelets<br>Liver function tests<br>Creatinine |
| Weekly | BhCG until negative if treatment a success | BhCG until negative if treatment a success | BhCG until negative if treatment a success |

[a]Give suggested dose of methotrexate if BhCG rises or decreases <15% compared to Day 4 concentrations
[b]Compare BhCG concentration to Day 11, if BhCG rises or decreases <15% then treatment is considered a failure

(47, 48). During the course of treatment, serum β-hCG concentrations are drawn on days 1, 3, 5, and 7 coinciding with the methotrexate dose. When the serum β-hCG concentrations decrease at least 15% over 48 h the treatment is considered successful and no further doses must be given (7). Serum β-hCG values are drawn weekly until they appear negative.

The desire to minimize the side-effects of the multidose protocol, and increase patient compliance, led to the development of the single-dose protocol (7). On day 1 of treatment, methotrexate (50 mg/m$^2$ intramuscularly) is given (Table 3) and a β-hCG concentration is drawn. A β-hCG concentration is drawn again on days 4 and 7 of the treatment cycle. If β-hCG values have not decreased 15% from day 4 to day 7, another dose of methotrexate is given on day 7. If β-hCG values have fallen more than 15% on day 7, then treatment is considered successful (45, 59) and a β-hCG concentration is drawn weekly until it reaches zero. If the β-hCG concentration plateaus or rises after day 7, an additional dose can be given at that time.

Determining which methotrexate protocol to use is a highly debated subject since the development of the single-dose protocol. A recent meta-analysis showed the success rate for the multidose protocol to be 92.7% and 88.1% for the single-dose (60). The odds ratio for failure with the single-dose, when β-hCG concentrations and cardiac activity were controlled for, was 4.74 compared to the multidose. Additionally, the multidose protocol is equally efficacious compared to laparoscopic salpingostomy but the single-dose is not (RR 0.83) (61).

The "single-dose" regimen is largely a misnomer and is not considerably more convenient than the multidose protocol. Since up to 40% of patients using the single-dose protocol require a second dose and almost 50% of patients using the multidose protocol get 4 doses, the optimum number of doses may fall between 1 and 4(60). Recently a hybrid 2-dose protocol has been proposed (62) to provide the convenience of the single-dose protocol and efficacy of the multidose protocol (Table 3). With this new protocol, the overall success rate was 87.1% and the satisfaction rate was 90.6%. A total of 53% of patients reported side-effects of which 64% were mild and 17.6% were moderate. Severe pain was experienced by 8.2% and there appeared to be no correlation between the side-effects and the number of doses.

### 5.3 Methotrexate: Clinical Course and Side Effects

Up to 60% of patients may experience increasing abdominal pain after methotrexate (59), the majority of whom can be successfully treated with NSAIDS (63). Only 13% may require hospitalization for pain. The pain is thought to be secondary to tubal abortion or hematoma formation (59). As 50% of patients successfully treated with methotrexate will show an increase in tubal diameter (64) and 30–100% will experience hemoperitoneum regardless of the success of the treatment (53, 63), serial ultrasound monitoring to detect rupture is not recommended. After methotrexate administration, β-hCG concentrations are expected to become undetectable after 20–35 days (59, 65–67) but it can take up to 109 days (65). Rupture occurs on an average of 14 days after treatment but may take up to 32 days (65). If β-hCG concentrations plateau or rise after two to three doses during the single-dose protocol, or after four doses during the multidose protocol, or if the patient becomes hemodynamically unstable, then operative management is warranted.

## 6 Surgical Management

Traditionally, exploratory laparotomy was the standard of care, and still is for patients who are hemodynamically unstable. More recently, an emphasis on minimizing costs and hospital stays, and advances in surgical technology have made laparoscopic salpingostomy (Fig. 2) the surgical treatment of choice (61). During initial comparisons, patients undergoing laparoscopic salpingostomy performed clinically as well as patients undergoing laparotomy (68–70), and demonstrated less blood loss during surgery, shorter hospital stays, faster recovery times and less postoperative adhesions (71). More recently laparoscopy was demonstrated to have a 3.6 times higher rate of persistent trophoblast activity postoperatively, and tubal rupture requiring further surgery (61). The presence of the persistent trophoblastic tissue is suggested by weekly post-operative β-hCG concentrations that do not fall and can be reduced with a single postoperative dose of methotrexate (1 mg/kg intramuscularly) (22, 72) with minimal side-effects (5.5%).

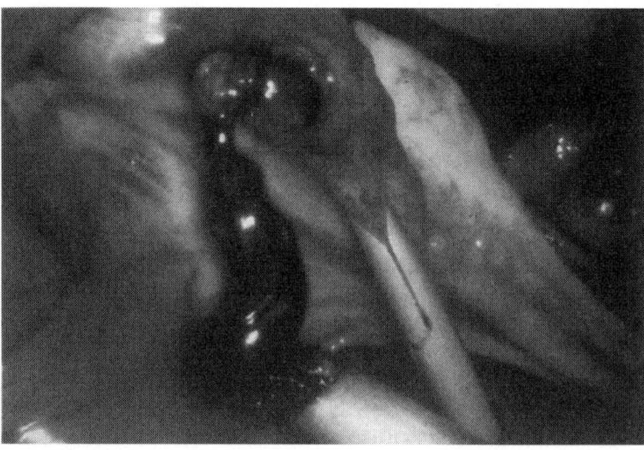

**Fig. 2** Laparoscopic salpingostomy on a tubal ectopic pregnancy. Courtesy of G. Frishman, M.D. and Shayne Plosker, M.D. Women and Infants Hospital of Rhode Island and Warren Alpert School of Medicine of Brown University

If laparoscopy is required to make the diagnosis, then surgical management is preferable at the time of surgical diagnosis. The decision to perform salpingostomy or salpingectomy depends on the patient's future reproductive desires and the extent of damage to the affected tube. Patients who undergo salpingostomy, regardless of laparoscopic or open approach, have better subsequent reproductive potential (61% vs. 38%) but slightly higher rates of ectopic pregnancy afterwards (15% vs. 10%) (73).

## 7 Nontubal Ectopic Pregnancies

### 7.1 Abdominal Pregnancies

Abdominal pregnancies present the greatest danger for both mother and fetus among all the ectopic pregnancies, with mortality rates ranging from 0.5 to 18% and 40 to 95%, respectively (74). They result from

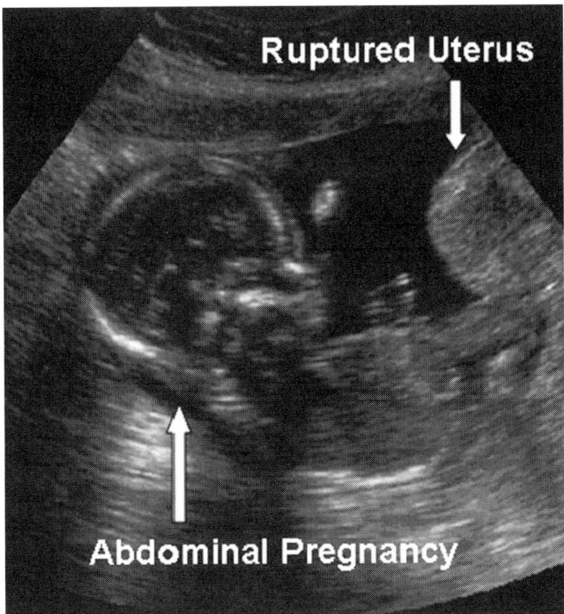


**Fig. 3** 18-Week ruptured cornual pregnancy with intra-abdominal growth. Courtesy of Courtney Woodfield, M.D. Rhode Island Hospital and Warren Alpert Medical School of Brown University

primary implantation in the abdomen or from secondary abdominal implantation after tubal rupture or extrusion (Fig. 3). Presenting symptoms and exam findings include abdominal pain (100%), nausea and vomiting (70%), abnormal fetal lie (70%), painful fetal movements (40%), displaced uterine cervix (40%) and general malaise (40%) (75). Due to the high rate of error with ultrasound, MR imaging is preferred. Laparoscopy still remains the gold standard (75) for diagnosis, and can be used in the management of early abdominal pregnancies; the more advanced abdominal pregnancies are to be managed by laparotomy. The placenta can be removed if doing so does not risk harming vascular and vital structures. Otherwise it can be left in place and can be treated with postoperative embolization or methotrexate to facilitate resorption (76).

## 7.2 *Cervical Ectopic Pregnancies*

Cervical ectopic pregnancies account for only 0.2% of ectopic pregnancies, making them rare. Methotrexate is the first line treatment with success rates ranging from 40% if embryonic cardiac activity exists and up to 90% if absent (77). Other factors predisposing patients to methotrexate failure include gestational age ≥9 weeks, serum β-hCG ≥10,000, or a crown-rump length greater than 10 mm (77). Patients with these factors may benefit from localized treatment using methotrexate, hyperosmolar glucose or potassium chloride (77), with reported success rates greater than 90% for local potassium chloride (78). Primary embolization is also a treatment option requiring methotrexate afterwards to treat residual trophoblasts (79). As many as 4–28% of patients may experience massive bleeding after systemic or local methotrexate treatment from failed involution of the pregnancy (77), warranting dilation and curettage in 13–43% (80). For this reason, patients who fail systemic methotrexate or localized treatment may have hypogastric artery embolization or laparoscopic ligation of the uterine arteries performed to reduce the risk of bleeding (79).

### 7.2.1 Heterotopic Pregnancy

The risk for heterotopic pregnancy, once considered extremely rare, may be as high as 1% in patients undergoing IVF (81). Pelvic ultrasound is the most sensitive imaging modality (82) for heterotopic pregnancy. The treatment modality employed depends on the patient's desire for intrauterine pregnancy. Methotrexate can be used in cases in which neither pregnancy is desired but is contraindicated when the intrauterine pregnancy is desired. While laparoscopy is considered the gold standard in management (83, 84), ultrasound guided injection of the extrauterine pregnancy with potassium chloride or hyperosmolar glucose can be effective in patients desiring their pregnancy. Risk of a rupture with local injection can be as high as 55% (85).

### 7.2.2 Interstitial (Cornual) Pregnancy

Interstitial (cornual) pregnancies are located in the proximal portion of the fallopian tube surrounded by myometrium and account for 2% of ectopic pregnancies (20, 21). The risk factors for interstitial (cornual) pregnancies include a history of prior ectopic pregnancy, salpingectomy, IVF and sexually transmitted

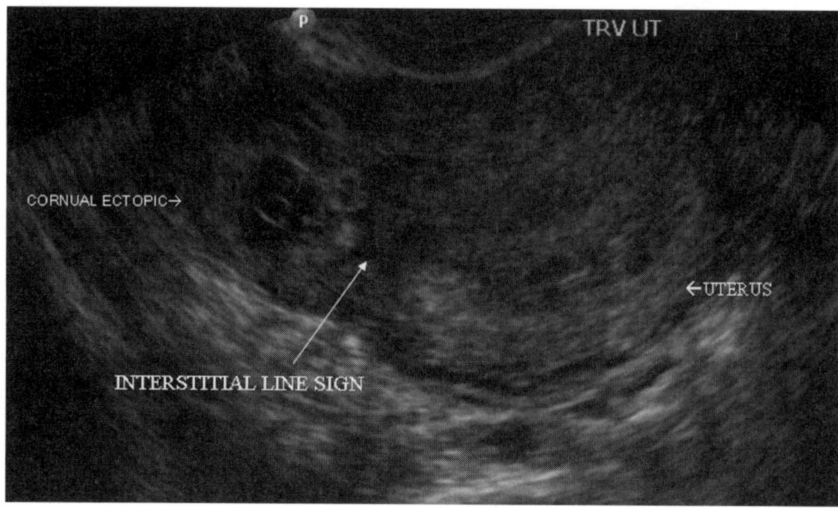


**Fig. 4** Interstitial line sign on pelvic ultrasound. Courtesy of Sandra Carson, M.D. Women and Infants Hospital of Rhode Island and Warren Alpert Medical School of Brown University

infections (86). Primarily, diagnosis is made with pelvic ultrasound and is highly suggested by the presence of an interstitial line sign (87) (Fig. 4) or the presence of Timor-Tritsch criteria (88). An interstitial line sign is the presence of an uninterrupted echolucent line between the gestational sac and the endometrium, suggesting that pregnancy is outside the uterine cavity proper. Timor-Tritsch criteria include: (1) an empty uterine cavity, (2) a chorionic sac seen separately and located >1 cm from the most lateral edge of the uterine cavity, and a (3) thin myometrial layer (<5 mm) surrounding the chorionic sac (88). In inconclusive cases MR imaging can be used; laparoscopy can be used for diagnosis as a last resort. Treatment of interstitial (cornual) ectopic pregnancies can be medical or surgical. The highest average mean gestational sac diameter for success with systemic methorexate is 23 mm or less (89) with an average success rate of 79%. If accessible, local injection with methotrexate or other agents such as hyperosmolar glucose or potassium chloride is another option that has been suggested for interstitial (cornual) pregnancies (90) with a success rate as high as 91% (89). In larger or more advanced pregnancies, however, laparoscopic management with an endo-loop or cornual resection has become the first choice (89, 91). Hysteroscopic approaches are investigational. Surgical management is better employed earlier than later, as catastrophic rupture of the uterus can occur earlier than 12 weeks (89, 91).

### 7.2.3 Ovarian Pregnancies

Ovarian pregnancies account for 0.2–3.2% of ectopic pregnancies (20, 21). The four criteria for an ovarian pregnancy were established by Spiegelberg in 1878: an intact ipsilateral tube separate from the ovary, a gestational sac occupying the position of the ovary, an ovary and gestational sac connected to the uterus by the utero-ovarian ligament, and histological presence of ovarian tissue in the gestational sac wall (92). The main risk factors for ovarian pregnancy include pelvic inflammatory disease, tubal surgery and oophoritis, and they tend to develop in younger patients with high parity (93). Up to 75% of ovarian pregnancies are mistaken for a ruptured corpus luteum cyst (94) and therefore may present as an abdominal pregnancy. Laparoscopic resection or oophorectomy is the preferred treatment; systemic methotrexate is still investigational (95).

### 7.2.4 Cesarean Scar Pregnancies

The incidence of Cesarean scar pregnancies has risen and although rare, now accounts for 1 in 2,000 pregnancies (96). Only 85% are diagnosed correctly by ultrasound due to their unusual location and often they are confused with cervical pregnancies or spontaneous abortions (97). MR imaging and Doppler can be used in inconclusive cases. As Cesarean scar pregnancy is still relatively rare, although increasing in incidence, no standard treatment regimen is defined. Systemic methotrexate has been employed with 100% success for patients with a β-hCG less than 5,000 and 50% success rate for all cases (96). Local administration of methotrexate, hyperosmolar glucose or potassium chloride can be employed, just as for interstitial (cornual) pregnancies (96). Laparotomy or laparoscopy remain the only other option, and a reasonable success rate can be expected (96).

## 8 Reproduction After Ectopic Pregnancy

Future fertility is comparable with all four main management methods employed to treat tubal ectopic pregnancy. The rates for tubal patency (75–81%), sub sequent pregnancy rates (52–61%) and ectopic pregnancy (8–13%) rates are similar for salpingostomy, multi-dose methotrexate, single-dose methotrexate and expectant management in properly selected cases (98).

## References


1. Goldner TE, Lawson HW, Xia Z, Atrash HK. Surveillance for ectopic pregnancy – United States, 1970–1989. In: CDC surveillance summaries. MMWR 1993; 42:73–85.
2. Current trends ectopic pregnancy – United States, 1990–1992, MMWR Morb Mortal Wkly Rep Jan 27, 1995; 44:46–8.
3. Centers for Disease Control (CDC). Selected behaviors that increase risk for HIV infection, other sexually transmitted diseases, and unintended pregnancy among high school students – United States, 1991. MMWR Morb Mortal Wkly Rep Dec 18 1992; 41:945–50.
4. Churgay CA, Apgar BS. Ectopic pregnancy: an update on technologic advances in diagnosis and treatment. Prim Care 1993; 20:629–38.
5. Ory SJ. New options for diagnosis and treatment of ectopic pregnancy. JAMA 1992; 267:534–7
6. Carson SA, Buster JE. Ectopic pregnancy. N Engl J Med 1993; 329:1174–81.
7. Stovall TG, Ling FW, Buster JE. Outpatient chemotherapy of unruptured ectopic pregnancy. Fertil Steril 1989; 51:435–8.
8. Grimes DA. Estimation of pregnancy-related mortality risk by pregnancy outcome, United States, 1991 to 1999. Am J Obstet Gynecol 2006; 194:92–4.
9. Stovall TG, Kellerman AL, Ling FW, Buster JE. Emergency department diagnosis of ectopic pregnancy. Ann Emerg Med 1990; 19:1098–103.
10. Mol BWJ, Ankum WM, Bossuyt PMM, Van der Veen F. Contraception and the risk of ectopic pregnancy: a meta-analysis. Contraception 1995; 52:337–41.
11. Ankum WM, Mol BW, Van der Veen F, Bossuyt PM. Risk factors for ectopic pregnancy: a meta-analysis. Fertil Steril 1996; 65:1093–9.
12. Barnhart KT, Sammel MD, Gracia CR, Chittams J, Hummel AC, Shaunik A. Risk factors for ectopic pregnancy in women with symptomatic first trimester pregnancies. Fertil Steril 2006; 86:36–43.
13. Butts S, Sammel M, Hummel A, Chittams J, Barnhart K. Risk factors and clinical features of recurrent ectopic pregnancy: a case control study. Fertil Steril 2003; 80:1340–4.
14. Mol BW, van der Veen F, Bossuyt PM. Symptom-free women at increased risk of ectopic pregnancy: should we screen? Acta Obstet Gynecol Scand 2002; 81:661–72.
15. Bouyer J, Coste J, Shojaei T et al. Risk factors for ectopic pregnancy: a comprehensive analysis based on a large case-control, population-based study in France. Am J Epidemiol 2003; 157:185–94.
16. Miller HG, Cain VS, Rogers SM, Gribble JN, Turner CF. Correlates of sexually transmitted bacterial infections among U.S. women in 1995. Fam Plann Perspect 1999; 31:4–9.
17. Menon S, Sammel MD, Vichnin M, Barnhart KT. Risk factors for ectopic pregnancy: a comparison between adults and adolescent women. J Pediatr Adolesc Gynecol 2007; 20:181–5.
18. Clayton HB, Schieve LA, Peterson HB, Jamieson DJ, Reynolds MA, Wright VC. Ectopic pregnancy risk with assisted reproductive technology procedures. Obstet Gynecol 2006; 107:595–604.
19. Clayton HB, Schieve LA, Peterson HB, Jamieson DJ, Reynolds MA, Wright VC. A comparison of heterotopic and intrauterine-only pregnancy outcomes after assisted reproductive technologies in the United States from 1999 to 2002. Fertil Steril 2007; 87:303–9.
20. Breen JL. A 21 year survey of 654 ectopic pregnancies. Am J Obstet Gynecol 1970; 106:1004–19.
21. Bouyer J, Coste J, Fernandez H, Pouly JL, Job-Spira N. Sites of ectopic pregnancy: a 10 year population-based study of 1,800 cases. Hum Reprod 2002; 17:3224–30.
22. Gracia C, Barnhart K. Diagnosing ectopic pregnancy: decision analysis comparing six strategies. Obstet Gynecol 2001; 97:464–70.
23. Yeh HC, Goodman JD, Carr L, Rabinowitz JG. Intradecidual sign: a US criterion of early intrauterine pregnancy. Radiology 1986; 161:463–7.
24. Bradley WG, Fiske CE, Filly RA. The double sac sign of early intrauterine pregnancy: use in exclusion of ectopic pregnancy. Radiology 1982; 143:223–6.
25. Russell SA, Filly RA, Damato N. Sonographic diagnosis of ectopic pregnancy with endovaginal probes: what really has changed? J Ultrasound Med 1993; 12:145–51.
26. Taylor KJ, Meyer WR. New techniques in the diagnosis of ectopic pregnancy. Obstet Gynecol Clin North Am 1991; 18:39–54.
27. Seeber B, Sammel M, Zhou L, Hummel A, Barnhart KT. Endometrial stripe thickness and pregnancy outcome in first-trimester pregnancies with bleeding, pain or both. J Reprod Med 2007; 52:757–61.
28. Goldstein SR, Snyder JR, Watson C, Danon M. Very early pregnancy detection with endovaginal ultrasound. Obstet Gynecol 1988; 72:200–4

29. Timor-Tritsch IE, Yeh MN, Peisner DB, Lesser KB, Salvik BS. The use of transvaginal ultrasound in the diagnosis of ectopic pregnancy. Am J Obstet Gynecol 1988; 161: 157–61
30. Barnhart KT, Kamelle SA, Simhan H. Diagnostic accuracy of ultrasound, above and below the beta-hCG discriminatory zone. Obstet Gynecol 1999; 94:583–7
31. Nagayama M, Watanabe Y, Okumura A, Amoh Y, Nakashita S, Dodo Y. Fast MR imaging in obstetrics. Radiographics 2002; 22:563–80.
32. Ha HK, Jung JK, Kang SJ et al. MR imaging in the diagnosis of rare formsof ectopic pregnancy. Am J Roentgenol 1993; 160:1229–32.
33. Nishino M, Hayakawa K, Iwasaku K, Takasu K. Magnetic resonance imaging findings in gynecologic emergencies. J Comput Assist Tomogr 2003; 26:756–61.
34. DeWitt C, Abbott J. Interstitial pregnancy: a potential for misdiagnosis of ectopic pregnancy with emergency department ultrasonography. Ann Emerg Med 2002; 40:106–9.
35. Kadar N, Caldwell BV, Romero R. A method of screening for ectopic pregnancy and its indications. Obstet Gynecol 1981; 58:162–6.
36. Seeber BE, Sammel MD, Guo W, Zhou L, Hummel A, Barnhart KT. Application of redefined human chorionic gonadotropin curves for the diagnosis of women at risk for ectopic pregnancy. Fertil Steril 2006; 86:454–9.
37. Barnhart K, Sammel MD, Chung K, Zhou L, Hummel AC, Guo W. Decline of serum human chorionic gonadotropin and spontaneous complete abortion: defining the normal curve. Obstet Gynecol 2004; 104:975–81.
38. McCord ML, Arheart KL, Muram DM, Stovall TG, Buster JE, Carson SA. Single serum progesterone as a screen for ectopic pregnancy: exchanging specificity and sensitivity to obtain optimal test performance. Fertil Steril 1996; 66:513–6.
39. Daponte A, Pournaras S, Zintzaras E et al. The value of a single combined measurement of VEGF, glycodelin, progesterone, PAPP-A, HPL and LIF for differentiating between ectopic and abnormal intrauterine pregnancy. Hum Reprod 2005; 20:3163–6.
40. Mueller MD, Raio L, Spoerri S, Ghezzi F, Dreher E, Bersinger NA. Novel placental and nonplacental serum markers in ectopic versus normal intrauterine pregnancy. Fertil Steril 2004; 81:1106–11.
41. Barnhart KT, Katz I, Hummel A, Gracia CR. Presumed diagnosis of ectopic pregnancy. Obstet Gynecol 2002; 100: 505–10.
42. Ries A, Singson P, Bidus M, Barnes JG. Use of the endometrial pipelle in the diagnosis of early abnormal gestations. Fertil Steril 2000; 74:593–5.
43. Barnhart KT, Gracia CR, Reindl B, Wheeler JE. Usefulness of pipelle endometrial biopsy in the diagnosis of women at risk for ectopic pregnancy. Am J Obstet Gynecol 2003; 188:906–9.
44. Lindahl B, Ahlgren M. Identification of chorion villi in abortion s pecimens. Obstet Gynecol 1986; 67:79–81.
45. ASRM Practice Committee. Treatment of ectopic pregnancy. Fertil Steril 2006; 86:96–102.
46. Kirk E, Condous G, Bourne T. The non-surgical management of ectopic pregnancy. Ultrasound Obstet Gynecol 2006; 27:91–100.
47. Calabresi P, Cahbner BA. Antineoplastic agents. In: Gilman A, Goodman LS and Goodman A (eds). The Pharmacologic Basis of Therapeutics, 8th edn. New York: Macmillan, 1990: 1275–6.
48. Berlin NI, Rall D, Mead JA et al. Folic acid antagonists: effects on the cell and the patient. Clinical staff conference at National Institutes of Health. Ann Intern Med 1963; 59:931–56.
49. Tanaka T, Hayashi H, Kutsuzawa T, Fujimoto S, Ichinoe K. Treatment of interstitial ectopic pregnancy with methotrexate: report of a successful case. Fertil Steril 1982; 37:851–2.
50. Walden PA, Bagshawe KD. Pregnancies after chemotherapy for gestational trophoblastic tumours. Lancet 1979; 2:1241.
51. Hajenius PJ, Engelsbel S, Mol BW, Van der Veen F, Ankum WM, Bossuyt PM, Hemrika DJ, Lammes FB. Randomised trial of systemic methotrexate versus laparoscopic salpingostomy in tubal pregnancy. Lancet 1997; 350:774–9.
52. Seeber BE, Barnhart KT. Suspected ectopic pregnancy. Obstet Gynecol 2006; 107:399–413.
53. Lipscomb GH, McCord ML, Stovall TG, Huff G, Portera SG, Ling FW. Predictors of success of methotrexate treatment in women with tubal ectopic pregnancies. New Engl J Med 1999; 341:1974–8.
54. Menon S, Colins J, Barnhart KT. Establishing a human chorionic gonadotropin cutoff to guide methotrexate treatment of ectopic pregnancy: a systematic review. Fertil Steril 2007; 87:481–4.
55. Tawfiq A, Agameya AF, Claman P. Predictors of treatment failure for ectopic pregnancy treated with single-dose methotrexate. Fertil Steril 2000; 74:877–80.
56. Dudley PS, Heard MJ, Sangi-Haghpeykar H, Carson SA, Buster JE. Characterizing ectopic pregnancies that rupture despite treatment with methotrexate. Fertil Steril 2004; 82:1374–8.
57. Rodi IA, Sauer MV, Gorrill MJ, Bustillo M, Gunning JE, Marshall JR, Buster JE. The medical treatment of unruptured ectopic pregnancy with methotrexate and citrovorum rescue: preliminary experience. Fertil Steril 1986; 46:811–3.
58. Ory SJ, Villanueva AL, Sand PK, Tamura RK. Conservative treatment of ectopic pregnancy with methotrexate. Am J Obstet Gynecol 1986; 154:1299–306.
59. Stovall TG, Ling FW. Single-dose methotrexate: an expanded clinical trial. Am J Obstet Gynecol 1993; 168:1759–62.
60. Barnhart KT, Gosman G, Ashby R, Sammel M. The medical management of ectopic pregnancy: a meta-analysis comparing "single dose" and "multidose" regimens. Obstet Gynecol 2003; 101:778–84.
61. Hajenius PJ, Mol BW, Bossuyt PM, Ankum WM, Van Der Veen F. Interventions for tubal ectopic pregnancy. Cochrane Database Syst Rev 2000; (2):CD000324.
62. Barnhart K, Hummel AC, Sammel MD, Menon S, Jain J, Chakhtoura N. Use of "2-dose" regimen of methotrexate to treat ectopic pregnancy. Fertil Steril 2007; 87:250–6.
63. Lipscomb GH, Puckett KJ, Bran D, Ling FW. Management of separation pain after single-dose methotrexate therapy for ectopic pregnancy. Obstet Gynecol 1999; 93:590–3.
64. Atri M, Bret PM, Tulandi T, Senterman MK. Ectopic pregnancy: evolution after treatment with transvaginal methotrexate. Radiology 1992; 185:749–53.
65. Lipscomb GH, Bran D, McCord ML, Portera JC, Ling FW. Analysis of three hundred fifteen ectopic pregnancies treated with single-dose methotrexate. Am J Obstet Gynecol 1998; 178:1354–8.

66. Saraj AJ, Wilcox JG, Najmabadi S, Stein SM, Johnson MB, Paulson RJ. Resolution of hormonal markers of ectopic gestation: a randomized trial comparing single-dose intramuscular methotrexate with salpingostomy. Obstet Gynecol 1998; 92:989–94.
67. Natale A, Busacca M, Candiani M, Gruft L, Izzo S, Felicetta I, Vignali M. Human chorionic gonadotropin patterns after a single dose of methotrexate for ectopic pregnancy. Eur J Obstet Gynecol Reprod Biol 2002; 100:227–30.
68. Vermesh M, Silva PD, Rosen GF, Stein AL, Fossum GT, Sauer MV. Management of unruptured ectopic gestation by linear salpingostomy: a prospective, randomized clinical trial of laparoscopy versus laparotomy. Obstet Gynecol 1989; 73:400–4.
69. Lundorff P, Thorburn J, Hahlin M, Kallfelt B, Lindblom B. Laparoscopic surgery in ectopic pregnancy. A randomized trial versus laparotomy. Acta Obstet Gynecol Scand 1991; 70:343–8.
70. Murphy AA, Nager CW, Wujek JJ, Kettel LM, Torp VA, Chin HG. Operative laparoscopy versus laparotomy for the management of ectopic pregnancy: a prospective trial. Fertil Steril 1992; 57:1180–5.
71. Lundorff P, Hahlin M, Kallfelt B, Thorburn J, Lindblom B. Adhesion formation after laparoscopic surgery in tubal pregnancy: a randomized trial versus laparotomy. Fertil Steril 1991; 55:911–5.
72. Graczykowski JW, Mishell DR Jr. Methotrexate prophylaxis for persistent ectopic pregnancy after conservative treatment by salpingostomy. Obstet Gynecol 1997; 89:118–22.
73. Yao M, Tulandi T. Current status of surgical and nonsurgical management of ectopic pregnancy. Fertil Steril 1997; 67:421–33.
74. Atrash HK, Friede A, Hogue CJ. Abdominal pregnancy in the United States: frequency and maternal mortality. Obstet Gynecol 1987; 69:333–7.
75. Rahman MS, Al-Suleiman SA, Rahman J, Al-Sibai MH. Advanced abdominal pregnancy – observations in 10 cases. Obstet Gynecol 1982; 59:366–72.
76. Rahaman J, Berkowitz R, Mitty H, Gaddipati S, Brown B, Nezhat F. Minimally invasive management of an advanced abdominal pregnancy. Obstet Gynecol 2004; 103:1064–8.
77. Hung TH, Shau WY, Hsieh TT, Hsu JJ, Soong YK, Jeng CJ. Prognostic factors for an unsatisfactory primary methotrexate treatment of cervical pregnancy: a quantitative review. Hum Reprod 1998; 13:2636–42.
78. Doubilet PM, Benson CB, Frates MC, Ginsburg E. Sono graphically guided minimally invasive treatment of unusual ectopic pregnancies. Radiology 1994; 191:773–5.
79. Kung FT, Lin H, Hsu TY et al. Differential diagnosis of suspected cervical pregnancy and conservative treatment with the combination of laparoscopy-assisted uterine artery ligation and hysteroscopic endocervical resection. Fertil Steril 2004; 81:1642–9.
80. Kung FT, Chang SY. Efficacy of methotrexate treatment in viable and nonviable cervical pregnancies. Am J Obstet Gynecol 1999; 181:1438–44.
81. Lemus JF. Ectopic pregnancy: an update. Curr Opin Obstet Gynecol 2000; 12:369–75.
82. Em F, Gersovich EO. High resolution ultrasound in the diagnosis of heterotopic pregnancy combined trans-abdominal and transvaginal approach. BJOG 1993; 100:871–2
83. Pisarska MD, Casson PR, Moise KJ Jr, DiMaio DJ, Buster JE, Carson SA. Heterotopic abdominal pregnancy treated at laparoscopy. Fertil Steril 1998; 70:159–60.
84. Wang PH, Chao HT, Tseng JY. Laparoscopic surgery for heterotopic pregnancies: a case report and a brief review. Eur J Obstet Gynecol Reprod Biol 1998; 80:267–71.
85. Goldstein JS, Ratts VS, Philpott T, Dahan MH. Risk of surgery after use of potassium chloride for treatment of tubal heterotopic pregnancy. Obstet Gynecol 2006; 107:506–8.
86. Tulandi T, Al-Jaroudi D. Interstitial pregnancy: results generated from the Society of Reproductive Surgeons Registry. Obstet Gynecol 2004; 103:47–50.
87. Ackerman TE, Levi CS, Dashefsky SM, Holt SC, Lindsay DJ. Interstitial line: sonographic finding in interstitial (cornual) ectopic pregnancy. Radiology 1993; 189:83–7.
88. Timor-Tritsch IE, Monteagudo A, Matera C, Veit CR. Sonographic evolution of cornual pregnancies treated without surgery. Obstet Gynecol 1992; 79:1044–9.
89. Lau S, Tulandi T. Conservative medical and surgical management of interstitial ectopic pregnancy. Fertil Steril 1999; 72:207–15.
90. Raughley MJ, Frishman GN. Local treatment of ectopic pregnancy. Semin Reprod Med 2007; 25:99–115.
91. Soriano D, Vicus D, Mashiach R, Schiff E, Seidman D, Goldenberg M. Laparoscopic treatment of cornual pregnancy: a series of 20 consecutive cases. Fertil Steril 2008; 90:839–43.
92. Spiegelberg O. Zur Casuistik der Ovarialschwangerschaft. Arch Gynaekol 1878; 13:73–9.
93. Hallatt JG. Primary ovarian pregnancy: a report of twenty-five cases. Am J Obstet Gynecol 1982; 143:55–60.
94. Jonathan S, Adashi BE, Hillard PA. Novak's Textbook of Gynaecology, 12th edn. Baltimore, MD: Williams & Wilkins, 1999: 512–3.
95. Mittal S, Dadhwal V, Baurasi P. Successful medical management of ovarian pregnancy. Int J Gynaecol Obstet 2003; 80:309–10.
96. Rotas MA, Haberman S, Levgur M. Cesarean scar ectopic pregnancies: etiology, diagnosis, and management. Obstet Gynecol 2006; 107:1373–81.
97. Vial Y, Petignat P, Hohlfeld P. Pregnancy in a cesarean scar. Ultrasound Obstet Gynecol 2000; 16:592–3.
98. Buster JE, Krotz S. Reproductive performance after ectopic pregnancy. Semin Reprod Med 2007; 25:131–3.

# Recent Advances in Fertility Preservation for the Female

Ozgur Oktem and Kutluk Oktay

**Abstract** Modern methods of the treatment of cancer have a significant negative impact on human reproduction. In this chapter we briefly overview recent cancer statistics and discuss premature ovarian failure and other adverse reproductive outcomes in female patients who receive chemotherapy and radiation. In addition to this, we also discuss and delineate the options to preserve their fertility.

**Keywords** Fertility preservation • Cancer • Chemotherapy • Gonadotoxicity • Xenografting • Vitrification • Cryopreservation

## 1 Introduction

Cancer continues to be a major health problem in the world. Of 1.5 million new cancer cases expected to occur in 2008 in the United States, 692,000 will be females. The most common cancers in females under the age of 40 are breast cancer, cancers of the lung and bronchus, colon and rectum, leukemia and lymphomas, and cervical cancer. The probability of being diagnosed with an invasive cancer for women under the age 40 is 2%. This rate increases to 9% by the age of 60. Among females, the leading cause of death due to cancer before the age of 20 years is leukemia. Breast cancer ranks first between the ages 20 and 59 years, and lung cancer ranks first between the age 60 and above. Overall, cancer is the leading cause of death among women between the ages 40 and 79 (1).

Cancer is also an important health issue for children and adolescents, being the second leading cause of death among children between ages 1 and 14 years in the United States. Leukemia, tumors of the central nervous system, neuroblastoma, Wilms tumor and non-Hodgkin lymphoma are the most common (1).

Over the last three decades there have been significant improvements in the 5-year relative survival rate for many cancer types due to advanced diagnostic modalities, improved surgical technique, combination chemotherapy, radiotherapy and supportive care. When cancers of all sites and all races are considered, the survival rate increased from 50% in 1970s to 66 in 2003 (1). Survival rates are more encouraging in children.

The 5-year relative survival rate among children for all cancer sites combined, improved from 58% for patients diagnosed in 1975 to 1977, to 80% for those diagnosed between 1996 and 2003.

Nevertheless modern combination chemotherapy and radiotherapy regimens have a substantial impact on reproduction. Premature ovarian failure and other poor reproductive outcomes subsequent to cancer therapies are being recognized. Furthermore, besides malignancies, treatment of certain pre-cancerous and benign conditions such as myelodysplasia, aplastic anemia, and systemic lupus erythematosus may necessitate administration of high dose chemotherapeutics with and without stem cell transplantation (2). Therefore preservation of gonadal function and fertility has become one of the major quality of life issues for cancer survivors at reproductive ages.

O. Oktem
Institute for Fertility Preservation, Center for Human Reproduction, NY, and Department of Obstetrics & Gynecology, New York Medical College-Westchester Medical Center, Valhalla, NY

K. Oktay (✉)
Institute for Fertility Preservation, Center for Human Reproduction, NY, and Department of Obstetrics & Gynecology, New York Medical College-Westchester Medical Center, Valhalla, NY
e-mail: koktay@fertilitypreservation.org

D.T. Carrell et al. (eds.), *Biennial Review of Infertility*, DOI: 10.1007/978-1-60327-392-3_6

Accordingly, clinical guidelines, have recently been issued by the American Society of Clinical Oncology encouraging fertility preservation among all young cancer survivors with interest in fertility. (3).

The gonads of both sexes are adversely affected by multi-agent chemotherapy regimens and radiotherapy. Ovaries are endowed with a finite, non-renewable number of eggs that are very sensitive to cytotoxic drugs and radiation. Ovarian reserve (reproductive life span) is determined by the number of quiescent primordial follicles in the ovary that are established before birth, even though this dogma has recently been challenged by two studies (4, 5). An accelerated and premature depletion of germ cells in the gonads caused by direct toxic insults to the oocyte, surrounding steroid-producing somatic cell layers (granulosa and theca cells), or both, are the main mechanism underlying gonadal failure induced by chemotherapy and radiation (6). The age of the patient, the type, dose and intensity of chemotherapy and/or radiotherapy are the main factors determining the magnitude of the damage in the ovary. Older patients have lower ovarian reserve compared to younger ones; therefore they have a higher risk of ovarian failure during or after chemotherapy or radiation. Furthermore, as noted in the adult survivors of childhood cancers, there are some other adverse *extragonadal* effects, such as abnormalities in the regulation of growth and endocrine functions, and other poor reproductive outcomes that appear later in life such as preterm births and miscarriages.

It is not within the scope of this chapter to review all published data on the effects of every chemotherapy agent and radiotherapy on reproductive function. Rather, the basic principles of gonadotoxicity associated with chemotherapy and radiation use, and the current strategies of preservation of reproductive function will be summarized.

## 2 Chemotherapy and Ovarian Damage

Chemotherapeutics have different mechanisms of action, therefore, they have different gonadotoxic potentials. Data on their gonadotoxic effects is largely collected from two important sources; clinical trials and animal studies.

In clinical studies, the magnitude of the impact of chemotherapy on human ovary is determined by assessing menstrual function in patients receiving that chemotherapy regimen. However, menstrual status may not be a good marker of fertility as shown previously in patients who were still menstruating despite their critically elevated FSH levels and diminished ovarian reserve (7). Furthermore, current modern cancer treatments commonly employ multi-agent chemotherapy drugs precluding assessment of individual gonadotoxicity of each drug in a combination regimen. While ovarian reserve markers such as FSH, estradiol, and anti-Mullerian hormone (AMH) measurements (7) as well as antral follicle counts (8) can give a better estimate of the ovarian reserve before and after chemotherapy, there are no comprehensive studies evaluating the impact of chemotherapy regimens with these markers nor are these markers direct measures of the ovarian reserve. More accurate information of gonadotoxicity on the human ovary can be obtained by real-time quantitative analysis of primordial follicle counts using histomorphological methods in ovarian samples, but it necessitates an operation because it cannot be done in clinical settings for ethical and practical reasons. Moreover, as new agents are introduced to adjuvant setting, their long-term impact on the human ovary is extremely difficult to determine from short-term studies.

Several animal studies, mainly in rodents, showed individual gonadotoxicity of certain cancer drugs such as cyclophosphamide and doxorubicin (9, 10). However, some discrepancies may exist between animal and human ovaries. Therefore by considering all these needs, we developed a human xenograft model (11). This model enabled us to characterize the course of time and the mechanism of action of gonadal damage induced by chemotherapy agents via quantitative histomorphometric analysis of primordial follicle counts and cell death assays.

According to both clinical and animal studies, chemotherapy agents of alkylating group appear to have more toxic effects in the gonads of both sexes and are therefore associated with the highest risk of infertility. Antineoplastic agents of alkylating category have different members, such as the nitrogen mustard family (cyclophosphamide, uramustine, chlorambucil and melphalan, mechlorethamine), alkyl sulfonates (busulfan), nitrosureas (carmustine, streptozocin), ethyleneimines and methylmelamines (hexamethylmelamine and thiotepa), triazenes (dacarbazine) and imidazotetrazines (temozolomide). Cyclophosphamide is one of the most commonly used antineoplastic drugs in the treatment of many solid and hematologic malignancies as well as certain auto-immune diseases (6). We recently characterized gonadotoxicity of cyclophosphamide in the human ovary using a xenograft model (11). Cyclophosphamide based regimens CEF, CMF, CAF, AC (combinations of cyclophosphamide with methotrexate, epirubicin, fluorouracil, doxorubicin) are commonly used in the adjuvant treatment of breast cancer. Cyclophosphamide and busulfan combination are administered at high doses for myeloablative conditioning prior to hematopoietic stem cell transplantation. CHOP (in combination with doxorubicin and vincristine) is another cyclophosphamide-based alkylating regimen commonly used in the treatment of leukemia and lymphomas. All these regimens are associated with a higher risk of permanent and premature ovarian failure, even at smaller doses, especially in patients at the age of 40 and older with diminished ovarian reserve. Patients who receive these combinations when younger than 39 may pose lower risk for gonadal failure due to their high ovarian reserve (3).

Data on the gonadal toxicity associated with the use of other antineoplastic agents are scarce. Cisplatin and Adriamycin poses intermediate risk for gonadotoxicity whereas administration of non-alkylating agents such as vincristine methotrexate, fluorouracil, Idarubicin or ABVD combination (doxorubicin/bleomycin/vinblastin/dacarbazine) may pose lower risk for ovarian failure due to the less harmful nature of the agents (2, 3). It should be kept in mind that newer drugs with unknown toxicity profile such as, Taxanes, Oxaliplatin, Irinotecan, monoclonal antibodies (trastuzumab, bevacizumab, cetuximab) or tyrosine kinase inhibitors (erlotinib, imatinib); or less cytotoxic agents when used at higher doses, longer duration of use or at more frequent intervals may be associated with higher risk for premature ovarian failure.

A recent study quantified the impact of chemotherapy on primordial follicle count in age-matched cancer patients undergoing ovarian freezing before and after chemotherapy administration by providing histological evidence for chemotherapy induced primordial follicle loss (12). The main mode of infertility and premature gonadal failure after chemotherapy is believed to be through follicular destruction. However, ovarian stromal cells may play a role in ovarian endocrine function and possibly in the restoration of ovulatory function post-chemotherapy (13). Therefore preservation of ovarian stromal function, may also be important in fertility preservation but further research is needed to prove this hypothesis. We showed that, in vitro, ovarian cortical pieces from individuals who were previously exposed to chemotherapy (chemotherapy group) produced significantly less estradiol compared to those who were not (control group) (12). Since the importance of stromal cells has been shown in other organs such as bone marrow, in which stromal cells previously exposed to cancer drugs suppress hematopoiesis from normal donor cells (14), studies to address if chemotherapy induced damage in ovarian stromal cells has importance in restoration of ovarian stromal function are needed.

## 3 Radiotherapy and Ovarian Failure

Abdominal, pelvic, or spinal irradiation are associated with increased risk of developing acute ovarian failure, especially if both ovaries are within the treatment field (15, 16). Direct actions on DNA are the predominant mechanism of damage for particle radiation, such as neutrons and particles. Indirect actions come from the interaction of radiation with other substances in the cell such as water leading to formation of free radicals and DNA damage. This mechanism is particularly true for sparsely ionizing radiation such as X-rays.

Gonadal damage occurs not only by direct exposure to radiation such as in the case of pelvic or low abdominal irradiation, but also scatters radiation which may cause significant damage even if gonads are outside of the radiation. The risk of premature ovarian failure is higher with increasing radiation doses. Single doses may have more toxic effects than fractionated dose (17). Recently, it was suggested that the LD 50, the radiation dose required to kill 50% of oocytes, is <2 Gray (Gy) in humans (17). The ovary of younger individuals is more resistant to permanent damage from irradiation than is the ovary of older individuals due to higher number of primordial follicles in younger ovaries (18, 19). For instance, 6 Gy may be sufficient to produce irreversible ovarian damage in women older than 40 years of age, in contrast to 10–20 Gy doses needed to induce permanent ovarian failure in the majority of females treated during childhood (20, 21). This is because younger patients harbor more primordial follicles in their ovaries; therefore they are more likely to retain some residual ovarian function after radiotherapy than do older patients. Sadly, the most extensive damage of radiation on the ovary occurs in patients who receive a stem cell transplant with high dose total body irradiation (TBI). One study showed that almost all the patients who had undergone a marrow transplant with TBI after the age of 10 developed acute ovarian failure, whereas approximately 50% of girls who had received a transplant before the age of 10 suffered acute loss of ovarian function (22). Total body irradiation, given as a single dose or fractionated (10–15 Gy), is often used in combination with gonadotoxic cyclophosphamide or melphalan. The use of cyclophosphamide in conjuction with radiation increases further the extent of the damage as exemplified by a study showing that all 144 patients receiving TBI with cyclophosphamide for bone marrow transplantation (BMT) developed amenorrhea in the first 3 years. Return of menses occurred 3–7 years post-transplant only in nine patients; all were younger than 25 years (23).

## 4 Other Adverse Reproductive Outcomes After Chemotherapy and Radiation

Due to extra-gonadal effects, there are some other long-term adverse outcomes in reproductive function especially among survivors of childhood cancer after exposure to chemotherapy and radiotherapy. It appears that the female sex is more commonly associated with higher treatment-related risks such as cognitive dysfunction after cranial irradiation, poor cardiovascular outcomes, obesity, radiation-associated differences in pubertal timing, development of primary hypothyroidism, breast cancer as a second malignant neoplasm and osteonecrosis (24). The timing of menarche may be altered in survivors of childhood cancer, especially in those exposed to cranial and craniospinal radiotherapy compared to those treated with chemotherapy alone. Therefore those exposed to cranial and craniospinal radiotherapy, especially at a young age, should be monitored closely for abnormal timing of menarche (25).

Uterine function is also often compromised by radiation-induced damage to uterine vascular and muscular structures resulting in decreased uterine blood flow, reduced uterine volume, decreased endometrial thickness, and loss of distensibility. Whole body irradiation (20–30 Gy) during childhood has been documented to cause mid-trimester miscarriages (26). Unfortunately women exposed to radiation postpubertally have larger uterus and greater likelihood of livebirth than those exposed prepubertally (27). Sadly, women with ovarian failure secondary to whole body irradiation (20–30 Gy) have significantly reduced uterine size with no improvement in blood flow and endometrial thickness in response to exogenous sex hormones (28). Another adverse effect of radiation therapy is lower birth weight in the offspring and a higher risk of miscarriage in childhood cancer survivors according to the report of the Childhood Cancer Survey Study (29). Restricted fetal growth and early births may occur as late effects among the off springs of female childhood cancer survivors, especially in those who had received pelvic irradiation (30).

Amenorrhea occurring post-exposure to radiation may be hypothalamic in origin rather than ovarian as seen in individuals receiving radiation at doses >30 Gy to the hypothalamic – pituitary unit (31).

## 5 Fertility Preservation Strategies

The options for fertility preservation in female cancer patients vary depending upon the patient's age, type of treatment, diagnosis, whether she has a partner, the time available and the potential that cancer has metastasized to her ovaries. Table 1 summarizes the main

**Table 1** Table compares the advantages and disadvantages of three main fertility preservation options

| | Ovarian tissue freezing | Oocyte freezing | Embryo freezing |
|---|---|---|---|
| Applicability in prepubertal patients | Yes | Limited | No |
| Applicability in patients with low ovarian reserve | Limited | Limited | Limited |
| Requires ovarian stimulation | No | Yes | Yes |
| Requires a delay in initiation of cancer therapy | No | Yes | Yes |
| Requires surgery | Yes | No | No |
| Risk of cancer seeding | Yes[a] | No | No |
| Live birth in human | Yes[b] | Yes | Yes |
| Restoration of endocrine function | Possible | No | No |

[a]Theoretically possible, but no documented case to date
[b]Obtained only in orthotopic transplants, but the origin of pregnancies could not be confirmed with 100% certainty

fertility preservation options in females and the *pros and cons* of each procedure.

## 5.1 Ovarian Tissue Cryopreservation

Ovarian tissue cryopreservation and transplantation studies date back to the 1950s in animals, but its application to human ovarian tissue is confined to the last decade (32). Feasibility of ovarian tissue freezing and transplantation has been documented and offsprings have been reproduced in several animal models, such sheep, mice, rat and primate (33). Ovarian cryopreservation maybe the only option for fertility preservation, especially in prepubertal children and those who do not have time to undergo ovarian stimulation for oocyte or embryo cryopreservation. The ovarian cortex contains quiescent primordial follicles with oocytes arrested in the diplotene of prophase of the first meiotic division. Banking of ovarian tissue relies on the relative resistance of primordial follicles to cryo-toxicity and ischemia due to their relatively high surface/volume ratio, low metabolic rate, the absence of zona pellucida, and lack of metaphase spindles compared to follicles at other developmental stages (34).

With the advent of effective modern cryoprotectants, such as ethylene glycol, DMSO and propanediol, and new sophisticated automated cryopreservation machines, studies show more encouraging results. In addressing the most optimum way of freezing human ovarian tissue several points need to be considered:

*Age of the patient* is one of the most important factors determining the success of ovarian freezing and transplantation procedure. More than 60% of primordial follicles are lost after transplantation during ischemic period until re-vascularization is established according to animal autograft (35) and human xenograft studies (11). An additional 7% appear to be lost during freezing and thawing. Since there is an age-related decline in primordial follicle counts (36), women older than 40 tend to have low follicle density and therefore may not be good candidates for the procedure. The losses are tolerated better in younger patients with higher ovarian reserve.

*Size of the cortical pieces* is another important factor. Even though we still don't know the optimum size of the pieces for freezing and grafting, long term survival and follicle growth are achieved in 0.5 × 0.5–1 cm pieces. Excessive tissue slicing may damage the primordial follicle reserve in the tissue and, small cortical pieces may not be manageable for future transplantation. Because of these considerations we have utilized ovarian cortical pieces with 0.5 × 1 cm long and 0.1–0.2 cm for cryopreservation.

*Cryoprotectant* of choice can be dimethyl sulfoxide (DMSO), propanediol or ethylene glycol. Glycerol is not as effective for ovarian tissue freezing and therefore should not be used (37). At present, the slow freezing technique appears to be the most suitable technique for ovarian tissue freezing and vitrification has not yet produced reliable results.

### 5.1.1 Ovarian Transplantation

Two main approaches have been developed to autotransplant ovarian cortical pieces in humans. *Orthotopic* transplants involve grafting these strips near the infundibulopelvic ligament or possibly on a postmenopausal ovary. In the *heterotopic* transplant, tissues can be grafted subcutaneously at various locations including forearm and abdominal wall.

We reported the first case of autologous ovarian transplantation with cryopreserved tissue in 2000 (37). The case was a 29-year old patient suffering from severe endometriosis and underwent orthotopic transplantation in which the grafts were sutured to a peritoneal pocket created in the left pelvic ovarian bursa. The grafts were stimulated with gonadotropins and ovulation was documented fifteen weeks postgrafting. Endocrine function continued up to 9 months post-transplantation. Likewise, we also reported the first cases of embryo generation and spontaneous pregnancies following subcutaneous transplantation of frozen banked tissue in 2004 and 2006, respectively (13, 38). In both cases the grafts were transplanted heterotopically beneath the skin of abdomen. In the first case ovarian tissue was cryopreserved from a 30-year-old woman with breast cancer before chemotherapy-induced menopause, and this tissue was transplanted beneath the skin of her abdomen six years later. Ovarian function returned in the patient three months after transplantation, as shown by follicle development and oestrogen production. The patient underwent eight oocyte retrievals percutaneously and 20 oocytes were retrieved. Of the eight oocytes suitable for in-vitro fertilization, one fertilized normally and developed into a four-cell embryo. The other patient was a Hodgkin lymphoma survivor who became menopausal for 2½ years following a homologous stem cell transfer. Interestingly, following a heterotopic ovarian transplantation the patient spontaneously conceived within 4 months of transplantation, concurrent with follicular activity in the ovarian transplant under her abdominal skin. She eventually delivered a healthy girl who is now two years old. This case clearly illustrates that spontaneous pregnancies can occur even in those who appear to be in menopause for years, and even after unilateral oophorectomy for ovarian cryopreservation. It also brings up a new research question as to whether ovarian transplants could play a role in the recovery of the damaged ovary by triggering regeneration of oocytes post-chemotherapy (13, 39).

More recently live births following autologous ovarian transplantation to pelvis have been reported. Even though these results are encouraging, some argued that it is not possible to confirm if the patients have ovulated from their pre-existing ovaries or from the transplanted tissues (40–42).

Overall, the experience with ovarian cryopreservation is still limited, the utilization rate of banked tissue is very low because the procedure itself is a relatively new technology and the patients are young and some are still undergoing cancer treatment and/or surveillance (43).

## 5.2 Embryo Freezing

In vitro fertilization (IVF) and embryo cryopreservation is the most established fertility preservation technique if the patient has a partner and sufficient amount of time before cancer treatment. It is not technically challenging and has been used for nearly two decades to store unused embryos from in vitro fertilization and embryo transfer cycles.

Low-temperature storage methods of embryos at the pronuclear, early cleavage stage, and more recently at the blastocyst stage, have been successfully established (44). It is not within the scope of this chapter to review literature and provide detailed technical information on embryo freezing; rather we will be mainly focusing on the ovarian stimulation protocol with aromatase inhibitors recently developed by us for IVF and embryo freezing as a means of fertility preservation in breast cancer patients.

An IVF cycle typically takes approximately two weeks to complete, and this time period may not be available to most cancer patients except breast cancer patients who have a six week period between surgery and initiation of adjuvant therapies. However, standard ovarian stimulation protocols are contraindicated in patients with breast cancer due to high estrogen levels. Since most of these tumors are estrogen receptor positive, supraphysiologic estrogen levels (typically greater than 1,000 pg/mL compared to peak levels of 200–350 pg/mL in natural cycles) attained with gonadotropin stimulation during ovarian stimulation in general is not considered safe.

We recently developed an ovarian stimulation protocol using aromatase inhibitors in combination with FSH for the purpose of preserving fertility via embryo or oocyte cryopreservation in breast cancer patients (45, 46). Tamoxifen and Letrozole appear to be the best candidate aromatase inhibitor drugs as they have a proven efficacy in the prevention of breast cancer recurrence and because, coincidentally, both have ovulation-inducing properties (47, 48). Ovarian stimulation especially with letrozole and FSH appears to be a cost-effective alternative for fertility preservation in breast cancer patients with reduced estrogen exposure, compared with standard IVF. If patients are referred promptly, they may undergo embryo or oocyte cryopreservation without a delay in chemotherapy (45).

## 5.3 Oocyte Freezing

Oocyte cryopreservation is an emerging option for young adolescents, women without partners, or women who do not wish to have their oocytes fertilized by sperm from a partner or anonymous donor. The first reported case of a human live birth after successful oocyte cryopreservation was followed by additional pregnancies and deliveries using a slow freeze, rapid thaw technique thereafter (49–51). However, in contrast to recent advances and encouraging results with IVF and embryo freezing, oocyte freezing is still associated with lower pregnancy rates. Low pregnancy rates relate to several technical challenges encountered during the freeze, including the thaw process and the in vitro maturation of immature oocytes.

Mature oocytes provide the best chance for pregnancy but have several characteristics that make them susceptible to cryodamage. As mature oocytes are arrested in metaphase II, the spindle apparatus is fully extended and prone to disassembly at lower temperature, with subsequent chromosome dispersion and aneuploidy (52–53). The oocyte's large size and high water content also make it vulnerable to ice crystal formation, rupture, and limited penetration of cryoprotectant solutions because of the low ratio of surface area to volume.

We recently conducted a meta-analysis to determine the efficiency of oocyte cryopreservation relative to IVF with unfrozen oocytes (54). In vitro fertilization success rates with slow-frozen oocytes are significantly lower when compared with the case of IVF with unfrozen oocytes. Although oocyte cryopreservation with the slow freeze method appears to be justified for preserving fertility when a medical indication exists, its value for elective applications remains to be determined. Pregnancy rates with VF appear to have improved, but further studies will be needed to determine the efficiency and safety of this technique.

## 6 Conclusions

Fertility preservation is an emerging new field and most techniques are still investigational. When choosing a fertility preservation technique, the patient's age, type of treatment, diagnosis, whether she has a partner, the time available and the potential that the cancer has metastasized to her ovaries have to be taken into account. Appropriate counseling and good communication with the oncologist is also vital to facilitate and perform the fertility preservation procedures safely and without delay.

## References


1. Jemal A, Siegel R, Ward E, et al. Cancer statistics, 2008. CA Cancer J Clin 2008;58:71–96.
2. Sonmezer M, Oktay K. Fertility preservation in female patients. Hum Reprod Update 2004;10:251–266.
3. Lee SJ, Schover LR, Partridge AH, et al. American Society of Clinical Oncology. American Society of Clinical Oncology recommendations on fertility preservation in cancer patients. J Clin Oncol 2006;24:2917–2931.
4. Johnson J, Bagley J, Skaznik-Wikiel M, et al. Oocyte generation in adult mammalian ovaries by putative germcells in bone marrow and peripheral blood. Cell 2005;122:303–315.
5. Johnson J, Canning J, Kaneko T, et al. Germline stem cells and follicular renewal in the postnatal mammalian ovary. Nature 2004;428:145–150.
6. Oktem O, Oktay K. Preservation of menstrual function in adolescent and young females. Ann N Y Acad Sci 2008;1135:237–243.
7. Oktay K, Oktem O, Reh A. Measuring the impact of chemotherapy on fertility in women with breast cancer. J Clin Oncol 2006;24:4044–4046.
8. Scheffer GJ, Broekmans FJ, Looman CW, et al. The number of antral follicles in normal women with proven fertility is the best reflection of reproductive age. Hum Reprod 2003;18:700–706.
9. Plowchalk DR, Mattison DR. Phosphoramide mustard is responsible for the ovarian toxicity of cyclophosphamide. Toxicol Appl Pharmacol 1991;107:472–481.
10. Morita Y, Perez GI, Paris F, et al. Oocyte apoptosis is suppressed by disruption of the acid sphingomyelinase gene or by sphingosine-1-phosphate therapy. Nat Med 2000;10:1109–1114.
11. Oktem O, Oktay K. A novel ovarian xenografting model to characterize the impact of chemotherapy agents on human primordial follicle reserve. Cancer Res 2007;67(21):10159–10162.
12. Oktem O, Oktay K. Quantitative assessment of the impact of chemotherapy on ovarian follicle reserve and stromal function. Cancer 2007;110:2222–2229.
13. Oktay K. Spontaneous conceptions and live birth after heterotopic ovarian transplantation: is there a germline stem cell connection? Hum Reprod 2006;21:1345–1348.
14. Schwartz GN, Warren MK, Rothwell SW, et al. Post-chemotherapy and cytokine pretreated marrow stromal cell layers suppress hematopoiesis from normal donor CD341 cells. Bone Marrow Transplant 1998;22:457–468.
15. Stillman RJ, Schinfeld JS, Schiff I, et al. Ovarian failure in long term survivors of childhood malignancy. Am J Obstet Gynecol 1981;139:62–66.
16. Sklar C. Maintenance of Ovarian function and risk of premature menopause related to cancer treatment. J Natl Cancer Inst Monogr 2005;34:25–27.
17. Wallace WHB, Thompson AB, Kelsey TW. Radiosensitivity of the human oocyte. Hum Reprod 2003;18:117–121.
18. Horning SJ, Hoppe RT, Kaplan HS, Rosenberg SA. Female reproductive potential after treatment for Hodgkin's disease. N Engl J Med 1981;304:1377–1382.
19. Lushbaugh CC, Casarett GW. The effects of gonadal irradiation in clinical radiation therapy: a review. Cancer 1976; 37:1111–1120.
20. Thibaud E, Ramirez M, Brauner R,. et al Preservation of ovarian function by ovarian transposition performed before pelvic irradiation during childhood. J Pediatr 1992;121:880–884.
21. Sarafoglou K, Boulad F, Gillio A, Sklar C. Gonadal function after bone marrow transplantation for acute leukemia during childhood. J Pediatr 1997;130:210–216.
22. Sklar C. Growth and endocrine disturbances after bone marrow transplantation in childhood. Acta Paediatr 1995; 411(suppl):57–61.
23. Sanders JE, Hawley J, Levy W, et al. Pregnancies following high-dose cyclophosphamide with or without high-dose busulfan or total-body irradiation and bone marrow transplantation. Blood 1996;87:3045–3052.

24. Armstrong GT, Sklar CA, Hudson MM, Robison LL. Long-term health status among survivors of childhood cancer: does sex matter? J Clin Oncol 2007;25:4477–4489.
25. Chow EJ, Friedman DL, Yasui Y, et al. timing of menarche among survivors of childhood acute lymphoblastic leukemia: a report from the childhood cancer survivor study. Pediatr Blood Cancer 2008;50:854–858.
26. Wallace W, Shalet SM, Crowne EC, Morris-Jones PH, Gattamaneni HR. Ovarian failure following abdominal irradiation in childhood: natural history and prognosis. Clin Oncol 1989;1:75–79.
27. Bath LE, Wallace WH, Critchley HO. Late effects of the treatment of childhood cancer on the female reproductive system and the potential for fertility preservation. BJOG 2002;1092:107–114.
28. Critchley HO, Wallace WH, Shalet SM, Mamtora H, Higginson J, Anderson DC. Abdominal irradiation in childhood: the potential for pregnancy. Br J Obstet Gynaecol 1992;99:392–394.
29. Green DM, Whitton JA, Stovall M, et al. Pregnancy outcome of female survivors of childhood cancer: a report from the Childhood Cancer Survivor Study. Am J Obstet Gynecol 2002;187:1070–1080.
30. Signorello LB, Cohen SS, Bosetti C, et al. Female survivors of childhood cancer: preterm birth and low birth weight among their children. J Natl Cancer Inst 2006;98: 1453–1461.
31. Sklar CA, Constine LS. Chronic neuroendocrinological sequelae of radiation therapy. Int J Radiat Oncol Biol Phys 1995;31:1113–1121.
32. Oktay K, Newton H, Aubard Y, Salha O, Gosden RG. Cryopreservation of immature human oocytes and ovarian tissue: an emerging technology? Fertil Steril 1998;69:1–7.
33. Shamonki MI, Oktay K. Oocyte and ovarian tissue cryopreservation: indications, techniques, and applications. Semin Reprod Med 2005;23:266–276.
34. Oktem O, Sonmezer M, Oktay K. Ovarian tissue cryopreservation and other fertility preserving strategies. In Gardner DK, Weismann A, Howles CM, Shoham Z eds. Textbook of Assisted Reproductive Techniques, 2nd Edition. Florida: Taylor & Francis 2004:315–327.
35. Baird DT, Webb R, Campbell BK, Harkness LM, Gosden RG. Long-term ovarian function in sheep after ovariectomy and transplantation of autografts stored at −196 C. Endocrinology 1999;140:462–471.
36. Oktay K. Ovarian cryopreservation and transplantation: preliminary findings and implications for cancer patients. Hum Reprod Update 2001;7:526–534.
37. Oktay K, Karlikaya G. Ovarian function after transplantation of frozen, banked autologous ovarian tissue. N Engl J Med 2000;342:1919.
38. Oktay K, Buyuk E, Veeck L, et al. Embryo development after heterotopic transplantation of cryopreserved ovarian tissue. Lancet 2004;363:837–840.
39. Oktay K, Oktem O. Regeneration of oocytes after chemotherapy: connecting the evidence from mouse to human. J Clin Oncol 2007;25:3185–3187.
40. Donnez J, Dolmans MM, Demylle D, et al. Livebirth after orthotopic transplantation of cryopreserved ovarian tissue. Lancet 2004;364:1405–1410.
41. Meirow D, Levron J, Eldar-Geva T, et al. Pregnancy after transplantation of cryopreserved ovarian tissue in a patient with ovarian failure after chemotherapy. N Engl J Med 2005;353:318–321.
42. Demeestere I, Simon P, Buxant F, et al. Ovarian function and spontaneous pregnancy after combined heterotopic and orthotopic cryopreserved ovarian tissue transplantation in a patient previously treated with bone marrow transplantation: case report. Hum Reprod 2006;21: 2010–2014.
43. Oktay K, Oktem O. Ovarian cryopreservation for fertility preservation and transplantation for fertility preservation for medical indications: report of an ongoing experience. Fertil Steril 2008 Nov 13. (Epub ahead of Print).
44. Borini A, Cattoli M, Bulletti C, Coticchio G. Clinical efficiency of oocyte and embryo cryopreservation. Ann N Y Acad Sci 2008;1127:49–58.
45. Oktay K, Hourvitz A, Sahin G, et al. Letrozole reduces estrogen and gonadotropin exposure in women with breast cancer undergoing ovarian stimulation before chemotherapy. J Clin Endocrinol Metab 2006;91:3885–3890.
46. Oktay K, Buyuk E, Libertella N, Akar M, Rosenwaks Z. Fertility preservation in breast cancer patients: a prospective controlled comparison of ovarian stimulation with tamoxifen and letrozole for embryo cryopreservation. J Clin Oncol 2005;23:4347–4353.
47. Fisher B, Costantino J, Redmond C, et al. A randomized clinical trial evaluating tamoxifen in the treatment of patients with node-negative breast cancer who have estrogen-receptor-positive tumors. N Engl J Med 1989;320:479–484.
48. Goss PE, Ingle JN, Martino S, et al. Arandomized trial of letrozole in postmenopausal women after five years of tamoxifen therapy for early-stage breast cancer. N Engl J Med 2003;349:1793–1802.
49. Chen C. Pregnancy after human oocyte cryopreservation. Lancet 1986;1:884–886.
50. Van Uem JFHM, Siebzehnruebl ER, Schuh B, et al. Birth after cryopreservation of unfertilized oocytes. Lancet 1987;1:752–753.
51. Chen C. Pregnancies after human oocyte cryopreservation. Ann N Y Acad Sci 1988;541:541–549.
52. Boiso I, Marti M, Santalo J, Ponsa M, Barri PN, Veiga A. A confocalmicroscopy analysis of the spindle and chromosome confi gurations of human oocytes cryopreserved at the germinal vesicle and metaphase II stage. Hum Reprod 2002;17:1885–1891.
53. Cobo A, Rubio C, Gerli S, Ruiz A, Pellicer A, Remohi J. Use of fluorescence in situ hybridization to assess the chromosomal status of embryos obtained from cryopreserved oocytes. Fertil Steril 2001;75:354–360.
54. Oktay K, Cil AP, Bang H. Efficiency of oocyte cryopreservation: a meta-analysis. Fertil Steril 2006;86:70–80.

# Section II
# Male Infertility

# Effect of Advanced Age on Male Infertility

Matthew Wosnitzer and Harry Fisch

**Abstract** Similar to females, males have biological clocks that affect the quality of their sperm, fertility levels, and hormone levels. Advanced paternal age increases the risk for occurrence of spontaneous abortion as well as genetic abnormalities in offspring due to multiple factors including DNA damage from abnormal apoptosis and reactive oxygen species. Increased paternal age is associated with a decrease in semen volume, percentage of normal sperm, and sperm motility. Males of advanced age must have a thorough physical examination with disclosure of sexual dysfunction and any medications that impair ejaculation or sperm formation. Men of advanced age should be counseled regarding the effects of paternal age on spermatogenesis and pregnancy. Future research will clarify novel treatments to increase fertility, reduce adverse genetic consequences, and increase the chance for a couple to have healthy children.

**Keywords** Male infertility • Paternal age • Spermatogenesis • Male biological clock

## 1 The Male Biological Clock

The concept of "biological clock" encompasses the decline in sex hormones, decline in fertility, and increased risk of pregnancy loss and congenital anomalies that are associated with advanced maternal age. Although typically associated with women, the biological clock is also applicable to men as advanced paternal age is linked with testosterone and fertility decline, as well as pregnancy loss (1). In this chapter, we review the effects of the male biological clock, and the association between advanced paternal age and decreased spermatogenesis and pregnancy rates. The approximately 1% per year decline in testosterone levels after the age of 30 has been documented in elderly men who have decreased concentrations of total and free testosterone (2, 3).

The most recent analysis, i.e., the Massachusetts Male Aging Study, a large population –based random-sample cohort, reported that 1,709 healthy men between ages 40 and 70 (mean age 55.2 years) had a mean total testosterone level of 520 ng/mL. With approximately 10 years of follow-up, this cohort included 1,156 healthy men (mean age 62.7 years) with a mean total testosterone level of 450 ng/mL. Feldman et al. quantified the decreasing testosterone levels as a cross-sectional decline of 0.8% per year of age and a longitudinal decline of 1.6% per year during follow-up. The rate of decline was not significantly different between healthy men and those with chronic illnesses or multiple co-morbidities (4). An estimated 2–4 million men in the United States suffer from such a decrease in testosterone ($T < 325$ ng/mL) (5).

The increasing prevalence of abnormally low testosterone levels in elderly men was also assessed as a part of the Baltimore Longitudinal Study on Aging, which determined that hypogonadal testosterone levels were present in approximately 20% of men over 60, 30% over 70, and 50% over 80 years of age (6). In this study, age was determined to be an independent predictor of longitudinal decline in both the total and free testosterone (2). The consequences of the correlation between age and decline in testosterone include decreased libido, muscle mass/strength, cognitive function as well

M. Wosnitzer and H. Fisch (✉)
Columbia University College of Physicians and Surgeons, Department of Urology, Columbia University Medical Center, 944 Park Avenue, New York, NY 10028, USA
e-mail: harryfisch@aol.com

D.T. Carrell et al. (eds.), *Biennial Review of Infertility,* DOI: 10.1007/978-1-60327-392-3_7

as increased incidence of erectile dysfunction, weight gain, type II diabetes, and cardiovascular disease including metabolic syndrome.

## 2 Advanced Paternal Age and Fertility

A reduction in fertility has been correlated with increasing paternal age. In women, a decline in estrogen production is associated with decreased oocyte production in the late thirties to early forties. Advanced maternal age also carries increased risk for genetic abnormalities in offspring. By contrast, there is no significant cessation of spermatogenesis in men with increasing age. There still remains the question regarding the effect of age on semen quality, risk of infertility, or congenital anomalies. Studies in the murine model have correlated histologic changes in testicular architecture with semen quality decline. At 18 months (defined as "older"), several age-related changes occur, including increased number of vacuoles in germ cells and thinning of seminiferous epithelium. At the age of 30 months, seminiferous epithelia with scant spermatocytes were identified. Overall, total sperm production was significantly reduced and mutation frequency was significantly increased in "older" mice (7–9).

Does such a correlation exist in humans? The effects of male aging on semen quality in men were described in a detailed review by Kidd et al. of all studies published between January 1980 and December 1999 (10). Parameters examined were semen volume, sperm concentration, sperm motility, sperm morphology, pregnancy rate, and time to pregnancy/subfecundity in the aging male. The literature (11 of 16 published studies) overall demonstrated a decrease in semen volume with advanced age. In two studies which adjusted for the confounder of abstinence duration, a decrease in semen volume of 0.15–0.5% was reported for each increase in year of age (11, 12). The semen volume of men aged 50 or older was decreased by 20–30% when compared with men younger than age 30 (10).

The correlation between sperm concentration and increasing age remains unclear (10). Of 21 studies examining this relationship, none documented a clear link between these parameters. Many of the studies did not adjust for duration of abstinence, so no clear association can be determined. The association of advanced paternal age and decreased sperm motility, however, is apparent in the literature. Kidd et al. reviewed 19 studies in this regard with the majority (13/19) studies identifying a decrease in sperm motility with increasing age. Five studies adjusted for the duration of abstinence and observed changes were statistically significant (12–16). A comparison of men age 50 or older to men younger than 30, revealed a 3–37% decline in motility. Decreased linear motion was identified in sperm of aging men in a study utilizing computer-assisted technology. This may indicate some reduction in fertility potential in older men despite normal appearing motility results during conventional semen analysis (17). The literature overall suggests that an inverse correlation exists between age and sperm motility.

Advanced paternal age is also correlated with abnormal sperm morphology. In 14 studies reviewed, 9 studies documented decrease in the % of normal sperm with increasing age and only 5 of these had a statistically significant finding. Two studies described that the % of normal sperm decreased by 0.2–0.9% per year of age when controlling for confounders of duration of abstinence and year of birth (11, 13). There were 5 studies that did not identify an association between % of normal sperm and age, but none of these reached statistical significance. The relationship between increasing age and decreasing semen volume, sperm motility, and sperm morphology support the conclusion that semen quality diminishes with increasing paternal age. Age-related changes to the germinal epithelium and prostate are one rationale for this impact on sperm parameters.

With the link between increased paternal age and adverse semen parameters, there remains the question regarding the effect of paternal age on fertility and offspring. The 9 out of 11 studies evaluating the association between male age and subfecundity identified a strong correlation between paternal age and time required for a couple to achieve pregnancy (10). Of the 9 studies, 7 demonstrated a statistically significant increase in time to pregnancy with increased male age. Increased risks of subfecundity with older age groups ranged from 11 to 250%. Of the studies conducted on the female partner's age (a well-established independent predictor affecting conception), fertility rate in males was greater, but for those above the age of 50 it was 23–38% lower than that of men younger than 30 years (15, 18). When stratified as 35 years or greater and less than 30 years, there was a 60% decrease in the chance of initiating pregnancy in the older group. The risk of delayed conception was validated in a study of 8,515 planned pregnancies in which older men were significantly less likely to impregnate their partners in less than 6 or less than 12 months compared with the younger comparison group. This result remained statistically significant after adjustment for various confounding factors. The odds ratio for conception within 6 months decreased by 2% per year of age and for conception within 12 months decreased by 3% per year of age. The probability that a fertile couple will take more than 12 months to conceive nearly doubles from 8% when younger than 25 years to 15% when greater than 35 years.

Overall there is the adjustment of potential confounders and age-group stratifications in literature, but no definitive conclusion regarding linearity of relationship between a man's age, semen parameters, or fertility can be proven.

## 3 Advanced Paternal Age and Pregnancy Outcomes

There now seems to be a significant increase in paternal age in the United States with postponement of childbearing by many couples until their mid-thirties to mid-forties. CDC birth statistics show the average maternal age in 2003 was 25.1 years, which is increased from the average maternal age of 21.4 years in 1974. Paternal age is simultaneously increasing among American men. The birth rate of children of men less than 25 years has been decreasing while the birth rate of children fathered by men 25–44 years has been increasing since the 1970s (19). Increasing paternal age seems to result in a higher incidence of spontaneous abortions, autosomal dominant disorders, trisomy 21, and schizophrenia. An understanding of the effects of increasing parental age on a developing fetus is required to properly counsel older couples who are considering childbearing. Data from recent studies confirms an association between advanced paternal age and the risk of spontaneous abortion. In the prospective study of 5,121 American women, the risk of spontaneous abortion increased with advanced paternal age (20). Pregnancies fathered by men 50 years or older had almost twice the risk of spontaneous abortion compared to pregnancies from younger fathers after adjustment for maternal age, reproductive history, and maternal lifestyle in a prospective analysis of 23, 821 women from the Danish National Birth Cohort (21).

There is still debate in current literature as to which trimester is at the greatest risk from advanced paternal age, even though the correlation between advanced paternal age and spontaneous abortion is very well demonstrated. A retrospective multi-center European study revealed that the affects of advanced paternal age and maternal age are cumulative. If both partners are advanced in age, the risk of spontaneous abortion is higher. Chromosomal abnormalities in the developing fetus are thought to be a significant underlying factor in this increased risk of spontaneous abortion (22).

As described earlier in this chapter, increasing paternal age is associated with a decrease in semen volume, percentage of normal sperm, and sperm motility. The genetic integrity of the sperm is also at risk with advanced paternal age (15). Age is associated with the number of Leydig cells and Sertoli cells, and an increase in arrested division of germ cells (23). Spermatozoa are continuously produced and undergo lifelong replication, meiosis, and spermatogenesis in contrast to oogenesis in the aging female (24). There are some spontaneous mutations within the parental cell line with continuous replication. An essential aspect of spermatogenesis that ensures selection of normal DNA is the process of apoptosis of sperm with damaged DNA (25). The rate of genetic abnormalities during spermatogenesis increases as men age. In humans, the frequency of numerical and structural aberrations in sperm chromosomes increases with increasing paternal age (26). The cause of such damage to DNA is undetermined at this time, but aberrant apoptosis and oxidative stress have both been implicated (27). Spermatozoa have low concentrations of antioxidant scavenging enzymes which makes them particularly susceptible to DNA damage from reactive oxygen species (28). A recent study of 98 fertile men (78 patients were younger than 40 years, and 20 patients were 40 years or older) recently identified that seminal reactive oxygen species levels are significantly elevated in healthy fertile men older than 40 years of age (27).

With advanced paternal age, aneuploidy errors in germ cell lines also occur at higher rates. A common aneuploidy error that affects newborns is trisomy 21 or Down syndrome at a rate of 1/800 to 1/1,000 births (29).

Advanced maternal age and trisomy 21 were first documented to be associated in 1933 (30). The trisomy 21 rate increases exponentially from the maternal age of 35 years according to the amniocentesis data from the European collaborative study of Ferguson-Smith and Yates (31). It is only more recently that the effects of advanced paternal age have also been documented. An increased risk of Down syndrome with a paternal age of 50 years or greater was found in the Medical Birth Registry of Norway from 1967 to 1978 which included 685,000 births with 693 cases of Down syndrome (32). A paternal age effect was apparent when paternal age was 35 years or greater and was most pronounced when the maternal age was 40 years or greater in the New York State Department of Health Congenital Malformation Registry which contained 3,419 trisomy 21 births from 1983 to 1997 (33). The rate of Down syndrome with a combined parental age greater than 40 years, was 60/10,000 births, which when compared with parents less than 35 years of age, was a six fold increase. Both advanced paternal age and advanced maternal age significantly increased the risk of trisomy 21 (34).

The age-related increase in sperm cells with highly damaged DNA results from both increased double strand DNA breaks and decreased apoptosis during spermatogenesis (35). Many autosomal dominant disorders such as Apert syndrome, achrondroplasia, osteogenesis imperfecta, progeria, Marfan syndrome, Waardenburg syndrome, and thanatophoric dysplasia are associated with advanced paternal age (36). Apert syndrome is the result of an autosomal dominant mutation on chromosome 10, mutating fibroblast growth factor receptor 2 (FGFR2). With increasing paternal age, the incidence of sporadic Apert syndrome increases exponentially with paternal age resulting in part from an increased frequency of FGFR2 mutations in the sperm of older men (37). An autosomal dominant mutation on FGFR3 results in achondroplasia. The clinical achondroplasia registry data reveals that 50 of affected children were born to men 35 years or older. There was an exponential increase in the rate of achondroplasia with increasing paternal age (38). An autosomal dominant mutation in FGFR3 results entirely from the paternal allele in the Muenke-type craniosynostosis (39). Men as young as 35 years of age are at higher risk for many autosomal dominant disorders, especially costochondrodysplasias.

Spontaneous mutations arising in paternal germ cells can be associated with schizophrenia. There is evidence for a genetic component for schizophrenia although it has an unclear etiology (40). In studies from the 1960s and 1970s there was a suggested association. This has been confirmed by recent studies showing the association between schizophrenia and advanced paternal age (41). Whereas maternal age demonstrated no affect on the development of schizophrenia, a 12-year evaluation of the Jerusalem Birth Registry and the Israel Psychiatric Registry, which includes 658 persons with schizophrenia, showed that the risk of schizophrenia increased monotonically with increasing paternal age (42). Another study from Israel found a significant association between the risk of autism and advancing paternal age (43). Offspring of men 40 years or older were 5.75 times more likely to have autism than the children of males younger than 30 years of age. Advancing age of the mother showed no association with autism when paternal age was adjusted (43).

Olshan et al. found 4,110 heart defects in the British Columbia Health Surveillance Registry from 1952 to 1973 (44). There was a suggestive general pattern of increased risk with increasing paternal age for atrial septal defects, ventricular septal defects, and patent ductus arteriosus. But the authors estimated that only 5% of cases might be the result of advanced paternal age greater than 35 years. They did find an increased risk of ventricular septal defects and atrial septal defects when the father was younger than 20 years of age. Either errors in division of germ cells over time, cigarette smoking, or alcohol may have contributed (44).

## 4 Medications and Comorbidities

The aging male who is taking multiple medications such as antihypertensive drugs, antidepressants, and hormonal agents may have a pharmacologically mediated infertility and some sexual dysfunction (45). Seminal emission can be blocked by alpha blocker medications, used for treatment of symptoms of the lower urinary tract. Gonadotropin-releasing hormone agonists, which are used for prostate cancer treatment, can directly affect sperm production. Severe disruption of sperm production occurs as a result of the castrate levels of testosterone. Whereas testosterone therapy used for hypo-gonadism impairs spermatogenesis, it is usually reversible. Extremely high doses of anabolic steroids or multiple agents, sometimes used for enhancement of performance and muscle enlargement, cause reduction of sperm production that may be permanent (45).

When drugs such as alpha-1 adrenoceptor antagonists or 5 alpha-reductase inhibitors are used individually or in combination, male reproductive problems can occur. Erectile dysfunction, ejaculatory disorders, and decreased libido can be caused by the 5-alpha-reductase inhibitors. Greatly reduced ejaculatory volume, or failure of seminal emission occurs in men with the use of alpha blockers (45). Ejaculatory volumes can decrease by 25% in men taking 5 mg of finasteride daily. In men taking 1 mg of finasteride daily for hair loss, there was no change in the semen parameters (45).

Aging and associated erectile dysfunction in some men has resulted in the use of oral phosphodiesterase inhibitors such as sildenafil, tadalafil, and vardenafil. Using computer-assisted semen analysis and acrosome-reaction testing by fluorescein staining, it was found that the number of progressively motile sperm was increased with sildenafil. There was also a significant increase in the proportion of acrosome-reacted sperm (46). In a study on the effects of taedalafil, chronic administration had no effects on semen volume, sperm concentration, morphology, or motility (47).

Sexual function and reproductive function can substantially decline in males treated for prostate cancer. Treatments such as radiotherapy, surgery or hormones, alone or in combination can result in these dysfunctions in younger males as well as those in the fourth and fifth decades of life (48, 49). Some aggressive prostate cancers have been reported to be associated with low testosterone and the initial presentation has been sexual dysfunction and impaired fertility (50–52). A recent report found that ultrasound-guided needle biopsy of the prostate was associated with some abnormal semen parameters (53). Since prostate biopsy is more common in men in the 50 years or older group, this can be an issue for some older men who wish to father children.

## 5 Conclusions

Similar to females, males have biological clocks that affect the quality of their sperm, fertility levels, and hormone levels. Advanced paternal age increases the risk for occurrence of spontaneous abortion as well as genetic abnormalities in offspring. The decreasing apoptotic rate, increase in reactive oxygen species, and constantly replicating spermatogonia are the probable causes of amplified errors in the male germ cell line with advanced age. An increase in chromosomal abnormalities in the aging male increases rates of spontaneous abortion, trisomy 21, schizophrenia and autosomal dominant disorders.

In older men, a complete medical history with attention to medications and prior surgical and medical history is critical. Medications that impair ejaculation, or sperm formation may need to be discontinued with the approval of their prescribing physician. Oral phosphodiesterase inhibitors may be required to improve erectile function. If the couple is to have IVF, preimplantation genetic screening is more readily available now, especially if there is a concern for a health risk issue in the fetus (54, 55). If a familial history of genetic defects exists, the couple should consult a geneticist regarding risks to the fetus and their decision to pursue a pregnancy.

With future studies, the effects of the male biological clock and advanced paternal age on fertility and birth defects will be further elucidated. Novel methods to reverse or slow down the male biologic clock will be discovered by improved understanding of the cellular and biochemical mechanisms of gonadal aging. This research will diminish potential adverse genetic consequences in the offspring and increase the couple's chance of having a healthy child (34).

## References

1. Lewis BH, Legato M, Fisch H. Medical implications of the male biological clock. JAMA 2006;296(19):2369–71.
2. Gray A, Berlin JA, McKinlay JB, Longcope C. An examination of research design effects on the association of testosterone and male aging: results of a meta-analysis. J Clin Epidemiol 1991;44(7):671–84.
3. Sparrow D, Bosse R, Rowe JW. The influence of age, alcohol consumption, and body build on gonadal function in men. J Clin Endocrinol Metab 1980;51(3):508–12.
4. Feldman HA, Longcope C, Derby CA, et al. Age trends in the level of serum testosterone and other hormones in middle-aged men: longitudinal results from the Massachusetts male aging study. J Clin Endocrinol Metab 2002;87(2):589–98.
5. Rhoden EL, Morgentaler A. Risks of testosterone-replacement therapy and recommendations for monitoring. N Engl J Med 2004;350(5):482–92.

6. Harman SM, Metter EJ, Tobin JD, Pearson J, Blackman MR. Longitudinal effects of aging on serum total and free testosterone levels in healthy men. Baltimore Longitudinal Study of Aging. J Clin Endocrinol Metab 2001;86(2): 724–31.
7. Serre V, Robaire B. Paternal age affects fertility and progeny outcome in the Brown Norway rat. Fertil Steril 1998;70(4):625–31.
8. Tanemura K, Kurohmaru M, Kuramoto K, Hayashi Y. Age-related morphological changes in the testis of the BDF1 mouse. J Vet Med Sci 1993;55(5):703–10.
9. Walter CA, Intano GW, McCarrey JR, McMahan CA, Walter RB. Mutation frequency declines during spermatogenesis in young mice but increases in old mice. Proc Natl Acad Sci U S A 1998;95(17):10015–9.
10. Kidd SA, Eskenazi B, Wyrobek AJ. Effects of male age on semen quality and fertility: a review of the literature. Fertil Steril 2001;75(2):237–48.
11. Andolz P, Bielsa MA, Vila J. Evolution of semen quality in North-eastern Spain: a study in 22,759 infertile men over a 36 year period. Hum Reprod 1999;14(3):731–5.
12. Fisch H, Goluboff ET, Olson JH, Feldshuh J, Broder SJ, Barad DH. Semen analyses in 1,283 men from the United States over a 25-year period: no decline in quality. Fertil Steril 1996;65(5):1009–14.
13. Auger J, Kunstmann JM, Czyglik F, Jouannet P. Decline in semen quality among fertile men in Paris during the past 20 years. N Engl J Med 1995;332(5):281–5.
14. Henkel R, Bittner J, Weber R, Huther F, Miska W. Relevance of zinc in human sperm flagella and its relation to motility. Fertil Steril 1999;71(6):1138–43.
15. Rolf C, Behre HM, Nieschlag E. Reproductive parameters of older compared to younger men of infertile couples. Int J Androl 1996;19(3):135–42.
16. Schwartz D, Mayaux MJ, Spira A, et al. Semen characteristics as a function of age in 833 fertile men. Fertil Steril 1983;39(4):530–5.
17. Sloter E, Schmid TE, Marchetti F, Eskenazi B, Nath J, Wyrobek AJ. Quantitative effects of male age on sperm motion. Hum Reprod 2006;21(11):2868–75.
18. Mathieu C, Ecochard R, Bied V, Lornage J, Czyba JC. Cumulative conception rate following intrauterine artificial insemination with husband's spermatozoa: influence of husband's age. Hum Reprod 1995;10(5):1090–7.
19. Hamilton BE, Martin JA, Sutton PD. Births: preliminary data for 2002. Natl Vital Stat Rep 2003;51(11):1–20.
20. Slama R, Bouyer J, Windham G, Fenster L, Werwatz A, Swan SH. Influence of paternal age on the risk of spontaneous abortion. Am J Epidemiol 2005;161(9):816–23.
21. Nybo Andersen AM, Hansen KD, Andersen PK, Davey Smith G. Advanced paternal age and risk of fetal death: a cohort study. Am J Epidemiol 2004;160(12):1214–22.
22. de la Rochebrochard E, Thonneau P. Paternal age and maternal age are risk factors for miscarriage; results of a multicentre European study. Hum Reprod 2002;17(6):1649–56.
23. Tsitouras PD. Effects of age on testicular function. Endocrinol Metab Clin North Am 1987;16(4):1045–59.
24. Evans HJ. Mutation and mutagenesis in inherited and acquired human disease. The first EEMS Frits Sobels Prize Lecture, Noordwijkerhout, The Netherlands, June 1995. Mutat Res 1996;351(2):89–103.
25. Roosen-Runge EC. Germinal-cell loss in normal metazoan spermatogenesis. J Reprod Fertil 1973;35(2):339–48.
26. Sartorelli EM, Mazzucatto LF, de Pina-Neto JM. Effect of paternal age on human sperm chromosomes. Fertil Steril 2001;76(6):1119–23.
27. Cocuzza M, Athayde KS, Agarwal A, et al. Age-related increase of reactive oxygen species in neat semen in healthy fertile men. Urology 2008;71(3):490–4.
28. Lewis SE, Boyle PM, McKinney KA, Young IS, Thompson W. Total antioxidant capacity of seminal plasma is different in fertile and infertile men. Fertil Steril 1995;64(4):868–70.
29. Cunningham FMP, Gant N, Leven K, Gilstrap C, Hankins G, et al. Williams Obstetrics. 21st edn. New York: McGraw-Hill; 1997.
30. Fisch H, Golden RJ, Libersen GL, et al. Maternal age as a risk factor for hypospadias. J Urol 2001;165(3):934–6.
31. Ferguson-Smith MA, Yates JR. Maternal age specific rates for chromosome aberrations and factors influencing them: report of a collaborative european study on 52 965 amniocenteses. Prenat Diagn 1984;4 Spec No:5–44.
32. Erickson JD, Bjerkedal TO. Down syndrome associated with father's age in Norway. J Med Genet 1981;18(1):22–8.
33. Fisch H, Hyun G, Golden R, Hensle TW, Olsson CA, Liberson GL. The influence of paternal age on down syndrome. J Urol 2003;169(6):2275–8.
34. Fisch H. The Male Biological Clock. New York: Free Press; 2005.
35. Singh NP, Muller CH, Berger RE. Effects of age on DNA double-strand breaks and apoptosis in human sperm. Fertil Steril 2003;80(6):1420–30.
36. Lian ZH, Zack MM, Erickson JD. Paternal age and the occurrence of birth defects. Am J Hum Genet 1986;39(5): 648–60.
37. Glaser RL, Broman KW, Schulman RL, Eskenazi B, Wyrobek AJ, Jabs EW. The paternal-age effect in Apert syndrome is due, in part, to the increased frequency of mutations in sperm. Am J Hum Genet 2003;73(4):939–47.
38. Orioli IM, Castilla EE, Scarano G, Mastroiacovo P. Effect of paternal age in achondroplasia, thanatophoric dysplasia, and osteogenesis imperfecta. Am J Med Genet 1995;59(2):209–17.
39. Rannan-Eliya SV, Taylor IB, De Heer IM, Van Den Ouweland AM, Wall SA, Wilkie AO. Paternal origin of FGFR3 mutations in Muenke-type craniosynostosis. Hum Genet 2004;115(3):200–7.
40. Kendler KS, Diehl SR. The genetics of schizophrenia: a current, genetic-epidemiologic perspective. Schizophr Bull 1993;19(2):261–85.
41. Hare EMP. Raised paternal age in psychiatric patients: evidence for the constitutional hypothesis. Br J Psychiatry 1979;134:169–77.
42. Malaspina D, Harlap S, Fennig S, et al. Advancing paternal age and the risk of schizophrenia. Arch Gen Psychiatry 2001;58(4):361–7.
43. Reichenberg A, Gross R, Weiser M, et al. Advancing paternal age and autism. Arch Gen Psychiatry 2006; 63(9):1026–32.
44. Olshan AF, Schnitzer PG, Baird PA. Paternal age and the risk of congenital heart defects. Teratology 1994;50(1):80–4.
45. Francis ME, Kusek JW, Nyberg LM, Eggers PW. The contribution of common medical conditions and drug exposures to

erectile dysfunction in adult males. J Urol 2007;178(2):591–6; discussion 6.
46. Glenn DR, McVicar CM, McClure N, Lewis SE. Sildenafil citrate improves sperm motility but causes a premature acrosome reaction in vitro. Fertil Steril 2007;87(5):1064–70.
47. Hellstrom WJ, Overstreet JW, Yu A, et al. Tadalafil has no detrimental effect on human spermatogenesis or reproductive hormones. J Urol 2003;170(3):887–91.
48. Lazarou S, Morgentaler A. The effect of aging on spermatogenesis and pregnancy outcomes. Urol Clin North Am 2008;35(2):331–9.
49. Sakr WA, Haas GP, Cassin BF, Pontes JE, Crissman JD. The frequency of carcinoma and intraepithelial neoplasia of the prostate in young male patients. J Urol 1993;150(2 Pt 1):379–85.
50. Hoffman MA, DeWolf WC, Morgentaler A. Is low serum free testosterone a marker for high grade prostate cancer? J Urol 2000;163(3):824–7.
51. Morgentaler A. Testosterone deficiency and prostate cancer: emerging recognition of an important and troubling relationship. Eur Urol 2007;52(3):623–5.
52. Penson DF, Chan JM. Prostate cancer. J Urol 2007;177(6): 2020–9.
53. Smith A SP, Nagle HM. Does Transrectal ultrasound guided needle biopsy of prostate affect semen parameters? J Urol 2007;177(3 Suppl):597.
54. Braude P, Pickering S, Flinter F, Ogilvie CM. Preimplantation genetic diagnosis. Nat Rev Genet 2002;3(12):941–53.
55. Collins JA. Preimplantation genetic screening in older mothers. N Engl J Med 2007;357(1):61–3.

# Genetic Variants in Male Infertility

Mounia Tannour-Louet and Dolores J. Lamb

**Abstract** Different types of genetic variants are present in the genome. Single nucleotide polymorphisms, or SNPs, are minor variations in the genetic sequence that differ between members of a species or even between paired chromosomes in an individual. There are common SNPs that occur in at least 1% of a population. These SNPs may be specific to an ethnic group or between individuals of a geographic region. There are also rare SNPs with minor allele frequencies of less than 1%. As will be seen in this chapter, these SNPs can be located in the non-coding regions of genes, such as the 5T allele in the cystic fibrosis transmembrane conductance regulator gene (CFTR) associated with congenital bilateral absence of the vas deferens, or within coding regions. Some SNPs are silent with no effect whereas others may act like a rheostat to influence disease susceptibility or severity, response to drugs or chemicals or immunological stimuli or infectious diseases. SNPs appear also to be very helpful in forensics to identify or exclude criminals based upon DNA evidence or in paternity testing. Copy number variants (CNVs) are gains or losses of large pieces of DNA consisting of 10,000–5 million nucleotides. Genetic diseases and even susceptibility to infections and complex diseases can be caused by CNVs. This chapter first describes SNPs and CNVs- their detection and importance and then focuses on SNPs in male infertility, including those impacting congenital disorders as well as reproductive function.

**Keywords** Male fertility • Single nucleotide polymorphism • Genetic variants • Mutation • Copy number variants (CNV)

M. Tannour-Louet and D.J. Lamb(✉)
Scott Department of Urology, Baylor College of Medicine, Houston, TX, 77030, USA
e-mail: dlamb@bmc.tmc.edu

## 1 A "Multifaceted" Genome

The 23 pairs of chromosomes that exist in each of our cells contain information that governs our physical appearance and traits, our susceptibility to develop diseases, as well as our responses to environmental influences. When the chromosomes of two distinct individuals are compared, genetic sequences encrypted by more than 6 billion of bases, display a remarkable degree of similarity. But at a rate of about one in every 1,200 bases (on average), the sequences will be slightly different. Several types of genetic variations exist: insertions, deletions or inversions, repetitions of elements and copy number variations. It is estimated that currently, nearly 12% of the human genome is "multifaceted" in this way (1). Most changes are not considered deleterious. However, others play a significant role in numerous human anomalies and syndromes.

As previously described, the genetic differences that affect one pair of bases either by substitution or by deletion or insertion of a base are known as single nucleotide polymorphisms, or SNPs (Fig. 1). These point changes are by far the most common type of genetic variation (http://www.ncbi.nlm.nih.gov/About/primer/snps.html). Indeed, approximately 10 million SNPs are estimated to commonly occur in the human genome. There are different types of SNPs (Fig. 2):

(a) *Synonymous SNP* that do not change the sequence of amino acids,
(b) *Not Synonymous SNP* (nsSNP) that change the amino acid causing polymorphism in a protein,
(c) *Regulatory SNP* (rSNP) that affect the expression or function of the protein in question.

The latter two types of SNPs (nsSNP and rSNP) are relatively rare compared to the total number of existing

D.T. Carrell et al. (eds.), *Biennial Review of Infertility,* DOI: 10.1007/978-1-60327-392-3_8

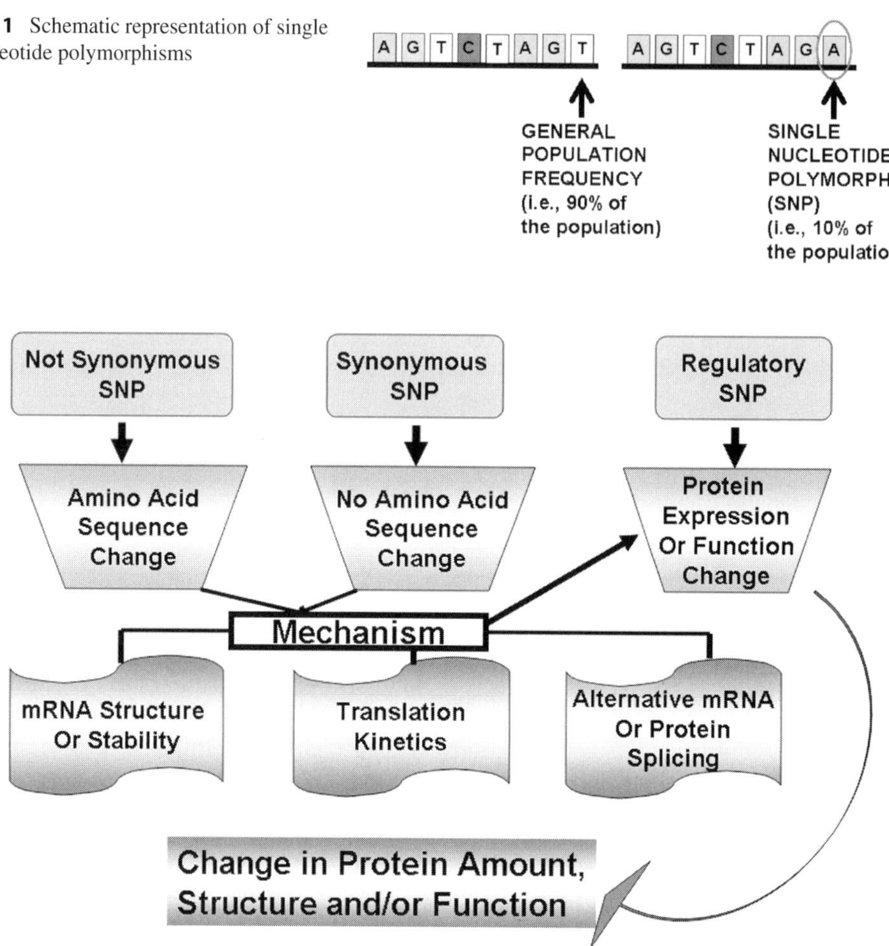


**Fig. 1** Schematic representation of single nucleotide polymorphisms

**Fig. 2** SNP categories and their action on mRNA structure, stability or processing ultimately affecting protein expression, amount, structure and/or function

SNPs in the human genome. Some of these variants might be involved in the occurrence of pathologies but it is still difficult to specify their impact depending simply on the basis of the nucleotide sequence, even if the variant does not change amino acid or does not disturb the structure of the protein.

CNVs represent a type of genetic variability not recognized until the development of G-banding karyotyping and later the advent of molecular cytogenetics. These variations are defined as deletions and duplications of DNA segments larger than 1,000 bases and up to several Mb when compared with a reference genome. Using a molecular karyotype (an array of bacterial artificial chromosomes (BACs) and later oligonucleotides) it was discovered that the human genome contains a large number of these CNVs distributed throughout the genome. These CNVs can affect the gene dosage and gene expression levels ultimately influencing phenotypic diversity, as well as disease susceptibility. Some CNVs can affect transcription over large genomic distances of as much as 5 Mb.

## 2 Strategies Used for SNP and CNV Detection

There are currently two main approaches commonly used for SNP detection: the candidate gene approach and the whole-genome scan. The candidate gene approach is the most widely used strategy and aims to investigate the role of one particular susceptibility gene in disease aetiology where gene polymorphisms are considered as a risk factor. Several reliable SNP genotyping technologies like SNaPShot, TaqMan, SNP-IT, Mass Array and Invader assay were developed for this specific use (2–7). Most of these technologies rely on polymerase chain reaction to amplify signals except the Invader. But, due to the ever growing number of SNPs identified and the need to simultaneously interrogate multiple SNPs to encrypt genetic signals associated with a specific clinical condition, multiplex genotyping systems were developed. Few SNPs (10–12 for Mass Array or SNPstream respectively) to thousands of SNPs (1,536 for Illumina's BeadArray and 25,000 for Molecular Inversion Probes from ParAllele) can then be easily detected (8–11). Low-end multiplexing systems are based on single-base extension assays while the others use allele-specific extension and ligation as the main biochemical reactions. All of these technologies depend on polymerase chain reaction to amplify signals for proper detection. Accordingly, when the knowledge of genes involved in a certain disease is limited, the alternative strategy of scanning the whole-genome appears more suitable. This approach allows scanning for multiple SNP markers distributed across several genes in the human genome using SNP arrays. These chips are high-density oligonucleotide-based arrays that comprise up to 500,000 SNPs. Each SNP probe, consisting of a 25-mer oligonucleotide, is represented on the array with both a sense and an antisense strands. The fluorescent probe intensities corresponding to the two possible alleles of the SNP reveal which of the three expected genotypes (for example, AA, BB or AB) is present. Two commercial platforms currently exist: the GeneChip system developed by Affymetrix and the Infinium assay developed by Illumina. The GeneChip system is based on the hybridization of amplified genomic DNA onto the SNP chips. Discrimination of single-base differences is based on the hybridization strength between the oligonucleotides on the chip and the genomic DNA. The Illumina assay performs an allele-specific extension and signal amplification on the chip instead of hybridization. Both assays provide high quality genotype data.

CNVs are detected today using comparative genomic hybridization arrays (CGH arrays) consisting of oligonucleotides that can span the entire genome with large numbers of 60-mer probes (40,000 or so) immobilized on a chip (Fig. 3). With reference DNA stained with a fluorescent green dye and patient DNA stained with a fluorescent red dye, the samples in equimolar concentration are mixed and hybridized to the array (Fig. 3). If the regions of DNA are present in the same concentration the individual loci will fluoresce yellow. A loss in the patient will fluoresce green and a gain will fluoresce red. These submicroscopic chromosome gains and losses can encompass many genes and/or regulatory sequences.

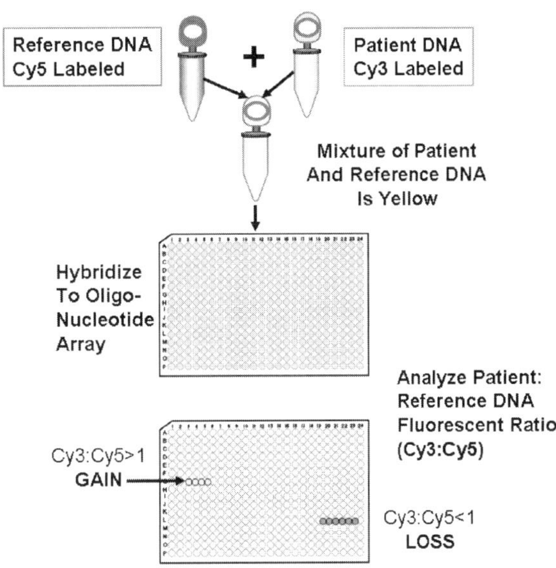


**Fig. 3** Comparative genomic hybridization (CGH) array provides one approach to identification of chromosome gains and losses. Shown in the *upper panel* is the basic approach to CGH array. Reference DNA from a gender matched control is labeled with a red fluorescent dye (Cy5) and the patient DNA is labeled with a green fluorescent dye, Cy3. The two stained DNA samples are mixed together resulting in a yellow fluorescence (equal amounts of red + green = yellow). After hybridization of the fluorescent labeled DNA to an oligonucleotide (or BAC) array, the chip is analyzed for the presence of green or red fluorescence. *Green fluorescence* indicates a Cy3:Cyr5 ratio greater than 1 denoting a chromosome gain. Multiple overlapping clones are positive for green fluorescence in the region. Similarly, when the C3:C5 ratio is less than 1 the spots *fluoresce red* denoting a region of chromosome loss in the patient. Again, multiple overlapping clones show the region of loss. The *lower panel* shows an actual analysis of gender mismatched DNA to illustrate the principles of the assay. In this study a BAC array was illustrate and female DNA patient DNA competed with male reference DNA and then hybridized to the CGH array. The array shows the loss of the entire Y chromosome in the XX female and the gain of an extra X chromosome. (*see Color Plates*)

**CGH Array (Female Patient: Male Reference) Shows**

**Principles of Analysis:**

- **Examines the genome at a resolution of 1 Mb intervals (or less)**
- **Detects abnormalities at a rate: ~12%**
- **Detects 99% of clinically significant abnormalities detected by karyotype**
  - XX Female shows X gain and absence of Y when tested against male reference DNA
- **High-throughput analysis using minimal amounts of DNA**

**Limitation**

**Unable to detect balanced translocations**

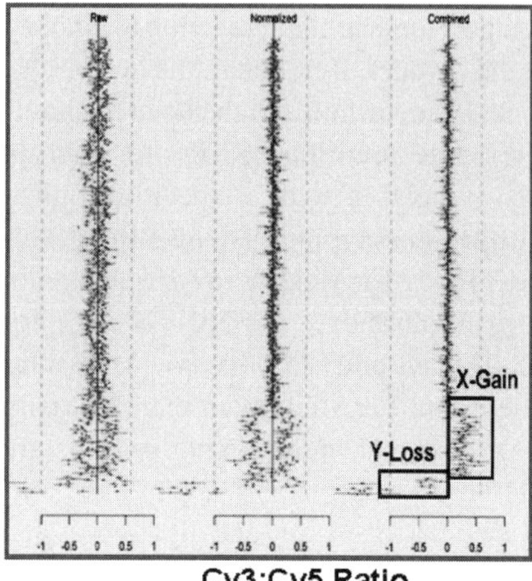


**Fig. 3** (continued) (*see Color Plates*)

## 3 Genome-Wide Genetic Variant Association Studies and Their Clinical Impact

SNPs are distributed uniformly throughout the genome and, as microsatellites, are used to build linkage cards. Indeed, genetic variants that are physically located close to each other tend to be inherited together. For instance, all individuals who have a G rather than an A at a specific location in a chromosome can have identical genetic variants at other SNPs in the chromosomal region surrounding the G. These regions of linked variants are known as haplotypes. By identifying most of the existing SNPs in populations from different parts of the world, the International HapMap Project is providing researchers precious information about how SNPs are organized on chromosomes (12). The number of "haplotype tag" SNPs (htSNPs) that uniquely characterize the common haplotypes, is estimated to be about 300,000–600,000 in one individual, which is far fewer than the 10 million common SNPs. Thus, an htSNP selected on the basis of linkage disequilibrium has the potential to reduce the amount of genotyping needed per gene for the identification of genetic variants associated with a specific clinical condition. Researchers only need to "genotype" the tag SNPs in affected patients and by association studies, compare the haplotypes in these affected individuals to the haplotypes of a control group of unaffected persons. If a particular haplotype or CNV occurs more frequently in affected individuals when compared with control groups of unaffected individuals, a gene influencing the disease may be located within or close to that haplotype (Fig. 4). An emerging number of genetic variants associated with common diseases are being discovered (13–15). Knowledge derived from these discoveries will have a significant potential for the establishment of new approaches for improving clinical prevention, patient diagnosis and disease treatment in many medical fields.

### *3.1 Genetic Variants Can Impact Patient Pharmacologic Treatment*

#### 3.1.1 A Clinical Example of SNP Importance

The discovery of clinically predictive genotypes and haplotypes together with the recent approval of genetic tests and incorporation of genetic information linked to the dosage in package inserts by the FDA were an

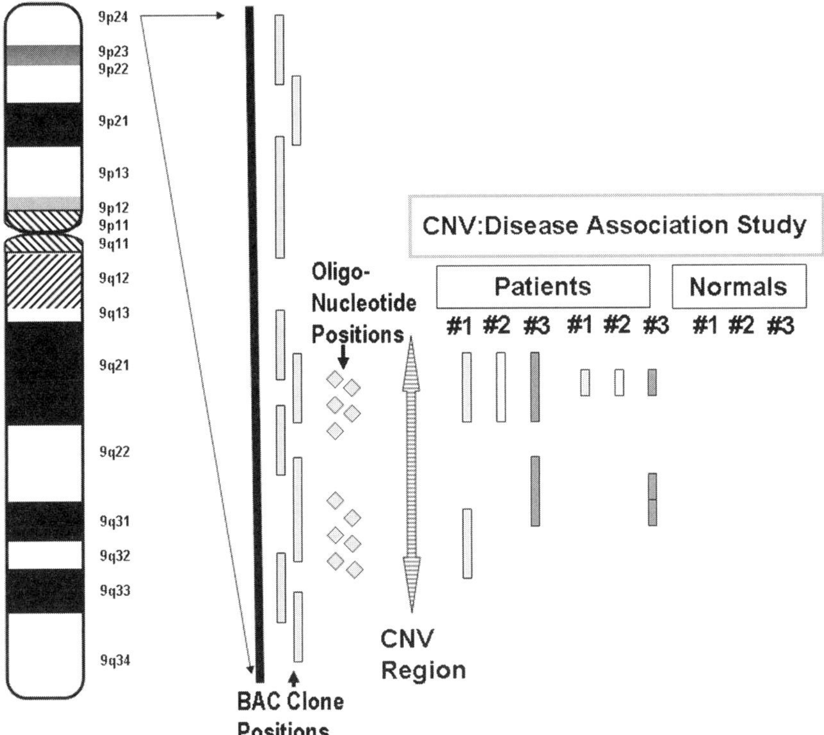


**Fig. 4** CNV: Disease associations are discovered by CGH array spanning all chromosomes. In this figure, analysis of chromosome 9 is depicted. Three Patients and three normal controls are analyzed using both a BAC array and an oligonucleotide array. The overlapping BAC clone positions spanning chromosome region 9p24 are shown. In the oligonucleotide array, the probe positions are clustered in two specific candidate regions. Analysis shows that the patients were positive for one specific genetic variant (the upper probes) while a variable CNV region shown below was also evident. These variable regions did not show areas of chromosome gain or loss in the normal controls. Adapted from http://projects.tcag.ca/variation from the database of Genomic Variants

important milestone (16–18). These actions provided the first step towards the clinical integration of the information provided by the SNP analysis with the treatment of the disease. The UGT1A genotype described below and its impact on the Irinotecan dosage in the cancer treatment is the most illustrative example of the potential for such SNP association studies to be integrated into clinical practice.

Irinotecan (CPT-11; Camptosar) is a camptothecin analogue approved for treatment of advanced colorectal cancer and lung, brain and breast tumors. The active form of Irinotecan, SN-38, can be inactivated through glucuronidation by a member of the UDP glucuronosyltransferase family, UGT1A1, an enzyme responsible for hepatic bilirubin glucuronidation. Variability in UGT1A1 expression leads to inter-individual variation in SN-38G formation (19–21). This variability is in part due to the presence of a polymorphic dinucleotide repeat identified in the UGT1A1 promoter TATA element which consists of 5, 6, 7, or 8 copies of a TA repeat [(TA)nTAA], with the $(TA)_6$TAA allele the considered wild-type. The longer the repeat allele, the lower is the corresponding level of UGT1A1 gene expression. The presence of more than 6 TA repeats in the UGT1A1 promoter region leads to less SN-38 being inactivated. Excess SN-38 is consequently retained in the cell, leading to severe toxicity, including potentially fatal neutropenia and diarrhea. In 2005, the FDA approved the inclusion of UGT1A1 genotype information in the Irinotecan package insert with dosing guidelines based on UGT1A1 genotype (22), (http://www.fda.gov/medwatch/safety/2005/jul_PI/Camptosar_PI.pdf). One month later, the FDA approved a clinical test for the most frequently reported variant of UGT1A1 allele (http://www.fda.gov/bbs/topics/NEWS/2005/NEW01220.html).

### 3.2 The Benefit of Defining Genetic Variants in Male Fertility

Building on these precedents, additional research has the potential to rapidly expand SNP and CNV studies in diverse clinical arenas, including male infertility (Table 1). Until now, the molecular basis of impaired spermatogenesis can only be explained in a very small subset of infertile patients, which is not surprising as male factor infertility is thought to be a complex disorder involving multiple genes as suggested by gene targeting studies in animal models (23–28). Clinicians treating male infertility would benefit greatly from the results of SNP and CNV association studies on patients presenting various reproductive anomalies including impaired spermatogenesis and/or a lack of testicular function. Strengthened by this knowledge, physicians could offer a more defined diagnosis, a better clinical prevention and a customized treatment to their infertile patients.

From another perspective, the definition of genetic determinants in male infertility is of great importance to aid in the care of infertile couples. Indeed, the assisted reproductive technologies have helped many infertile men to father children and transmit their genetic information to their offspring. But, while natural selection prevented transmission of mutations leading to infertility, today medically assisted conception contributes in a significant manner to the risk involved and of a future increase in genetic causes of infertility. Thus, defining the contribution of genetic variants in male fertility appears crucial.

## 4 Male Infertility Associated SNPs Affecting Genitourinary Development

### 4.1 Cryptorchidism and Mutations of Insl3 and Lgr8 Genes

Cryptorchidism is a risk factor for infertility because of the deleterious effects on spermatogenesis (29). In addition, the cryptorchid testis is at high risk of malignancy. During development, gubernaculum growth is under the control of Insl3 (insulin-like hormone 3) (30). This hormone is produced by Leydig cells of the fetal testis. It is not found in the ovary. A mutation in the gene of this hormone or in its receptor, Lgr8, results in cryptorchidism in humans and mice

**Table 1** Current understanding of the relationship of genetic variants to male infertility

| | Genes | Nature of the variants |
|---|---|---|
| **Genetic variants linked to male infertility** | CFTR | • Deletion of 3 nucleotides ΔF508<br>• Repeat length variant of a polypirimidine tract (allele 5T)<br>• Repetition of 9–13 TG nucleotides |
| | Androgen receptor | • Polymorphic sequence of CAG triplets coding for polyglutamines in the first exon<br>• Length of a GGN segment |
| | Insl3-Lgr8 | • 2 not synonymous SNP T222P and R223K in Lgr8 |
| **Genetic variants with a potential link to male infertility** | Folate-related enzymes | • MTFHR (C677T)<br>• Methionine synthase (A2756G)<br>• Methionine synthase reductase (A666G) |
| | DAZL | • SNP in exon 3 (A386G) |
| | FSHR | |
| | Estrogen receptor α | • Xba I and Pvu II intron 1 variants<br>• Variable repeated elements (TA)n within the promoter region<br>• SNP C325G in exon 4 |
| | Region 11p15 | • SNPs in ZNF214, ZNF215, RBMXL2, NALP14 |
| | c-kit and KIT ligand | |
| | SPO11 | |
| | MEI1 | |
| | Hrb, GOBC, CsnK2a2 | |
| **Genetic variants with no association to male infertility** | TNP1 and 2<br>Protamines (PRM1 and PRM2)<br>H1FNT gene | |

(31). The genetic basis of most cases of cryptorchidism, like many genetic defects, is thought to be multifactorial (32). Indeed, in some cases, defects of androgen biosynthesis, androgen receptor function or signaling pathways may cause cryptorchidism. Some cases may reflect an abnormal endocrine milieu or even maternal exposure to endocrine disruptors/hormone mimics. In others, the cause is idiopathic. Accordingly, most cryptorchid cases are not due to a mutation of Insl3 gene, which reflects the genetic diversity of this condition. Two polymorphisms not synonymous T222P and R223K in the gene Lgr8 were reported in several cryptorchid patients (33). SNP association studies of large groups of patients and controls with advanced epidemiological analysis will ultimately be required to determine their significance. Ultimately, this is true for many (but not all) of the other SNPs described below.

## 4.2 Congenital Bilateral Absence of the Vas Deferens (CBAVD) and CFTR

CBAVD is a form of cystic fibrosis where the patients usually exhibit only the genital form of the disease manifested by the absence of the vas deferens. The CFTR (cystic fibrosis transmembrane conductance regulator) encodes a chloride ion channel regulating the transport of water and salt across the plasma membrane of epithelial cells (34). CFTR is found in many organs including the lung, liver, pancreas, skin, digestive and vas deferens. The gene encoding CFTR is located on the human chromosome 7, on the long arm at position q31.2. Over one thousand mutations are known including more than 120 polymorphic sites (35). Mutations mainly cause two genetic disorders, congenital bilateral agenesis of the vas deferens (CBAVD) and cystic fibrosis, an autosomal recessive disease of variable severity (affecting one child in 2,500–3,000) (36).

Nearly half of patients with CBAVD carry a common and severe CFTR mutation (delta F508) in heterozygous state whereas the frequency of these alleles is much lower (3–4%) in the general population (37). This specific mutation consists of a deletion of three nucleotides resulting in a loss of the amino acid phenylalanine at the 508th position on the protein. The resulting CFTR protein does not fold normally and is more quickly degraded resulting in an overall count of less CFTR protein in the cell. In addition, the CBAVD men are often carriers of another polymorphism on the second allele aggravating or worsening the effect of the first mutation.

In 1995, Chillon, et al., (38), Costes, et al., (39), and Jarvi, et al., (40) reported that a repeat length variant of a polypyrimidine tract (called IVS8-5T allele) was found in about 13–44% of men with CBAVD and showed inter-individual variability with incomplete penetrance. This variant is located at the splice acceptor site of exon 8 and impacts mRNA processing (41, 42). In the same individual, there is a great variability in the maturation of CFTR messenger between the tissues with less efficiency in the epididymal epithelium than the respiratory tract. This could explain why individuals with a 5T allele, in association with a mutation on the other allele, would only develop CBAVD without expressing any lung symptoms. Another determining factor for the penetrance of the 5T allele is the existence of another polymorphism consisting of a repetition of 9–13 TG nucleotides (37, 43). The alleles TG11 and TG12 multiply by respectively 2.8 and 6 the proportion of exon 9 deleted mRNAs compared to the allele TG10. Moreover, 5T alleles in CBAVD patients are more often associated with long repeats, TG12 or TG13, than 5T alleles in healthy individuals. Thus, the combination of polymorphisms together can alter further the ultimate amount of CFTR protein synthesized.

Spermatogenesis of the CBAVD patients is often normal, providing the potential for a medically assisted reproduction using sperm collected surgically from epidydimis. The prognosis for the offspring is actually dependent on the genotype of the mothers whom the risk of being heterozygous is of 1/25 in the absence of any familial history of cystic fibrosis. Thus, it is important that the female partner of the CBAVD patient will be tested for CFTR mutations if they desire to achieve a pregnancy. When a couple both carry an anomaly in the CFTR gene, preimplantation or prenatal genetic diagnosis of the embryo or fetus is advisable. Paradoxically, the situation is more complicated when no CFTR anomaly is found in a CBAVD male patient while his partner is carrying a mutation: cystic fibrosis due to the fetal transmission of the mutated maternal allele is still possible because the paternal allele could still be perhaps carrying an undetected mutation. Most clinical laboratories only test for about 30–50 of the most common mutations (out of 1,300 known) that cause cystic fibrosis. In this case, analysis of the complete sequence of CFTR is indicated.

## 5 Male Infertility Associated SNPs Affecting Spermatogenesis

Analysis of polymorphisms CNV of genes involved in spermatogenesis revealed numerous variants associated with the occurrence of male infertility. Several examples will be presented here. It is important to note that, thus far, results of association studies are not always consistent because of several important confounders: the size and composition of the studied populations (especially the control groups), ethnicity and geographical differences contributing to the genetic variation, the type of polymorphisms studied and techniques used, as well as the multifactorial and phenotypic heterogeneity of male infertility. The phenotypic effects of polymorphisms are themselves modulated by other genetic factors and by environmental factors, thus rendering the analysis complex. Nevertheless, several SNPs are important for male fertility.

### *5.1 Androgen Receptor Polyglutamine Tract in Exon 1 and Male Infertility*

Androgens, mainly testosterone and 5-alpha-dihydrotestosterone, act through specific binding to a nuclear steroid receptor, the androgen receptor (AR), which controls specific gene expression in androgen-responsive targets through regulation of gene expression and the initiation of a complex cascade of events that ultimately affect cell function (44). The human AR gene is located on the long arm of chromosome X at the locus Xq11-q12. It covers about 90 kb and consists of 8 exons. More than 600 mutations have been described for this receptor mainly associated with androgen insensitivity syndrome (45). This gene also contains a polymorphic sequence of CAG triplets coding for polyglutamines in the first exon that impact androgen action (46, 47).

Exon 1 of the androgen receptor gene is characterized by two polymorphic regions; the first consists of a string of CAG repeats encoding a stretch of glutamines in the transactivation domain of the receptor. The average number of repeats varies by ethnic and geographic location (48–55). In 1991, La Spada et al., (56) observed that expansions of this polyglutamine stretch beyond 40 copies was associated with spinal bulbar and muscular atrophy, an autosomal dominant neurodegenerative triplet repeat disease of aging (57). This phenotype has been replicated in a mouse model (58). As the repeat length increases, the transcriptional regulatory competence and expression of the androgen receptor is reduced (59–61). This disease is due to the neurodegeneration of motor neurons. A weakness of proximal muscles appears gradually in men between 30 and 40 years accompanied with oligo or azoospermia and deficient masculinization. One manifestation of spinal bulbar and muscular atrophy is testicular atrophy with male infertility with aging. Although the expanded CAG region changes the structure of the androgen receptor and results in reduced AR transcriptional activity, it is unclear how the altered protein disrupts nerve cells. It is believed that a fragment of the androgen receptor containing the CAG repeats accumulates within motor neurons and interferes with normal cell functions. This buildup leads to the gradual loss of nerve cells in the brain and spinal cord that control muscle movement.

Within the normal polymorphic range of polyglutamine repeats, an association of the increased repeat tract length with male infertility has been reported (51, 61–64), although not all authors agree (65–68). Indeed, studies performed in Singapore, Australia, North America and Japan observe an association between the length of CAG triplets and male infertility, reporting substantially longer CAG tracts in infertile males than in controls (51, 61, 62, 69–71). In contrast, European studies found no correlation between the number of AR-CAG repeats and impaired spermatogenesis (66, 67, 72–75). These discordant results may reflect differences in the ethnicity and the geographical location of the recruited patients. Indeed, distribution of the number of CAG triplets is low among African Americans, intermediate among Europeans and high in Asians. Importantly, Casella et al., (64) reported that the CAG repeat length corresponded directly to the testicular histology of azoospermic men with men having the longest repeat lengths. Thus, the etiology of the male's infertility and the bias of patient selection could impact the results. Other explanations for these contradictory observations might be the size of the studied samples, the choice of the control groups and the criteria for the inclusion of the patients in the study. Despite all these confounders, a recent meta-analysis on a survey of the literature confirmed that longer CAG repeat tract length in exon 1 of the androgen receptor is associated with male infertility (76).

Finally, a recent study analyzed the impact of the combination of the length changes of the CAG and the GGC tracts (GGC encodes polyglycine). This investigation showed that some haplotypes modulate the function of the androgen receptor, resulting in a significant susceptibility to infertility. Indeed, the length of the GGN segment, in combination with CAG repeat size, might, in some ethnic groups, modify the AR protein function, leading to varying degrees of impaired spermatogenesis (74, 75). It seems that the combination of more than 21 CAG and 18 GGC confers an increased risk for infertility. However a causal association between GGN repeats number and failure of spermatogenesis is lacking (61, 74, 75, 77).

### 5.2 The Estrogen Receptor Alpha (ESR1)

The physiological response to estrogens is mediated by two functional isoforms of the same receptor (ER alpha and ER beta), encoded by two distinct genes. An association between ER alpha polymorphism and infertility men is suggested. ER alpha has several polymorphic regions. The most studied ones are PvuII and XbaI restriction enzymes sites polymorphisms at the intron 1; variable repeated elements (TA)n within the promoter region, and a polymorphism C/G at the codon 325 in exon 4. In a Greek study, an association was found for the intronic XbaI variant but not PvuII (78), while in Spain, an association was found only for the polymorphism PvuII (23). Another Japanese study analyzing the exon 4 reported a significant difference in the distribution of allelic frequencies between azoospermic males and controls (79). Finally, the [TA]n polymorphism seems to have an impact on sperm concentration, although their frequencies are identical in infertile patients and controls (80).

### 5.3 SNPs of the Human Gonadotropin (FSH and LH) Receptor Genes

The FSH receptor is expressed in the Sertoli cell and its main function is signal transduction through activation of adenylate cyclase upon ligand binding leading to increased intracellular levels of cyclic AMP. It plays an important, albeit not clearly understood role in regulating the function of the Sertoli cell. The LH receptor is expressed in the Leydig cell and LH induces steroidogenesis and androgen biosynthesis. SNPs have been identified in the FSH receptor with several allelic variants found, but their functional significance is largely unknown (81) as they were not related to measures of male reproductive characteristics such as testicular volume, serum FSH or inhibin B levels.

### 5.4 Chromosome Region 11p15

Recently, the 11p15 region was linked to a lack of spermatogenesis. In this region, several genes coexist and are predominantly expressed in the testis. Among them, ZNF214 (Zinc Finger 214), ZNF215 (Zinc Finger 215) and RBMXL2 (heterogeneous nuclear ribonucleoprotein GT) genes were mutated in some infertile patients (82, 83). NALP14 represents another 11p15 gene exclusively expressed in the testis, specifically in the germ cells. This protein may play a regulatory role in the innate immune system as similar family members belong to the signal-induced multiprotein complex, the inflammasome that activates the pro-inflammatory caspases, caspase-1 and caspase-5. An analysis of 157 patients presenting a severe azoo/oligozoospermia clearly defined five mutations in this gene that are not found in the control group of 158 men with a normal sperm count. One of these mutations introduces a premature stop codon in the coding sequence and led to a truncated protein (84).

### 5.5 C-KIT and KIT Ligand

The receptor tyrosine kinase c-KIT and its ligand KITLG are involved in the survival and proliferation of germ cells. In humans, a c-KIT gene polymorphism (rs3819392) was associated with idiopathic male infertility in a population of 167 infertile patients (sperm count < 5 million spz/mL) compared to a control group consisting of individuals originating from the same geographical region (85).

## 5.6 Polymorphisms of the DNA Repair Genes

Of particular interest are the polymorphisms in DNA mismatch repair genes, as these genes are involved not only in DNA repair but also in meiotic recombination. MLH3 is a member of this family of proteins, but unlike several other members of this family, deletions reveal that the protein is not involved in microsatellite instability but does result in male infertility due to meiotic arrest (86). SPO11, a type II topoisomerase, is required for double strand breaks (DSB) formation and the eventual synapsis of chromosomes during meiotic recombination. A genetic screening study identified two nonobstructive azoospermic men with missense mutations in exon 1 and exon 9 of the SPO11 gene and 16 SNPs in intronic regions (87). One of the missense mutations identified corresponds to an amino acid residue shown to play a crucial role in DSB formation. Three of the SNPs were located in the 3′ untranslated region, which could have an effect on transcription of this gene.

## 5.7 Folate-Related Enzyme Polymorphisms

Polymorphisms of genes required for folate metabolism are of interest because of their key roles in DNA synthesis and methylation within cells. This pathway serves to maintain a stable pool of circulating folate and methionine and to prevent increased homocysteine concentration. Analysis of methylenetetrahydrofolate reductase (MTHFR), methionine synthase and methionine synthase reductase genes for male infertility related polymorphisms showed that in addition to the presence of a methylenetetrahydrofolate reductase variant, Cytosine 677 Thymidine, an Adenosine 2,756 Guanine variant of methionine synthase and a methionine synthase reductase variant adenosine 666 guanine were independently associated with male infertility (88). 20% of male patients consulting for infertility are homozygous for the MTHFR 677TT polymorphism, which is twice more the frequency found in the control population (89). The MTHFR mutation C677T causes a decrease of the enzymatic activity by 30% in (CT) and 80% in homozygotes (TT). Bentivoglio et al. have reported an improvement in the quality of sperm in patients taking folate (90). Irrespective to the status of fertility, sperm concentration increases significantly in patients 677CC after treatment with folic acid and zinc sulfate, while CT heterozygous and homozygous TT do show no improvement (91).

## 5.8 MEI1 Polymorphic Alleles are Associated with Meiotic Arrest

In the mouse, the mei1 gene defects were identified in infertile mice with meiotic arrest. Sato et al., (92) examined a series of 27 men with a complete early maturation arrest for coding SNPs in MEI1. Four SNPs were examined in more detail in 26 azoospermic men and 121 normal American and Israeli men. Two of these SNPs were associated with azoospermia in the Americans but not the Israeli.

## 5.9 Y Chromosome SNPs: Diversity of the Y Chromosome

The Y chromosome has a region specific to male individuals named MSY or male-specific region that includes nearly 95% of the chromosome. This region is flanked by two pseudo-autosomal regions PAR1 and PAR2. A non-coding heterochromatic region exists at the end of the long arm of this chromosome and consists of a large number of repeated units belonging to two families, DYZ1 and DYZ2. Each unit is formed by hundreds of repeated elements in tandem. In the general population, this region presents a great polymorphism, although none of these variations has been linked to any phenotype. Outside this region, the remainder of the Y chromosome is euchromatic, ie containing coding sequences, but with a very high proportion (50–70%) of various repeated elements (Alu, LINE, SINE).

Because of the lack of recombination between the Y chromosome and the X chromosome, any structural change (mutation, deletion, duplication, insertion or inversion) occurring in the Y chromosome, outside the two pseudo-autosomal regions, tends to be "stabilized" and transmitted from generation to generation.

The use of SNP as genetic markers on the male-specific region MSY of the Y chromosome has helped to identify several distinct Y chromosomes (93, 94). Each mutation defines one haplotype. These haplotypes have a paternal transmission and change only when a mutation occurs. It then becomes possible to establish a paternal genealogy, to build haplogroups and to establish a phylogenetic tree for the human Y chromosome and estimate the occurrence of evolutionary events using mutation rates. By far, more than 150 different Y chromosome haplogroups have been characterized (see Y chromosome consortium website: http://ycc.biosci.arizona.edu/), reflecting the diversity and the extension of the human species on the entire planet. Thus, the male-specific region MSY has become a far more useful tool than the autosomal chromosomes for studying the human genetic history.

The study of SNPs in the male-specific region of the Y chromosome provides the opportunity to obtain specific information on spontaneous mutation rates in a given population, without any interference from inter-allelic processes occurring in the other chromosomes. Numerous diseases have already been linked to the genetic background of the Y chromosome. Male reproductive function was the first clinical condition linked to the Y polymorphisms: indeed, several studies have involved haplogroup individuals in reduced sperm count (53, 95). Other disorders, including cardiovascular disease were also correlated to a polymorphism in Y chromosome (96, 97). However, the over-representation of haplogroups in some infertile men must be compared to a control group because it could be linked to the geographical diversity of the chromosome Y haplogroups rather than the clinical phenotype.

### *5.10 DAZL*

DAZL (Deleted in AZoospermia Like), located on chromosome 3, is expressed in germ cells and encodes a RNA binding protein. Transposition and amplification of the autosomal DAZ gene family during primate evolution gave rise to the DAZ gene cluster on the Y chromosome. There is no mutation described at the moment except the description of two SNPs in exon 2 (A260G) and exon 3 (A386G). The first polymorphism A260G, described in patients in Taiwan was found at a similar frequency in infertile men and in controls (98). The second A386G polymorphism, which involves a change in the 54th amino acid Thr → Ala (T54A), was significantly associated with severe spermatogenic failure and male infertility (98). However, other studies made in Italy, Germany and Japan and in India have not confirmed these results (99–102).

## 6 SNPs Affecting Sperm Development or Function

### *6.1 The Sperm Nuclear Proteins*

The protamines are highly basic DNA-binding proteins in the sperm nucleus that play an important role in packaging the DNA in the sperm head during spermiogenesis. Several groups have focused specifically on protamines 1 and 2 (PRM1, PRM2). There are four SNPs in the coding region of PRM1 and 2 in the coding region of PRM2, with other SNPs observed in the non-coding regions (103). Although these sequences were largely similar in populations of fertile and infertile men, a SNP was identified in a single man that produced a nonsense codon resulting in translation termination (103, 104).

The transition nuclear proteins (TNP)1 and TNP2 gene sequences were assessed as well and a series of SNPs identified in TNP2 (105). A deletion of 15 base pairs in the 5′ promoter region was identified and thought to be of importance because the diminished expression of TNP1 and TNP2 in mouse models was associated with infertility in at least some of the males (106). Of note, the significance of TNP1 in human spermatogenesis is not yet fully understood.

Targeted deletion of the h-HANP1 gene, which encodes a H1-like protein, resulted in male infertility in a mouse model characterized by teratozoospermia and abnormal function; however, the 5 SNPs evaluated in a group of fertile and infertile men in the coding region did not reveal a difference (107).

### *6.2 Globozoospermia*

In a case report, Christensen et al., (108) reported polymorphisms in three genes, Hrb (encoding the cytosolic surface of proacrosomic transport vesicles), GOBC (a PDZ domain protein interacting with $Csnk_2a_2$ that is found in the trans-Golgi region of round spermatids in the mouse) and CsnK2a2 (encoding the catalytic alpha subunit of casein kinase II, a serine/threonine kinase) in men with globozoospermia, commonly known as round headed sperm syndrome. In this syndrome, the acrosome, a vesicle containing the hydrolytic enzymes needed for fertilization, is either absent or largely deficient with remnants possibly present. The syndrome is rare in the infertile male population accounting for about 0.1% of male infertility and even rarer in the general population. In this case, definitive gene mutations were not clearly linked to the globozoospermia and functional studies were not possible to define the consequences of the SNP variants observed. This study in particular highlights the challenges faced in the study of SNPs in male infertility. As the incidence of globozoospermia is very rare, collection of sufficient numbers of patients for statistically significant analysis is difficult.

## 7 Conclusion

The realization that genetic variants, such as SNPs and CNVs, exist provides further insight into both genetic disorders and normal human phenotypic diversity. However, the current challenges for associating a genetic variant with a clinical disorder remains sizeable. The technologies available today for SNP or CNV definition are expensive and cumbersone. Analysis of complex data represents a significant problem and this area of genetics represents an excellent example of the application of an advanced technology to clinical diagnosis prior to a complete understanding of the biologic implications of the genetic variants found. Additional research into clinical phenotypes, genetic disorders and normal human diversity is clearly warranted.

**Acknowlegement** Reproductive biology and cancer studies in the Lamb laboratory are supported in part by the National Institutes of Health grants NIH 5 P01 HD36289, NIH 1 R01 DK078121, NIH 5 T32 DK00763, and the Department Of Defense, U.S. Army Materiel Command PC061154.

## References

1. Redon R, Ishikawa S, Fitch KR, et al. Global variation in copy number in the human genome. Nature 2006;444(7118):444–54.
2. Kwok PY. Methods for genotyping single nucleotide polymorphisms. Annu Rev Genomics Hum Genet 2001;2:235–58.
3. Kwok PY, Chen X. Detection of single nucleotide polymorphisms. Curr Issues Mol Biol 2003;5(2):43–60.
4. Livak KJ. Allelic discrimination using fluorogenic probes and the 5′ nuclease assay. Genet Anal 1999;14(5–6):143–9.
5. Miller RD, Phillips MS, Jo I, et al. High-density single-nucleotide polymorphism maps of the human genome. Genomics 2005;86(2):117–26.
6. Buetow KH, Edmonson M, MacDonald R, et al. High-throughput development and characterization of a genomewide collection of gene-based single nucleotide polymorphism markers by chip-based matrix-assisted laser desorption/ionization time-of-flight mass spectrometry. Proc Natl Acad Sci U S A 2001;98(2):581–4.
7. Kwiatkowski RW, Lyamichev V, de Arruda M, Neri B. Clinical, genetic, and pharmacogenetic applications of the Invader assay. Mol Diagn 1999;4(4):353–64.
8. Syvanen AC. Toward genome-wide SNP genotyping. Nat Genet 2005;37 Suppl:S5–10.
9. Bell PA, Chaturvedi S, Gelfand CA, et al. SNPstream UHT: ultra-high throughput SNP genotyping for pharmacogenomics and drug discovery. Biotechniques 2002;Suppl:70–2, 4, 6–7.
10. Fan JB, Oliphant A, Shen R, et al. Highly parallel SNP geno-typing. Cold Spring Harb Symp Quant Biol 2003;68:69–78.
11. Hardenbol P, Yu F, Belmont J, et al. Highly multiplexed molecular inversion probe genotyping: over 10,000 targeted SNPs genotyped in a single tube assay. Genome Res 2005;15(2):269–75.
12. The International HapMap Project. Nature 2003;426(6968): 789–96.
13. Hirschhorn JN, Daly MJ. Genome-wide association studies for common diseases and complex traits. Nat Rev Genet 2005;6(2):95–108.
14. McCarthy MI, Abecasis GR, Cardon LR, et al. Genome-wide association studies for complex traits: consensus, uncertainty and challenges. Nat Rev Genet 2008;9(5):356–69.
15. Kruglyak L. The road to genome-wide association studies. Nat Rev Genet 2008;9(4):314–8.
16. Woodcock J. Pharmacogenetics: on the road to 'personalized medicine'. FDA Consum 2005;39(6):44.
17. Meadows M. Genomics and personalized medicine. FDA Consum 2005;39(6):12–7.
18. Service RF. Pharmacogenomics. Going from genome to pill. Science 2005;308(5730):1858–60.
19. Ciotti M, Chen F, Rubaltelli FF, Owens IS. Coding defect and a TATA box mutation at the bilirubin UDP-glucuronosyltransferase gene cause Crigler-Najjar type I disease. Biochim Biophys Acta 1998;1407(1):40–50.
20. Innocenti F, Ratain MJ. Irinotecan treatment in cancer patients with UGT1A1 polymorphisms. Oncology (Williston Park) 2003;17(5 Suppl 5):52–5.
21. Iyer L, Hall D, Das S, et al. Phenotype-genotype correlation of in vitro SN-38 (active metabolite of irinotecan) and bilirubin glucuronidation in human liver tissue with UGT1A1 promoter polymorphism. Clin Pharmacol Ther 1999;65(5):576–82.
22. FDA releases final guidance for pharmacogenomic data. Pharmacogenomics 2005;6(3):209.
23. Galan JJ, Buch B, Cruz N, et al. Multilocus analyses of estrogen-related genes reveal involvement of the ESR1 gene in male infertility and the polygenic nature of the pathology. Fertil Steril 2005;84(4):910–8.

24. Grootegoed JA, Baarends WM, Roest HP, Hoeijmakers JH. Knockout mouse model and gametogenic failure. Mol Cell Endocrinol 1998;145(1–2):161–6.
25. Hackstein JH, Hochstenbach R, Pearson PL. Towards an understanding of the genetics of human male infertility: lessons from flies. Trends Genet 2000;16(12):565–72.
26. Venables JP, Cooke HJ. Lessons from knockout and transgenic mice for infertility in men. J Endocrinol Invest 2000;23(9):584–91.
27. Matzuk MM, Lamb DJ. Genetic dissection of mammalian fertility pathways. Nat Cell Biol 2002;4 Suppl:s41–9.
28. Ferlin A, Raicu F, Gatta V, Zuccarello D, Palka G, Foresta C. Male infertility: role of genetic background. Reprod Biomed Online 2007;14(6):734–45.
29. Virtanen HE, Bjerknes R, Cortes D, et al. Cryptorchidism: classification, prevalence and long-term consequences. Acta Paediatr 2007;96(5):611–6.
30. Agoulnik AI. Relaxin and related peptides in male reproduction. Adv Exp Med Biol 2007;612:49–64.
31. Virtanen HE, Toppari J. Epidemiology and pathogenesis of cryptorchidism. Hum Reprod Update 2008;14(1):49–58.
32. Foresta C, Zuccarello D, Garolla A, Ferlin A. Role of hormones, genes and environment in human cryptorchidism. Endocr Rev 2008;29(5):560–80.
33. Bogatcheva NV, Ferlin A, Feng S, et al. T222P mutation of the insulin-like 3 hormone receptor LGR8 is associated with testicular maldescent and hinders receptor expression on the cell surface membrane. Am J Physiol Endocrinol Metab 2007;292(1):E138–44.
34. Chen TY, Hwang TC. CLC-0 and CFTR: chloride channels evolved from transporters. Physiol Rev 2008;88(2):351–87.
35. MacDonald KD, McKenzie KR, Zeitlin PL. Cystic fibrosis transmembrane regulator protein mutations: 'class' opportunity for novel drug innovation. Paediatr Drugs 2007;9(1):1–10.
36. Cuppens H, Cassiman JJ. CFTR mutations and polymorphisms in male infertility. Int J Androl 2004;27(5):251–6.
37. Claustres M. Molecular pathology of the CFTR locus in male infertility. Reprod Biomed Online 2005;10(1):14–41.
38. Chillon M, Casals T, Mercier B, et al. Mutations in the cystic fibrosis gene in patients with congenital absence of the vas deferens. N Engl J Med 1995;332(22):1475–80.
39. Costes B, Girodon E, Ghanem N, et al. Frequent occurrence of the CFTR intron 8 (TG)n 5T allele in men with congenital bilateral absence of the vas deferens. Eur J Hum Genet 1995;3(5):285–93.
40. Jarvi K, Zielenski J, Wilschanski M, et al. Cystic fibrosis transmembrane conductance regulator and obstructive azoospermia. Lancet 1995;345(8964):1578.
41. Viel M, Leroy C, Des Georges M, Claustres M, Bienvenu T. Novel length variant of the polypyrimidine tract within the splice acceptor site in intron 8 of the CFTR gene: consequences for genetic testing using standard assays. Eur J Hum Genet 2005;13(2):136–8.
42. Chu CS, Trapnell BC, Curristin S, Cutting GR, Crystal RG. Genetic basis of variable exon 9 skipping in cystic fibrosis transmembrane conductance regulator mRNA. Nat Genet 1993;3(2):151–6.
43. Disset A, Michot C, Harris A, Buratti E, Claustres M, Tuffery-Giraud S. A T3 allele in the CFTR gene exacerbates exon 9 skipping in vas deferens and epididymal cell lines and is associated with Congenital Bilateral Absence of Vas Deferens (CBAVD). Hum Mutat 2005;25(1):72–81.
44. Claessens F, Denayer S, Van Tilborgh N, Kerkhofs S, Helsen C, Haelens A. Diverse roles of androgen receptor (AR) domains in AR-mediated signaling. Nucl Recept Signal 2008;6:e008.
45. Gottlieb B, Beitel LK, Wu JH, Trifiro M. The androgen receptor gene mutations database (ARDB): 2004 update. Hum Mutat 2004;23(6):527–33.
46. Palazzolo I, Gliozzi A, Rusmini P, et al. The role of the polyglutamine tract in androgen receptor. J Steroid Biochem Mol Biol 2008;108(3–5):245–53.
47. Rajender S, Singh L, Thangaraj K. Phenotypic heterogeneity of mutations in androgen receptor gene. Asian J Androl 2007;9(2):147–79.
48. Manning JT. The androgen receptor gene: a major modifier of speed of neuronal transmission and intelligence? Med Hypotheses 2007;68(4):802–4.
49. Erenpreiss J, Tsarev I, Giwercman A, Giwercman Y. The impact of androgen receptor polymorphism and parental ethnicity on semen quality in young men from Latvia. Int J Androl 2008;31(5):477–82.
50. Zitzmann M, Nieschlag E. The CAG repeat polymorphism within the androgen receptor gene and maleness. Int J Androl 2003;26(2):76–83.
51. Mifsud A, Sim CK, Boettger-Tong H, et al. Trinucleotide (CAG) repeat polymorphisms in the androgen receptor gene: molecular markers of risk for male infertility. Fertil Steril 2001;75(2):275–81.
52. Li JW, Yuan D, Li H, Liang XW, Lu WH, Gu YQ. [Effect of (CAG) n polymorphism of androgen receptor gene on hormonal male contraception]. Zhonghua Nan Ke Xue 2008;14(2):126–30.
53. Krausz C, Quintana-Murci L, Rajpert-De Meyts E, et al. Identification of a Y chromosome haplogroup associated with reduced sperm counts. Hum Mol Genet 2001;10(18):1873–7.
54. Eckardstein SV, Schmidt A, Kamischke A, Simoni M, Gromoll J, Nieschlag E. CAG repeat length in the androgen receptor gene and gonadotrophin suppression influence the effectiveness of hormonal male contraception. Clin Endocrinol (Oxf) 2002;57(5):647–55.
55. Sampson ER, Yeh SY, Chang HC, et al. Identification and characterization of androgen receptor associated coregulators in prostate cancer cells. J Biol Regul Homeost Agents 2001;15(2):123–9.
56. La Spada AR, Wilson EM, Lubahn DB, Harding AE, Fischbeck KH. Androgen receptor gene mutations in X-linked spinal and bulbar muscular atrophy. Nature 1991;352(6330):77–9.
57. MacLean HE, Gonzales M, Greenland KJ, Warne GL, Zajac JD. Age-dependent differences in androgen binding affinity in a family with spinal and bulbar muscular atrophy. Neurol Res 2005;27(5):548–51.
58. McManamny P, Chy HS, Finkelstein DI, et al. A mouse model of spinal and bulbar muscular atrophy. Hum Mol Genet 2002;11(18):2103–11.
59. Mhatre AN, Trifiro MA, Kaufman M, et al. Reduced transcriptional regulatory competence of the androgen receptor in X-linked spinal and bulbar muscular atrophy. Nat Genet 1993;5(2):184–8.
60. Choong CS, Kemppainen JA, Zhou ZX, Wilson EM. Reduced androgen receptor gene expression with first exon CAG repeat expansion. Mol Endocrinol 1996;10(12):1527–35.

61. Tut TG, Ghadessy FJ, Trifiro MA, Pinsky L, Yong EL. Long polyglutamine tracts in the androgen receptor are associated with reduced trans-activation, impaired sperm production, and male infertility. J Clin Endocrinol Metab 1997;82(11): 3777–82.
62. Dowsing AT, Yong EL, Clark M, McLachlan RI, de Kretser DM, Trounson AO. Linkage between male infertility and trinucleotide repeat expansion in the androgen-receptor gene. Lancet 1999;354(9179):640–3.
63. Yoshida KI, Yano M, Chiba K, Honda M, Kitahara S. CAG repeat length in the androgen receptor gene is enhanced in patients with idiopathic azoospermia. Urology 1999;54(6): 1078–81.
64. Casella R, Maduro MR, Misfud A, Lipshultz LI, Yong EL, Lamb DJ. Androgen receptor gene polyglutamine length is associated with testicular histology in infertile patients. J Urol 2003;169(1):224–7.
65. Giwercman YL, Xu C, Arver S, Pousette A, Reneland R. No association between the androgen receptor gene CAG repeat and impaired sperm production in Swedish men. Clin Genet 1998;54(5):435–6.
66. Dadze S, Wieland C, Jakubiczka S, et al. The size of the CAG repeat in exon 1 of the androgen receptor gene shows no significant relationship to impaired spermatogenesis in an infertile Caucasoid sample of German origin. Mol Hum Reprod 2000;6(3):207–14.
67. Van Golde R, Van Houwelingen K, Kiemeney L, et al. Is increased CAG repeat length in the androgen receptor gene a risk factor for male subfertility? J Urol 2002;167(2 Pt 1):621–3.
68. Tse JY, Liu VW, Yeung WS, Lau EY, Ng EH, Ho PC. Molecular analysis of the androgen receptor gene in Hong Kong Chinese infertile men. J Assist Reprod Genet 2003;20(6):227–33.
69. Patrizio P, Leonard DG, Chen KL, Hernandez-Ayup S, Trounson AO. Larger trinucleotide repeat size in the androgen receptor gene of infertile men with extremely severe oligozoospermia. J Androl 2001;22(3):444–8.
70. Wallerand H, Remy-Martin A, Chabannes E, Bermont L, Adessi GL, Bittard H. Relationship between expansion of the CAG repeat in exon 1 of the androgen receptor gene and idiopathic male infertility. Fertil Steril 2001;76(4):769–74.
71. Mengual L, Oriola J, Ascaso C, Ballesca JL, Oliva R. An increased CAG repeat length in the androgen receptor gene in azoospermic ICSI candidates. J Androl 2003;24(2): 279–84.
72. Thangaraj K, Joshi MB, Reddy AG, Gupta NJ, Chakravarty B, Singh L. CAG repeat expansion in the androgen receptor gene is not associated with male infertility in Indian populations. J Androl 2002;23(6):815–8.
73. Lund A, Tapanainen JS, Lahdetie J, Savontaus ML, Aittomaki K. Long CAG repeats in the AR gene are not associated with infertility in Finnish males. Acta Obstet Gynecol Scand 2003;82(2):162–6.
74. Ferlin A, Bartoloni L, Rizzo G, Roverato A, Garolla A, Foresta C. Androgen receptor gene CAG and GGC repeat lengths in idiopathic male infertility. Mol Hum Reprod 2004;10(6):417–21.
75. Ruhayel Y, Lundin K, Giwercman Y, Hallden C, Willen M, Giwercman A. Androgen receptor gene GGN and CAG polymorphisms among severely oligozoospermic and azoospermic Swedish men. Hum Reprod 2004;19(9): 2076–83.
76. Davis-Dao CA, Tuazon ED, Sokol RZ, Cortessis VK. Male infertility and variation in CAG repeat length in the androgen receptor gene: a meta-analysis. J Clin Endocrinol Metab 2007;92(11):4319–26.
77. Rajender S, Rajani V, Gupta NJ, Chakravarty B, Singh L, Thangaraj K. No association of androgen receptor GGN repeat length polymorphism with infertility in Indian men. J Androl 2006;27(6):785–9.
78. Kukuvitis A, Georgiou I, Bouba I, et al. Association of oestrogen receptor alpha polymorphisms and androgen receptor CAG trinucleotide repeats with male infertility: a study in 109 Greek infertile men. Int J Androl 2002;25(3):149–52.
79. Suzuki Y, Sasagawa I, Itoh K, Ashida J, Muroya K, Ogata T. Estrogen receptor alpha gene polymorphism is associated with idiopathic azoospermia. Fertil Steril 2002;78(6): 1341–3.
80. Guarducci E, Nuti F, Becherini L, et al. Estrogen receptor alpha promoter polymorphism: stronger estrogen action is coupled with lower sperm count. Hum Reprod 2006;21(4): 994–1001.
81. Simoni M, Nieschlag E, Gromoll J. Isoforms and single nucleotide polymorphisms of the FSH receptor gene: implications for human reproduction. Hum Reprod Update 2002;8(5):413–21.
82. Gianotten J, van der Veen F, Alders M, et al. Chromosomal region 11p15 is associated with male factor subfertility. Mol Hum Reprod 2003;9(10):587–92.
83. Westerveld GH, Gianotten J, Leschot NJ, van der Veen F, Repping S, Lombardi MP. Heterogeneous nuclear ribonucleoprotein G-T (HNRNP G-T) mutations in men with impaired spermatogenesis. Mol Hum Reprod 2004;10(4):265–9.
84. Westerveld GH, Korver CM, van Pelt AM, et al. Mutations in the testis-specific NALP14 gene in men suffering from spermatogenic failure. Hum Reprod 2006;21(12):3178–84.
85. Galan JJ, De Felici M, Buch B, et al. Association of genetic markers within the KIT and KITLG genes with human male infertility. Hum Reprod 2006;21(12):3185–92.
86. Ferras C, Zhou XL, Sousa M, Lindblom A, Barros A. DNA mismatch repair gene hMLH3 variants in meiotic arrest. Fertil Steril 2007;88(6):1681–4.
87. Christensen GL, Ivanov IP, Atkins JF, Mielnik A, Schlegel PN, Carrell DT. Screening the SPO11 and EIF5A2 genes in a population of infertile men. Fertil Steril 2005;84(3): 758–60.
88. Lee HC, Jeong YM, Lee SH, et al. Association study of four polymorphisms in three folate-related enzyme genes with non-obstructive male infertility. Hum Reprod 2006;21(12):3162–70.
89. Bezold G, Lange M, Peter RU. Homozygous methylenetetrahydrofolate reductase C677T mutation and male infertility. N Engl J Med 2001;344(15):1172–3.
90. Bentivoglio G, Melica F, Cristoforoni P. Folinic acid in the treatment of human male infertility. Fertil Steril 1993;60(4): 698–701.
91. Ebisch IM, van Heerde WL, Thomas CM, van der Put N, Wong WY, Steegers-Theunissen RP. C677T methylenetetrahydrofolate reductase polymorphism interferes with the effects of folic acid and zinc sulfate on sperm concentration. Fertil Steril 2003;80(5):1190–4.

92. Sato H, Miyamoto T, Yogev L, et al. Polymorphic alleles of the human MEI1 gene are associated with human azoospermia by meiotic arrest. J Hum Genet 2006;51(6):533–40.
93. Jobling MA, Tyler-Smith C. The human Y chromosome: an evolutionary marker comes of age. Nat Rev Genet 2003;4(8):598–612.
94. Garrigan D, Hammer MF. Reconstructing human origins in the genomic era. Nat Rev Genet 2006;7(9):669–80.
95. Kuroki Y, Iwamoto T, Lee J, et al. Spermatogenic ability is different among males in different Y chromosome lineage. J Hum Genet 1999;44(5):289–92.
96. Ellis JA, Stebbing M, Harrap SB. Association of the human Y chromosome with high blood pressure in the general population. Hypertension 2000;36(5):731–3.
97. Charchar FJ, Tomaszewski M, Padmanabhan S, et al. The Y chromosome effect on blood pressure in two European populations. Hypertension 2002;39(2 Pt 2):353–6.
98. Teng YN, Lin YM, Sun HF, Hsu PY, Chung CL, Kuo PL. Association of DAZL haplotypes with spermatogenic failure in infertile men. Fertil Steril 2006;86(1):129–35.
99. Bartoloni L, Cazzadore C, Ferlin A, Garolla A, Foresta C. Lack of the T54A polymorphism of the DAZL gene in infertile Italian patients. Mol Hum Reprod 2004;10(8):613–5.
100. Tschanter P, Kostova E, Luetjens CM, Cooper TG, Nieschlag E, Gromoll J. No association of the A260G and A386G DAZL single nucleotide polymorphisms with male infertility in a Caucasian population. Hum Reprod 2004;19(12):2771–6.
101. Yang XJ, Shinka T, Nozawa S, et al. Survey of the two polymorphisms in DAZL, an autosomal candidate for the azoospermic factor, in Japanese infertile men and implications for male infertility. Mol Hum Reprod 2005;11(7): 513–5.
102. Thangaraj K, Deepa SR, Pavani K, et al. A to G transitions at 260, 386 and 437 in DAZL gene are not associated with spermatogenic failure in Indian population. Int J Androl 2006;29(5):510–14.
103. Tanaka H, Miyagawa Y, Tsujimura A, Matsumiya K, Okuyama A, Nishimune Y. Single nucleotide polymorphisms in the protamine-1 and -2 genes of fertile and infertile human male populations. Mol Hum Reprod 2003;9(2): 69–73.
104. Iguchi N, Yang S, Lamb DJ, Hecht NB. An SNP in protamine 1: a possible genetic cause of male infertility? J Med Genet 2006;43(4):382–4.
105. Miyagawa Y, Nishimura H, Tsujimura A, et al. Single-nucleotide polymorphisms and mutation analyses of the TNP1 and TNP2 genes of fertile and infertile human male populations. J Androl 2005;26(6):779–86.
106. Meistrich ML, Mohapatra B, Shirley CR, Zhao M. Roles of transition nuclear proteins in spermiogenesis. Chromosoma 2003;111(8):483–8.
107. Tanaka H, Matsuoka Y, Onishi M, et al. Expression profiles and single-nucleotide polymorphism analysis of human HANP1/H1T2 encoding a histone H1-like protein. Int J Androl 2006;29(2):353–9.
108. Christensen GL, Ivanov IP, Atkins JF, Campbell B, Carrell DT. Identification of polymorphisms in the Hrb, GOPC, and Csnk2a2 genes in two men with globozoospermia. J Androl 2006;27(1):11–5.

# Sperm Chromatin Abnormalities and Reproductive Outcome

Peter N. Schlegel

**Abstract** The clinical relevance of abnormal sperm DNA integrity to human reproduction has been the source of substantial research over the past decade. A recent, rigorous meta-analysis of published studies has shown that abnormal sperm DNA integrity will adversely affect IVF and ICSI outcomes. Although this is the only sperm-related parameter documented to adversely affect ICSI success, the magnitude of this effect is not adequate to require routine sperm DNA testing prior to assisted reproduction. For subsets of infertility patients, sperm DNA integrity testing may be relevant. The limited data on treatment of patients with abnormal sperm DNA integrity is presented. This subject remains an expanding field with conflicting data.

**Keywords** Sperm DNA integrity • Sperm chromatin • Systematic review • Meta-analysis • Likelihood ratio • Treatment • Male infertility • Assisted reproduction • ICSI • IVF

## 1 Introduction

Available literature relating sperm DNA integrity to reproductive outcomes of IVF and ICSI were recently summarized in an article by Drs. Collins, Barnhart, and myself reporting a meta-analysis of existing published literature on this subject (1). With the permission of the other authors, I have summarized the findings of that article here and introduce evolving concepts of the potential treatment of abnormal sperm DNA integrity.

The integrity of sperm DNA is required for transmission of the paternal genomic complement (1). Tests of sperm DNA integrity, often reported as percent of sperm with substantial DNA fragmentation, generally correlate with routine semen variables including impaired sperm concentration or motility (2, 3). The proportion of sperm with abnormal DNA integrity correlates with time to natural pregnancy, and, at least in some studies, with results of treatment for infertility using intrauterine insemination (IUI), in vitro fertilization (IVF) or intracytoplasmic sperm injection (ICSI) (4–7). Sperm DNA integrity may also correlate with spontaneous abortion rates after assisted reproduction (8), and the proportion of patients with abnormal sperm DNA integrity is higher in couples with recurrent spontaneous miscarriage. New diagnostic tests for male infertility would be clinically useful because standard tests (sperm concentration, percent motility, and percent normal morphology) are not accurate enough to discriminate between infertile men whose partners will or will not conceive (9, 10). Indeed, no standard semen parameter correlates well with success or failure of IVF or ICSI.

The theoretical basis for analysis of sperm DNA integrity is sound. In its normal state, DNA in the mature spermatozoon is a condensed, compact structure. Up to 85% of DNA is bound to protamine in complexes that are more compact than the DNA–histone complexes in somatic cells (8). In this condensed, insoluble form, sperm DNA is protected from damage while the sperm is transported through the male and female reproductive tracts. If sperm DNA damage does occur, impaired fertility could be a natural consequence.

P.N. Schlegel
Starr 900, Department of Urology, New York Presbyterian/Weill Cornell Medical Center, 525 East 68th Street, New York, NY, 10021, USA
e-mail: pnschleg@med.cornell.edu

D.T. Carrell et al. (eds.), *Biennial Review of Infertility,* DOI: 10.1007/978-1-60327-392-3_9

Causes of DNA damage are numerous and the mechanisms for damage have not all been well elucidated. Protamine deficiency or mutation, genetic disorders that are more common in infertile men, impairs the protection of DNA (11). Oxidative stress due to leukocytosis or varicocele is associated with sperm DNA damage (12). DNA repair systems are thought to be less active in the later stages of spermatogenesis, allowing sperm with DNA strand breaks to reach the ejaculate (6). Also, increased apoptotic activity in older men and those with abnormal semen parameters may contribute to DNA damage (13). Interestingly, sperm DNA abnormalities for a population of sperm may predict the fertility potential of sperm in that semen specimen that do not have defined DNA damage. Therefore, selection of sperm, which occurs with standard semen processing techniques during assisted reproduction in an attempt to isolate spermatozoa "without DNA damage", may not obviate the effects of a patient's abnormal sperm DNA integrity (13).

Among assays developed to assess DNA damage, the most frequently used in published clinical studies is the sperm chromatin structure assay (SCSA) (8). SCSA measures the stability of sperm chromatin in hot or acid media with acridine orange. The dye gives rise to green fluorescence when bound to intact DNA and red when bound to fragmented DNA (14). The proportion of sperm with fragmented DNA is determined by flow cytometric analysis and expressed as a DNA fragmentation index (DFI) (15). Another common assay is the deoxy-nucleotidyl transferase-mediated dUTP nick end labelling (TUNEL) test (16). The TUNEL method labels the strand breaks of cleaved DNA, making them visible as brown in color; it is a widely used method for detecting DNA damage in somatic cells at various stages of apoptosis.

The SCSA and TUNEL methods are used in the majority of current studies on infertility. Other sperm DNA integrity assays include the single-cell electrophoresis assay (COMET), the sperm chromatin dispersion test (SCD) and the acridine orange test (AO). The COMET assay quantifies single- and double-strand breaks using electrophoresis of DNA-fluorochrome-stained single sperm cells (17). The SCD test identifies sperm with fragmented DNA because they fail to produce the characteristic halo when mixed with aqueous agarose following acid/salt treatment, which removes nuclear proteins and fragmented DNA (18). The AO test is an inexpensive method based on the same fluorescence reaction as the SCSA, but lacks the precise measurement system that is integral to the SCSA (19).

In clinical studies, sperm DNA integrity tests correlate with fertile status (infertile versus fertile males) and poor semen quality (6, 20, 21). Two time-to-pregnancy studies showed, among normal couples discontinuing the use of family planning in order to conceive, that SCSA test results were significantly associated with the probability of pregnancy (14, 22). In IVF and ICSI studies, however, associations between sperm DNA integrity results and fertilization rates or pregnancy rates have been less consistent (6, 8, 23). Even when associations between sperm DNA damage and markers of infertility are significant, associations may not be sufficient to discriminate reliably, as a diagnostic test must do, between couples who will or will not conceive.

## 2 Meta-Analysis of Previous Studies

To effectively identify the contemporary role of DNA integrity tests in reproductive medicine, we undertook a systematic review of published literature to clarify whether routine testing for sperm DNA integrity is clinically worthwhile for infertile couples undergoing IVF and ICSI treatment (1). The primary question addressed was: among infertile couples considering IVF or ICSI treatment, do the results of sperm DNA integrity testing predict pregnancy? The secondary question addressed in this study was whether sperm DNA integrity test results differed by treatment groups (IVF or ICSI) and sperm DNA integrity analysis technique (SCSA vs. TUNEL).

### 2.1 *Search Strategy for Meta-Analysis*

The search strategy used the terms (sperm DNA) and (pregnancy[Title/Abstract]) and humans (198 citations). Citations were included from the first clinical publication on this topic in 1999 (14) until 15 December 2006. Studies were eligible if they (a) assayed sperm DNA integrity in fresh ejaculated sperm, (b) had pregnancy or live birth among the reported outcomes, and (c) reported DNA integrity and pregnancy results in a manner that allowed the creation of two-by-two tables from the study data. Meeting abstracts were not included. The search was not restricted by language but it was limited to Medline citations and additional studies that were identified from the study reference lists.

## 2.2 Selection of Studies

Relevance was initially evaluated from titles and then determined from abstracts. Full reports were reviewed for all potentially pertinent citations. Where more than one study was reported from the same centre, authors were contacted to avoid inclusion of studies with the same patients (24–27).

## 2.3 Data Extraction

Data were abstracted from eligible studies on dates of accrual, whether accrual was consecutive, country of origin of study, direction of data collection, treatment type, type of assay, cut point, number of cycles or patients, and number of pregnancies relative to abnormal or normal test results. The outcomes recorded were clinical pregnancy, ongoing pregnancy, delivery and live birth. If a 2 × 2 table was not reported, it was reconstructed from sensitivity, specificity, prevalence and total sample size. Where results were available for more than one cut point, the cut point recommended by the authors or the cut point nearest to the most frequently reported cut point was chosen (SCSA DFI ≤30%, TUNEL ≤40%). From the two-by-two tables of test results by pregnancy, the following test properties were calculated for each study: sensitivity, specificity, accuracy (sensitivity plus specificity), likelihood ratios (positive and negative), the proportion of abnormal tests and the diagnostic odds ratio.

## 2.4 Analysis

The initial steps of the analysis were to provide, for each included study, a summary of the important methodological features (Table 1) and to show the key diagnostic properties as reported or calculated (Table 2). The next step was to determine whether diagnostic accuracy depended on the methodological features of the studies. Following that, we estimated heterogeneity and determined which diagnostic test properties could be combined into a summary measure of accuracy. The meta-analysis then estimated a summary effect of diagnostic accuracy and finally, the meta-analysis was repeated within predetermined subgroups to assess whether diagnostic accuracy differed between tests (SCSA and TUNEL) and patient groups (IVF and ICSI) (37).

Specifically, the effects of study methodology on diagnostic accuracy were assessed by means of stepwise multiple regression with the natural log of the diagnostic odds ratio as the dependent variable. Sensitivity and specificity were plotted in a receiver operating characteristics (ROC) curve of true positive values on false-positive values (38). Heterogeneity of reported sensitivity, specificity and other diagnostic test properties was assessed by visually examining ROC curves and by the Cochran's Q test for heterogeneity (39). Between-study heterogeneity was judged to be excessive when the $p$-value for the Q-statistic was less than 0.10. Heterogeneity was quantified by $I^2$, the proportion of variability across studies that is due to heterogeneity rather than chance (40).

In the meta-analyses, weighted average summary estimates were calculated with weights equal to the inverse variance. The random effects model is more appropriate when homogeneity is threatened; in all analyses except the LR (+), the P-value for the Q-statistic was <0.10 and $I^2$ was greater than 40%. Since heterogeneity was prevalent, only random effects models are presented in the results (41). The primary meta-analysis combined the log diagnostic odds ratio (DOR). DOR is the odds of an abnormal test result in diseased cases over the odds of an abnormal test result in non-disease cases and it can be estimated from sensitivity and specificity (42). The computation of the DOR is the same as the odds ratio (ad/bc). Publication bias was explored by funnel plot and analyzed by the Begg and Mazumdar rank correlation test (43, 44). Potential sources of heterogeneity from assay type and treatment type were evaluated by categorical analysis which partitions heterogeneity into the components from the model (groups) and the residual error in a manner which is analogous to the partitioning of variance in ANOVA (45). Sensitivity analyses evaluated the effects on the summary measure of diagnostic accuracy from adding back excluded studies for which two-by-two table data could be extracted.

**Table 1** Methodological features: studies of the association between sperm DNA fragmentation and pregnancy

| References | Treatment | Assay | Normal range | Cycles | Pregnancy outcome | Outcome rates (%) |
|---|---|---|---|---|---|---|
| Boe-Hanson et al. (28) | IVF | SCSA | DFI <27% | 139 | Clinical | 28 |
| | ICSI | SCSA | DFI <27% | 47 | Clinical | 30 |
| Borini et al. (29) | IVF | TUNEL | <10% | 82 | Clinical | 22 |
| | ICSI | TUNEL | <10% | 50 | Clinical | 24 |
| Bungum et al. (26) | IVF | SCSA | DFI <30% | 388 | Delivery | 28 |
| | ICSI | SCSA | DFI <30% | 223 | Delivery | 38 |
| Check et al. (30) | IVF | SCSA | DFI <30% | 106 | Ongoing | 17 |
| Gandini et al. (31) | ICSI | SCSA | DFI <30% | 22 | Full term | 41 |
| Host et al. (32) | IVF | TUNEL | ≤40% | 175 | Biochemical | 29 |
| | ICSI | TUNEL | ≤40% | 61 | Biochemical | 34 |
| Huang et al. (33) | IVF | TUNEL | ≤40% | 217 | Pregnancy | 55 |
| | ICSI | TUNEL | ≤40% | 86 | Pregnancy | 51 |
| Larson et al. (24) | IVF, ICSI | SCSA | DFI <27% | 24 | Pregnancy | 29 |
| Larson-Cook et al. (25) | IVF, ICSI | SCSA | DFI <27% | 89 | Clinical | 31 |
| Payne et al. (34) | IVF, ICSI | SCSA | DFI <27% | 94 | Clinical | 33 |
| Seli et al. (13) | IVF, ICSI | TUNEL | <20% | 49 | Clinical | 47 |
| Virro et al. (35) | IVF, ICSI | SCSA | DFI <30% | 249 | Ongoing | 41 |
| Zini et al. (36) | ICSI | SCSA | DD ≤30% | 60 | Clinical | 52 |

*SCSA*, sperm chromatin structure assay; *TUNEL*, Terminal deoxynucleotidyl transferase-mediated deoxyuridine triphosphate-biotin nick end labeling assay; *DFI*, DNA fragmentation index; *DD*, sperm DNA denaturation

**Table 2** Diagnostic test properties: studies of the association between sperm DNA fragmentation and pregnancy

| References | Treatment | Sens | Spec | Sens + Spec | Abnormal tests (%) | DOR | 95% CI |
|---|---|---|---|---|---|---|---|
| Boe-Hanson et al. (28) | IVF | 0.06 | 0.97 | 1.03 | 5 | 2.04 | 0.38, 11.0 |
| | ICSI | 0.36 | 0.57 | 0.94 | 38 | 0.76 | 0.21, 2.73 |
| Borini et al. (29) | IVF | 0.17 | 0.89 | 1.06 | 16 | 1.57 | 0.38, 6.51 |
| | ICSI | 0.71 | 0.75 | 1.46 | 60 | 6.55 | 1.77, 24.3 |
| Bungum et al. (26) | IVF | 0.17 | 0.85 | 1.02 | 16 | 1.16 | 0.64, 2.12 |
| | ICSI | 0.30 | 0.63 | 0.93 | 33 | 0.74 | 0.42, 1.31 |
| Check et al. (30) | IVF | 0.30 | 0.83 | 1.13 | 27 | 1.90 | 0.61, 5.89 |
| Gandini et al. (31) | ICSI | 0.38 | 0.44 | 0.83 | 45 | 0.52 | 0.10, 2.74 |
| Host et al. (32) | IVF | 0.34 | 0.80 | 1.14 | 30 | 1.91 | 0.93, 3.91 |
| | ICSI | 0.58 | 0.38 | 0.96 | 59 | 0.84 | 0.29, 2.43 |
| Huang et al. (33) | IVF | 0.22 | 0.83 | 1.04 | 19 | 1.30 | 0.66, 2.56 |
| | ICSI | 0.64 | 0.50 | 1.14 | 57 | 1.78 | 0.76, 4.16 |
| Larson et al. (24) | IVF, ICSI | 0.58 | 0.94 | 1.59 | 42 | 10.17 | 1.77, 58.4 |
| Larson-Cook et al. (25) | IVF, ICSI | 0.17 | 0.98 | 1.16 | 11 | 5.08 | 1.24, 20.8 |
| Payne et al. (34) | IVF, ICSI | 0.16 | 0.71 | 0.87 | 20 | 0.44 | 0.15, 1.27 |
| Seli et al. (13) | IVF, ICSI | 0.46 | 0.61 | 1.07 | 43 | 1.32 | 0.43, 4.07 |
| Virro et al. (35) | IVF, ICSI | 0.35 | 0.81 | 1.17 | 29 | 2.27 | 1.30, 3.96 |
| Zini et al. (36) | ICSI | 0.17 | 0.81 | 0.98 | 18 | 0.87 | 0.24, 3.19 |

*Sens*, sensitivity; *Spec*, specificity; *DOR*, diagnostic odds ratio

## 2.5 Results of Meta-Analysis: Studies Selected

Of the initial 198 citations retrieved, review of the titles and abstracts indicated that 168 were not relevant. Full papers were obtained for the remaining 30 citations (Fig. 1). One study (26) using the DFI 27% cut point was later replaced by an updated report which included all the earlier patients and used a DFI 30% cut point (27). After reviewing the 30 papers, eight were excluded because: the couples were not infertile ($n = 3$); the study did not involve sperm DNA integrity ($n = 2$); the study was an intervention among men with high levels of sperm DNA fragmentation rather than a diagnostic study ($n = 2$); or the study did not have pregnancy as an outcome ($n = 1$).

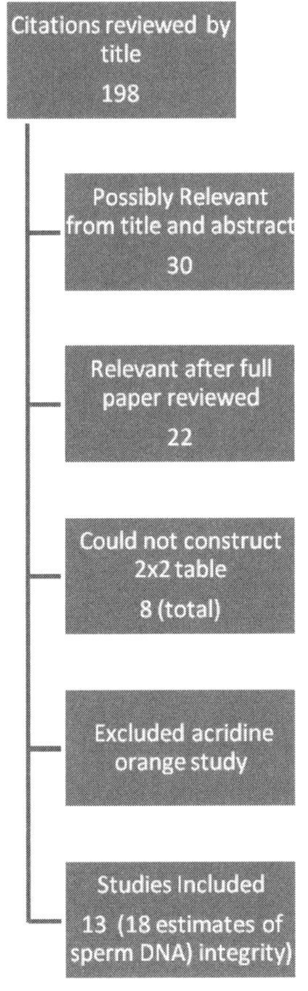


**Fig. 1** Flow chart for citations

In the 22 eligible reports, a two-by-two table could not be constructed from the data in eight studies involving 717 cycles of treatment. The number of pregnancies by test results was uncertain or missing (46–49): or pregnancy was reported only according to mean sperm DNA test results (50–53). All the studies that used COMET or SCD assays were in this group of eight excluded studies. Two of the eight studies did report sensitivity and specificity: 76 and 25% with TUNEL (46), 75 and 43% with TUNEL (47), and 60 and 58% with acridine orange (47).

In the remaining 14 studies, only one did not use either the SCSA or TUNEL assay. In order to reduce clinical heterogeneity, we excluded that otherwise eligible study, which made use of the acridine orange test in 183 ICSI cycles. The sensitivity and specificity were 64 and 30% (54). After that exclusion, 13 studies involving 2,162 cycles of treatment remained for analysis, of which nine involved the SCSA assay (24, 25, 27, 28, 30, 31, 34–36) and four the TUNEL assay (13, 29, 32, 33). (Table 1) When results were available for patients receiving more than one type of treatment, data were abstracted for each treatment group, yielding 18 estimates of diagnostic accuracy: six for IVF treatment, seven for IVF with ICSI and five from studies where IVF and ICSI results were mixed.

## 2.6 Study Characteristics of Evaluated Literature

The characteristics of the 13 studies are shown in Table 1. None were case control studies, sampling appeared to be consecutive in six (13, 27, 28, 30, 32, 36) and only two involved retrospective data collection (25, 35). All studies had pregnancy as the reference standard, although definitions ranged from biochemical pregnancy to delivery. Some studies allowed more than one entry per patient. In the cycles involved in the 18 estimates of sperm DNA integrity, the overall pregnancy rates ranged from 17 to 55%. None of the study methodology characteristics were associated with diagnostic accuracy in a stepwise multiple regression analysis.

## 2.7 Study Observations

Selected diagnostic test properties for the individual studies are shown in Table 2. Sensitivity and specificity can be seen to be mutually dependent (higher sensitivity is associated with lower specificity and vice versa). The correlation between sensitivity and specificity was significant ($r = -0.53$, $p = 0.024$). The sum of sensitivity and specificity, which ideally would approach 2.0, ranges from 0.83 to 1.59. The proportion of tests that were abnormal, which depends on the cut point within each study, ranges from 5 to 65%. Diagnostic odds ratios ranged from 0.44 to 10.1 and in only four of the eighteen estimates were these significantly different from unity.

Likelihood ratios are shown in Table 3. The likelihood ratios for an abnormal test (LR (+), the ratio of true positive to false-positive results) range from 0.54 to 9.8. For all but one estimate (1.90, 95% CI 1.04, 3.68) (35), the lower 95% confidence interval was less than one, implying that false-positive results could be more common than true positives. The likelihood ratios

**Table 3** Likelihood ratios: studies of the association between sperm DNA fragmentation and pregnancy

| References | Treatment | LR (+) | 95% CI | LR (−) | 95% CI |
|---|---|---|---|---|---|
| Boe-Hanson et al. (28) | IVF | 2.34 | 0.27, 20.1 | 0.96 | 0.05, 18.1 |
| | ICSI | 0.85 | 0.24, 3.03 | 1.11 | 0.56, 2.22 |
| Borini et al. (29) | IVF | 1.55 | 0.31, 7.72 | 0.93 | 0.28, 3.08 |
| | ICSI | 2.84 | 0.65, 12.5 | 0.39 | 0.27, 0.54 |
| Bungum et al. (26) | IVF | 1.14 | 0.61, 2.11 | 0.98 | 0.56, 1.71 |
| | ICSI | 0.82 | 0.46, 1.45 | 1.11 | 0.76, 1.60 |
| Check et al. (30) | IVF | 1.77 | 0.47, 6.65 | 0.85 | 0.48, 1.50 |
| Gandini et al. (31) | ICSI | 0.69 | 0.12, 3.89 | 1.38 | 0.51, 3.79 |
| Host et al. (32) | IVF | 1.68 | 0.77, 3.69 | 0.83 | 0.56, 1.23 |
| | ICSI | 0.93 | 0.32, 2.74 | 1.12 | 0.63, 1.98 |
| Huang et al. (33) | IVF | 1.25 | 0.63, 2.45 | 0.95 | 0.53, 1.69 |
| | ICSI | 1.29 | 0.54, 3.06 | 0.71 | 0.49, 1.05 |
| Larson et al. (24) | IVF, ICSI | 9.33 | 0.46, 190 | 0.44 | 0.27, 0.74 |
| Larson-Cook et al. (25) | IVF, ICSI | 9.82 | 0.55, 174 | 0.85 | 0.23, 3.13 |
| Payne et al. (34) | IVF, ICSI | 0.54 | 0.19, 1.50 | 1.19 | 0.41, 3.41 |
| Seli et al. (39) | IVF, ICSI | 1.18 | 0.38, 3.68 | 0.88 | 0.51, 1.53 |
| Virro et al. (35) | IVF, ICSI | 1.90 | 1.04, 3.47 | 0.79 | 0.58, 1.10 |
| Zini et al. (36) | ICSI | 0.89 | 0.24, 3.31 | 1.03 | 0.28, 3.77 |

*LR (+)*, likelihood ratio of a positive (abnormal) test result; *LR (−)*, likelihood ratio of a normal test result

for a normal test (LR (−), the ratio of false negatives to true negatives), ranged from 0.39 to 1.38. Only two in the effective range below 0.5 were significantly different from unity and six LR(−) estimates were actually greater than unity.

## 2.8 Meta-Analysis

### 2.8.1 Primary Analysis

In the ROC curve, seven of the 18 points lie below the diagonal line, which marks where a guess would be correct in 50% of the cases (Fig. 2). Few of the other points approach the left upper corner where there would be good discrimination between the likelihood of success or failure with respect to pregnancy. Sensitivity and specificity values were heterogeneous (P-values for the Q-statistic in each case were <0.0001). This heterogeneity, together with the correlation between sensitivity and specificity, argues against combining sensitivity or specificity. Therefore, the meta-analyses combined the logs of the diagnostic odds ratios and the likelihood ratios, which are derived from sensitivity and specificity. The random effects model summary diagnostic odds ratio was 1.44 (95% CI 1.03, 2.03, $p = 0.045$). The funnel plot and the rank-correlation test ($z = 1.504$;

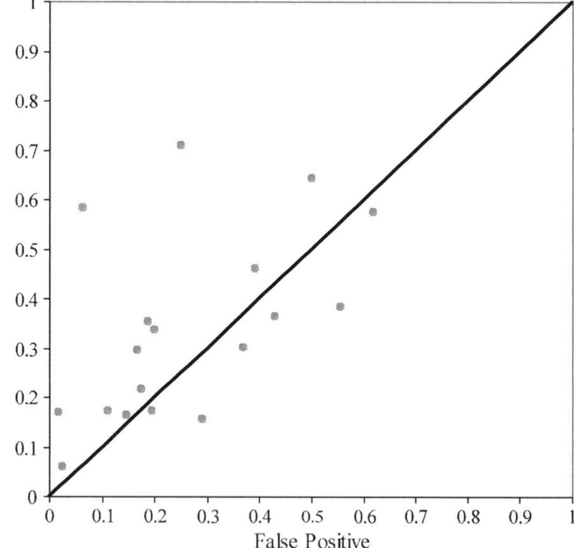


**Fig. 2** Receiver operating characteristics (ROC) curve: sperm DNA integrity and pregnancy

**Table 4** Subgroup analyses among studies of sperm DNA integrity and pregnancy

| | Number of studies | Number of cycles | DOR | 95% CI | *p*-Value |
|---|---|---|---|---|---|
| Treatment | | | | | |
| IVF | 6 | 1,107 | 1.53 | 0.77, 3.02 | 0.41 |
| ICSI | 7 | 549 | 1.12 | 0.59, 2.15 | |
| IVF, ICSI | 5 | 505 | 1.91 | 0.79, 4.57 | |
| Assay type | | | | | |
| SCSA | 11 | 1,441 | 1.31 | 0.81, 2.11 | 0.48 |
| TUNEL | 7 | 720 | 1.67 | 0.89, 3.11 | |

$p$ = 0.13) indicated that there was no significant publication bias. The random effects summary LR (+) was 1.23, 95% CI 0.98, 1.54, and the LR (−) was 0.81, 95% CI 0.67, 0.98).

### 2.8.2 Categorical Analyses

Categorical weighted average random effects model summary DORs are shown in Table 4. The DORs for each treatment group have confidence intervals that broadly overlap and the P-value indicates no significant difference according to treatment type. Although there is a nonsignificant trend to a higher diagnostic odds ratio in IVF cycles than in ICSI cycles, sperm DNA integrity test results were not significantly associated with pregnancy in 1,107 IVF cycles, and if it were significant, the association would not be strong (DOR = 1.53). In five studies that did not distinguish between IVF and ICSI cycles, the summary DOR (1.91) was inexplicably higher than in either of the defined treatment groups and might represent a stronger association or merely chance, as the lower 95% confidence interval lies below unity.

Weighted average random effects model summary DORs are also shown in Table 4 according to the type of sperm DNA assay that was used. There were no important differences in the summary estimates between studies using SCSA and TUNEL to estimate sperm DNA integrity.

*Sensitivity analysis.* Including the acridine orange study of ICSI cycles did not materially change the results: the revised diagnostic odds ratio was 1.53, 95% CI 1.07–2.19 (54).

## 2.9 Meta-Analysis Overview

In this systematic review of 13 studies involving 2,161 cycles of IVF and ICSI treatment, assessment of sperm DNA integrity was significantly associated with pregnancy (DOR = 1.44, 95% CI 1.03, 2.03). A diagnostic odds ratio greater than 1.0 means that with abnormal DNA integrity test results, the chance of disease (in this case, nonpregnancy) with IVF or ICSI is higher. This association was not adequate by itself to discriminate which couples would conceive after treatment. Sensitivity and specificity of the test in different studies were scattered around the nondiscriminatory diagonal of the ROC space. In general, likelihood ratios less than 0.5 or greater than 2.0 are needed for the prediction of disease or nondisease to be clinically important. The LRs in this study (LR+ = 1.23, LR− = 0.81) are not in a range that would prevent the application of assisted reproductive treatment (55). However, an LR of 1.2 or 0.8 will have a measurable impact (for example, decreasing expected pregnancy rates from 50 to 40% in some cases (60)). Subgroup analyses showed that test accuracy was not materially affected by test type or in the different types of patients who would have IVF or ICSI cycles.

One of the strengths of a systematic review is the improved precision of the summary diagnostic odds ratio estimates compared with the individual studies. Thus, although the diagnostic odds ratio was not large, the combined estimate was significantly different from unity, indicating that DNA integrity results have some effect on IVF and ICSI outcomes. No systematic review can be better, however, than the component studies and in this evaluation, the study quality varied. The data collection in 11/13 cohort studies was said to be prospective, which is a good feature because random allocation would not be expected in studies of diagnostic accuracy. The number of patients in each study was a limitation of this systematic review: average group size per estimate was just over 100 cycles (2,161/18); also, the diagnostic effects were generally small; and few studies provided a sample size statement. In only six of 13 studies was accrual of couples reported to be consecutive (13, 27, 28, 30, 32, 36). Also, few studies controlled for female age, a prognostic factor that might have altered the predictive value of sperm DNA integrity on IVF and ICSI pregnancy rates and thereby limited the ability of the meta-analysis to predict reproductive outcome. We did not detect significant publication bias but this is not surprising: publication bias usually means that small studies with negative results may be missing, while this analysis included six small studies with diagnostic odds ratios less than unity.

### 2.10 Conclusions of Meta-Analysis

The finding of a clinically significant but limited association between sperm DNA integrity and IVF or ICSI outcome is consistent with the results of other studies. In two studies that were otherwise eligible for this review for which a two-by-two table could not be constructed, three evaluations of sensitivity and specificity were within the range of the 18 estimates from the 13 studies that were included in the analysis (46, 47). Also, a subgroup analysis indicated no significant heterogeneity between summary estimates from SCSA and TUNEL studies, suggesting that both the measures of DNA integrity had similar predictive value. Moreover, inclusion of a study using the acridine orange method in the sensitivity analysis did not materially alter the summary diagnostic odds ratio. Variability in the association with pregnancy is unlikely to reflect intra- and interlaboratory variability or imprecision in the SCSA; this sperm DNA assay is adequately standardized between laboratories and statistically robust with limited intra- and interlaboratory variability (8). It is possible, of course, that better diagnostic performance might be observed in subgroups of infertility patients undergoing IVF or ICSI or in patient populations undergoing other treatments such as IUI, evaluation of which was not an objective of this study. Results of one large IUI study using SCSA suggested a strong effect of abnormal DNA integrity on pregnancy (27), while another IUI study found no difference in sperm chromatin dispersal results between pregnant and nonpregnant groups (49).

The sperm DNA integrity results are reminders that correlations can only describe how much of an outcome (e.g., pregnancy after IVF or ICSI) is explained by the variability in a "predictive test" (e.g., sperm DNA integrity testing.) Diagnosis and prediction in clinical practice are more demanding and require that the test results accurately discriminate between disease and nondisease states (55). Thus, the sperm DNA integrity assay results discriminate only between pregnancy rates of 23 and 30%, which may have limited utility for couples even if the prediction were precise.

The findings of this systematic review suggest a limited relation between sperm DNA integrity and IVF/ICSI outcome that may provide direction for further research. More clinical studies are needed to further evaluate other clinical groups of infertility patients such as those undergoing IUI to determine whether tests of DNA damage would be worthwhile with this treatment (56). Also, although the current literature does not identify subgroups of couples undergoing IVF or ICSI beyond those with recurrent spontaneous abortion who might have clinical characteristics that would merit the use of DNA integrity testing, the lack of strong predictors other than female age for ICSI success suggests that additional studies are needed to identify possible subgroups in which sperm DNA integrity testing might have greater value. Since TUNEL and SCSA are continuous variables, it is possible that "highly abnormal" sperm DNA integrity values (e.g., >50% DNA fragmentation) could have a more dramatic negative effect on IVF/ICSI outcome than that reported in this meta-analysis.

## 3 Treatment Options for Abnormal Sperm DNA Integrity

There are no treatments for abnormal sperm DNA integrity that are documented to be of clinical benefit. This may reflect the possibility that several different causes of sperm DNA fragmentation exist, so a "one size fits all" approach to treatment may not work. Alternatively, treatments that have been suggested to date may be inadequately effective or incompletely tested.

Abnormal sperm DNA integrity is hypothesized to occur because of intrinsic sperm defects (e.g., lack of protamine, ineffective sperm DNA packaging, etc.), after spermatogenesis (e.g., during sperm transport or as an effect of the paratesticular environment, such as heat from a varicocele, or from excess reactive oxygen species (ROS) effects on sperm, delayed sperm transport (such as in a partially obstructed epididymis or other region of the male reproductive tract) or from other unknown effects. Treatment has been directed toward these conditions that may cause abnormal sperm DNA integrity, or to "rescue" sperm before these effects manifest with sperm DNA fragmentation (e.g., testicular sperm extraction.) Relevant studies can be summarized in the following three different categories of treatment.

### 3.1 Varicocele Repair

Two published studies have examined the effect of varicocele repair on abnormal sperm DNA integrity. In these case series, men with abnormal SCSA results were selected for varicocelectomy and postoperative sperm DNA testing was compared to preoperative levels. No controls were provided in either of these studies. Zini et al. reported on patients with abnormal DNA integrity who underwent varicocele repair. A statistically significant, but perhaps clinically irrelevant, decrease of DNA fragmentation from 27.7 to 24.6% was observed (61). Werthman et al. reported on 11 men with abnormal sperm DNA integrity who underwent varicocele repair. Out of the 11 patients, ten men had decreased sperm DNA integrity postoperatively, and, based on the figures in this study, overall sperm DNA integrity appeared to decrease from 39 to 29% postoperatively (57). The Zini and Werthman studies support the observation that varicocele may contribute to abnormal DNA integrity, but the role of varicocelectomy in the treatment of these patients has not yet been definitively demonstrated.

### 3.2 Antioxidant Therapy

On the basis of the potential role of reactive oxygen species on sperm DNA fragmentation, the use of antioxidants could have utility in the treatment of men with abnormal sperm DNA fragmentation. Unfortunately, randomized controlled studies are very limited. Many case series have suggested that the use of antioxidants is associated with a decrease in sperm DNA integrity, but it is not clear if this observation is "regression to the mean" of a biological variable (e.g., sperm DNA integrity) or a true treatment effect. One randomized controlled study reported a randomized, controlled double-blind study of "Menevit," an antioxidant compound containing lycopene 6 mg, vitamin E 400 IU, vitamin C 100 mg, zinc 25 mg, selenium 26 mg, folate 0.5 mg, and garlic 1,000 mg (58). Sixty severe male factor couples with abnormal sperm DNA fragmentation were randomized to antioxidant treatment or placebo prior to IVF/ICSI. Unfortunately, sperm DNA fragmentation was not retested after antioxidant vitamin therapy. Couples where the man was treated with antioxidants had a higher embryo implantation rate (38.5 vs. 16% in those receiving placebo), but the pregnancy rate was not statistically significant for these groups. Greco et al. (62) treated 64 men with oral antioxidants (1 gm vitamin C, 1 gm vitamin E) and showed marked improvement in sperm DNA fragmentation (decreased from 22 to 9%). In another group of patients treated by the same authors, antioxidant treatment of men providing sperm for ICSI was associated with an increased pregnancy rate (7 to 48%) despite no effect on fertilization and cleavage rates (63). Unfortunately, we also do not know if the treatment actually changed sperm DNA fragmentation, as this was not tested during treatment. A trial of antioxidants may be reasonable to consider in couples where consistently abnormal sperm DNA integrity is detected, but repeat sperm DNA testing may be necessary to detect a beneficial effect of treatment.

### 3.3 Testicular Sperm Retrieval

As the testis is rich in antioxidant enzymes, it is possible that sperm are "protected" while in the testis and retrieval of sperm from the testis could provide sperm that have not yet undergone sperm DNA damage. Greco et al. reported on a series of 18 couples who had undergone at least two failed IVF cycles and had sperm DNA fragmentation >15% (59). Repeat ICSI cycles were done with both ejaculated and testicular sperm. Testicular sperm had lower DNA fragmentation (4.8 vs. 23.4%), and pregnancy rates were higher using testicular sperm (44 vs. 5.6%). Although this study suggested a benefit of testicular sperm extraction, only two couples in this series had abnormal sperm DNA integrity using the criteria typically applied in similar studies (sperm DNA fragmentation >30%.) Therefore, it is not clear if these results can be translated to the typical patient with abnormal sperm DNA integrity seen in clinical practice.

## 4 Clinical Summary

Abnormal sperm DNA integrity is associated with adverse reproductive outcomes after IVF/ICSI, although the magnitude of effect is not adequate to require sperm DNA integrity testing prior to assisted reproduction.

The summary DOR was 1.44 (95% CI 1.03, 2.03), indicating a statistically significant adverse effect of abnormal sperm DNA integrity on IVF/ICSI outcome. However, a secondary outcome measure of the meta-analysis, the summary likelihood ratios (LR) were not statistically predictive of pregnancy outcome (LR+ = 1.23, 95% CI 0.98, 1.54, LR− = 0.81, 95% CI 0.67, 0.98). Neither SCSA nor TUNEL tests were more predictive of pregnancy outcome after IVF/ICSI, and DNA integrity testing was not more predictive for IVF than ICSI. Treatments for abnormal DNA integrity, including varicocele repair, retrieval of testicular sperm, and antioxidant treatments have been investigated, but their role for management of this condition is still evolving. In summary, SCSA results affect the outcome of IVF/ICSI but the magnitude of effect is limited.

## References


1. Collins JA, Barnhart KT, Schlegel PN. Do sperm DNA integrity tests predict pregnancy with in vitro fertilization? Fertil Steril 2008; 89:823–31.
2. Sharma RK, Said T, Agarwal A. Sperm DNA damage and its clinical relevance in assessing reproductive outcome. Asian J Androl 2004; 6:139–48.
3. Alvarez JG. DNA fragmentation in human spermatozoa: significance in the diagnosis and treatment of infertility. Minerva Ginecol 2003; 55:233–9.
4. Agarwal A, Allamaneni SS. The effect of sperm DNA damage on assisted reproduction outcomes. A review. Minerva Ginecol 2004; 56:235–45.
5. O'Brien J, Zini A. Sperm DNA integrity and male infertility. Urology 2005; 65:16–22.
6. Lewis SE, Aitken RJ. DNA damage to spermatozoa has impacts on fertilization and pregnancy. Cell Tissue Res 2005; 322:33–41.
7. Erenpreiss J, Spano M, Erenpreisa J, Bungum M, Giwercman A. Sperm chromatin structure and male fertility: biological and clinical aspects. Asian J Androl 2006; 8:11–29.
8. Liu M-H, Lee KR, Li SH, Lu CH, Sun FJ, Hwu YM. Sperm chromatin structure assay parameters are not related to fertilization rates in in vitro fertilization and intracytoplasmic sperm injection, but might be related to spontaneous abortion rates. Fertil Steril 2008; 90:352–9.
9. Adamson GD, Baker VL. Subfertility: causes, treatment and outcome. Best Pract Res Clin Obstet Gynaecol 2003; 17:169–85.
10. Steures P, van der Steeg JW, Mol BW, et al. Prediction of an ongoing pregnancy after intrauterine insemination. Fertil Steril 2004; 82:45–51.
11. Carrell DT, Liu L. Altered protamine 2 expression is uncommon in donors of known fertility, but common among men with poor fertilizing capacity, and may reflect other abnormalities of spermiogenesis. J Androl 2001; 22:604–10.
12. Saleh RA, Agarwal A, Sharma RK, Said TM, Sikka SC, Thomas AJ, Jr. Evaluation of nuclear DNA damage in spermatozoa from infertile men with varicocele. Fertil Steril 2003; 80:1431–6.
13. Seli E, Gardner DK, Schoolcraft WB, Moffatt O, Sakkas D. Extent of nuclear DNA damage in ejaculated spermatozoa impacts on blastocyst development after in vitro fertilization. Fertil Steril 2004; 82:378–83.
14. Evenson DP, Jost LK, Marshall D, Zinaman MJ, Clegg E, Purvis K, et al. Utility of the sperm chromatin structure assay as a diagnostic and prognostic tool in the human fertility clinic. Hum Reprod 1999; 14:1039–49.
15. Evenson DP, Larson KL, Jost LK. Sperm chromatin structure assay: its clinical use for detecting sperm DNA fragmentation in male infertility and comparisons with other techniques. J Androl 2002; 23:25–43.
16. Sun JG, Jurisicova A, Casper RF. Detection of deoxyribonucleic acid fragmentation in human sperm: correlation with fertilization in vitro. Biol Reprod 1997; 56:602–7.
17. Irvine DS, Twigg JP, Gordon EL, Fulton N, Milne PA, Aitken RJ. DNA integrity in human spermatozoa: relationships with semen quality. J Androl 2000; 21:33–44.
18. Fernandez JL, Muriel L, Rivero MT, Goyanes V, Vazquez R, Alvarez JG. The sperm chromatin dispersion test: a simple method for the determination of sperm DNA fragmentation. J Androl 2003; 24:59–66.
19. Darzynkiewicz Z, Traganos F, Sharpless T, Melamed MR. Thermal denaturation of DNA in situ as studied by acridine orange staining and automated cytofluorometry. Exp Cell Res 1975; 90:411–28.
20. De Jonge C. The clinical value of sperm nuclear DNA assessment. Hum Fertil 2002; 5:51–3.
21. Sergerie M, Laforest G, Bujan L, Bissonnette F, Bleau G. Sperm DNA fragmentation: threshold value in male fertility. Hum Reprod 2005; 20:3446–51.
22. Spano M, Bonde JP, Hjollund HI, Kolstad HA, Cordelli E, Leter G. Sperm chromatin damage impairs human fertility. The Danish First Pregnancy Planner Study Team. Fertil Steril 2000; 73:43–50.
23. Agarwal A, Allamaneni SS. Sperm DNA damage assessment: a test whose time has come. Fertil Steril 2005; 84:850–3.
24. Larson KL, DeJonge CJ, Barnes AM, Jost LK, Evenson DP. Sperm chromatin structure assay parameters as predictors of failed pregnancy following assisted reproductive techniques. Hum Reprod 2000; 15:1717–22.
25. Larson-Cook KL, Brannian JD, Hansen KA, Kasperson KM, Aamold ET, Evenson DP. Relationship between the outcomes of assisted reproductive techniques and sperm DNA fragmentation as measured by the sperm chromatin structure assay. Fertil Steril 2003; 80:895–902.

26. Bungum M, Humaidan P, Spano M, Jepson K, Bungum L, Giwercman A. The predictive value of sperm chromatin structure assay (SCSA) parameters for the outcome of intrauterine insemination, IVF and ICSI. Hum Reprod 2004; 19:1401–8.
27. Bungum M, Humaidan P, Axmon A, Spano M, Bungum L, Erenpreiss J, et al. Sperm DNA integrity assessment in prediction of assisted reproduction technology outcome. Hum Reprod 2007; 22:174–9.
28. Boe-Hansen GB, Fedder J, Ersboll AK, Christensen P. The sperm chromatin structure assay as a diagnostic tool in the human fertility clinic. Hum Reprod 2006; 21:1576–82.
29. Borini A, Tarozzi N, Bizzaro D, Bonu MA, Fava L, Flamigni C, et al. Sperm DNA fragmentation: paternal effect on early post-implantation embryo development in ART. Hum Reprod 2006; 21:2876–81.
30. Check JH, Graziano V, Cohen R, Krotec J, Check ML. Effect of an abnormal sperm chromatin structural assay (SCSA) on pregnancy outcome following (IVF) with ICSI in previous IVF failures. Arch Androl 2005; 51:121–4.
31. Gandini L, Lombardo F, Paoli D, Caruso F, Eleuteri P, Leter G, et al. Full-term pregnancies achieved with ICSI despite high levels of sperm chromatin damage. Hum Reprod 2004; 19:1409–17.
32. Host E, Lindenberg S, Smidt-Jensen S. The role of DNA strand breaks in human spermatozoa used for IVF and ICSI. Acta Obstet Gynecol Scand 2000; 79:559–63.
33. Huang CC, Lin DP, Tsao HM, Cheng TC, Liu CH, Lee MS. Sperm DNA fragmentation negatively correlates with velocity and fertilization rates but might not affect pregnancy rates. Fertil Steril 2005; 84:130–40.
34. Payne JF, Raburn DJ, Couchman GM, Price TM, Jamison MG, Walmer DK. Redefining the relationship between sperm deoxyribonucleic acid fragmentation as measured by the sperm chromatin structure assay and outcomes of assisted reproductive techniques. Fertil Steril 2005; 84:356–64.
35. Virro MR, Larson-Cook KL, Evenson DP. Sperm chromatin structure assay (SCSA) parameters are related to fertilization, blastocyst development, and ongoing pregnancy in in vitro fertilization and intracytoplasmic sperm injection cycles. Fertil Steril 2004; 81:1289–95.
36. Zini A, Meriano J, Kader K, Jarvi K, Laskin CA, Cadesky K. Potential adverse effect of sperm DNA damage on embryo quality after ICSI. Hum Reprod 2005; 20:3476–80.
37. Irwig L, Macaskill P, Glasziou P, Fahey M. Meta-analytic methods for diagnostic test accuracy. J Clin Epidemiol 1995; 48:119–30.
38. Hanley J, McNeil B. The meaning and use of the area under a receiver operating characteristic (ROC) curve. Radiology 1982; 143:29–36.
39. Greenland S. Quantitative methods in the review of epidemiologic literature. Epidemiol Rev 1987; 9:1–30.
40. Higgins JPT, Thompson SG, Deeks JJ, Altman DG. Measuring inconsistency in meta-analyses. BMJ 2003; 327:557–60.
41. Deeks JJ, Altman DG, Bradburn MJ. Statistical methods for examining heterogeneity and combining results from several studies in meta-analysis. In: Egger M, Davey Smith G, Altman DG, eds. Systematic Reviews in Health Care: Meta-analysis in Context, 2 ed. London: BMJ; 2001. p. 285–312.
42. Glas AS, Lijmer JG, Prins MH, Bonsel GJ, Bossuyt PM. The diagnostic odds ratio: a single indicator of test performance. J Clin Epidemiol 2003; 56:1129–35.
43. Egger M, Davey Smith G, Schneider M, Minder C. Bias in meta-analysis detected by a simple graphical test. BMJ 1997; 315:629–34.
44. Begg CB, Mazumdar M. Operating characteristics of a rank correlation test for publication bias. Biometrics 1994;50:1088–101.
45. Hedges LV, Olkin I. Statistical Methods for Meta-Analysis. Orlando: Academic; 1985.
46. Benchaib M, Braun V, Lornage J, Hadj S, Salle B, Lejeune H, et al. Sperm DNA fragmentation decreases the pregnancy rate in an assisted reproductive technique. Hum Reprod 2003; 18:1023–8.
47. Henkel R, Hajimohammad M, Stalf T, Hoogendijk C, Mehnert C, Menkveld R, et al. Influence of deoxyribonucleic acid damage on fertilization and pregnancy. Fertil Steril 2004; 81:965–72.
48. Morris ID, Ilott S, Dixon L, Brison DR. The spectrum of DNA damage in human sperm assessed by single cell gel electrophoresis (Comet assay) and its relationship to fertilization and embryo development. Hum Reprod 2002; 17:990–8.
49. Muriel L, Meseguer M, Fernandez JL, Alvarez J, Remohi J, Pellicer A, et al. Value of the sperm chromatin dispersion test in predicting pregnancy outcome in intrauterine insemination: a blind prospective study. Hum Reprod 2006; 21:738–44.
50. Duran EH, Morshedi M, Taylor S, Oehninger S. Sperm DNA quality predicts intrauterine insemination outcome: a prospective cohort study. Hum Reprod 2002; 17:3122–8.
51. Saleh RA, Agarwal A, Nada EA, El-Tonsy MH, Sharma RK, Meyer A, et al. Negative effects of increased sperm DNA damage in relation to seminal oxidative stress in men with idiopathic and male factor infertility. Fertil Steril 2003; 79 Suppl 3:1597–605.
52. Tomlinson MJ, Moffatt O, Manicardi GC, Bizzaro D, Afnan M, Sakkas D. Interrelationships between seminal parameters and sperm nuclear DNA damage before and after density gradient centrifugation: implications for assisted conception. Hum Reprod 2001; 16:2160–5.
53. Tomsu M, Sharma V, Miller D. Embryo quality and IVF treatment outcomes may correlate with different sperm comet assay parameters. Hum Reprod 2002; 17:1856–62.
54. Virant-Klun I, Tomazevic T, Meden-Vrtovec H. Sperm single-stranded DNA, detected by acridine orange staining, reduces fertilization and quality of ICSI-derived embryos. J Assist Reprod Genet 2002; 19:319–28.
55. Jaeschke R, Guyatt G, Lijmer J. Diagnostic tests. In: Guyatt G, Rennie D, eds. Users' Guides to the Medical Literature: A Manual for Evidence-Based Practice. Chicago: The American Medical Association; 2002. p. 121–40.
56. Loft S, Kold-Jensen T, Hjollund NH, Giwercman A, Gyllemborg J, Ernst E, et al. Oxidative DNA damage in human sperm influences time to pregnancy. Hum Reprod 2003; 18:1265–72.
57. Werthman P, Wixon R, Kasperson K, Evenson DP. Significant decrease in sperm deoxyribonucleic acid fragmentation after varicocelectomy. Fertil Steril 2007; 90(5):1800–4.

58. Tremellen K, Miari G, Froiland D, Thompson J. A randomised control trial examining the effect of an antioxidant (Menevit) on pregnancy outcome during IVF-ICSI treatment. Aust N Z J Obstet Gynaecol 2007; 47: 216–221.
59. Greco E, Scarselli F, Iacobelli M, Rienzi L, Ubaldi F, Ferrero S, Franco G, Anniballo N, Mendoza C, Tesarik J. Efficient treatment of infertility due to sperm DNA damage by ICSI with testicular spermatozoa. Hum Reprod 2005; 20:226–300.
60. Grimes DA, Schulz KF. Refining clinical diagnosis with likelihood ratios. Lancet 2005;365:1500–5.
61. Zini A, Blumenfeld A, Libman J, Willis J. Beneficial effect of microsurgical varicocelectomy on human sperm DNA integrity. Hum Reprod. 2005;20:1018–21.
62. Greco E, Iacobelli M, Rienzi L, Ubaldi F, Ferrero S, Tesarik J. Reduction of the incidence sperm DNA fragmentation by oral antioxidant treatment. J Androl 2005;26:349–53.
63. Greco E, Romano S, Iacobelli M, Ferrero S, Baroni E, Minasi MG, Ubaldi F, Rienzi L, Tesarik J, ICSI in cases of sperm DNA damage: beneficial effect of oral antioxidant treatment. Hum Reprod 2005;20:2590–4.

# Section III
# Assisted Reproduction Techniques

# Selecting the Most Competent Embryo

S. Temel Ceyhan, Katharine V. Jackson, and Catherine Racowsky

**Abstract** With improvements in implantation potential, and the compelling need to reduce the likelihood of multiple pregnancies resulting from in vitro fertilization (IVF), efforts have continued to focus on developing methods to select the most competent embryo for transfer. For the first 15 years or so of human IVF, embryo selection methodologies exclusively involved morphological assessment of the embryo at a single time-point, immediately prior to transfer. Despite considerable efforts to define those characteristics predictive of high implantation potential, the implantation rate of selected embryos is typically only around 30%. More recent attempts to improve selection have assessed characteristics of the oocyte along with those of the embryo at specific times during culture in order to derive a cumulative score. However, these studies have led to conflicting results regarding the worth of cumulative scoring. These conflicting results are likely associated with various study limitations including small sample sizes, a preponderance of retrospective studies combined with variation in timing of evaluations and, in some cases, the use of transfer cohorts in which not all embryos have known implantation fate. While culture to the blastocyst stage has been used in attempts to improve selection, this approach is beneficial for only selected, good prognosis patients, and it is unlikely that even the best current culture media precisely mimic the uterine environment.

Given the accepted limitations of morphological approaches, alternative selection methodologies are under development involving targeted analyses or profiling approaches. Targeted analyses involve quantification of known markers in the medium. While these analyses hold some promise, technologies are either cumbersome with turnaround times too long for prospective application, and/or have relatively low predictive value. Of greater potential, metabolomic profiling using spectroscopic analyses of spent media have rapid turnaround, require very small volumes of medium for analysis and may provide superior selection as compared with morphological assessment alone.

While we still depend on morphological assessment as our first line approach to embryo selection, it is likely that this may be used in conjunction with metabolomic profiling in the future. As we continue to strive towards identifying the single most competent embryo in any cohort, the aim will be to interface such technologies with the cutting-edge areas of genomic and proteomics research. These are exciting times in the field of IVF, and much future research is required to fine-tune these promising technologies.

**Keywords** Noninvasive embryo selection • Implantation • Morphology scoring • Spectroscopic metabolomic profiling

## 1 Introduction

The single most important challenge for the success of in vitro fertilization (IVF) is the identification of the most developmentally competent embryo in every cohort. Once this challenge has been met, we will be positioned to transfer that one identified embryo in each and every cycle, thereby performing single embryo transfer (SET) to all of our patients. Nevertheless, even when so positioned, our expectations for the probability of a live birth from SET must be realistically set against

S.T. Ceyhan, K.V. Jackson and C. Racowsky (✉)
Department of Obstetrics and Gynecology,
ASB 1 + 3, Rm 082, Brigham and Women's Hospital,
75 Francis Street, Boston, MA, 02115, USA
e-mail: temelceyhen@yahoo.com

D.T. Carrell et al. (eds.), *Biennial Review of Infertility,* DOI: 10.1007/978-1-60327-392-3_10

the background rate of natural conception. The chance of an in vivo fertilized oocyte reaching term is approximately 20–30% (1), which is not dissimilar to the implantation rate achieved after SET in unselected patients (2).

Although there have been significant developments in IVF during the last three decades, approaches for embryo selection and assessment remain limited. Indeed, despite active research in the fields of genomics, proteomics and metabolomics, we still depend on morphological assessment as our first line approach when evaluating embryos. Initially, in order to compensate for our deficiencies in embryo selection, more than one embryo was typically transferred in the hope that at least one viable embryo was included. The consequence was unacceptably high multiple rates from IVF, and the attendant risks to fetal and maternal health.

Principles underlying embryo selection techniques should take into consideration potential adverse effects to the embryo, the level of skill required to perform the selection technique, turn-around to avoid need for freezing, cost and need for specialized equipment and, lastly, the amount of information obtained. The approaches used fall into the two broad categories of noninvasive and invasive. In this chapter, we will focus exclusively on the noninvasive approaches (see the chapters discussing preimplantation genetic screening (PGS) for coverage of the invasive techniques). We will start by considering assessment of oocyte quality since it is generally considered that this is the primary driver behind embryo quality. We will then proceed to consider the various approaches used in the evaluation of the embryo itself and the relative efficacies of the evaluation procedures. Finally, we will offer an objective appraisal of the current literature regarding selection of the most competent embryo with respect to morphological approaches on the one hand, and developing technologies to screen spent culture media on the other.

As we consider these topics, we must continually bear in mind that numerous variables impact upon the ability of embryos to develop to their full potential in vitro. These variables include, but undoubtedly are not limited to, maternal age, infertility diagnosis, ovarian stimulation, and endometrial receptivity, in addition to the lab technologies and successful intrauterine placement of the embryos at transfer. Each of these variables independently and collectively will inevitably impact when evaluating efficacy of the selection techniques used. Any evaluation technique will obviously only have use for selection when more embryos are available than will be transferred.

## 2 Oocyte Morphological Assessment

### *2.1 Gross Morphology*

With the introduction of intracytoplasmic sperm injection (ICSI) (3, 4), it became possible to identify the meiotic status of freshly retrieved oocytes and to assess, in some detail, the morphology of both intracellular and extracellular structures. In contrast, assessment of oocytes destined for standard IVF is only possible at the fertilization check after removal of the cumulus and corona cells as the oocyte is prepared for pronuclear evaluation. Early work suggested a relationship between the degree of expansion of corona-cumulus complex and oocyte maturity (5). However, the oocyte-cumulus complex needs to be spread for accurate assessment of meiotic status, which may compromise viability. Furthermore, such an approach provides little information regarding the actual quality of mature, metaphase-II (MII) oocytes [i.e., those with an extruded first polar body (PBI)]. Indeed, the results of further studies support general agreement that there is poor correlation between the quality and degree of expansion of corona-cumulus complex and oocyte maturity (6–8).

Several studies have attempted to correlate morphological characteristics of the oocyte with meiotic maturity and quality, such as overall shape, the color and granularity of the cytoplasm, the zona pellucida thickness, the size of the perivitelline space (PVS), the presence of vacuoles, the presence or absence of the germinal vesicle, and the shape of the PBI when present (9–13) (see Chapter "Human Oocyte Abnormalities: Basic Analyses and Clinical Applications" for an excellent review). Indeed, morphological abnormalities have been classified into those that are extracytoplasmic and those that are intracytoplasmic (9–14; Table 1). In contrast to these abnormal characteristics, morphologically normal oocytes are those considered to be spherical in shape exhibiting an unfragmented PBI,

**Table 1** Classification of oocyte abnormalities

| Oocyte abnormalities | |
|---|---|
| Intracytoplasmic | Extracytoplasmic |
| Granular cytoplasm | Fragmented PBI |
| Centrally located granular area | Abnormal PBI (large and/or cytoplasmic abnormalities) |
| Vacuoles | Abnormal zona pellucida (thick and/or dark) |
| SER clusters | Large perivitelline space |
| Refractile bodies | Abnormal oocyte shape |

*SER* smooth endoplasmic reticulum
Characteristics compiled from (9–14)

smooth cytoplasm with no inclusions, a uniform PVS, and a transparent zona pellucida (Fig. 1) Interestingly, zona thickness decreases both with increasing days in culture (average thickness of 17.7 μm on day 1, 16.3 μm, and 14.9 μm on day 3), and with increasing patient age (15).

Several studies have demonstrated an association between oocyte quality and one or more of the above abnormalities. For example, the presence of vacuoles, an abnormal PBI, and a large perivitelline space each have been related to a lower fertilization rate (12, 14, 16, 17). Moreover, cytoplasmic abnormalities appear to be tightly associated with oocyte quality, and reflective of poorer embryo quality (18). Based on these observations, Rienzi et al. (14) derived a MII oocyte morphological score (MOMS) by identifying relationships among oocyte appearance, fertilization status, PN score, and day 2 embryo quality. As shown in Table 2, abnormal morphology of the PBI, a large perivitelline space, increased cytoplasmic granularity, the presence of a centrally located granular area, and vacuoles at MII stage were each associated with a decreased potential of the oocyte to fertilize, cleave, and/or develop into a viable embryo. However, earlier studies showed no relationship between embryo morphology (10) and any oocyte abnormality except for the refractile body which was associated with a lower, albeit insignificantly reduced, fertilization rate (19).

Clearly, although gross oocyte morphology may give us important information about fertilization potential and subsequent developmental fate, there are some inconsistencies in the findings, and evaluation at this stage is unlikely to be as powerful for selection as observations acquired at later stages of culture.

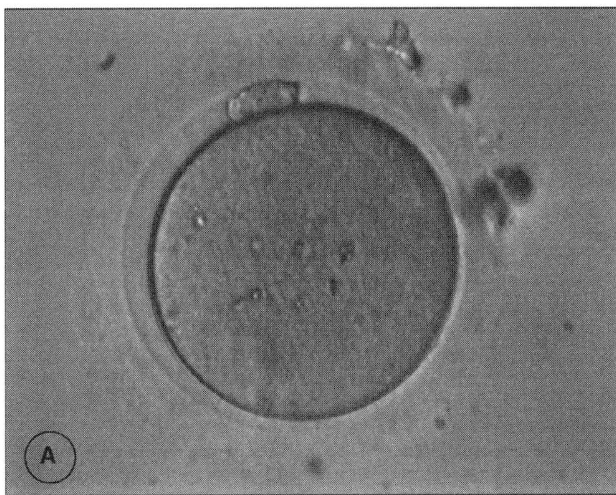


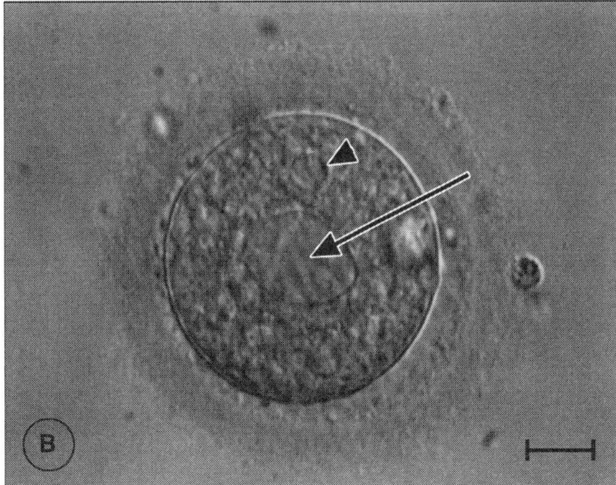


**Fig. 1** Micrographs of oocytes showing normal and abnormal gross morphology. (**a**) Normal oocyte with a smooth cytoplasm, an intact PB with clear zona pellucida of uniform thickness; (**b**) An oocyte showing abnormal morphology with severely pycnotic cytoplasm with a large central vacuole (*arrow*) and a smaller inclusion (*arrowhead*), and a rough zona pellucida overlying a perivitelline space with inclusions along the inner zona surface. The *bar* represents 20 μm

**Table 2** Metaphase II oocyte morphology scoring system (MOMS)

| | Points |
|---|---|
| *Extracytoplasmic features* | |
| Abnormal I polar body | 2.0 |
| Large perivitelline space | 1.4 |
| *Cytoplasmic features* | |
| Granular cytoplasm | 1.4 |
| Centrally located granular area | 2.7 |
| Vacuoles | 2.1 |

Reprinted from (14), (Table 4), with permission, Elsevier

## 2.2 The First Polar Body

Formation of the PBI occurs at the end of the first meiotic division and is dependent upon precise formation of the meiotic spindle under delicate structural and functional control of microtubule formation. Since the extruded and otherwise to be discarded haploid set of chromosomes give rise to PBI, it is not surprising that the appearance of PBI may provide insight regarding the ploidy status of the oocyte and its overall viability. Accordingly, much effort has focused on assessing the relationship between the PBI characteristics and embryo quality.

The absence of the PBI indicates that the oocyte is likely to have failed to progress to MII, although the rare possibility exists that the oocyte may have undergone rapid maturation to MII with subsequent degeneration and disappearance of the PBI before examination (20). For those oocytes retrieved at metaphase-I (MI), a portion will complete meiotic maturation in vitro, reaching MII. Fertilization rates are maximized in such oocytes if ICSI is performed at least 2 h after PBI emission (21, 22).

Ebner et al. (23) graded the oocyte according to PBI morphology into three grades: (1) Ovoid or round, smooth surface; (2) Ovoid or round, rough surface; (3) Fragmented, with a fourth grade including oocytes with a large perivitelline space. These investigators found that ICSI of oocytes with an intact, well-shaped PBI (grade 1 or 2) yielded higher fertilization rates and also higher quality embryos than those oocytes with a fragmented PBI or having a large perivitelline space. Collectively, the results showed that embryo selection on the basis of PBI morphology resulted in improved implantation rates and pregnancy rates. In contrast, other studies relating PBI morphology to oocyte quality have failed to reveal this correlation (24–27), except for a lower viability associated with a large PBI (24). In fact, aneuploidy rate of MII oocytes may be unrelated to the morphology of the PBI (26).

## 2.3 The Meiotic Spindle

During the very early phase of transition from MI to MII of meiosis, the meiotic spindle is formed with a highly dynamic structure of microtubules. It is located radially, at the oocyte periphery, with one pole attached to the cell cortex. The meiotic spindle controls chromosome movement through the different stages of meiosis and is involved in various functions that are essential for fertilization and early post-fertilization events, recognized as crucial for ensuring correct chromosome segregation and genomic stability after oocyte activation. For these reasons, integrity and positioning of the spindle may provide valuable markers for predicting oocyte quality.

The polarized light microscope (PolScope™) (see Chapter "Human Oocyte Abnormalities: Basic Analyses and Clinical Applications") has been used to screen metaphase II oocytes for quality by assessing the presence, position, and integrity of the birefringent spindle (see 28, for review). Although the PolScope™ is expensive, this real-time approach does not require fixation or staining of the oocytes. Furthermore, this imaging system provides a noninvasive approach, therefore apparently not rendering the oocyte nonviable, as is the case with confocal microscopy (29, 30). Visualization of the bifringent spindle can predict fertilization potential, embryo development and clinical outcome (31–35). Indeed, absence of the spindle has been associated with lower probability of fertilization, lower likelihood of embryo cleavage and blastocyst formation (31), and lower implantation rates (33). Of interest, despite a significantly higher proportion of abnormal spindles in older women (36), is the fact that surprisingly there appears to be no relationship between the extent of spindle retardance and patient age (27). While several authors have suggested that the PolScope may be used to reduce spontaneous abortions by screening out the oocytes with chromosomal aberrations (37), no rigorous studies have been performed to confirm this possibility. Nevertheless, detection of the position of the spindle may avoid damage from ICSI since spindle location does not always correlate with PBI position (32).

## 2.4 Zona Pellucida

During oogenesis, a glycoprotein coat- the zona pellucida (ZP)- is laid down around the developing oogonium. This structure is comprised of three layers (see 38, for review) and plays a fundamental role in the fertilization process. The structure is also thought to provide a protective coating to the embryo as it traverses the reproductive tract (39), prior to release of the embryo during the "hatching" process, with subsequent interaction between the trophectoderm and uterine epithelium at implantation. Because of the wide variation in thickness and also appearance of the ZP (Fig. 2), studies have investigated the relationship between zona appearance and developmental competency. Twenty years ago, Cohen et al. (40) studied the association between the extent of ZP variation within an embryo (Z variation) and its implantation potential. This study, which showed that implantation rates were significantly increased with increasing variation in thickness, laid the foundation for other studies assessing the relationship between ZP thickness and embryo viability. While the results of one study showed that zona thickness was inversely related to the likelihood of pregnancy (41), a more recent analysis revealed that adding Z variation to embryo selection was only beneficial in embryos of poor morphological grade (42). Consistent with the Cohen study, pregnancy rates were positively associated with Z variation after transfer of poor quality embryos. Shen et al. (43), have further analyzed the relationship between implantation potential, ZP thickness, and the structure of the three overt ZP layers using the Polscope™,. They found that thickness was significantly increased, and the mean magnitude of light retardance was nearly 30% higher in the inner ZP layer of oocytes contributing to conception cycles compared to non conception cycles. They offer this technique as a new option in oocyte selection.

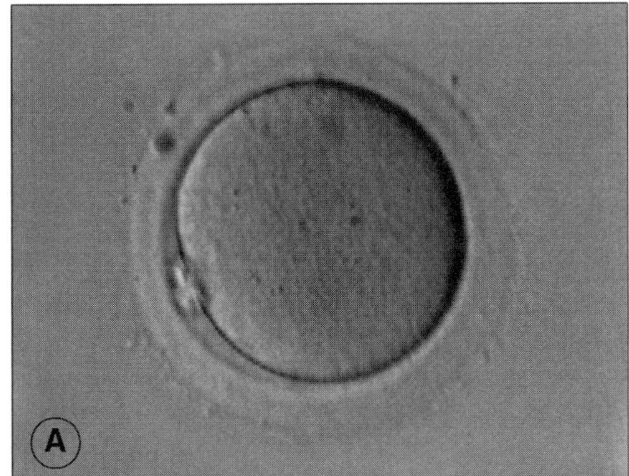


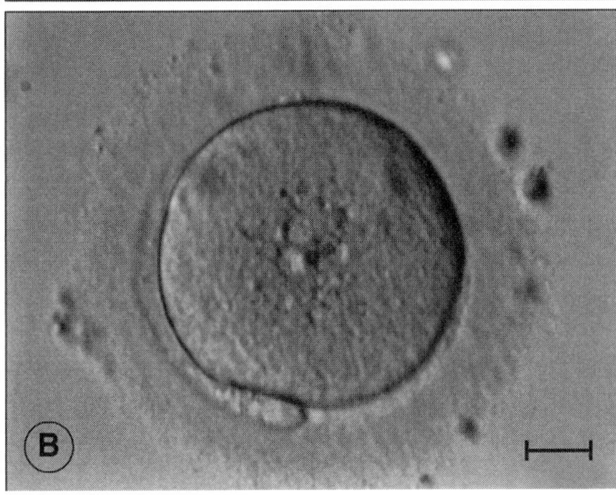


**Fig. 2** Micrographs of oocytes with zonae pellucidae of varying thickness and appearance. (**a**) An oocyte with a zona of average thickness (~17 μm) and smooth outer edge; (**b**) An oocyte with a thick zona (~30 μm) and a rough outer edge. The *bar* represents 20 μm

## 2.5 Summary

Based on the above discussion, it is clear that numerous studies have attempted to correlate morphological appearance of the oocyte with embryo developmental competency. Despite the recognized shortfalls of correlating oocyte appearance with cytoplasmic maturity, findings from several studies do support some relationship between oocyte abnormalities and compromised embryonic development. In addition, there is some data in support of an association between implantation potential and Z variation, and/or retardance of the inner zonal layer. However, further work is required to assess the true benefit of oocyte assessment in selecting the best embryo. In this context, sperm morphology ,and in particular integrity of sperm chromatin is a critical consideration.

# 3 Embryo Morphology

## 3.1 Single-Day Scoring

### 3.1.1 Pronuclear Stage Embryos

Oocytes are typically evaluated for fertilization status 14–16 h after ICSI and 16–18 h after standard insemination. At the fertilization check, the presence and number of pronuclei (PNs) are recorded. A diploid zygote will exhibit 2PN, while other variants include those failing to fertilize (0PN), or having either a single PN, or more than 2PN.

After sperm entry into the ooplasm, the oocyte resumes meiosis to release the second polar body at telophase II. The retained female haploid chromatids form the female PN and the sperm DNA decondenses to form the male pronucleus. Within the pronuclei, the nuclear precursor bodies (NPB; the sites for rRNA synthesis) become visible. These dynamic structures vary in size, shape, and number as they migrate within the nucleus, eventually merging to reduce the overall number. Due to the importance of the NPB's in development, many studies have investigated a possible association between implantation potential and their disposition (44, 45). These studies have given rise to various PN scoring systems that reflect the size, number, and position of the NPBs in each of the PNs.

## PN Scoring Systems

The original PN scoring system as devised by Tesarik and Greco (44), correlated NPB size, number, and distribution with implantation potential. Six patterns of PN morphology were distinguished; 0 (normal): the number of NPB in both PN never differed by more than three; (1) Big difference (>3) in the number of NPB in both PN, (2) Small number (<7) of NPB without polarization in at least one PN, (3) Large number (>7) of NPB with polarization in at least one PN, (4) Very small number (<3) of NPB in at least one PN, (5) Polarized distribution of NPB in one PN and nonpolarized in the other. They found that pattern 0 was associated with higher pregnancy rates than patterns 1–5 (50% vs. 9% clinical pregnancy rate, respectively), although the differences did not reach statistical significance.

Subsequent to the establishment of the above scoring system, Scott et al. (45) advanced another scoring system based more on nuclei size and alignment, although also including NPB number and distribution. Using these criteria, four categories were developed: Z-1, Z-2, Z-3, and Z-4. The Z-1 zygotes exhibited polarized NPBs, with each PN having the same number; Z-2 zygotes exhibited equal numbers and sizes of NPBs which were equally scattered in the two nuclei; Z-3 zygotes had either equal numbers of NPBs in each PN but with polarization only evident in one, or unequal numbers or sizes of NPBs between the two PNs; Z-4 zygotes had unequal numbers of NPBs with or without PN alignment. Examples of zygotes exhibiting various Z-scores are shown in Fig. 3. Results showed an equivalent increase of 1.6-fold in implantation rates when this Z-scoring system was included in embryo selection.

Numerous other studies have assessed whether the PN scores are correlated with improved outcomes. The balance of publications shows a relationship between PN scoring (with or without day 3/day 5 grading) and improved embryo development (46–48), and/or increased pregnancy and implantation potential (49–51; reviewed by 52). Further, several studies have reported that PN morphology also predicts blastocyst formation (45) and embryo chromosomal constitution (53–55). Inconsistent with these findings, however, Salumets et al. (56) failed to show a relationship between zygote scores and embryo quality or implantation, and Payne et al. (57) found that use of a Z-scoring model provided no additional benefit to embryo selection as compared with a standard cleavage stage embryo morphology model. Moreover, when analyses were performed exclusively with transfers involving embryos with unique zygote scores, no significant differences in live birth rates were observed among embryos having Z-1, Z-2, or Z-3 scores (58).

It is unclear why the utility of the Z-score for embryo selection varies among investigators. However, several possibilities exist: (a) Given the dynamic nature of PN formation (59), including NPB distribution, migration, coalescence, and dissolution, the timing of evaluation is of critical importance; (b) Zygotes formed from ICSI reveal their PNs approximately 4 h earlier than those formed by routine insemination (60), indicating that the method of fertilization must be taken into consideration when evaluating pronuclear embryos; and (c) Accurate assessment of the 3-dimensional disposition and number of NPBs is challenged not only by the difficulty of visually memorizing spatial organization of the structures through multiple focal planes, but also because the procedure must be performed rapidly to avoid prolonged exposure of the zygote to light, and to temperature and pH shifts.

## The Cytoplasmic Halo

In addition to the disposition and appearance of the pronuclei, attention has also been given to the cytoplasmic "halo". This refers to the clear ring-like region, located

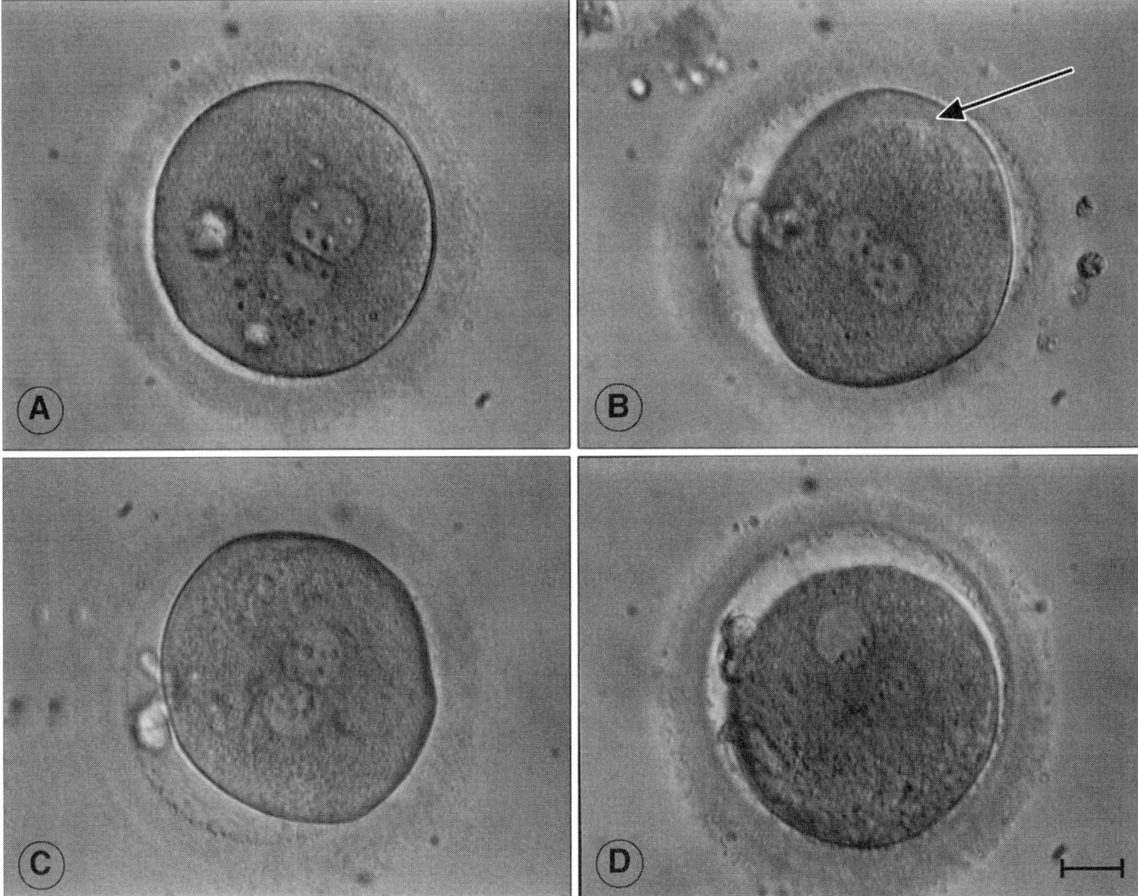


**Fig. 3** Micrographs of zygotes showing various Z-scores (Scott, 44). (**a**) A Z-1 zygote showing polarized NPBs of equal number; (**b**) a Z-2 zygote showing equal numbers and sizes of NPBs, equally scattered in the PNs; note also the clear cytoplasmic region (*arrow*), representing the "cytoplasmic halo"; (**c**) a Z-3 zygote showing unequal numbers and sizes of NPBs between the two PNs; and (**d**) a Z-4 zygote with non-alignment of the PNs and unequal number and distribution of NPBs. The *bar* represents 20 μm

immediately under the oolemma, which represents cytoplasmic streaming as organelles [particularly mitochondria (61)] are translocated towards the center of the zygote (Fig. 3b). Similar to the conflicting results regarding relevance of the Z-score for embryo selection, disagreement exists with respect to the utility of using the cytoplasmic halo as a marker of embryo quality. Some studies report improved quality of embryos derived from zygotes having a halo (56), with increased blastocyst formation (62), and implantation (63). Interestingly, however, in cases of extreme halo visualization, there appears to be a negative effect on blastocyst development (48). The few studies attempting to relate the presence of a halo to pregnancy have also produced conflicting data; Salumets et al. (56) found no relationship; in contrast, Stalf et al. (64) found a positive association.

### 3.1.2 Cleavage Stage Embryo

#### First Mitotic Division ("Early Cleavage")

The timing of human embryos through the first mitotic division occurs over a wide interval, ranging from 20 to beyond 27 h after zygote formation (65, 66), with a majority entering this division between 25 and 27 h. Within this timeframe, one can expect four classes of embryo (67): (a) those still at the 2PN stage; (b) those at the 0PN stage (i.e. that have undergone syngamy, breakdown of the PN membranes and their subsequent fusion; (c) those at the 2-cell stage; and (d) those exhibiting more than 2 cells.

In view of the variance in developmental kinetics among embryos, considerable attention has focused on the possibility that those zygotes that complete this first division first, have the highest developmental competence. Over 10 years ago, Shoukir et al. (68) designated those embryos that had reached the 2-cell stage by 25-h post-insemination as having undergone "early cleavage". These investigators found that more clinical pregnancies were associated with transfers of "early cleavage" embryos as compared with those not involving "early cleavage" embryos (33.3% vs. 14.7%; $p = 0.04$).

Following this first report, the time to first cell division has been extensively studied as a predictor of improved pregnancy outcomes. However, precise timing for evaluating zygotes for early cleavage remains to be definitively established. Majority of studies have selected a 25–27 h time window (69–71), with only a few taking into consideration a possible earlier developmental programming of ICSI zygotes (e.g. 25–26 h vs. 26–27 h, respectively; 72). Regardless, most investigations have confirmed the findings of Shoukir et al. that early cleavage is associated with increased developmental potential, as assessed by blastocyst formation (73) and clinical pregnancy rates (70, 74). However, at least one study has failed to show any such relationship when examining only mononucleated 4-cell embryos on day 2 (75).

It is unknown why early cleavage stage embryos appear to yield embryos of high quality. However, it may be hypothesized that (a) they have improved synchronization of cytoplasmic and nuclear maturation, and overall higher metabolic fitness; and/or (b) that sperm quality is implicated, as reflected by superior contribution of centrioles to the oocyte since these are required for entry into the first mitotic division (71).

While very few studies have addressed a possible relationship between morphological features of the 2-cell embryos and quality of cleavage stage embryos, it has recently been concluded that 2-cell embryos with blastomeres of even size result in more "top" quality day 2 embryos than those with blastomeres of "uneven" size (77% vs. 46.3%, $p < 0.0001$; (72)).

## Second and Third Mitotic Divisions

### *Cell Number*

Development of the 1-cell zygote progresses through the early mitotic divisions to reach the 8-cell stage on day 3 of culture (Fig. 4). However, determination of precise developmental timeline for human embryos can only be accurately assessed using time-lapse cinematography. Unfortunately, such an approach has not been

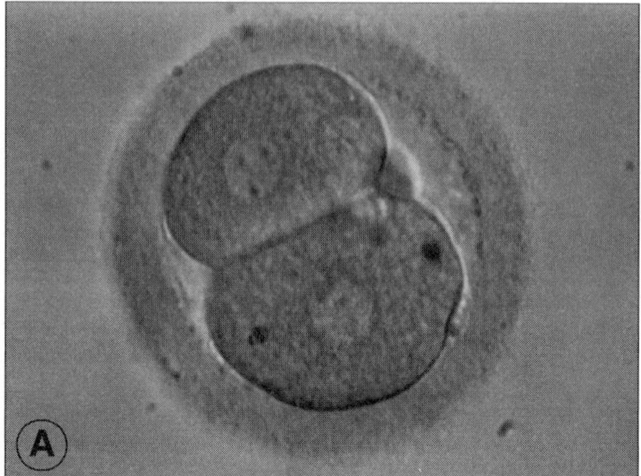


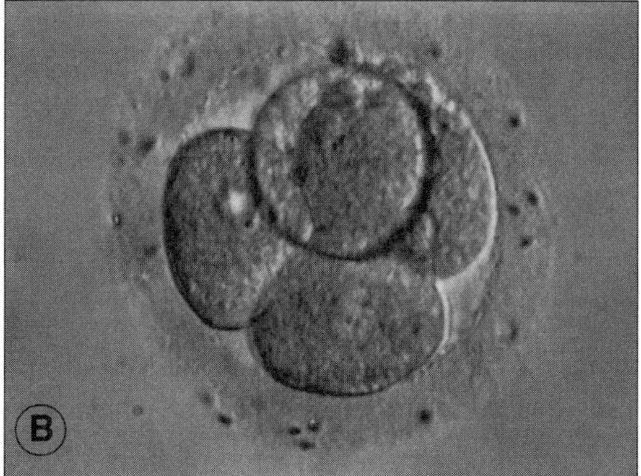


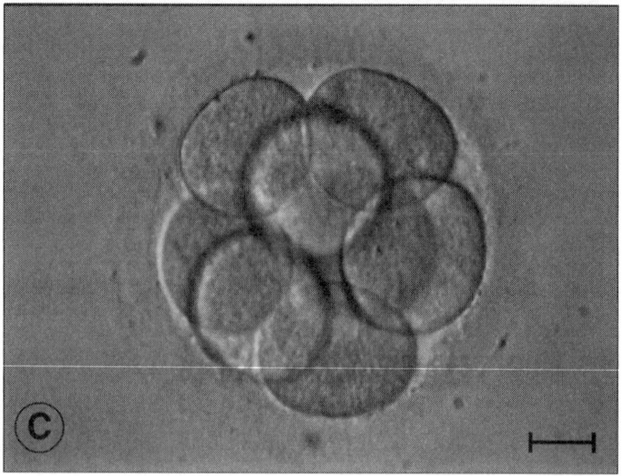


**Fig. 4** Micrographs showing (**a**) a 2-cell embryo; note the mononucleated blastomeres, each exhibiting a single nucleus; (**b**) a 4-cell embryo; note that the blastomeres are slightly asymmetric and that one of them exhibits a single nucleus (*arrowhead*); (**c**) an 8-cell embryo showing perfectly symmetric blastomeres and no fragmentation. The *bar* represents 30 μm

used in the clinical IVF setting due, presumably, to the attendant risks to the embryos (e.g. maintenance of a stable environment without prolonged light-exposure etc.). The next best way to develop growth curves for human embryos is to perform intermittent evaluations from which timelines can be derived. More than 25 years ago, this methodology was used by Edwards et al. (76). Their findings showed that normal human embryos progress through pre-implantation development along a predictable timeline, with 95% of them estimated to reach the 2-cell stage by 33.2 h, the 4-cell stage by 49.0 h, the 8-cell stage by 64.8 h, and the 16-cell stage by 80.7 h after insemination. From the data, an "average" growth curve was generated for normal development of the human embryo up to the 16-cell stage (Fig. 5).

Consistent with these early observations of Edwards and his colleagues, many studies have reported the existence of optimal cleavage rates, with those embryos cleaving either too quickly or too slowly being associated with compromised development (77–79). Numerous studies have shown a direct correlation between the number of cells in day 3 embryos (up to 8) and implantation rates following day 3 transfer (80, 81). Carillo et al. (82) demonstrated that embryos with at least 8 cells on day 3 resulted in significantly higher pregnancy rates when compared to embryos with <8 cells, and Racowsky et al. (83) demonstrated that those embryos with exactly 8 cells on day 3 had the highest implantation rates. Interestingly, these authors found that embryos having more than 8 cells had a significantly lower implantation rate than those with 8 cells (18.1% vs. 24.9%; $p < 0.01$). This reduced developmental competency of the faster cleaving embryos may relate to their increased incidence of aneuploidy (84). Some authors have also associated cell number on day 3 with blastocyst formation rate (85), suggesting that an optimal number of blastomeres on day 3 is a key developmental feature for further developmental progression. Of interest is the observation by Alikani et al.that embryos having 7–9 cells on day 3 converted to blastocysts at a significantly higher rate than day 3 embryos with <7 cells or >9 cells (79).

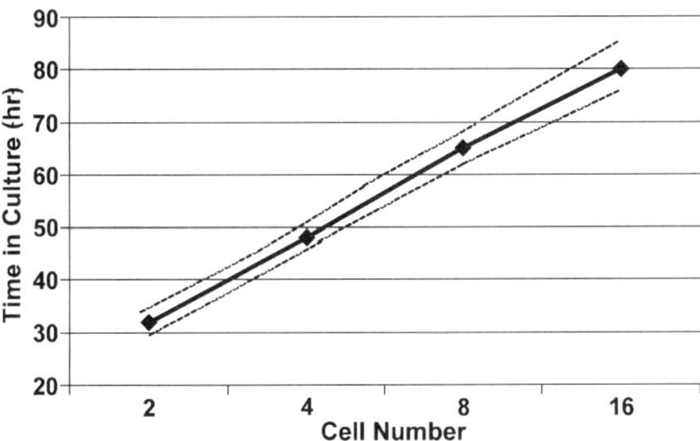


**Fig. 5** The estimated "growth" curve of development of human embryos in culture. The *solid line* represents the average developmental timeline; the *dashed lines* indicate that 95% confidence limits. Reproduced from Fig. 3, with permission from Elsevier (76)

### *Fragmentation*

Human embryos - those of at least some of the other higher primates- exhibit the unique feature of extracellular cytoplasmic structures not associated with blastomeres *per se*. These structures are typically classified as fragments, although it is clear that some may indeed, be normal "blebs" that occur transiently during cell division (86). True fragmentation has many phenotypes characterized by differences in size of fragments, percentage of the volume of the embryo occupied by fragments, and the disposition of this anomaly among the blastomeres (Fig. 6; 87). Fragmentation is thought to be secondary to abnormalities in cell metabolism or cell division, that may reflect apoptosis (88, 89) or anomalies in chromosomal segregation (90, 91). These abnormalities may arise from intrinsic problems within the embryo, and/or from developmental aberrations caused by poor culture conditions (92). Regardless, the etiology of fragmentation appears to lie in abnormalities in the link between nuclear and cytoplasmic cell division (see 93, for review).

There are numerous scoring systems for fragmentation. The simplest system describes solely the percentage of the volume of the embryo occupied by fragments (e.g. Score 0 = 0%; Score 1 = < 10%; Score 2 = 10–25%; Score 3 = > 25%) (83). Alternatively, some systems provide more detailed information, that reflects the size and location of fragments relative to the size and position of nucleated cell (Table 3; 87).

Fragmentation has been considered a primary marker of embryo developmental potential (78, 87). Numerous studies have shown that highly fragmented cleavage stage embryos have severely compromised implantation rates (83), and one study showed an association between high fragmentation and an increased incidence of neonatal malformations (94). There is a close relationship between the extent of fragmentation on day 3 and implantation following day 3 transfer on

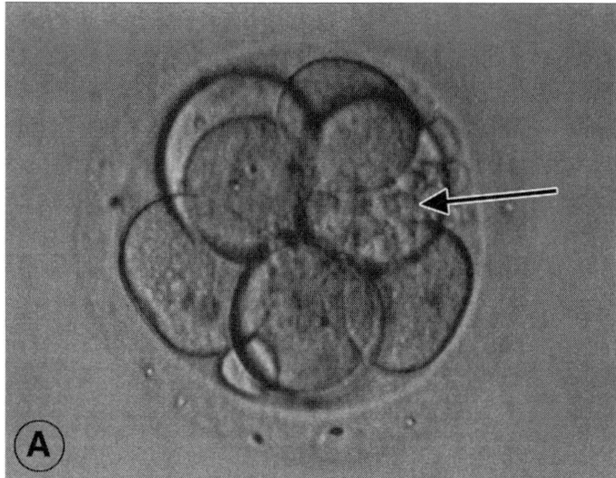


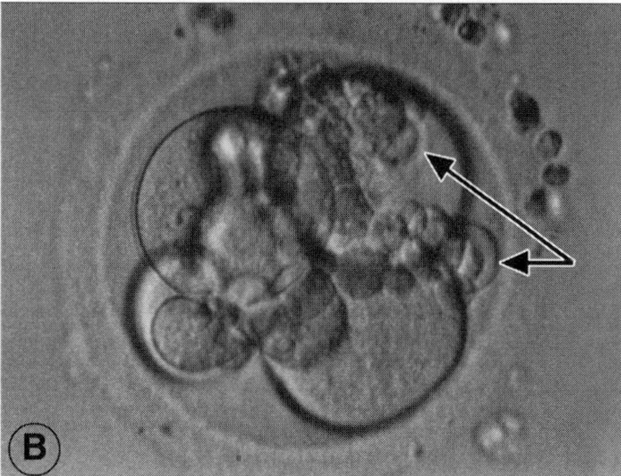


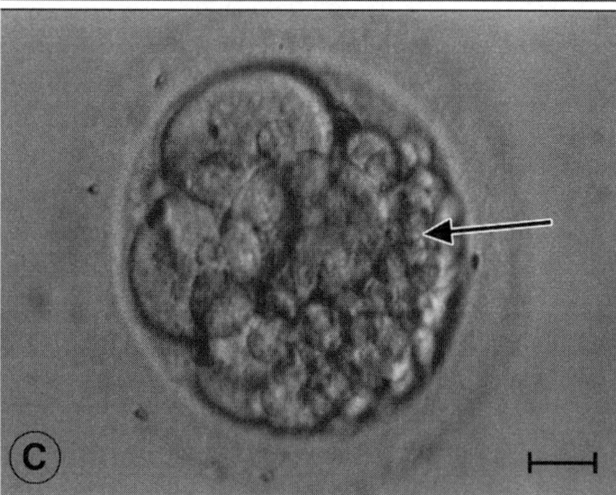


**Fig. 6** Micrographs showing embryos with various patterns and degrees of fragmentation. (**a**) An 8-cell embryo with <10% fragmentation involving fragments of similar size and localized to only one blastomere (*arrow*); (**b**) A 4-cell embryo showing 10–24% fragmentation involving fragments of various sizes, dispersed among the blastomeres (*arrows*); (**c**) A 5-cell embryo showing >50% fragmentation involving fragments of various sizes (*arrow*). The *bar* represents 30 μm

the one hand (83), and the likelihood of progressing to blastocyst formation and subsequent implantation on the other (95–97). Nevertheless, Alikani et al. (87) showed that microsurgical removal of small fragments can improve implantation potential of embryos by restoring spatial relationship of cells within the embryo and prevention of secondary degeneration.

### *Symmetry*

As a characteristic for assessing embryo quality, symmetry typically refers to the size and shape of the blastomeres, rather than an abnormal disposition of the blastomeres in the embryo, giving rise to a nonspherical overall shape (Fig. 7). In embryos with an even number of blastomeres (i.e. 4, 6, or 8 cells), and which exhibit asymmetry, the asymmetry likely arises from an uneven distribution of proteins, mRNA, and various organelles, including mitochondria, between the two sister cells (98). In embryos having an uneven number of blastomeres (i.e. 5 or 7 cells), the asymmetry is more likely to reflect an asynchrony in cell division than an uneven distribution of cytoplasm. In general, these distinctions are not made when evaluating the relationship between asymmetry and implantation potential.

As compared with cell number or fragmentation, fewer studies have assessed the relationship between asymmetry and implantation potential. Nevertheless, where investigated, embryos with marked cellular asymmetry have been shown to have substantially reduced implantation rates (22.4% vs. 1.4%; $p < 0.0001$ (83); 36.4% vs. 23.9%; $p = 0.003$ (99)), and this association has been found to hold up even after controlling for cell number and percent fragmentation (77). Interestingly, embryos displaying uneven cleavage also had a higher incidence of aneuploidy as compared with those having even cleavage (29.4% vs. 8.5%; $p = 0.014$, 99). It remains to be definitively determined whether the spatial arrangement of the blastomeres bears any relationship to developmental competency. However, one study failed to show any significance in a multiple logistic regression analysis (100).

### *Multinucleation*

The nuclear status of the blastomeres and the presence of mononucleation provide an additional means of

**Table 3** Fragmentation system, as proposed by Alikani (87)

| Pattern | | Degree | |
|---|---|---|---|
| Type 1 | Minimal in volume, and fragments are associated typically with one blastomere | W1 | 0–5% |
| Type 2 | Localized fragments predominantly occupying the perivitelline space | W2 | 6–15% |
| Type 3 | Small, scattered fragments may be in the cleavage cavity or peripherally positioned | W3 | 16–25% |
| Type 4 | Large fragments distributed through the embryonic mass and are associated with asymmetric cells | W4 | 26–35% |
| Type 5 | Fragments appear necrotic, with characteristic granularity and cytoplasmic contraction within the intact blastomeres | W5 | >35% |

assessment in the 4-cell embryo. Multinucleation has also been correlated with other morphological characteristics of early cleaving embryos such as fragmentation and cleavage rate (101). Jackson et al. (102) found that multinucleation is associated with decreased embryo development potential, implantation, clinical pregnancy, and live birth rates and suggested it should be included in embryo scoring system. Several more recent studies have confirmed these earlier findings for day 2 transfers. Saldeen et al. (103) found that equal sized, mononucleated blastomeres in four-cell embryo were associated with significantly higher implantation rates as compared to those with 0–3 mononucleated blastomeres (42% vs. 22%; $p < 0.0005$). Interestingly, although standard morphologic features were used to guide embryo grading, mononucleation of all four blastomeres was the only morphologic sign that was associated with implantation in this study. These investigators suggested that four mononucleated blastomeres are important markers for selecting an embryo for transfer. Consistent with this conclusion, embryos with multinucleated blastomeres have been associated with a higher rate of aneuploidy and chromosomal abnormalities (104, 105), and a lower rate of blastocyst formation (73, 106) when compared to embryos with mononucleated blastomeres (101).

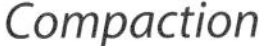

### *Compaction*

As with symmetry, relatively few studies have considered compaction in cleavage stage embryos as a potential

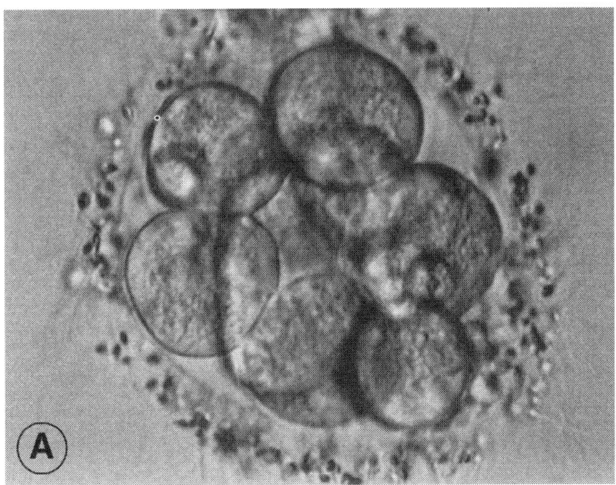


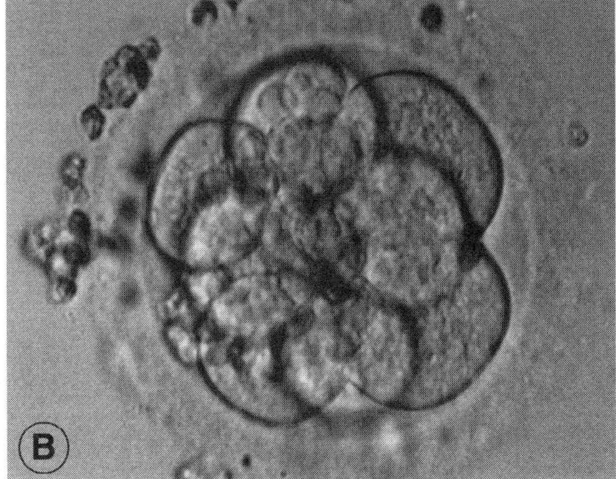


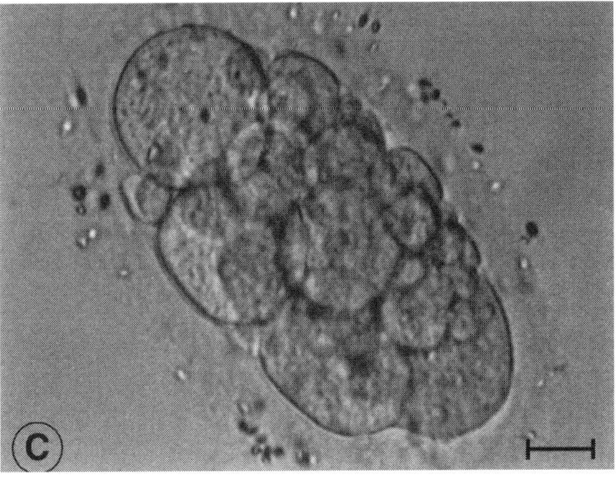


**Fig. 7** Micrographs showing embryos with various degrees of asymmetry. (**a**) A 10-cell embryo exhibiting blastomeres moderately asymmetrical in size and shape (note the supernumerary sperm attached to the zona pellucida); (**b**) An 8-cell embryo exhibiting blastomeres severely asymmetrical in size and shape; (**c**) An 8-cell embryo exhibiting severe distortion of blastomere spatial arrangement, in addition to having severely asymmetric blastomeres (a few supernumerary sperm are attached to the zona pellucida). The *bar* represents 30 μm

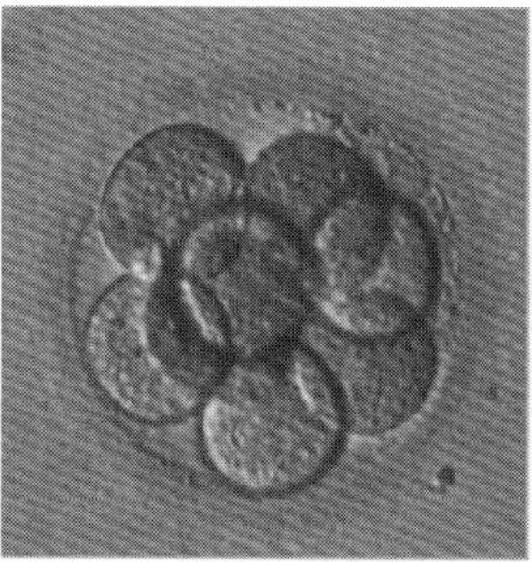
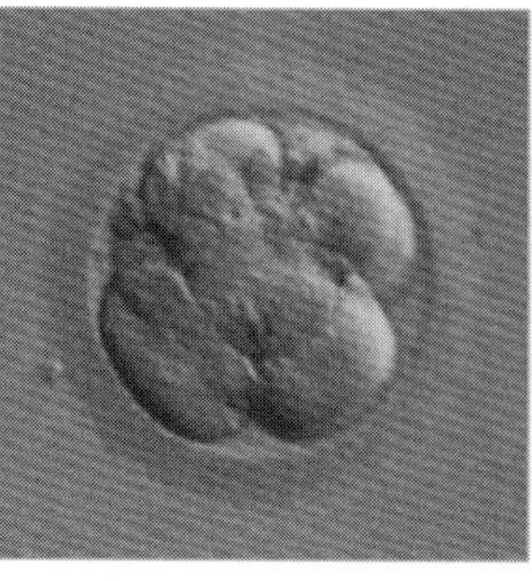
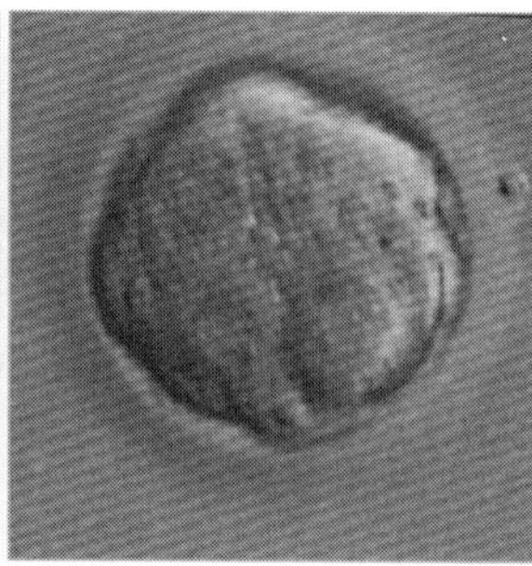

**Fig. 8** Micrographs showing embryos with various degrees of compaction. (**a**) An 8-cell embryo exhibiting minimal compaction; the blastomere membranes are readily discernible; (**b**) A 6-cell embryo showing moderate compaction; blastomere membranes are less distinct; (**c**) A embryo showing a high degree of compaction making it difficult to count the blastomeres; the blastomere membranes are fusing as tight junction formation gets underway

predictor for implantation potential. This phenomenon begins as early as the 8–16 cell stage on day 3, although is typically observed as a prelude to morula formation on day 4. Since the degree of compaction in day 4 embryos, is associated with implantation potential (107), the possibility exists that "early compaction" on day 3 may also be an important positive predictor of development. The process of compaction is characterized by gradual decreased resolution of the blastomere membranes as cell to cell adherence proceeds and tight junctions form (108) (Fig. 8).

The presence of compaction was used in a combined embryo grading score on day 3 by Desai et al. (109). Although pregnancy rate was found to increase with the transfer of a compacting embryo, no statistical association between compaction and pregnancy was obtained. In contrast, in a study by Skiadas et al. (110), "early compaction" was significantly associated with implantation depending upon the degree of fragmentation. In embryos having ≥8 cells and displaying <10% fragmentation, early compaction was associated with a significantly higher implantation rate, whereas, in embryos with ≥10% fragmentation, early compaction was negatively associated with implantation.

### 3.1.3 Morula

In contrast to the numerous studies assessing the relevance of morphological characteristics in cleavage stage embryos for selection, relatively little attention has been given to grading embryos on day 4 at the morula or early blastocyst stage. Nevertheless, at least two studies have shown that criteria such as degree of compaction, extent of fragmentation, and cytoplasmic vacuolization are useful markers for developmental competency when selecting at these stages (107, 111). For example, the Feil (111) scoring system on day 4 is as follows: Grade 1: early blastocyst, with cavitation or compacted embryo; Grade 2: grade 1 compacted morula with one or more morphological anomaly; Grade 3: partially compacted embryo with vacuoles or excessive fragmentation present, or embryo with 8 cells or more and without any sign of compaction; Grade 4: embryos with 8 cells or more, with no signs of compaction and having vacuoles or excess fragments, or embryos with less than eight cells, and with no sign of compaction.

### 3.1.4 Blastocyst

#### Development of Systems for Blastocyst Culture

Support for the sustainability of mitotic activity and normal embryo metabolism is crucial for blastocyst development in vitro. Blastocyst culture was first reported by Steptoe et al. (112) and then, 20 years later, live births, following transfer on day 5, were documented (113). However, the live-birth rate was only 10%, and the application of blastocyst transfer did not become routine until the late 1990's following improved understanding of the metabolic needs of the blastocyst and the physiological changes which may occur in the human reproductive tract.

While sequential media, designed to mimic the environments of the fallopian tube and uterus, paved the way for establishing blastocyst culture and transfer as a routine option in the IVF laboratory (114, 115), several other single media have since been proven to have comparable efficacy (116; see 117, for review). However, despite these developments, it is likely that none of these systems precisely mimics the oviduct conditions (117). Furthermore, practical implementation of blastocyst culture also involves consideration of the increased costs of culture media, increased embryologist time required to set-up and maintain these extended cultures, and the increased risk of monozygotic (118), as well as monochorionic (119) twinning.

#### Patient Selection

Despite the current availability of media that support reasonable blastocyst formation rates of around 40–50% in good prognosis patients, it is still not known to what extent we make concessions in terms of implantation capacity or, especially, viability through the extended culture duration. Specifically, it remains to be clarified how many of the embryos that sustain their development under in vivo conditions would be able to reach the blastocyst stage under in vitro conditions. Indeed, at least with the culture media available a decade ago, extending culture to day 5 significantly reduced the likelihood of pregnancy in those patients with no 8-cell embryos, as compared with those who underwent a day 3 transfer (120).

Despite the above caveats regarding blastocyst culture and transfer, studies have shown that this approach results in improved implantation rates compared with cleavage stage transfer (121, 122), and also improved pregnancy rates either in unselected patients (122) or only in select, good prognosis patients (121). In this setting, good prognosis patients include those having at least 10 follicles (121) or oocytes (123), or at least four embryos (124) or a minimum of at least three 8-cell embryos (120).

There are three primary reasons underlying the potential benefit of day 5 transfer: (a) Extended culture may assist in determination of the most competent embryo (125; see 126, for review) by the introduction of the paternal transcript and activation of the embryonic genome which occurs around the 4–8 cell stage (127). Indeed, the probability of normal embryonic genome expression is higher among embryos that form blastocyst (128), although some aneuploid embryos are capable of reaching the blastocyst stage (129); (b) In blastocyst transfer, there is shorter exposure of the embryo before implantation to possible deleterious adverse conditions in the uterus induced by supraphysiological concentrations of gonadotropins (130, 131); and (c) when the transfer is performed at this relatively later stage, uterine contractions may be dampened leading to a reduced risk of embryo expulsion and higher implantation rates (132).

The above potential advantages of blastocyst transfer aside, some studies have revealed comparable implantation rates between day 3 and day 5 transfer (47, 133). Moreover, whether blastocyst culture and transfer is beneficial for poorer prognosis patients (such as those with repeated implantation failure, or having exclusively bad quality embryos on day 2 or day 3) remains to be confirmed despite a few studies demonstrating some benefit (134, 135).

#### Blastocyst Scoring System

Since the two cell lineages in the blastocyst perform unique roles (the trophectoderm giving rise to the embryonic component of the placenta, while the inner cell mass forming the embryo per se), it is not surprising that the scoring system for assessment of blastocyst quality appraises both cell types. The system advanced by Gardner et al. (136), is that most typically used for blastocyst selection. It takes into consideration the size of the blastocoelic cavity and whether the blastocyst is hatching, in addition to assessment of the organization and number of cells within the inner cell mass and the trophectoderm (Fig. 9).

### 3.2 Multi-Day Scoring

It is well established that a large proportion of human pre-implantation embryos undergo deviant development, failing to follow expected normal developmental timeline (76, 138) by either cleaving too slowly or too quickly. This fact has provided the rationale for investigating whether multiple evaluations through early pre-implantation development may improve selection compared with a single evaluation, performed shortly before transfer. Indeed, a large number of studies have been performed in recent years in which various

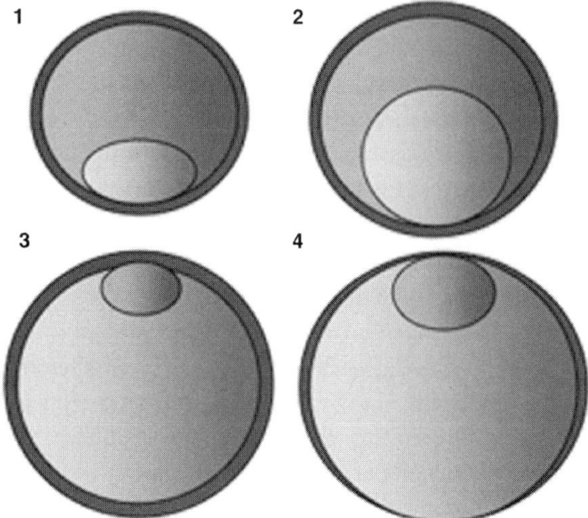


**Fig. 9** Scoring system for human blastocyst. Blastocysts are initially given a numerical score from 1 to 6 based upon their degree of expansion and hatching status: (plus 1) Early blastocyst, the blastocoel occupies less than half the volume of the embryo; (plus 2) Expanding blastocyst, the blastocoel occupies half the volume of the embryo or more; (plus 3) Full blastocyst, the blastocoel completely the embryo, but the zona is not thinned; (plus 4) Expanded blastocyst, the blastocoel volume is now larger than that of the early embryo and the zona is thinning; (plus 5) Hatching blastocyst, the blastocyst has completely escaped from the zona. The second step in the scoring procedure involves grading those blastocysts with a Score of 3–6 for development of each of the trophectoderm and inner cell mass as indicated in the figure. Reproduced from Fig. 7.1 in (137), with permission from Taylor & Francis, London

combinations of days for scoring have been chosen (see 139, for review), and systems for evaluation have been proposed.

Appraisal of this literature shows that there is no consensus on (a) the optimum day(s) for evaluation; (b) the statistical methods used for data analyses and interpretation; or (c) the scoring system to use for selection. Nevertheless, many systems have been advanced (Table 4), and several of these have been adopted for widespread use (see 139, for review). However, the need for even more sensitive morphological approaches has become apparent, as pressures to perform SET have increased (see Chapter "Elective Single Embryo Transfer").

There are numerous reasons for the lack of an established morphological grading system. First and foremost, many studies have involved datasets in which the developmental fate of each embryo was not traceable to a viable implantation (109, 143–146). The assumption in these studies has been that the predicted "best" embryo, was the one that implanted in the case of singleton pregnancies, when more than one embryo is transferred. However, without proof that the identified "best" embryo was indeed, the one that successfully gave rise to the fetus, the conclusions must be interpreted with caution. Secondly, the vast majority of scoring systems have been derived from retrospective analyses, with only a handful reporting prospective assessment with demonstrated improvement in selection (147, 148). Thirdly, a "numerical scoring system" for selection is frequently based on assignment of seemingly arbitrarily weighted values without multivariate analyses being performed (47, 109, 149); such multivariate analyses or Spearman rank order correlation are necessary for developing a model in which prediction for implantation is precisely reflected by the score (100, 150). Fourthly, many studies have involved datasets involving both day 3 and day 5 transfers (145, 147), an approach likely to reduce utility of the analyses due to various confounders relating to patient selection bias, culture influences (e.g. probable improved overall quality of embryos cultured to day 5, possible loss of developmentally competent day 3 embryos not supported by extended culture conditions), and variances in uterine receptivity. Fifthly, datasets involving transfer of more than one embryo may introduce further confounding due to possible inter-embryo cooperation/interaction whereby a poorer quality embryo may either increase or decrease the likelihood of a better quality embryo implanting or, conversely, a better quality embryo may enhance the independent implantation potential of one considered of poorer quality (151). Sixthly, possible confounding caused by inter-embryologist variance in grading (particularly for those embryos of marginal quality) may reduce the accuracy of a system (149). Lastly, data is sparse regarding rigorous prospective testing of any specific selection algorithm to prove that its implementation does, indeed, improve embryo selection.

Collectively, published studies in this field show that derivation of selection algorithms have used various paradigms regarding the days and times for scoring, morphological characteristics recorded, and the transformation and statistical analyses of the data. The utility of any of these subjective evaluations is likely tempered by several factors including: (a) the unique morphological phenotype of each embryo; (b) the dynamic nature of early development, thereby highlighting the

**Table 4** Examples of various scoring systems proposed for embryo selection

| Author | Name | Day of assessment | System type | Scoring range | Best embryo | Cell number | Frag | Symm | Compaction/ expansion | Cytoplasm features | Cleavage rate | Multi nucleation |
|---|---|---|---|---|---|---|---|---|---|---|---|---|
| Cummins (138) | Embryo quality score (EQS)/ embryo development rating (EDR) | 2 or 3 | Score | 1–4 | Score 4 | | + | + | | + | + | |
| Puissant (81) | Embryo scoring | 2 | Grade | 1–4 | Grade 4 | + | + | + | | | | |
| Veeck (140) | Morphological grading | 3 | Grade | I–IV | Grade I | + | + | + | | | | |
| Steer(80) | Cumulative embryo score (CES) | 3 | Grade | 1–4 | Grade 4 | + | + | + | | | | |
| Giorgetti (141) | 4 point embryo score | 2 | Point | 1–4 | 4 Point | + | + | + | | | + | |
| Ziebe (78) | Embryo quality score | 2 | Symm or frag score with cell | Symm: 1.0–2.0 Frag: 2.1, 2.2, 3.0, 4.0 | ≥4 cell + 2.1 | + | + | + | | | | |
| Van Royen (142) | Top quality embryo | 2 and 3 | Score | Frag:A, B, C | Top quality | + | + | | | | | + |
| Desai (109) | Embryo quality score (D3EQ) | 3 | Score | 1–10 | Score 10 | + | + | + | +/+ | Pitting vacuole | | |

+ indicates characteristic included in assessment system. *Frag* fragmentation; *Symm* symmetry

need to evaluate embryos within discrete time windows; (c) the lack of precise correlation between aneuploidy and morphology (152); and (d) the difficulties associated with categorical grouping of continuous variables (e.g. fragmentation).

### 3.3 Summary

The balance of studies shows that one or more morphological parameter on any one day of culture independently provides predictive value in embryo selection. Whether multi-day, as compared with single day, scoring consistently aids in embryo selection remains to be definitively proven. The central question is, to what extent does appearance on one day reflect appearance at a previous stage of development? Moreover, any potential advantage of multi-day scoring must be weighed against possible detrimental effects of environmental perturbations (light exposure, temperature and pH shifts etc), caused by serial evaluations. Finally, precision and consistency of scoring among embryologists within and across laboratories must be taken into consideration.

Logic would dictate that, an embryo showing normal development on day 3, is likely also to have exhibited normal development earlier in culture; this concept is supported by the finding that there is, indeed, a link between day 1 and day 3 morphologies (153, 154). It may well be, therefore, that only one morphological assessment, immediately before transfer, is sufficient to select the developmentally most competent day 3 embryo. The burden of proof rests on demonstrating, unequivocally, that more than this single observation improves selection. This can only be accomplished using multivariate analysis of a pristine dataset of embryos of known developmental fate, and preferably involving only SETs to rule out any influence of inter-embryo interactions. Using such an approach, preliminary data from our group has shown that no additional benefit is accrued from early cleavage and day 2 assessments over that obtained exclusively from evaluation on day 3 (Racowsky et al. unpublished data). However, there is considerable overlap in the morphological appearance of those embryos that successfully implant versus those that fail, indicating that, as concluded by Guerif et al. (69) other methods for embryo selection must be developed.

## 4 Analysis of Spent Culture Medium

Although morphological grading certainly contributes to prediction of implantation potential, the data obtained has limitations, indicating the need for new selection methods with greater sensitivity. Two different broad approaches are being investigated: that of spent culture media assays, which are low risk and give insight regarding the proteomic and metabolomic profiles of the embryos, and biopsy of polar bodies, blastomeres or trophectoderm, which may have attendant high risks to embryo health and provide information regarding the genomic and transcriptional status (see 155, for review; Table 5).

Spent culture media analyses can be considered to fall into two broad classes: targeted analyses on the one hand, and "profiling" approaches on the other (Fig. 10; see (156), for review). While the profiling approach of "finger printing" (i.e. assessment of the intracellular compartment) might provide a more accurate reflection of embryo viability, current technologies would require blastomere

**Table 5** Comparison of various strategies for embryos selection, based on risk, nearness to phenotype, and amount of information obtained (Risk increases from left to right, nearness to phenotype increases from top to bottom)

| | Culture medium assays | Oocyte PB/TE biopsy | Cleavage embryo biopsy |
|---|---|---|---|
| Genomic | N | Aneuploidy screening | Aneuploidy screening |
| Transcriptomic | N | Qualitative RT-PCR; quantitative RT-PCR; mRNA amplification + microarrays[a,b] | Qualitative RT-PCR; quantitative RT-PCR; mRNA amplification + microarrays[a,b] |
| Protein | Human leukocyte antigen-G | N | N |
| Metabolites | Amino acids;[a] infrared analyses;[a] mass spectroscopy[a] | N | N |

*PB* polar body; *RT-PCR* reverse transcription polymerase chain reaction; *TE* trophectoderm; *N* not possible, at least with current technology

[a]Systems biology approaches; [b]technologies that are theoretically possible but not yet demonstrated in principle

Modified from (155), (Table 1), with permission from Reproductive Biomedicine Online

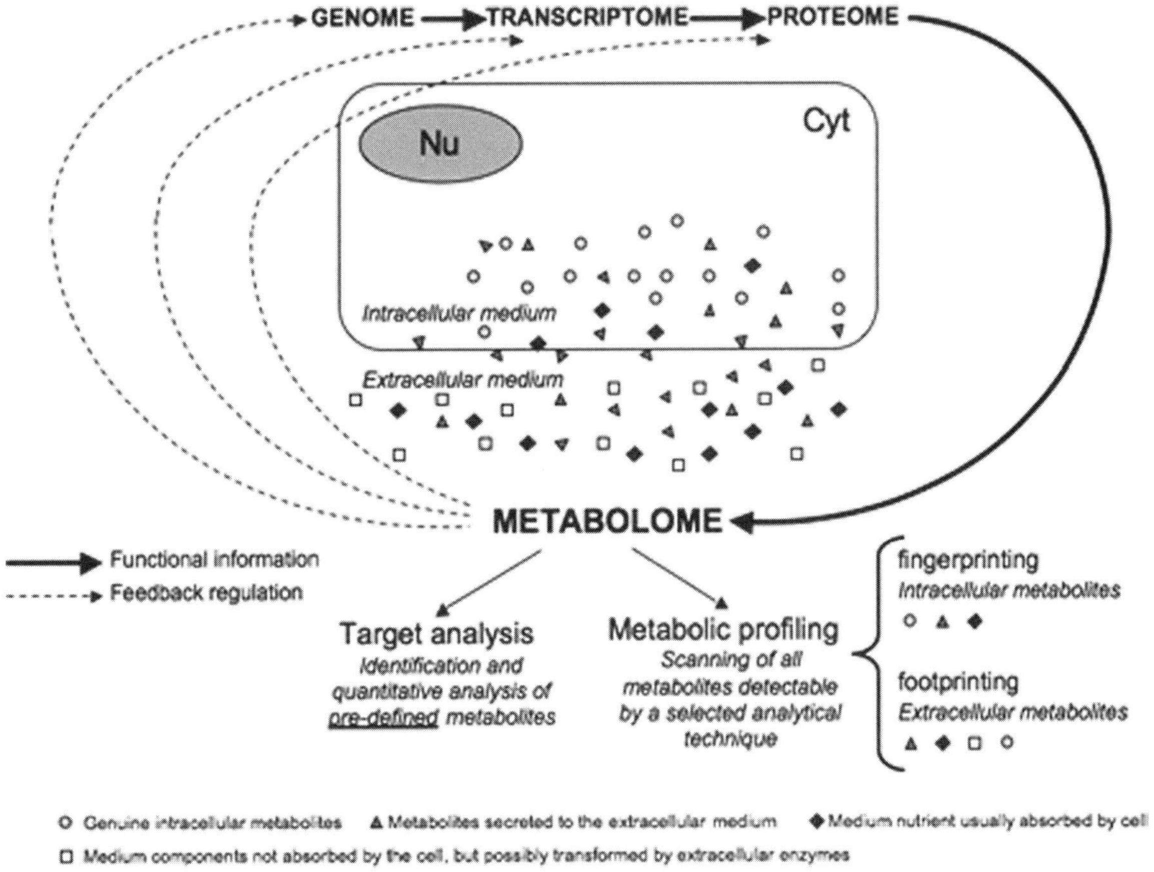

**Fig. 10** Different strategies to study the metabolome in the context of functional genomics. *Nu*, nucleus; *Cyt*, cytoplasm. Reproduced from (156), with permission from Wiley

destruction. Therefore, "footprinting" (i.e. assessment of the extracellular compartment), is currently the approach being used. Regardless, the overall goal is to obtain information on the metabolism of each embryo, which can then be used either alone, or in conjunction with, morphological evaluation to assist in selection.

## 4.1 Targeted Analyses

Targeted analyses involve identification and quantification of defined metabolites that are related to a specific pathway or to intersecting pathways of pre-implantation embryos with their in vitro conditions (156). Such analyses provide insight into aberrations in genetic (157, 158) or cellular metabolism and rely on measurement of substances either taken up or secreted into the medium (Fig. 11), (137).

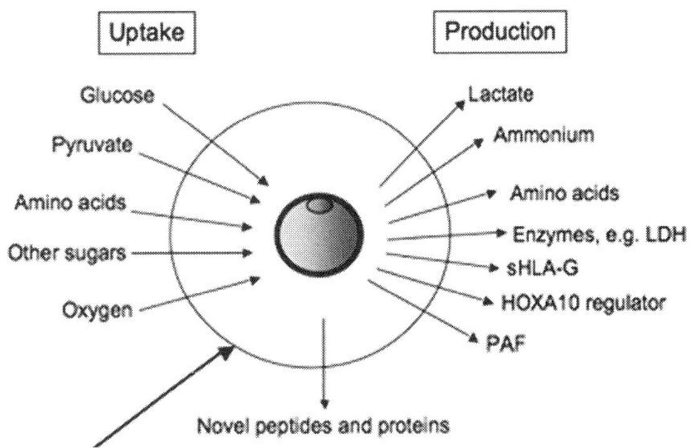


**Fig. 11** Uptake and secretion of specific nutrients by the embryo. Diagram depicting examples of nutrients that either decrease or increase in concentration depending upon their uptake or secretion by the embryo in culture. LDH, lactate dehydrogenase; sHLA-G, soluble histocompatability antigen class I G; HOXA10, homeobox platelet activating factor. Reproduced from Fig. 7.5 in (137) with permission from Taylor & Francis, London

### 4.1.1 Pyruvate and Glucose

Leese et al. (159) has proposed that "quiet" metabolism rather than "active" metabolism is associated with increased embryo viability. This quiet metabolism is proposed to reflect a basal state in which there is a minimal or reduced rate of oxygen consumption and nutrient uptake (159, 160). In embryos developing to the blastocyst stage, pyruvate uptake occurs through day 4, while uptake of glucose continues through day 5 and exceeds that of pyruvate (161, 162). Based on these early findings, several studies have measured pyruvate and glucose uptake in relation to blastocyst formation and quality (161–163, 163–165). Since absolute uptake of pyruvate by embryos during the first 3 days varies over a wide range (165), any correlation with viability is tricky. Not surprisingly, therefore, conflicting data exists. While some studies show that uptake of both energy substrates appears related to blastocyst formation (162, 164), others have failed to reveal such a relationship either for pyruvate (166) alone, or for both pyruvate and glucose (167).

Taken together, while there may be a relationship between pyruvate and/or glucose uptake and embryo quality, the data appears somewhat conflicting and few, if any, laboratories are using these assays for routine embryo selection.

### 4.1.2 Amino Acids

It is well established that amino acids play an important role in cellular metabolism in terms of energy expenditure (ATP production, protein synthesis, as osmolytes, and for maintaining intracellular pH). Not surprisingly, therefore, studies have assessed the relationship between amino acid concentrations in spent culture media as related to embryo viability (168, 169). A relationship between depletion of several amino acids from the culture medium has been associated with blastocyst formation, with leucine being the most consistent marker in this regard (169); conversely, of those most consistently produced, alanine was present at the highest level through development. Interestingly, although the concentrations of glycine, asparagines, and leucine correlated with pregnancy and live-birth, those for two of them (glycine and leucine) were significantly lower in the medium of those embryos that implanted, while that for asparagine was increased. Moreover, the only amino acid concentration that was associated with embryo quality was glutamine (168). Based on the above findings, the authors suggested that amino acid turnover measurement in spent culture medium could aid in selection of the most viable embryo for transfer. However, the high performance liquid chromatography systems employed are unlikely to provide a practical screening method for routine use in IVF laboratories due to the long turnaround.

### 4.1.3 Soluble Human Leukocyte Antigen-G (sHLA-G)

Several recent investigations have assessed the efficacy of sHLA-G as a marker of implantation potential (170–172). The rationale for these studies rests on the facts that: (a) sHLA-G is thought to play a critical role at the maternal-embryonic interface as implantation proceeds (173, 174); and (b) the cytokine is synthesized primarily by trophoblast (175). Jurisicova et al. (176) were the first to report that the extent of HLA-G mRNA expression was associated with increased cleavage rate in human embryos, and that this molecule may therefore play an important role in human pre-embryo development. Consistent with this possibility, Fuzzi et al. (172) showed implantation to occur only in women having embryos transferred with sHLA-G detection in culture supernatants, and Noci et al. (170) and Fisch et al. (177), respectively, found that pregnancies only occurred in women who had at least one or two transferred embryo that secreted sHLA-G. Interestingly, however, neither of these groups found a direct correlation between embryo morphology and sHLA-G levels, and at least one other investigation failed to detect any sHLA-G in human embryo spent culture media (178). In contrast, a more recent study by Desai et al. (171) observed that expression of sHLA-G was, indeed, associated not only with implantation potential, but also with increasing cell stage.

Collectively, the contrasting results described above reflect the technical difficulties associated with measuring sHLA-G in spent culture media (see 179, for review). A multitude of assay systems have been employed with a wide range of sHLA-G concentrations being reported. Whether sHLA-G is a useful non-invasive biomarker for embryo viability awaits further clarification that may be dependent on development of more sensitive assays.

### 4.2 Profiling Studies

Only within the last couple of years have profiling studies been performed for analysis of the "metabolome" of the spent culture media (see 180, for review). The metabolome is defined as the low molecular weight metabolites (typically <3,000 *m/z*) that represent the end products of cell regulatory processes. Moreover, unlike analysis of mRNA (i.e. assessment of the transcriptome), proteins and metabolites are functional entities within the cell (181). Thus, metabolomic analysis gives information of the cellular function, and defines the phenotype of the cell based on the genotype and in response to a variety of nutrient or environmental changes (156).

While changes in the levels of individual enzymes may be expected to have little effect on metabolic fluxes, they can and do have significant effects on the concentrations of the variety of individual metabolites. In addition, as the downstream result of gene expression, changes in the metabolome are amplified relative to changes in the transcriptome and the proteome, which is likely to allow for increased sensitivity. Finally, it is known that metabolic fluxes are regulated not only by genetic expression, but also by post-transcriptional and post-translational events, together implying that the metabolome is an accurate reflection of the phenotype (182).

The profiling approach does not require identification and quantification of specific metabolites. Rather, it involves the analysis of a wide range of metabolites with the objective of identifying one or more that is associated with a specific biological outcome (in our case, viable embryos). Comparisons of the amount of one or more metabolite in spent medium of viable embryos are made with that in the spent medium of nonviable, unsuccessful embryos to enable distinction of unique metabolic characteristics of viable vs. nonviable embryos. Clearly, replication of profiles within the two embryo classes (viable and nonviable) is critical if the approach has validity in embryo selection.

To date, near infrared spectroscopy (183, 184) RAMAN spectroscopy (183, 185), and Fourier transform infrared spectroscopy (155) have all been used to screen embryo spent culture media. Following such spectroscopic analyses, mean spectra associated with viable and nonviable embryos have been obtained, from which identifiers of viability have been derived (the "viability index" (185), or a "discriminant function" (155). Of interest, the spectral regions most predictive of outcome (ROH, -SH, C = C, –CH, –NH, and –OH groups) are sensitive to reactive oxygen species. As such, these findings indicate that oxidative modification may be reflected in embryo viability. However, as expected, there is some over-lap between the indices for viable and nonviable embryos (183), and there is considerable inter-patient and inter-embryo variation regarding the embryo viability score (184). Nevertheless, this technology appears to have a higher degree of accuracy for selecting viable embryos, relative to that obtained exclusively from morphological evaluation (53.6% vs. 38.5%; 184).

### 4.3 Summary

In theory, there is great attraction for developing a new noninvasive technique for embryo selection that has practical application in the IVF clinic. This technique must have a proven high sensitivity and specificity, be reasonably priced and easy to use, and involve a short turnaround for selection of embryos for fresh transfers. While several target analyses have been explored, to date, none of these fulfill all these prerequisites. Of more promise, profiling approaches using metabolomic techniques such as near infrared spectroscopy and RAMAN spectroscopy may provide the high throughput technologies needed and which meet these criteria. However, available data are preliminary, no application of any algorithm has been applied for prospective embryo selection in the clinic, and larger prospective trials are needed to prove overall efficacy.

## 5 Clinical Applications Summary

The over-arching goal of embryo selection is to identify that embryo within a cohort with the highest implantation potential and with no genetic or epigenetic defects. To this end, morphological associations continue to be studied, while genomic, proteomic and metabolomic technologies are all under investigation. However, until efficacy is proven with these newer technologies, morphological assessments will remain the first-line approach for noninvasive embryo evaluation.

Several oocyte gross morphological characteristics, in addition to presence of a birefringent spindle, have been associated with implantation potential of the embryo. However, the application of these characteristics is limited not only by our incomplete understanding of what constitutes a normal oocyte, but also by the obvious exclusion of sperm contribution to embryo quality. In the absence of identified standard genomic or proteomic markers for oocyte quality (e.g. in associated follicular fluid or cumulus granulosa cells) any inclusion of oocyte markers in an algorithm for embryo selection will remain of limited value.

A wide range of studies have been conducted in attempts to identify not only the best day for embryo evaluation, but also which morphological markers provide the greatest power for predicting implantation potential. While numerous studies show that one or more morphological parameter on any one day has independent predictive value, the association among these independent predictors, both within and across days, has not been clearly elucidated. Currently, there is no consensus regarding an algorithm for embryo selection. Furthermore, the efficacy of any selection algorithm may vary from one IVF program to another, since a multitude of variables, in addition to embryo quality, may impact on whether an embryo will implant. Aside from the health of the gametes (as affected by parental age, genetic backgrounds and lifetime environmental exposures), the ovarian stimulation along with culture conditions/embryo manipulations, the day of transfer and uterine receptivity issues all play a role (Fig. 12). Therefore, we recommend that each program should develop its own algorithm for morphological scoring.

The prevailing need is to identify a marker(s) that reflects the cellular phenotype of viable embryos. Targeted approaches to screen spent culture media have been investigated since study of a single target (e.g. sHLA-G, or amino acid turnover) provides some insight as to the overall phenotype. However, none of these approaches are ready for prime time due to problems associated with inadequate sensitivity, specificity, need for specialized, expensive equipment, and/or staffing expertise. Of great promise, metabolomic profiling may provide the much searched for technique, by enabling accurate insight into the cellular phenotype of the embryo, which can then be applied to develop a genetic algorithm for embryo selection. However, efficacy of this approach is not proven and there is a critical need for prospective testing in trials with large numbers of patients. Whether metabolomic profiling, either alone or in conjunction with morphological grading, becomes the routine method for embryo selection ,awaits the test of time.

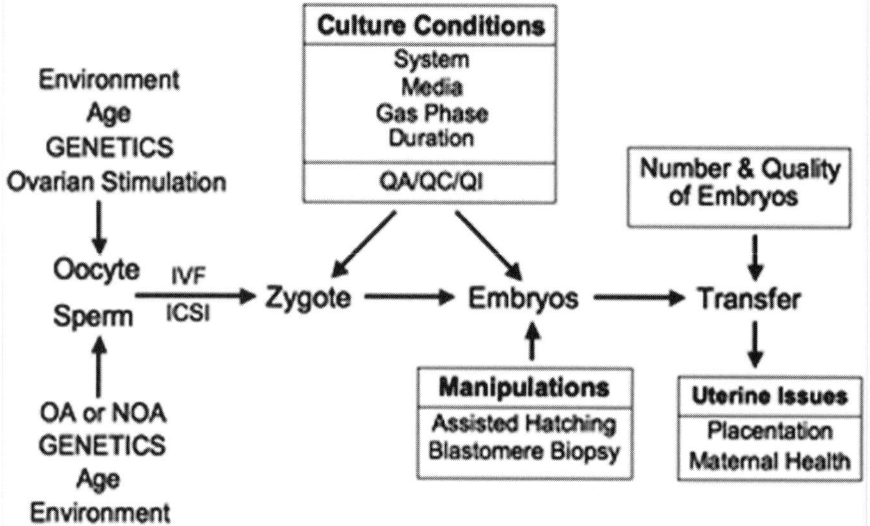


**Fig. 12** Diagram showing the multitude of variables that impact upon the probability of an embryo implanting. *OA* obstructed azoospermia; *NOA* non-obstructed azoospermia

**Acknowledgements** We thank Dr. Gena Ratiu for assistance in taking the photographic images, and Mr. Brian C. Bator for preparation of the photographic plates.

## References

1. Boiso I, Veiga A, Edawards RG. Fundamentals of human embryonic growth in vitro and the selection of high-quality embryos for transfer. Reprod Biomed Online 2002;5(3): 328–350.
2. Söderström-Anttila V, Vilska S. Five years of single embryo transfer with anonymous and non-anonymous oocyte donation. Reprod Biomed Online 2007;15(4):428–433.
3. Palermo G, Joris H, Devroey P. Pregnancies after intracytoplasmic injection of single spermatozoon into an oocyte. Lancet 1992;340(8810):17–18.
4. Van Steirteghem A, Nagy Z, Joris H. High fertilization and implantation rates after intracytoplasmic sperm injection. Hum Reprod 1993;8(7):1061–1066.
5. Veeck LL. The morphologic estimation of mature oocytes and their preparation for insemination. In: Jones HW Jr, Jones GS, Hodgen GD, and Rosenwack Z, eds. In Vitro Fertilization-Norfolk. Baltimore: Williams & Wilkins, 1986:81.
6. Rattanachaiyanont M, Leader A, Léveillé MC. Lack of correlation between oocyte-corona-cumulus complex morphology and nuclear maturity of oocytes collected in stimulated cycles for intracytoplasmic sperm injection. Fertil Steril 1999;71(5):937–940.
7. Laufer N, Tarlatzis BC, DeCherney AH, Master JT, Haseltine FB, MacLusky N, Naftolin F. Asynchrony between human cumulus-corona cell complex and oocyte maturation after human menopausal gonadotropin treatment for in vitro fertilization. Fertil Steril 1984;42(3):366–372.
8. Khamsi F, Roberge S, Lacanna IC, Wong J, Yavas Y. Effects of granulosa cells, cumulus cells, and oocyte density on in vitro fertilization in women. Endocrine 1999;10(2):161–166.
9. Borini A, Lagalla C, Cattoli M, Sereni E, Sciajno R, Flamigni C, Coticchio G. Predictive factors for embryo implantation potential. Reprod Biomed Online 2005;10(5):653–668.
10. Balaban B, Urman B, Sertac A, Alatas C, Aksoy S, Mercan R. Oocyte morphology does not affect fertilization rate, embryo quality and implantation rate after intracytoplasmic sperm injection. Hum Reprod 1998;13(12):3431–3433.
11. Balaban B, Urman B. Effect of oocyte morphology on embryo development and implantation. Reprod Biomed Online 2006;12(5):608–615.
12. Xia P. Intracytoplasmic sperm injection: correlation of oocyte grade based on polar body, perivitelline space and cytoplasmic inclusions with fertilization rate and embryo quality. Hum Reprod 1997;12(8):1750–1755.
13. Mikkelsen AL, Lindenberg S. Morphology of in-vitro matured oocytes: impact on fertility potential and embryo quality. Hum Reprod 2001;16(8):1714–1718.
14. Rienzi L, Ubaldi F, Iacobelli M, Minasi M, Romano S, Ferrero S, Sapienza F, Baroni E, Litwicka K, Greco E. Significance of metaphase II human oocyte morphology on ICSI outcome. Fertil Steril 2008;90(5):1692–700, PMID: 18249393.
15. Garside WT, Loret de Mola J, Bucci JA, Tureck RW, Heyner S. Sequential analysis of zona thickness during in vitro culture of human zygotes: correlation with embryo quality, age, and implantation. Mol Reprod Dev 1997;47(1):99–104.
16. Loutradis D, Drakakis P, Kallianidis K, Milingos S, Dendrinos S, Michalas S. Oocyte morphology correlates with embryo quality and pregnancy rate after intracytoplasmic sperm injection. Fertil Steril 1999;72(2): 240–244.
17. Serhal PF, Ranieri DM, Kinis A, Marchant S, Davies M, Khadum IM. Oocyte morphology predicts outcome of intracytoplasmic sperm injection. Hum Reprod 1997;12(6):1267–1270.
18. Kahraman S, Yakin K, Dönmez E, Samli H, Bahçe M, Cengiz G, Sertyel S, Samli M, Imirzalioglu N. Relationship between granular cytoplasm of oocytes and pregnancy outcome following intracytoplasmic sperm injection. Hum Reprod 2000;15(11):2390–2393.
19. De Sutter P, Dozortsev D, Qian C, Dhont M. Oocyte morphology does not correlate with fertilization rate and embryo quality after intracytoplasmic sperm injection. Hum Reprod 1996;11(3):595–597.
20. Eichhenlaub-Ritter U, Schmiady H, Kentenich H, Soewarto D. Recurrent failure in polar body formation and premature chromosome condensation in oocytes from a human patient: indicators of asynchrony in nuclear and cytoplasmic maturation. Human Reprod 1995;10(9):2343–2349.
21. Balakier H, Sojecki A, Motamedi G, Librach C. Time-dependent capability of human oocytes for activation and pronuclear formation during metaphase II arrest. Hum Reprod 2004;19(4):982–987.
22. Hyun CS, Cha JH, Son WY, Yoon SH, Kim KA, Lim JH. Optimal ICSI timing after the first polar body extrusion in in vitro matured human oocytes. Hum Reprod 2007;22(7):1991–1995.
23. Ebner T, Yaman C, Moser M, Sommergruber M, Feichtinger O, Tews G. Prognostic value of first polar body morphology on fertilization rate and embryo quality in intracytoplasmic sperm injection. Hum Reprod 2000;15(2):427–430.
24. Fancsovits P, Tothne ZG, Murber A, Takacs FZ, Papp Z, Urbancek J. Correlation between first polar body morphology and further embryo development. Acta Biol Hung 2006;57(3):331–338.
25. Ciotti PM, Notarangelo L, Morselli-Labate AM, Felletti V, Porcu E, Venturoli S. First polar body morphology before ICSI is not related to embryo quality or pregnancy rate. Hum Reprod 2004;19(10):2334–2339.
26. Verlinsky Yury, Lerner S, Illkevitch N, Kuznetsov V, Kuznetsov I, Cieslak J, Kuliev A. Is there any predictive value of first polar body morphology for embryo genotype or developmental potential? Reprod Biomed Online 2003;7(3):336–341.
27. De Santis L, Cino I, Rabellotti E, Calzi F, Borini A, Coticchio G. Polar body morphology and spindle imaging as predictors of oocyte quality. Reprod Biomed Online 2005;11(1): 36–42.
28. Keefe D, Liu L, Wang W, Silva C. Imaging meiotic spindles by polarization light microscopy: principles and applications to IVF. Reprod Biomed Online 2003;7(1):24–29.

29. Oldenbourg R, Salmon ED, Tran PT. Birefringence of single and bundled microtubules. Biophys J 1998;74(1):645–654.
30. Liu L, Oldenbourg R, Trimarchi JR, Keefe DL. A reliable, noninvasive technique for spindle imaging and enucleation of mammalian oocytes. Nat Biotechnol 2000;18(2):223–225.
31. Wang WH, Meng L, Hackett RJ, Keefe DL. Developmental ability of human oocytes with or without birefringent spindles imaged by Polscope before insemination. Hum Reprod 2001;16(7):1464–1468.
32. Wang WH, Meng L, Hackett RJ, Odenbourg R, Keefe DL. The spindle observation and its relationship with fertilization after intracytoplasmic sperm injection in living human oocytes. Fertil Steril 2001;75(2):348–353.
33. Madaschi C, Carvalho de Souza Bonetti T, Paes de Almeida Ferreira Braga D, Pasqualotto F, Iaconelli A, Jr, Borges E, Jr. Spindle imaging: a marker for embryo development and implantation. Fertil Steril 2008;90(1):194–198.
34. Cohen Y, Malcov M, Schwartz T, Mey-Raz N, Carmon A, Cohen T, Lessing JB, Amit A, Azem F. Spindle imaging: a new marker for optimal timing of ICSI? Human Reprod 2004;19(3):649–654.
35. Moo JH, Hyun CS, Lee SW, Son WY, Yoon SH, Lim JH. Visualization of the metaphase II meiotic spindle in living human oocytes using the Polscope enables the prediction of embryonic developmental competence after ICSI. Human Reprod 2003;18(4):817–820.
36. Battaglia DE, Goodwin P, Klein NA, Soules MR. Influence of maternal age on meiotic spindle assembly in oocytes from naturally cycling women. Hum Reprod 1996;11(10): 2217–2222.
37. Shen Y, Betzendahl I, Tinneberg H, Eichenlaub-Ritter U. Enhanced polarizing microscopy as a new tool in aneuploidy research in oocytes. Mutat Res 2008;12:651(1–2):131–140.
38. Green DPL. Three-dimensional structure of the zona pellucida. Rev Reprod 1997;2(3):147–156.
39. Herrler A, Beier HM. Early embryonic coats: morphology, function, practical applications. An overview. Cells Tissues Organs 2000;166(2):233–246.
40. Cohen J, Inge KL, Suzman K, Wiker SG, Wright G. Videocinematography of fresh and cryopreserved embryos: a retrospective analysis of embryonic morphology and implantation. Fertil Steril 1989;51(5):820–827.
41. Garside WT, Loret de Mola JR, Bucci JA, Tureck RW, Heyner S. Sequential analysis of zona thickness during in vitro culture of human zygotes: correlation with embryo quality, age, and implantation. Mol Reprod Dev 1997;47(1):99–104.
42. Gabrielsen A, Lindenberg S, Petersen K. The impact of the zona pellucida thickness variation of human embryos on pregnancy outcome in relation to suboptimal embryo development. A prospective randomized controlled study. Hum Reprod 2001;16(10):2166–2170.
43. Shen Y, Stalf T, Mehnert C, Eichenlaub-Ritter, Tinneberg HR. High magnitude of light retardation by the zona pellucida is associated with conception cycles. Hum Reprod. 2005;20(6):1596–1606.
44. Tesarik J, Greco E. The probability of abnormal preimplantation development can be predicted by a single static observation on pronuclear stage morphology. Hum Reprod 1999;14(5):1318–1323.
45. Scott L, Alvero R, Leondires M, Miller B. The morphology of human pronuclear embryos is positively related to blastocyst development and implantation. Human Reprod 2000;15(11):2394–2403.
46. Balaban B, Urman B, Isklar A, Alatas C, Aksoy S, Mercan R, Mumcu A, Nunhglu A. The effects of pronuclear morphology on embryo quality parameters and blastocyst transfer outcome. Hum Reprod 2001;16(11):2357–2361.
47. Rienzi L, Ubaldi F, Iacobelli M, Ferrero S, Minasi MG, Martinez F, Tesarik J, Greco E. Day 3 embryo transfer with combined evaluation at the pronuclear and cleavage stages compares favourably with day 5 blastocyst transfer. Hum Reprod 2002;17(7):1852–1855.
48. Zollner U, Zollner KP, Hartl G, Dietl J, Steck T. The use of a detailed zygote score after IVF/ICSI to obtain good quality blastocysts: the German experience. Hum Reprod 2002;17(5):1327–1333.
49. Ludwig M, Schopper B, Al-Hasani S, Diedrich K. Clinical use of a pronuclear stage score following intracytoplasmic sperm injection: impact on pregnancy rates under the conditions of the German embryo protection law. Hum Reprod 2000;15(2):325–329.
50. Wittemer C, Bettahar-Lebugle K, Ohl J, Rongieres C, Nisand I, Gerlinger P. Zygote evaluation: an efficient tool for embryo selection. Hum Reprod 2000;15(12): 2591–2597.
51. Montag M, van der Ven H. Evaluation of pronuclear morphology as the only selection criterion for further embryo culture and transfer: results of a prospective multicentre study. Hum Reprod 2001;16(11):2384–2389.
52. Zollner U, Zollner KP, Steck T, Dietl J. Pronuclear scoring: time for international standardization. J Reprod Med 2003(5);48:365–369.
53. Kahraman S, Kumtepe Y, Sertyel S, Donmez E, Benkhalifa M, Findikli N, Vanderzwalmen P. Pronuclear morphology scoring and chromosomal status of embryos in severe male infertility. Hum Reprod 2002;17(12):3193–3200.
54. Balaban B, Yakin K, Urman B, Isiklar A, Tesarik J. Pronuclear morphology predicts embryo development and chromosome constitution. Reprod Biomed Online 2004;8(6):695–700.
55. Gianarolli L, Magli MC, Ferrareti AP, Fortini D, Grieco N. Pronuclear morphology and chromosomal abnormalities as scoring criteria for embryo selection. Fertil Steril 2003; 80(2):341–349.
56. Salumets A, Hydén-Granskog C, Suikkari AM, Tiitinen A, Tuuri T. The predictive value of pronuclear morphology of zygotes in the assessment of human embryo quality. Hum Reprod 2001;16(10):2177–2181.
57. Payne J, Raburn D, Couchman G, Price T, Jamison M, Walmer D. Relationship between pre-embryo pronuclear morphology (zygote score) and standard day 2 or 3 embryo morphology with regard to assisted reproductive technique outcomes. Fertil Steril 2005;84(4):900–909.
58. James AN, Hennessy S, Reggio B, Wiemer K, Larsen F, Cohen J. The limited importance of pronuclear scoring of human zygotes. Hum Reprod 2006;21(6):1599–1604.
59. Tesarik J, Kopecyn V. Development of human male pronucleus: ultrastructure and timing. Gamete Res 1989;24(2): 135–149.

60. Nagy ZP, Janssenswillen C, Janssens R, De Vos A, Staessen C, Van de Velde H, Van Steirteghem AC. Timing of oocyte activation, pronucleus formation and cleavage in humans after intracytoplasmic sperm injection (ICSI) with testicular spermatozoa and after ICSI or in-vitro fertilizationn on sibling oocytes with ejaculated spermatozoa. Hum Reprod 1998;13(6):1606–1612.
61. Van Blerkom J, Davis P, Alexander S. Differential mitochondrial distribution in human pronuclear embryos leads to disproportionate inheritance between blastomeres: relationship to microtubular organization, ATP content and competence. Hum Reprod 2000;15(13):2621–2633.
62. Scott L. Pronuclear scoring as a predictor of embryo development. Reprod Biomed Online 2003;6(2):201–214.
63. Ebner T, Moser M, Sommergruber M, Gaiswinkler U, Wiesinger R, Puchner M, Tews G. Presence, but not type or degree of extension, of a cytoplasmic halo has a significant influence on preimplantation development and implantation behaviour. Hum Reprod 2003;18(11):2406–2412.
64. Stalf T, Herrero J, Mehnert C, Manolopoulos K, Lenhard A, Gips H. Influence of polarization effects in ooplasma and pronuclei on embryo quality and implantation in an IVF program. J Assist Reprod Genet 2002;19(8):355–362.
65. Balakier H, MacLusky NJ, Casper RF. Characterization of the first cell cycle in human zygotes: implications for cryopreservation. Fertil Steril 1993;59(2):359–365.
66. Trounson A, Mohr LR, Woos C, Leeton JF. Effect of delayed insemination on in-vitro fertilization, culture and transfer of human embryos. J Reprod Fertil 1982;64(2):285–294.
67. Terriou P, Giorgetti C, Hans E, Salzmann J, Charles O, Cignetti L, Avon C, Roulier R. Relationship between even early cleavage and day 2 embryo score and assessment of their predictive value for pregnancy. Reprod Biomed Online 2007;14(3):294–299.
68. Shoukir Y, Campana A, Farley T, Sakkas D. Early cleavage of in-vitro fertilized human embryos to the 2-cell stage: a novel indicator of embryo quality and viability. Hum Reprod 1997;12(7):1531–1536.
69. Guerif F, Le Gouge A, Giraudeau B, Poindron J, Bidault R, Gasnier O, Royere D. Limited value of morphological assessment at days 1 and 2 to predict blastocyst development potential: a prospective study based on 4042 embryos. Hum Reprod 2007;22(7):1973–1981.
70. Windt ML, Kruger TF, Coetzee K, Lombard CJ. Comparative analysis of pregnancy rates after the transfer of early dividing embryos versus slower dividing embryos. Hum Reprod 2004;19(5):1155–1162.
71. Lundin K, Bergh C, Hardarson T. Early embryo cleavage is a strong indicator of embryo quality in human IVF. Human Reprod 2001;16(12):2652–2657.
72. Hesters L, Prisant N, Fanchin R, Méndez Lozano D, Feyereisen E, Frydman R, Tachdjian G, Frydman N. Impact of early cleaved zygote morphology on embryo development and in vitro fertilization-embryo transfer outcome: a prospective study. Fertil Steril 2008;89(6):1677–1684.
73. Fenwick J, Platteau P, Murdoch AP, Herbert M. Time from insemination to first cleavage predits developmental competence of human preimplantation embryos in vitro. Human Reprod 2002;17(2):407–412.
74. Petersen CG, Mauri AL, Ferreira R, Baruffi RLR, Frango JG. Embryo selection by the first cleavage parameter between 25 and 27 hours after ICSI. J A Reprod Gen 2001;18(4): 209–212.
75. Sundström P, Saldeen P. Early embryo cleavage and day 2 mononucleation after intracytoplasmatic sperm injection for predicting embryo implantation potential in single embryo transfer cycles. Fertil Steril 2008;89(2):475–477.
76. Edwards RG, Purdy JM, Steptoe PC, Walters DE. The growth of human preimplantation embryos in vitro. Am J Obstet Gynecol 1981;141(4):408–416.
77. Giorgetti C, Terriou P, Auquier P, Hans E, Spach JL, Salzmann J, Roulier R. Embryo score to predict implantation after in-vitro fertilization: based on 957 single embryo transfers. Hum Reprod 1995;10(9):2427–2431.
78. Ziebe S, Petersen K, Lindenberg S, Andersen AG, Gabrielsen A, Andersen AN. Embryo morphology or cleavage stage: how to select the best embryos for transfer after in-vitro fertilization. Hum Reprod 1997;12(7):1545–1549.
79. Alikani M, Calderon G, Tomkin G, et al. Cleavage anomalies in early human embryos and survival after prolonged culture in-vitro. Hum Reprod 2000;15(12):2634–2643.
80. Steer C, Mills C, Tan S, et al. The cumulative embryo score: a predictive embryo scoring technique to select the optimal number of embryos to transfer in an in-vitro fertilization and embryo transfer program. Hum Reprod 1992;7:117–119.
81. Puissant F, Van Rysselberge M, Barlow P, et al. Embryo scoring as a prognostic tool in IVF treatment. Hum Reprod 1987;2:705–708.
82. Carillo A, Lane B, Pridham D, et al. Improved clinical outcomes for in vitro fertilization with delay of embryo transfer from 48 to 72 hours after oocyte retrieval: use of glucose- and phosphate-free media. Fertil Steril 1998;69: 329–334.
83. Racowsky C, Combelles C, Nureddin A, et al. Day 3 and day 5 morphological predictors of embryo viability. Reprod Biomed Online 2003;6:323–331.
84. Munne S, Alikani M, Tomkin G, Grifo J, Cohen J. Embryo morphology, developmental rates, and maternal age are correlated with chromosome abnormalities. Fertil Steril 1995;64(2):382–391.
85. Jones G, Trounson A, Lolatgis N, et al. Factors affecting the success of human blastocyst development and pregnancy following in vitro fertilization and embryo transfer. Fertil Steril 1998;70:1022–1029.
86. Antczak M, Van Blerkom J. Temporal and spatial aspects of fragmentation in early human embryos: possible effects on developmental competence and association with the differential elimination of regulatory proteins from polarized domains. Hum Reprod 1999;14(2):429–447.
87. Alikani M, Cohen J, Tomkin G, Garrisi GJ, Mack C, Scott RT. Human embryo fragmentation in vitro and its implications for pregnancy and implantation. Fertil Steril 1999;71(5): 836–842.
88. Jurisicova A, Varmuza S, Casper RF. Programmed cell death and human embryo fragmentation. Mol Hum Reprod 1996;2(2):93–98.
89. Perez GI, Tao XJ, Tilly JL. Fragmentation and death (a.k.a. apoptosis) of ovulated oocytes. Mol Hum Reprod 1999;5(5): 414–420.

90. Pellestor F, Girardet A, Andréo B, Arnal F, Humeau C. Relationship between morphology and chromosomal constitution in human preimplantation embryo. Mol Reprod Dev 1994;39(2):141–146.
91. Munné S, Alikani M, Cohen J. Monospermic polyploidy and atypical embryo morphology. Hum Reprod 1994;9(3): 506–510.
92. Sorimachi K, Naora H, Akimoto K, Niwa A, Naora H. Multinucleation and preservation of nucleolar integrity of macrophages. Cell Biol Int 1998;22(5):351–357.
93. Alikani M. The origins and consequences of fragmentation in mammalian eggs and embryos. In Human Preimplantation Embryo Selection. Elder K and Cohen J, eds. Informa Healthcare, London, UK, 2007:51–77.
94. Ebner T, Yaman C, Moser M, Sommergruber M, Pölz W, Tews G. Embryo fragmentation in vitro and its impact on treatment and pregnancy outcome. Fertil Steril 2001;76(2):281–285.
95. della Ragione T, Verheyen G, Papanikolaou EG, Van Landuyt L, Devroey P, Van Steirteghem A. Developmental stage on day-5 and fragmentation rate on day-3 can influence the implantation potential of top-quality blastocysts in IVF cycles with single embryo transfer. Reprod Biol Endocrinol 2007;5(2):1–8.
96. Stone B, Greene J, Vargyas J, Ringler G, Marrs R. Embryo fragmentation as a determinant of blastocyst development in vitro and pregnancy outcomes following embryo transfer. Am J Obstet Gynecol 2005;192(6):2014–2019.
97. Sathananthan H, Gunasheela S, Menezes J. Mechanics of human blastocyst hatching in vitro. Reprod Biomed Online 2003;7(2):228–234.
98. Rienzi L. Significance of morphological attributes of the early embryo. Reprod BioMed Online 2005;10(5):669–681.
99. Hardarson T, Hanson C, Sjogren A, Lundin K. Human embryos with unevenly sized blastomeres have lower pregnancy and implantation rates: indications for aneuploidy and multinucleation. Hum Reprod 2001;16:313–318.
100. Holte J, Berglund L, Milton K, Garello C, Gennarelli G, Revelli A, Bergh T. Construction of an evidence-based integrated morphology cleavage embryo score for implantation potential of embryos scored and transferred on day 2 after oocyte retrieval. Hum Reprod 2007;22(2):548–557.
101. Van Royen E, Mangelschots K, Vercruyssen M, De Neubourg D, Valkenburg M, Ryckaert G, Gerris J. Multinucleation in cleavage stage embryos. Hum Reprod 2003;18(5):1062–1069.
102. Jackson KV, Ginsburg ES, Hornstein MD, Rein MS, Clarke RN. Multinucleation in normally fertilized embryos is associated with an accelerated ovulation induction response and lower implantation and pregnancy rates in in vitro fertilization-embryo transfer cycles. Fertil Steril 1998;70(1):60–66.
103. Saldeen P, Sundstrom P. Nuclear status of four-cell preembryos predicts implantation potential in in vitro fertilization treatment cycles. Fertil Steril 2005;84(3):584–589.
104. Kligman I, Benadiva C, Alikani M, Munne S. The presence of multinucleated blastomeres in human embryos is correlated with chromosomal abnormalities. Hum Reprod 1996;11:1492–1498.
105. Munne S, Cohen J. Unsuitability of multinucleated human blastomeres for preimplantation genetic diagnosis. Human Reprod 1993;8:1120–1125.
106. Moriwaki T, Suganuma N, Hayakawa M, Hibi H, Katsumata Y, Oguchi H, Furuhashi M. Embryo evaluation by analysing blastomere nuclei. Hum Reprod 2004;19(1):152–6.
107. Tao J, Tamis R, Fink K, et al. The neglected morula/compact stage embryo transfer. Hum Reprod 2002;17(6): 1513–1518.
108. Nikas G, Ao A, Winston RML, Handyside AH. Compaction and surface polarity in the human embryo in vitro. Biol Reprod 1996;55(1):32–37.
109. Desai N, Goldstein J, Rowland DY, Goldfarb MJ. Morphological evaluation of human embryos and derivation of an embryo quality scoring system specific for day 3 embryos: a preliminary study. Hum Reprod 2000;15 (10):2190–2196.
110. Skiadas C, Jackson K, Racowsky C. Early compaction on day 3 may be associated with increased implantation potential. Fertil Steril 2006;86:1386–1391.
111. Feil D, Henshaw RC, Lane M. Day 4 embryo selection is equal to Day 5 using a new embryo scoring system validated in single embryo transfers. Hum Reprod 2008;23(7):1505–1510.
112. Steptoe PC, Edwards RG, Purdy JM. Human blastocyst grown culture. Nature 1971;229:132–133.
113. Bolton VN, Wren ME, Parsons JH. Pregnancies after in vitro fertilization and transfer of human blastocysts. Fertil Steril 1991;55(4):830–832.
114. Gardner DK, Lane M, Calderon I, Leeton J. Environment of the preimplantation human embryo in vivo: metabolite analysis of oviduct and uterine fluids and metabolism of cumulus cells. Fertil Steril 1996;65(2):349–353.
115. Ménézo YJR, Hamamah S, Hazout A, Dale B. Time to switch from co-culture to sequential defined media for transfer at the blastocyst stage. Hum Reprod 1998;13(8): 2043–2044.
116. Biggers JD, Racowsky C. The development of fertilized human ova to the blastocyst stage in KSOM(AA) medium: is a two-step protocol necessary? Reprod Biomed Online 2002;5(2):133–140.
117. Summers MC, Biggers JD. Chemically defined media and the culture of mammalian preimplantation embryos: historical perspective and current issues. Hum Reprod Update 2003;9(6):557–582.
118. Behr B, Fisch J, Racowsky C, Miller K, Pool T, Milki A. Blastocyst-ET and monozygotic twinning. J Assist Reprod Genet 2000;17:349–351.
119. Skiadas CC, Missmer SA, Benson CB, Gee RE, Racowsky C. Risk factors associated with pregnancies containing a monochorionic pair following assisted reproductive technologies. Hum Reprod 2008;23(6):1366–1371.
120. Racowsky C, Jackson KV, Cekleniak NA, Fox JH, Hornstein MD, Ginsburg ES. The number of eight-cell embryos is a key determinant for selecting day 3 or day 5 transfer. Fertil Steril 2000;73(3):558–564.
121. Gardner DK, Schoolcraft WB, Wagley L, Schlenker T, Stevens J, Hesla J. A prospective randomized trial of blastocyst culture and transfer in in-vitro fertilization. Hum Reprod 1998;13(12):3434–3440.
122. Marek D, Langley M, Gardner DK, Confer N, Doody KM, Doody KJ. Introduction of blastocyst culture and transfer for all patients in an in vitro fertilization program. Fertil Steril 1999;72(6):1035–1040.

123. Schoolcraft WB, Gardner DK, Lane M, Schlenker T, Hamilton F, Meldrum DR. Blastocyst culture and transfer: analysis of results and parameters affecting outcome in two in vitro fertilization programs. Fertil Steril 1999;72(4):604–609.
124. Papanikolaou EG, D'haeseleer E, Verheyen G, Van de Velde H, Camus M, Van Steirteghem A, Devroey P, Tournaye H. Live birth rate is significantly higher after blastocyst transfer than after cleavage-stage embryo transfer when at least four embryos are available on day 3 of embryo culture. A randomized prospective study. Hum Reprod 2005;20(11):3198–3203.
125. Milki AA, Hinckley MD, Gebhardt J, Dasig D, Westpal L, Behr B. Accuracy of day 3 criteria for selecting the best embryos. Fertil Steril 2002;77(6):1191–1195.
126. Ebner T, Moser M, Sommergruber M, Tews G. Selection based on morphological assessment of oocytes and embryos at different stages of preimplantation development: a review. Hum Reprod Update 2003;9(3):251–262.
127. Braude P, Bolton V, Moore S. Human gene expression first occurs between the four- and eight-cell stages of preimplantation development. Nature 1988;332(6163):459–461.
128. Sakkas D. The use of blastocyst culture to avoid inheritance of an abnormal paternal genome after ICSI. Hum Reprod 1999;14(1):4–5.
129. Sandalinas M, Sadowy S, Alikani M, Calderon G, Cohen J, Munné S. Developmental ability of chromosomally abnormal human embryos to develop to the blastocyst stage. Hum Reprod 2001;16(9):1954–1958.
130. Shi W, Haaf T. Aberrant methylation patterns at the two-cell stage as an indicator of early developmental failure. Mol Reprod Dev 2002;63:329–334.
131. Ertzeid G, Storeng R. The impact of ovarian stimulation on implantation and fetal development in mice. Hum Reprod 2001;16(2):221–225.
132. Fanchin R, Ayoubi JM, Righini C, Olivennes F, Schönauer LM, Frydman R. Uterine contractility decreases at the time of blastocyst transfers. Hum Reprod 2001;16(6):1115–1119.
133. Bungum M, Bungum L, Humaidan P, Yding Andersaen C. Day 3 versus day 5 embryo transfer: a prospective randomized study. Reprod Biomed Online 2003;7(1):98–104.
134. Cruz JR, Dubey AK, Patel J, Peak D, Hartog B, Gindoff PR. Is blastocyst transfer useful as an alternative treatment for patients with multiple in vitro fertilization failures? Fertil Steril 1999;72(2):218–220.
135. Balaban B, Urman B, Alatas C, Mercan R, Aksoy S, Isiklar A. Blastocyst-stage transfer of poor-quality cleavage-stage embryos results in higher implantation rates. Fertil Steril 2001;75(3):514–518.
136. Gardner D, Lane M, Stevens J, Schlenker T, Schoolcraft WB. Blastocyst score affects implantation and pregnancy outcome: towards a single blastocyst transfer. Fertil Steril 2000;73(6):1155–1158.
137. Gardner DK, Stevens J, Sheehan CB, Schoolcraft W. Analysis of blastocyst morphology. In Human Preimplantation Embryo Selection. Elder K and Cohen J, eds. Informa Healthcare, London, UK, 2007:79–87.
138. Cummins JM, Breen TM, Harrison KL, Shwan JM, Wilson LM, Hennessey JF. A formula for scoring human embryo growth rates in in vitro fertilization: its value in predicting pregnancy and in comparison with visual estimates of embryo quality. J In Vitro Fert Embryo Transf 1986;3(5):284–295.
139. Skiadas CC, Racowsky C. Developmental rate, cumulative scoring, and embryo viability. In Human Preimplantation Embryo Selection. Elder K and Cohen J, eds. Informa Healthcare, London, UK, 2007:101–121.
140. Veeck LL. Atlas of the human oocyte and early conceptus. Vol 2 Baltimore: Williams and Wilkins, 1991:427–444.
141. Giorgetti C, Terriou P, Auquier P, Hans E, Spach JL, Salzmann J, Roulier R. Embryo score to predict implantation after in-vitro fertilization: based on 957 single embryo transfers. Hum Reprod 1995;10(9):2427–2431.
142. Van Royen E, Mangelschots K, De Neubourg D, Valkenburg M, Van de Meerssche M, Ryckaert G, Eestermans W, Gerris J. Characterization of a top quality embryo, a step towards single-embryo transfer. Hum Reprod 1999;14(9):2345–2349.
143. Van Royen E, Mangelschots K, De Neubourg D, Laureys I, Ryckaert G, Gerris J. Calculating the implantation potential of day 3 embryos in women younger than 38 years of age: a new model. Human Reprod 2001;16(2):326–332.
144. Terriou P, Sapin C, Giorgetti C, Hans E, Spach JL, Roulier R. Embryo score is a better predictor of pregnancy than the number of transferred embryos or female age. Fertil Steril 2001;75(3):525–531.
145. Scott L, Finn A, O'Leary T, McLellan S, Hill J. Morphologic parameters of early cleavage-stage embryos that correlate with fetal development and delivery: prospective and applied data for increased pregnancy rates. Human Reprod 2007;22(1):230–340.
146. Peterson CM, Reading JC, Hatasaka HH, Parker Jones K, Udoff LC, Adashi EY, Kuneck PH, Erickson LD, Malo JW, Campbell BF, Carrell D. Use of outcomes-based data in reducing high-order multiple pregnancies: the role of age, diagnosis, and embryo score. Fertil Steril 2004;81(6):1534–1541.
147. Fisch J, Sher G, Adamowicz M, et al. The graduated embryo score predicts the outcome of assisted reproductive technologies better than a single day 3 evaluation and achieves results associated with blastocyst transfer from day 3 embryo transfer. Fertil Steril 2003;80:1352–1358.
148. Sakkas D, Percival G, D'Arcy Y, Sharif K, Afnan M. Assessment of early cleaving in vitro fertilized human embryos at the 2-cell stage before transfer improves embryo selection. Fertil Steril 2001;76(6):1150–1156.
149. Carrell DT, Peterson CM, Jones KP, Hatasaka HH, Udoff LC, Cornwell CE, Thorp C, Kuneck P, Erickson L, Campbell B. A simplified coculture system using homologous, attached cumulus tissue results in improved human embryo morphology and pregnancy rates during in vitro fertilization. J Assist Reprod Genet 1999;16(7):344–349.
150. Sjöblom P, Menezes J, Cummins L, Mathiyalagan B, Costello MF. Prediction of embryo developmental potential and pregnancy based on early stage morphological characteristics. Fertility Sterility 2006;86(4):848–861.
151. Hunault CC, Eijkemans MJ, Pieters MH, te Velde ER, Habbema JD, Fauser BC, Macklon NS. Aprediction model for selecting patients undergoing in vitro fertilization for elective single embryo transfer. Fertil Steril 2002;77(4):725–732.

152. Hardarson T, Caisander G, Sjögren A, Hanson C, Hamberger L, Lundin K. A morphological and chromosomal study of blastocysts developing from morphologically suboptimal human pre-embryos compared with control blastocysts. Hum Reprod 2003;18(2):399–407.
153. Ciray H, Karagenc L, Ulug U, et al. Early cleavage morphology affects the quality and implantation potential of day 3 embryos. Fertil Steril 2006;85:358–365.
154. Lan KC, Huang FJ, Lin YC, Kung FT, Hsieh CH, Huang HW, Tan PH, Chang SY. The predictive value of using a combined Z-score and day 3 embryo morphology score in the assessment of embryo survival on day 5. Hum Reprod 2003;18(6):1299–1306.
155. Brison DR, Hollywood K, Arnesen R, Goodacre R. Predicting human embryo viability: the road to non-invasive analysis of the secretome using metabolic footprinting. Reprod Biomed Online 2007;15(3):296–302.
156. Villas-Bôas S, Mas S, Åkesson M, Smedsgaard J, Nielsen J. Mass spectrometry in metabolome analysis. Mass Spect Rev 2005;24(5):613–646.
157. Khosla S, Dean W, Reik W, Feil R. Culture of preimplantation embryos and its long-term effects on gene expression and phenotype. Hum Reprod Update 2001;7(4):419–427.
158. Khosla S, Dean W, Brown D, Reik W, Feil R. Culture of preimplantation mouse embryos affects fetal development and the expression of imprinted genes. Biol Reprod 2001;64(3):918–926.
159. Leese HJ, Sturmey RG, Baumann CG, McEvoy TG. Embryo viability and metabolism: obeying the quiet rules. Hum Reprod 2007;22(12):3047–3050.
160. Lane M, Gardner DK. Understanding cellular disruptions during early embryo development that perturb viability and fetal development. Reprod Fertil Dev 2005;17(3):371–378.
161. Hardy K, Hooper MAK, Handyside AH, Rutherford AJ, Winston RML, Leese HJ. Non-invasive measurement of glucose and pyruvate uptake by individual human oocytes and preimplantation embryos. Hum Reprod 1989;4(2):188–191.
162. Gott AL, Hardy K, Winston RML, Leese HJ. Non-invasive measurement of pyruvate and glucose uptake and lactate production by single human preimplantation embryos. Hum Reprod 1990;5(1):104–108.
163. Conaghan J, Hardy K, Handyside AH, Winston RM, Leese HJ. Selection criteria for human embryo transfer: a comparison of pyruvate uptake and morphology. J Assist Reprod Genet 1993;10(1):21–30.
164. Gardner D, Lane M, Stevens J, Schoolcraft WB. Noninvasive assessment of human embryo nutrient consumption as a measure of developmental potential. Fertil Steril 2001;76(6):1175–1180.
165. Turner K, Martin KL, Woodward BJ, Lenton EA, Leese HJ. Comparison of pyruvate uptake by embryos derived from conception and non-conception natural cycles. Hum Reprod 1994;9(12):2362–2366.
166. Devreker F, Hardy K, Van den Bergh M, Vannin AS, Emiliani S, Englert Y. Noninvasive assessment of glucose and pyruvate uptake by human embryos after intracytoplasmic sperm injection and during the formation of pronuclei. Fertil Steril 2000;73(5):947–954.
167. Jones GM, Trounson AO, Vella PJ, Thouas GA, Lolatgis N, Wood C. Glucose metabolism of human morula and blastocyst-stage embryos and its relationship to viability after transfer. Reprod Biomed Online 2001;3(2):124–132.
168. Brison DR, Houghton FD, Falconer D, Roberts SA, Hawkhead J, Humpherson PG, Lieberman BA, Leese HJ. Identification of viable embryos in IVF by non-invasive measurement of amino acid turnover. Hum Reprod 2004;19(10):2319–2324.
169. Houghton FD, Hawkhead JA, Humpherson PG, Hogg JE, Balen AH, Rutherford AJ, Leese HJ. Non-invasive amino acid turnover predicts human embryo developmental capacity. Hum Reprod 2002;17(4):999–1005.
170. Noci I, Fuzzi B, Rizzo R, Melchiorri L, Criscuoli L, Dabizz S, Biagiotti R, Pellegrini S, Menicucci A, Baricordi OR. Embryonic soluble HLA-G as a marker of developmental potential in embryos. Hum Reprod 2005;20(1):138–146.
171. Desai N, Fillipovits J, Goldfarb J. Secretion of soluble HLA-G by day 3 human embryos associated with higher pregnancy and implantation rates: assay of culture media using a new ELISA kit. Reprod Biomed Online 2006;13(2):272–277.
172. Fuzzi B, Rizzo R, Criscuoli L, Noci I, Melchiorri L, Scarselli B, Bencini E, Menicucci A, Baricordi OR. HLA-G expression in early embryos is a fundamental prerequisite for the obtainment of pregnancy. Eur J Immunol 2002;32(2):311–315.
173. Bjorkman PJ, Saper MA, Samraoui B, Bennett WS, Strominger JL, Wiley DC. The foreign antigen binding site and T cell recognition regions of class I histocompatibility antigens. Nature 1987;329(6139):512–518.
174. Roussev RG, Coulam CB. HLA-G and its role in implantation. J Assist Reprod Genet 2007;24(7):288–2953 Review.
175. Chu W, Fant ME, Geraghty DE, Hunt JS. Soluble HLA-G in human placentas: synthesis in trophoblasts and interferon-gamma-activated macrophages but not placental fibroblasts. Hum Immunol 1998;59(7):435–442.
176. Jurisicova A, Casper RF, MacLusky NJ, Mills GB, Librach CL. HLA-G expression during preimplantation human embryo development. Proc Natl Acad Sci U S A 1996;9;93(1):161–165.
177. Fisch J, Keskintepe L, Ginsburg M, Adamowicz M, Sher G. Graduated Embryo Score and soluble human leukocyte antigen-G expression improve assisted reproductive technology outcomes and suggest a basis for elective single-embryo transfer. Fertil Steril 2007;87(4):757–763.
178. Sageshima N, Shobu T, Awai K, Hashimoto H, Yamashita M, Takeda N, Odawara Y, Nakanishi M, Hatake K, Ishitani A. Soluble HLA-G is absent from human embryo cultures: a reassessment of sHLA-G detection methods. J Reprod Immunol 2007;75(1):11–22.
179. Sargent I, Swales A, Ledee N, Kozma N, Tabiasco J, Le Bouteiller P. sHLA-G production by human IVF embryos: can it be measured reliably? J Reprod Immunol 2007;75 (2):128–132.
180. Bromer JG, Seli E. Assessment of embryo viability in assisted reproductive technology: shortcomings of current approaches and the emerging role of metabolomics. Curr Opin Obstet Gynecol 2008;20(3):234–241.
181. Raamsdonk LM, Teusink B, Broadhurst D, Zhang N, Hayes A, Walsh MC, Berden JA, Brindle KM, Kell DB, Rowland JJ, Westerhoff HV, van Dam K, Oliver SG.

A functional genomics strategy that uses metabolome data to reveal the phenotype of silent mutations. Nat Biotechnol 2001;19(1):45–50.
182. Hollywood K, Brison DR, Goodacre R. Metabolomics: current technologies and future trends. Proteomics 2006;6(17):4716–4723.
183. Seli E, Sakkas D, Scott R, Kwok SC, Rosendahl SM, Burns DH. Noninvasive metabolomic profiling of embryo culture media using Raman and near-infrared spectroscopy correlates with reproductive potential of embryos in women undergoing in vitro fertilization. Fertil Steril 2007;88(5):1350–1357.
184. Vergouw CG, Botros LL, Roos P, Lens JW, Schats R, Hompes PG, Burns DH, Lambalk CB. Metabolomic profiling by near-infrared spectroscopy as a tool to assess embryo viability: a novel, non-invasive method for embryo selection. Human Reprod 2008;23(7): 1499–1504.
185. Scott R, Seli E, Miller K, Sakkas D, Scott K, Burns DH. Noninvasive metabolomic profiling of human embryo culture media using Raman spectroscopy predicts embryonic reproductive potential: a prospective blinded pilot study. Fertil Steril 2008;90(1):77–83.

# Elective Single-Embryo Transfer

Jan Gerris and Petra De Sutter

**Abstract** In the early days of IVF, replacement of several embryos in order to compensate for low implantation rates in the human was considered good clinical practice. Lack of funding, suboptimal embryo culture and selection techniques and pressure from patients led to a staggering 50% of all children born after IVF/ICSI belonging to a set of multiples. The first step towards a more reasonable approach came when it was shown that transferring two or three embryos did not influence the pregnancy rate but only the triplet rate. Unfortunately, this step in the right direction did n ot result in a decrease of twins. Although the challenge of a triplet pregnancy is much greater than that of a twin, the epidemic size of iatrogenic twinning results in a more widespread negative effect on neonatal, perinatal and maternal outcome. The challenge is to combine excellent pregnancy rates with a reduction in twinning rate from 25–30% to 5–10%. The second step has received much attention but little following: elective single-embryo transfer (eSET). Published data indicate the feasibility to perform judicious eSET. This is definitely the case in good prognosis patients (less than 36 years of age, first or second IVF/ICSI trial) and if there is a choice from several embryos. Embryo selection, still on the basis of an optimized morphology assessment using strict criteria and time intervals, is essential. Apart from the preventive effect on the complications associated with many (but not all) twin pregnancies, both health-economic considerations and neonatal outcome considerations also underpin the value of SET. Cryopreservation is a useful tool in an optimal strategy and management of all oocyte harvests.

**Keywords** IVF/ICSI • Multiple pregnancy • Complications • Single-embryo transfer • Embryo selection

## 1 Introduction

Twins can be dizygotic (70%) or monozygotic (30%). Monozygotic twinning used to occur at a stable incidence of around 1/250 (0.4%) births worldwide. An increase in MZ twinning reaching 2–3% has been recorded since the early days of ART (1). Complications are more frequent in the later stages of separation of monozygotic twins and dizygotic twins; because there are many more twins than triplets in absolute number, more complications are the consequence of twins than of triplets. However, because of their much higher absolute numbers, dizygotic twins are the major cause of complications. The increase in twinning after ART is mainly an exponential rise in dizygotic twins, directly related to the fact that more than one embryo is transferred in IVF/ICSI (2). The effect of increased age, at which women bear children in modern societies, is responsible for about one quarter of this increase. In addition, many multiple pregnancies (MPs) are the result of so-called controlled ovarian hyperstimulation (3). High-order multiple pregnancies (HOMPs) are also strongly increased after ART and the complications are even more severe. It has been silently accepted that a high proportion of iatrogenic twins and HOMPs was the price to be paid for a reasonable success rate of a treatment that is physically and emotionally demanding and often expensive. An increased financial cost for multiple pregnancies, deliveries and neonatal care has

J. Gerris (✉) and P. De Sutter
Center for Reproductive Medicine, Women's Clinic, University Hospital Ghent, Belgium
e-mail: jan.gerris@uzgent.be

D.T. Carrell et al. (eds.), *Biennial Review of Infertility,* DOI: 10.1007/978-1-60327-392-3_11

been demonstrated (4–8) and severe emotional stress has been reported by parents of multiple births (9, 10).

MPs cause several pathologies (11–23), comprising both maternal and foetal/neonatal risks and complications. The main risk involved is prematurity. In singletons, prematurity occurs in 6–7% of births; in twins the incidence is >50% and in higher multiples it is >90%. Prematurity results in increased neonatal and infant mortality, a higher incidence of low and very low birth weight neonates, and more intraventricular haemorrhage, neonatal enterocolitis, respiratory distress syndrome and sepsis. Cerebral palsy is five times more frequent in twins than in singletons. Maternal risks are also increased and comprise pre-eclampsia, gestational diabetes, myocardial infarction, heart failure, venous thrombo-embolism, pulmonary oedema, postpartum haemorrhage and an increased chance for caesarean section and caesarean hysterectomy (24–27). These medical risks are accompanied by long-term complications: subtle neuro-linguistic development disorders, parenting stress and sibling-stress. All of these adverse outcomes have to be paid for by patients, insurers and society (28–30). It is becoming gradually accepted that the incidence of iatrogenic twinning should be kept within reasonable limits. A philosophical argument has focussed on the fact that we have responsibility for our children's health from the start of their lives (31, 32).

## 2 Clinical Data on Set

### 2.1 *Published Randomized Trials Comparing Outcome of Infertility Treatment*

Five truly prospective randomized trials have been published, four European studies, of which two utilised day 3 SET (33, 34) and two mostly day 2 SET (35, 36), and one American study using single blastocyst transfers (37) (Table 1). In our own study, patients were randomised between receiving one vs. two top quality embryos, strictly defined as an embryo with <20% fragmentation, four or five blastomeres on day 2 and ≥7 blastomeres on day 3 after fertilisation and no multinucleation in any of the blastomeres. Such embryos were shown to have an ongoing implantation potential of ~40% (38). A Finnish study concluded that a 32.4% pregnancy rate after SET is not significantly different from a 47.1% pregnancy rate after double embryo transfer (DET) (34). In a Scandinavian study, women <36 years of age in their first or second attempt were randomized to receive either one excellent fresh embryo *and* one frozen/thawed embryo in case no pregnancy occurred (Group 1+1) vs. two fresh embryos (Group +2) (35). It showed that a strategy of 1+1 transfer (39.7%) did not result in a substantial

**Table 1** Randomized studies and cohort studies comparing SET with DET

| Author | *N* cycles | PR SET (%) | Twins (%) | PR DET (%) | Twins (%) |
|---|---|---|---|---|---|
| *Randomised trials* | | | | | |
| Gerris et al. (33) | 53 | 10/26 (38.5) | 1/10 | 20/27 (73) | 6/20 (30.0) |
| Martikainen et al. (34) | 144 | 24/74 (32.4) | 1/24 | 33/70 (46.1) | 6/33 (18.2) |
| Gardner et al. (37) | 48 | 14/23 (64.9) | 0/14 | 19/25 (75) | 9/19 (46.4) |
| Thurin et al. (35) | 661 | 91/330 (27.6) | 1/91 | 144/331 (42.5) | 52/144 (36.1) |
| | + cryo | 131/330 (39.7) | 1/131 | | |
| Van Montfoort et al. (36) | 308 | 51/154 (33.) | 0/51 | 73/154 (46.4) | 13/73 (17.8) |
| Total | 906 | 190/607 (31.3) | 3/190 (1.58) | 289/607 (46.6) | 86/289 (29.8) |
| *Cohort studies* | | | | | |
| Reference | *N* cycles | PR SET (%) | Twins (%) | PR DET (%) | Twins +HOMPs(%) |
| Gerris et al. (60) | 1152 | 105/299 (35.1) | 1/124 | 309/853 (36.2) | 105 + /309 (35.6) |
| De Sutter et al. (62, 63) | 2898 | 163/579 (28.2) | 1/163 | 734/2319 (31.7) | 219 + 4/734 (30.4) |
| Tiitinen et al. (61) | 1494 | 162/470 (34.5) | 2/162 | 376/1024 (36.7) | 113/376 (30.1) |
| Catt et al. (96) | 385 | 49/111 (43.1) | 1/49 | 161/274 (56.8) | 71/161 (43.1) |
| Gerris et al. (28) | 367 | 83/206 (41.3) | 0 | 65/161 (41.4) | 20/65 (30.8) |
| Martikainen et al. (34) | 1111 | 107/308 (34.7) | 1/107 | 255/803 (31.8) | n.a. |
| | | 187/308 (64.7) | | | |
| Total | 7407 | 669/1,973 (33.9) | 6/591 (1.0) | 1,900/5,434 (35.0) | 537/1,645 (32.6) |

(Data for the Martikainen 2001 study and the Thurin 2004 study show both the fresh and the cryoaugmented pregnancy rates)

reduction in ongoing pregnancy rate when compared with 2-embryo transfer (43.5%). The fresh PR was 91/330 = 27.6% after SET vs. 142/330 = 43% after DET (OR= 1.56; 95%CI = 1.26–1.93). An American study compared the transfer of one with two day 5 embryos in a selected good prognosis group. Higher pregnancy rates were found in the DET-group but the pregnancy rate in the SET group was very high (~60%) (~37). In a Dutch study, eSET was compared in unselected patients with DET; all twins were prevented in the SET group but the pregnancy rate after DET was twice as high (40.3%) as after SET (20.4%). The mean rate of fresh pregnancy after SET in the four studies was 31.3% with 1.58% twins and 47.6% after DET with 29.8% twins. A formal Cochrane meta-analysis came to a similar conclusion (39).

## 2.2 Published Cohort Studies Describing Fertility Treatment Outcome After SET and DET

The mean pregnancy rate in a total of 7,407 cycles after SET was 33.9% with 1.0% twins vs. 35.0% after DET with 32.6% multiple pregnancies (Table 1). In most of these studies, SET was elective, i.e. was performed only if an excellent quality embryo was available in a cohort of embryos. These data suggest that elective SET (transfer of a high competence embryo) yields the same pregnancy rate as indiscriminate two-embryo transfer. This is because the high success rate after the transfer of two high competence embryos is balanced down by the low success rate after the transfer of two poor quality embryos. Recently, excellent results have been published from prospective nonrandomized studies in selected patients in Australia, the USA, India and the UK (39, 40–42) where use has been made of single blastocyst transfer in selected good-prognosis patients.

## 2.3 Opinion Papers

Some authors have spoken in support of single-embryo transfer, while others have expressed arguments against the application of single-embryo transfer. Single-embryo transfer has received support in the US (43). Others have stressed the importance of counselling and educating patients as well as staff members (44). On the other hand, some have argued that according to US guidelines, eSET appears to represent an appropriate transfer option for only a small minority of IVF patients. They consider indiscriminate SET (not advocated by any author) to be unrealistic and that it should be reconsidered (45). Arguments against SET are mostly of a non-medical nature and are related to values and circumstances characteristic for the societal context rather than to evidence. Reviews have shown arguments to optimize, not maximize IVF results (46–48).

## 2.4 A Balanced Appraisal of Published Results

Published data illustrate two points of paramount importance with respect to SET. First, cryopreservation is a very important tool in reducing twins after IVF/ICSI. Second, transferring the "two best" embryos always yields more pregnancies than transferring "the" best embryo. This is clearly shown when comparing the results after SET vs. DET between the randomised and the cohort studies. In the randomized there is a clear difference between both (DET: 216/453 vs. SET: 139/453; OR = 1.55; 99% CI = 1.24–1.94). In the non-randomized there is no difference. The fine point in *elective* SET is that it is closely tied up with optimal embryo selection and that it should only be applied if an embryo with putative high competence is available (38). The essential point that should not be missed is that optimized embryo selection, however and for whomever it is performed, is a tool that can be used in two opposite directions. It can be used to perform SET in a substantial proportion of patients, maintaining an overall PR in the vicinity of the natural conception rate for a normally fertile couple (~30%) but lowering the twinning rate substantially. Or it can be used to perform optimised two-embryo transfer in that same patient population, increasing the overall PR to well over 30% but "accepting" a substantially elevated twinning rate. The decision is a matter of judgement, a trade-off between outcome and complications and very much dependent on societal values and circumstances.

## 2.5 The European Experience with eSET

Belgium has resorted to a legal regulation regarding eSET (49). Six attempts of IVF/ICSI are covered by the government but the maximum number of embryos that can be transferred has been set, depending on the age of the woman and on the rank of the trial. The crux is that savings (mainly neonatal) from the reduction in twins and the disappearance of triplets make up for the money needed to cover six cycles, thus providing access to treatment to all who need it and at the same time ensuring quality outcome (49). There is also compulsory on-line registration of all cycles. Pivotal in the whole exercise is the judicious application of SET. Depending on the woman's age and the rank of the trial, the maximum number of embryos to transfer is regulated. All women <36 years of age in their first cycle receive one embryo, independent of its morphological assessment. In older women or in subsequent cycles, the number of embryos to transfer never exceeds two except in women >39 years of age, where there is no imposed maximum.

Table 2 shows data from the Belgian Registry of Artificial Reproduction (BELRAP) on the first year after the funding regulation. There has been a rise in the number of SET cycles and a drastic reduction of twins. Twins have dropped from ~25 to ~10%. The evolution of the number of embryos transferred and of singleton and multiple pregnancies over a longer period of time for the whole of Belgium is illustrated in Figs. 1–2. In Finland, SET has been applied widely for several years. On a national level, the incidence of IVF/ICSI twins has significantly decreased and even the total national birth registry shows a decrease in the proportion of twins (50). SET has been combined very successfully with cryopreservation (51) and was shown to be very successful in oocyte donation (52). In Sweden, the practice seems to be in concordance with the regulation of the National Board on Health and Welfare stating that in principle only one embryo should be replaced apart from exceptional circumstances, which seem to be loosely defined. The incidence of twinning after IVF/ICSI has dropped in these countries from >20 to <10%. With increasing eSET being performed, cryopreservation has become more important (51, 53) and the criterion for success after IVF/ICSI is now considered to be the *cumulative* rather than the per transfer chance for a *singleton* pregnancy, multiples being considered as a risk, a complication, or even as a failure. In Germany, the Embryo Protection Act rules that no more than three oocytes can be cultured further than the two pronuclear (2PN)-stage and no embryos can be frozen. This compels the German embryologists to select the embryos for transfer at the 2PN-stage, which hinders the application of SET. Switzerland and Austria have a similar ruling. In Italy, no more than three oocytes can be fertilised *and* all the embryos that result *have to* be replaced. Ethical concerns about respect of human life and protection of the family and offspring have the deplorable effect of burdening women with a legislation that is not reflecting biomedical reality (54). Dutch IVF centres seem convinced of the value of SET as testified by an increasing number of Dutch publications addressing clinical or health-economic aspects of SET (36, 55, 56). In the UK, there is at present legal restriction of two to the number of embryos to transfer, except in exceptional circumstances. The British Human Fertilization and

**Table 2** Results from the BELRAP showing results after the first full year of implementation of the reimbursement regulation in Belgium (July 2003-June 2004)

| | <36 years | | | | 36–40 years | | | |
|---|---|---|---|---|---|---|---|---|
| Rank | 1 | 2 | 3–6 | 7 | | | | |
| No. of cycles | 5,728 | 2,033 | 732 | 183 | 1,497 | 594 | 278 | 92 |
| No. of transfers (94%) | 5,384 | 1,921 | 691 | 170 | 1,371 (93%) | 546 | 259 | 87 |
| No. of embryos transferred | | | | | | | | |
| 1 | 4,918 | 807 | 98 | 71 | 344 | 135 | 55 | 13 |
| 2 | 426 | 1,103 | 581 | 82 | 968 | 382 | 114 | 58 |
| 3 | 28 | 7 | 12 | 14 | 50 | 28 | 86 | 13 |
| No cycles with +hCG | 1,880 | 697 | 213 | 74 | 419 | 135 | 66 | 34 |
| % per cycle | 33 | 34 | 29 | 40 | 28 | 23 | 24 | 37 |
| % per ET | 35 | 36 | 31 | 43 | 31 | 25 | 26 | 39 |

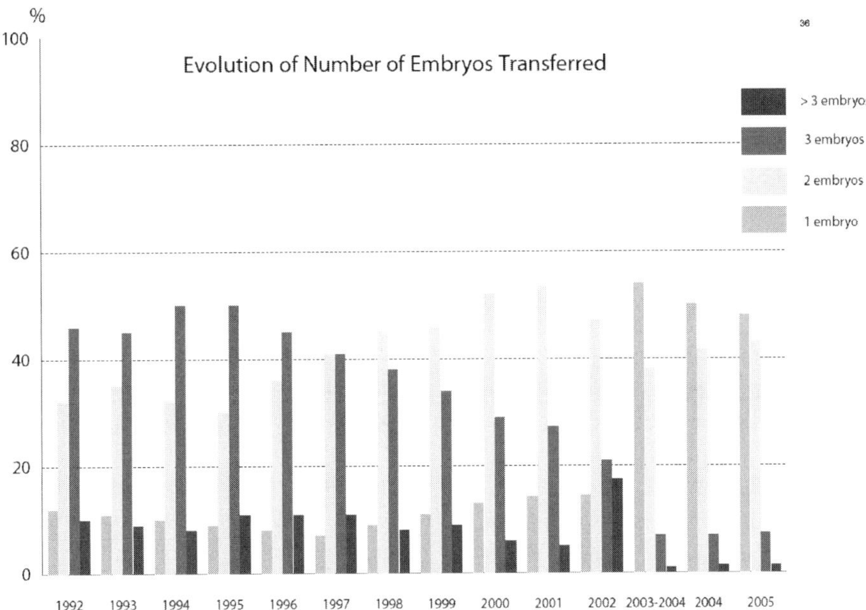


**Fig. 1** Evolution of the number of embryos replaced over the years 1992–2005 in Belgium

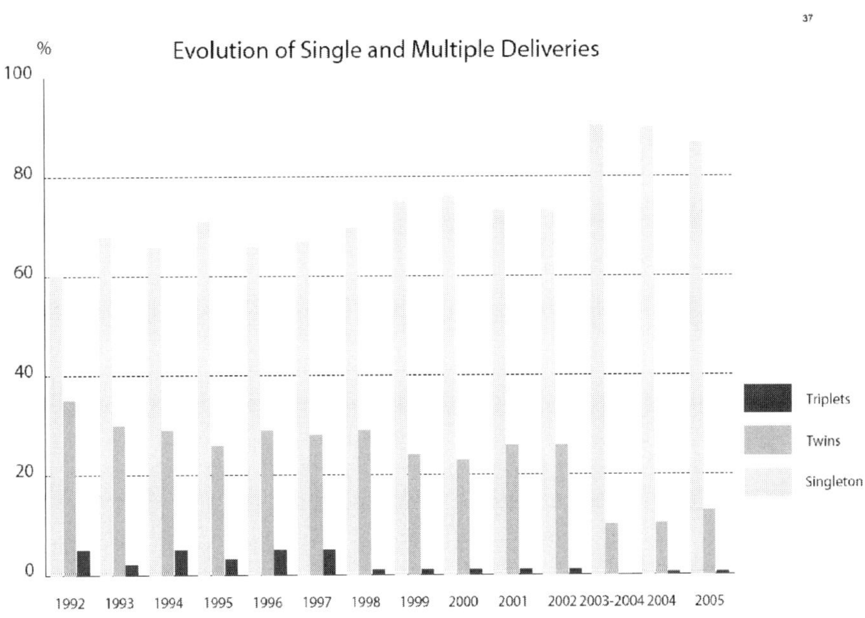


**Fig. 2** Evolution of the number of singleton, twin and triplet deliveries over the years 1992–2005 in Belgium. Because funding legislation started per 1st of June 2003, changes in twin percentages are to be viewed per year since June 2003

Embryology Authority (HFEA) has stated that it would like to move to SET and has installed a SET working group which is studying how and when to implement SET. Several recent papers from British authors support the introduction of SET (48, 57). Southern European countries (France, Spain, Portugal, Greece), to date, have neither produced clear evidence of a substantial proportion of SET cycles nor have legislation in place to limit the maximum number of embryos to transfer.

## 3 Indications and Exceptions: Set for Whom?

The essential prerequisites to introduce elective SET are simple. There must be a high base-line ongoing PR of the program in the group of good prognosis patients (e.g. first and second cycles in women <38 years of age) in combination with a compellingly high MP rate, and there must be an efficient cryopreservation program. There is a distinction between compulsory, medical and elective SET. In compulsory single-embryo transfer (cSET), the only available embryo is often of poor quality and the mean implantation rates in published series of cSET are low (Table 3) (58, 59, 64–67). There are women in whom a multiple pregnancy represents an *a priori* increased risk [e.g. those with congenital anomalies of the uterus, bad obstetrical history, previous loss of a twin, previous severe prematurity in a singleton, insufficiency of the cervical isthmus, severe systemic disease (e.g. insulin dependent diabetes)], which constitute absolute contraindications against two-embryo transfer. By definition, elective SET means that there is choice from among two or more embryos suitable for transfer, with the purpose of transferring only one embryo. The challenge is to define the subgroup of patients who should receive one embryo.

A number of retrospective studies examined which clinical factors correlate with the chance for pregnancy or MP (60–62). These were based on the transfer of two or more embryos. Most of the factors that were found to correlate (age being the single most important), are in fact themselves correlated with intrinsic embryo implantation potential (e.g. number of oocytes, number of normally fertilised 2PN-zygotes, number of "good looking" embryos, low dose of FSH needed, good ovarian response), emphasizing the dominant impact of the embryo factor as compared to the patient (uterine?) factor. Others have approached the problem using theoretical mathematical prediction models (68, 69) or made recommendations towards two-embryo transfer (70–74). One study tried to identify patients most suitable for SET on the basis of a multivariate analysis of >2,000 IVF/ICSI cycles with two-embryo transfers. These were found to be women <35–37 years of age in their first or second treatment cycles, with at least two embryos and without tubal pathology as an indication for IVF (75). A specific group that should be actively counselled towards SET are women who obtained a non-ongoing pregnancy in a first IVF/ICSI cycle (76, 77). In some countries SET is performed up to 38 or even 40 years of age. Above that age, transfer of more than one embryo is more liberal.

## 4 Set and Embryo Selection

Documented ongoing implantation is the gold standard for a particular embryo's competence. Published data show it to be a gradual biological variable, varying between 0% for the "worst" and ~60% for the "best" embryos. Labelling an embryo as a "top quality embryo" or a "high implantation potential embryo" or a "putative high competence embryo" remains clinically useful, when communicating with patients, but intrinsically oversimplified this gradual implantation potential.

Is has been previously shown that embryos with multinucleated blastomeres have very low implantation rates of ~5% (78–83). Morphological and functional

**Table 3** Published results of compulsory single embryo transfers. IR: implantation rate; LBR: live birth rate

| Reference | No of compulsory SETs | No of implantations | IR (%) | No of live births | LBR (%) |
|---|---|---|---|---|---|
| Giorgetti et al. (58) | 858 | 88 | 10.3 | 62 | 7.2 |
| Vilska et al. (59) | 94 | 19 | 20.2 | 15 | 16.0 |
| Gerris et al. (60) | 86 | 26 | 30.2 | 19 | 22.1 |
| Tiitinen et al. (61) | 205 | 39 | 19.0 | 31 | 15.1 |
| De Sutter et al. (62) | 211 | 21 | 10.0 | 19 | 9.0 |
| Total | 1454 | 193 | 13.3 | 146 | 10.1 |

characteristics that have been studied comprise of the following: morphology of the oocyte; ATP content and mitochondrial distribution in oocytes; pronuclear membrane breakdown; number and symmetry of distribution of nucleolar bodies in zygote pronuclei; early (25–27 h after fertilisation) or late first cleavage for day 2 embryos; number and symmetry of blastomeres, fragmentation and presence or absence of multinucleation in early cleaving embryos; number of blastomeres undergoing compaction and the morphology of the compaction process in day 4 morulae and blastocyst morphology in day 5 or day 6 embryos. Dynamic characteristics such as pyruvate and glucose metabolism or amino acid turnover have also been studied but not in an immediate clinical context.

Morphology alone cannot disclose whether a particular embryo will implant or not, because we are looking at a statistical correlation, not at an individual measurement and because morphology alone cannot disclose all the information contained in the embryo. Studies utilizing day 5 embryo transfers usually report highly selected patients (37, 39, 40). Culturing several high quality day 3 embryos, if available, to blastocysts may add selective power, increasing the chance to transfer *the* best embryo available, but this subgroup of patients is limited to those with at least four good quality embryos on day 3 (84). No single static observation gives all the information contained in an embryo's morphology. It is more logical to consider that a combination of *different* observations, preferably reflecting *different* aspects of implantation potential, should be used. Although some centres proclaim excellent results after single blastocyst transfer, others found the merit of blastocyst transfer not to exist for the overall population (85–91). It should be underlined that to obtain a high ongoing pregnancy, numerous factors impact on embryo competence in the IVF/ICSI treatment chain, including ovarian stimulation, optimized laboratory conditions at oocyte retrieval and embryo transfer, transfer technique and endometrial receptivity.

## 5 The Role of Cryopreservation

One benefit of SET is an increase in the number of embryos available for cryopreservation. Optimized cryopreservation of embryos after SET is part of the strategy to decrease multiple pregnancies (92). It increases the cumulative PR per oocyte harvest and ideally allows patients who "desire" a twin pregnancy to have their "delayed" twin. In a group of 127 Finnish patients, cryopreservation increased the PR per patient to 62.4% and the delivery rate to 52.8% (51, 67). In the Scandinavian study (35), the transfer of one frozen/thawed embryo after a failed fresh cycle was able to increase the cumulative PR (39.5%) to that observed after the transfer of two embryos (43.5%). In the Dutch study (56), the cumulative ongoing PR rose from 24 to 34% in SET patients and from 34 to 38% after DET, loosing significance between SET and DET. An Australian group performed a fresh transfer of either a single blastocyst or two blastocysts (pregnancy rates of 44% and 59%, respectively) followed by a frozen/thaw cycle involving transfer of a maximum of two embryos, rising the PR per patient to 74% in the SET group and 70% in the DET group, respectively (93). The twinning rates were 2% vs. 44% for the fresh SET vs. the fresh DET and 5% vs. 28% after cryoaugmentation. A small recent Japanese study of 66 patients (94) obtained a fresh PR of 44.9% in 66 fresh SET cycles and a cryoaugmented PR of 72.4% after 29 patients underwent a subsequent transfer of one frozen/thawed blastocyst. In this study embryos had been cryopreserved by vitrification. Further development of cryotechnology and increasing application of frozen/thawed cycles is becoming an integral part of every IVF/ICSI program applying SET.

## 6 eSET: Not Only Less Twins But Also Better Singletons

It has been shown (23, 95) that the outcome of singletons but not of twins after IVF/ICSI in a standard-two-embryo program is worse than that of naturally conceived singleton or twins. Recently, we found that ongoing IVF/ICSI pregnancies showing first trimester blood loss had an inferior obstetrical and neonatal outcome than if no first trimester blood loss occurred (96). A correlation was found between the incidence of first-trimester bleeding and the number of embryos transferred. This provides a further argument in favour of eSET. We also found that birth weight of singletons born after eSET (3324.6 ± 509.7 g) was higher than after two-embryo transfer (3204.3 ± 617.5) ($p<0.01$)

(97); that the incidence of prematurity <37 weeks was 6.2% for singletons after SET vs. 10.4% after DET (adjusted odds 1.77; 95% *CI* = 1.06–2.94); and that the incidence of low birth weight (<2,500 g) was lower for singletons after SET (4.2%) vs. DET (11.6%) (adjusted odds = 3.38; 95% *CI* = 1.86–6.12). These observations are in line with the fact that there appear to be more vanishing twins after IVF than previously suspected (98) and that in utero competition for implantation may play a role in the outcome of these pregnancies. Hence, eSET does not only prevent the complications of twins but also improves the outcome of singleton pregnancies.

## 7 Health-Economic Considerations

Although the main reason to apply SET is the health of the children at the start of their lives, financial considerations are also paramount. The increased utilisation of hospital care in ART-children is the consequence of MP (6). The estimated cost for an IVF singleton after IVF was calculated to be three times less than that of a twin (5); an American group found a twin twice and a triplet fifteen times as expensive as a singleton (4). Others have used a health-economic model to establish that SET and DET are financially equivalent per live born child. SET needs more cycles and yields less children per cycle but DET yields higher obstetrical and mainly neonatal costs per child (8, 99) and these effects balance out each other. A Dutch retrospective cost analysis showed that an IVF twin pregnancy costs on average (10,000 more than an IVF singleton pregnancy (55). In a real-life prospective comparison between elective SET vs. DET in women <38 years of age in their first IVF/ICSI cycle, elective SET of one high competence embryo was as efficient as two-embryo transfer (40% PR on both groups), but the cost per child was only approximately half after elective SET (100).

An international survey of IVF costs revealed huge differences both in accessibility and cost per cycle among countries (101). In the USA, the existence of (partial) insurance coverage had a decreasing effect on the number of embryos transferred (101). Funding may serve as a leverage to overrule short-sighted considerations for quick success. In Belgium, it has been calculated that the money saved by avoiding half of the MP would suffice to finance all IVF/ICSI cycles in a year (102). This is the basis for the Belgian reimbursement system. A British study also found that redirection of money saved by implementation of a mandatory "two embryo transfer" policy into increased provision of IVF treatment could double the number of NHS-funded IVF treatment cycles at no extra cost and further savings could be made if a selective "single-embryo transfer" policy were to be adopted (95).

## 8 The Patient's Perspective: Information and Counselling

Patients need accurate and complete information (28, 63) about the fact that prevention of MP is possible without serious decline in the chances for pregnancy, especially if combined with cryopreservation. This is particularly true if results are expressed (and patients or health insurers charged) per oocyte harvest and not per cycle or per transfer. Differences among patients, embryologists and clinicians in their perceptions of the desirability of MP (103) originate in a mix of objective and subjective factors. Effective counselling involves insight as to how patients think, or feel, about their chances of success, and about risks they do not always understand (104). A British study investigated whether patients' willingness to accept a hypothetical policy of SET changed with the method of providing information (105) and found that counselling could easily change patients' views. A Danish group found that the delivery of a child with very low birth weight and hence morbidity was predictive of high acceptance of SET (106). They concluded that SET requires extensive counselling. The importance of full counselling of patients was also stressed by an Australian group (44).

## 9 How to Implement eSet in Practice?

For a particular centre to implement eSET, several prerequisites must be fulfilled:

1. The pregnancy rate for the centre must be excellent
2. Clinicians must be willing to decrease a high multiple pregnancy rate at the expense of a slightly lower overall pregnancy rate

3. Investment in the optimisation of a freeze/thaw programme
4. Compatibility with specific societal circumstances in which the centre works

There are the five pillars on which eSET rests to make it work:

1. Creating awareness among physicians, midwives, nurses, mental health practitioners, clinical embryologists, laboratory technicians, insurers, politicians, ethicists and all who are directly or indirectly involved in promoting good clinical outcome after ART.
2. Marketing the idea of eSET in order to maintain pressure on the kettle of ethical medicine.
3. Coming to a formal international agreement on patient and embryo characteristics compatible with eSET that can be used in all routine clinical IVF units throughout the world. The development of sophisticated methods of embryo selection for SET is to be welcomed. However, to make eSET work on a large scale, the focus is on easy, cheap and reproducible methods, which at present rely on light microscopic observation of cleavage rate and morphology.
4. Organizing in-depth counselling by understanding, in a cross-cultural way, factors that determine the perception of multiple pregnancies all over the world, factors that impede eSET and effective methods to inform patients orally and in writing regarding the risks and complications of multiple pregnancies.
5. Creating appropriate funding through any means compatible with national health care systems so as to strike the balance between reasonable access to treatment for all who need it and an acceptable percentage of complications.

## 10 Conclusion and Future Perspectives

Elective SET, combined with subsequent transfer of frozen/thawed embryos, can maintain a high PR with a dramatic decrease in MP rate. It has been argued that in the near future, SET should be the default policy for good prognosis IVF/ICSI patients: if at least one high competence embryo is available only one should be transferred. This is probably the way to go on a global scale and we should welcome that evolution. On the other hand, there will always remain a substantial subgroup of patients in whom the transfer of more than one embryo remains unavoidable, acceptable or even desirable. Ovarian stimulation schemes might be adapted towards a lower dose approach, without compromising on the possibility of choice. To find the optimal trade-off between ongoing PR and twinning rate is the foremost clinical challenge for each IVF centre. Clinical judgements regarding SET differ between centres and countries. It should be underlined that it has been not been anyone's intention to implement SET in *all* or even in the large majority of IVF/ICSI cycles, as insinuated by some authors (45). It is also clear that in large parts of the world, none of the players are "ripe" for SET. This is the best reason to continue the search for optimized embryo selection and to exchange clinical experience with SET among different types of medical practice both within and across countries (107–111).

## References


1. Edwards R, Mettler L, Walters D. Identical twins and in vitro fertilization. J. In Vitro Fert Embryo Transf 1986;3: 114–117.
2. Blondel B, Kaminski M. Trends in the occurrence, determinants, and consequences of multiple births. Semin in Perinatol 2002; 26:239–249.
3. Fauser BC, Devroey P, Macklon NS. Multiple birth resulting from ovarian stimulation for subfertility treatment. Lancet 2005;365:1807–1816.
4. Hidlebaugh DA, Thompson IE, Berger MJ. Cost of assisted reproductive technologies for a health maintenance organization. J Reprod Med 1997;42:570–574.
5. Wølner-Hanssen P, Rydhstroem H. Cost-effectiveness analysis of in-vitro fertilization: estimated costs per successful pregnancy after transfer of one or two embryos. Hum Reprod 1998;13:88–94.
6. Ericson A, Nygren KG, Otterblad Olausson P, Källén B. Hospital care utilization of infants born after IVF. Hum Reprod 2002;17:929–932.
7. Garceau L, Henderson J, Davis LJ, Petrou S, Henderson LR, Mc Veigh DH, Barlow DH, Davidson LL. Economic implications of assisted reproductive techniques: a systematic review. Hum Reprod 2002;17:3090–3109.
8. De Sutter P, Gerris J, Dhont M. A health-economic decision-analytic model comparing double with single embryo transfer in IVF/ICSI. Hum Reprod 2002:17;2891–2896.
9. Ostfeld BM, Smith RH, Hiatt M, Hegyi T. Maternal behavior toward premature twins: implications for development. Twin Res 2000;3:234–241.

10. Glazebrook C, Sheard C, Cox S, Oates M, Ndukwe G. Parenting stress in first-time mothers of twins and triplets conceived after in vitro fertilization. Fertil Steril 2004;81:505–511.
11. Wennerholm UB, Bergh C. Obstetric outcome and follow-up of children born after in vitro fertilisation (IVF). Hum Reprod 2000;3:52–64.
12. Wennerholm UB. Obstetric risks and neonatal complications of twin pregnancy and higher-order multiple pregnancy. In: Gerris J, Olivennes F and De Sutter P (eds), Assisted Reproduction Technologies. Quality and Safety. New York: The Parthenon Publishing Group, 2004: 23–38.
13. Wennerholm UB, Bergh C. Outcome of IVF pregnancies. Fetal Mater Med Rev 2004;15:27–57.
14. Dhont M, De Sutter P, Ruyssinck G, Martens G, Bekaert A. Perinatal outcome of pregnancies after assisted reproduction: A case-control study. Am J Obstet Gynecol 1999;181: 688–695.
15. Senat M-V, Ancel P-Y, Bouvier-Colle M-H, Bréart G. How does multiple pregnancy affect maternal mortality and morbidity? Clin Obstet Gynaecol 1998;41:79–83.
16. Bergh T, Ericson A, Hillensjö T, Nygren KG, Wennerholm UB. Deliveries and children born after in-vitro fertilization in Sweden 1982–95: a retrospective cohort study. Lancet 1999;453:1579–1585.
17. Koudstaal J, Braat DDM, Bruinse HW, Naaktgeboren N, Vermeiden JPW, Visser GHA. Obstetric outcome of singleton pregnancies after in-vitro fertilization: a matched control study in four Dutch University hospitals. Hum Reprod 2000;15:1819–1825.
18. Rydhstroem H, Heraib F. Gestational duration, and fetal and infant mortality for twins vs. singletons. Twin Res 2001;4:227–231.
19. Klemetti R, Gissler M, Hemminski E. Comparison of perinatal health of children born from IVF in Finland in the early and late 1990s. Hum Reprod 2002;17:2192–2198.
20. Lynch A, McDuffie Jr R, Murphy J, Faber K, Orleans M. Preeclampsia in multiple gestation: the role of assisted reproductive technologies. Obstet Gynecol 2002;99: 445–451.
21. Strömberg B, Dahlquist G, Ericson A, Finnström O, Köster M, Stjernqvist K. Neurological sequelae in children born after in-vitro fertilization: a population-based study. Lancet 2002;359:461–465.
22. Wang JX, Norman RJ, Kristiansson P. The effect of various infertility treatments on the risk of preterm birth. Hum Reprod 2002;17:945–949.
23. Helmerhorst FM, Perquin DAM, Donker D, Keirse MJNC. Perinatal outcome of singletons and twins after assisted conception: a systematic review of controlled studies. BMJ 2004;328:261–264.
24. Waterstone M, Bewley S, Wolfe C. Incidence and predictors of severe obstetric morbidity: case-control study. Br Med J 2001;332:1089–1093.
25. Walker MC, Murphy KE, Pan S, Yang Q, Wen SW. Adverse maternal outcomes in multifetal pregnancies. Br J Obstet Gynecol 2004;111:1294–1296.
26. Scher AI, Petterson B, Blair E. The risk of mortality or cerebral palsy in twins: a collaborative population-based study. Pediatr Res 2002;52:671–681.
27. Smithers PR, Halliday J, Hale L, Talbot JM, Breheny S, Healy D. High frequency of cesarean section, antepartum hemorrhage, placenta previa, and preterm delivery in in-vitro fertilization twin pregnancies. Fertil Steril 2003;80:666–668.
28. Gerris J, De Sutter P, De Neubourg D. A real-life prospective health economic study of elective single embryo transfer versus two-embryo transfer in first IVF/ICSI cycles. Hum Reprod 2004;19:917–923.
29. Kjellberg AT, Carlsson P, Bergh C. Randomized single versus double embryo transfer: obstetric and paediatric outcome and a cost-effectiveness analysis. Hum Reprod 2006;21:210–216.
30. Fiddelers AAA, van Montfoort APA, Dirksen CD. Single versus double embryo transfer: cost-effectiveness analysis alongside a randomized clinical trial. Hum Reprod 2006;21:2090–2097.
31. Pennings G. Multiple pregnancies: a test case for the moral quality of medically assisted reproduction. Hum Reprod 2000;15:2466–2469.
32. ESHRE Task Force on Ethics and Law. Ethical issues related to multiple pregnancies in medically assisted procreation. Hum Reprod 2003;18:1976–1979.
33. Gerris J, De Neubourg D, Mangelschots K, Van Royen E, Van de Meerssche M, Valkenburg M. Prevention of twin pregnancy after in-vitro fertilization or intracytoplasmic sperm injection based on strict embryo criteria: a prospective randomized clinical trial. Hum Reprod 1999;14: 2581–2587.
34. Martikainen H, Tiitinen A, Tomàs C, Tapanainen J, Orava M, Tuomivaara L, Vilska S, Hydèn-Granskog C, Hovatta O. One versus two embryo transfers after IVF and ICSI: randomized study. Hum Reprod 2001;16:1900–1903.
35. Thurin A, Hausken J, Hillensjö T, Jablonowska B, Pinborg A, Strandell A, Bergh C. Elective single embryo transfer in IVF, a randomized study. N Engl J Med 2004;351: 2392–2402.
36. van Montfoort APA, Fiddelers AAA, Janssen JM, Derhaag JG, Dirksen CD, Dunselman GAJ, Land JA, Geraedts JPM, Evers JLH, Dumoulin JCM. In unselected patients, elective single embryo transfer prevents all multiples, but results in significantly lower pregnancy rates compared with double embryo transfer: a randomized controlled trial. Hum Reprod 2006;21:338–343.
37. Gardner DK, Surrey E, Minjarez D, Leitz A, Stevens J, Schoolcraft W. Single blastocyst transfer: a prospective randomized trial. Fertil Steril 2004;81:551–555.
38. Van Royen E, Mangelschots K, De Neubourg D, Valkenburg M, Van de Meerssche M, Ryckaert G, Eestermans W, Gerris J. Characterization of a top quality embryo, a step towards single-embryo transfer. Hum Reprod 1999;14: 2345–2349.
39. Pandian Z, Templeton A, Serour G, Bhattacharya S. Number of embryos for transfer after IVF and ICSI: a Cochrane review. Hum Reprod 2005;20:2681–2687.
40. Henman M, Catt JW, Wood T, Bowman MC, de Boer KA, Jansen RPS. Elective transfer of single fresh blastocysts and later transfer of cryostored blastocysts reduces the twin pregnancy rate and can improve the in vitro fertilization live birth rate in younger women. Fertil Steril 2005;84: 1620–1627.

42. Criniti A, Thyer A, Chow G, Lin P, Klein N, Soules M. Elective single blastocyst transfer reduces twin rates without compromising pregnancy rates. Fertil Steril 2005;84: 1613–1619.
43. Khalaf Y, El-Toukhy T, Coomarasamy A, Kamal A, Bolton V, Braude P. Selective single blastocyst transfer reduces the multiple pregnancy rate and increases pregnancy rates: a pre- and postintervention study. BJOG 2008;115:385–390.
44. Sadasivam N, Sadasivam NM. Selective single blastocyst transfer study: 604 cases in 6 years. J Hum Reprod Sci 2008;1:10–14.
45. Flisser E, Licciardi F. One at a time. Fertil Steril 2006;85:555–558.
46. Wang J, Lane M, Norman RJ. Reducing multiple pregnancy from assisted reproduction treatment: educating patients and medical staff. MJA 2006;184:180–181.
47. Gleicher N, Barad D. The relative myth of elective single embryo transfer. Hum Reprod 2006;21:1337–1344.
48. Bergh C. Single embryo transfer: a mini-review. Hum Reprod 2005;20:323–327.
49. Gerris J. Single embryo transfer and IVF/ICSI outcome: a balanced appraisal. Hum Reprod Update 2005;11:105–121.
50. El-Toukhy T, Yacoub Khalaf, Braude P. IVF results: Optimize not maximize. Am J Obstet Gynecol 2006;194:322–331.
51. Royal Decree of 4 June 2003. Belgisch staatsblad/Moniteur Belge 16 June 2003, 32127. http://www.juridat.be/cgi_loi/loi_N.pl?cn=2003060431.
52. Ombelet W, De Sutter P, Van der Elst J, Martens G. Multiple gestation and infertility treatment: registration, reflection and reaction – the Belgian project. Hum Reprod Update 2005;11:3–14.
53. Vilska S, Tiitinen A. National experience with elective single-embryo transfer: Finland. In Gerris J, Olivennes F and De Sutter P (eds), Assisted Reproduction Technologies. Quality and Safety. New York: The Parthenon Publishing Group, 2004:106–112.
54. Tiitinen A, Halttunen M, Härkki P, Vuoristo P, Hyden-Granskog C. Elective embryo transfer: the value of cryopreservation. Hum Reprod 2001;16:1140–1144.
55. Söderström-Anttila V, Vilska S, Mäkinen S, Foudila T, Suikkari AM. Elective single embryo transfer yields good delivery rates in oocyte donation. Hum Reprod 2003;18:1858–1863.
56. Le Lannou D, Griveau J, Laurent M, Gueho A, Veron E, Morcel K. Contribution of embryo cryopreservation to elective single embryo transfer in IVF-ICSI. RBM Online 2006;13:368–375.
57. Roberston JA. Protecting embryos and burdening women: assisted reproduction in Italy. Hum Reprod 2004;19: 1693–1696.
58. Giorgetti C, Terriou P, Auquier P, Hans E, Spach J-L, Salzmann J, Roulier R. Embryo score to predict implantation after in-vitro fertilization: based on 957 single embryo transfers. Hum Reprod 1995;10:2427–2431.
59. Vilska S, Tiitinen A, Hydèn-Granskog C, Hovatta O. Elective transfer of one embryo results in an acceptable pregnancy rate and eliminates the risk of multiple birth. Hum Reprod 1999;14:2392–2395.
60. Gerris J, De Neubourg D, Mangelschots K, Van Royen E, Vercruyssen M, Barudy-Vasquez J, Valkenburg M, Ryckaert G. Elective single day-3 embryo transfer halves the twinning rate without decrease in the ongoing pregnancy rate of an IVF/ICSI programme. Hum Reprod 2002;17: 2621–2626.
61. Tiitinen A, Unkila-Kallio L, Halttunen M, Hydén-Granskog C. Impact of elective single embryo transfer on the twin pregnancy rate. Hum Reprod 2003;18:1449–1453.
62. De Sutter P, Van der Elst J, Coetsier T, Dhont M. Single embryo transfer and multiple pregnancy rate reduction after IVF/ICSI: a 5-year appraisal. RBM Online 2003;18: 464–469.
63. De Sutter P, Gerris J, Dhont M. A health-economic decision-analytic model comparing double with single embryo transfer in IVF/ICSI: a sensitivity analysis. Hum Reprod 2003;18:1361.
64. Lukassen HGM, Schönbeck Y, Adang EMM, Braat DDM, Zielhuis GA, Kremer JAM. Cost analysis of singleton versus twin pregnancies after in vitro fertilization. Fertil Steril 2004;81:1240–1246.
65. van Montfoort APA, Janssen JM, Fiddelers AAA, Derhaag JG, Dirksen CD, Evers JLH, Dumoulin JCM. Single versus double embryo transfer: a randomized study. Hum Reprod 2004;19 (suppl 1):i134.
66. Ledger WL, Anumba D, Marlow N, Thomas CM, Wilson ECF. The costs to the NHS of multiple births after IVF treatment in the UK. BJOG 2006;113:21–25.
67. Gerris J, Van Royen E, De Neubourg D, Mangelschots K, Valkenburg M, Ryckaert G. Impact of single embryo transfer on the overall and twin-pregnancy rates of an IVF/ICSI programme. RBM Online 2001;2:172–177.
68. Staessen C, Camus M, Bollen N, Devroey P, Van Steirteghem A. The relationship between embryo quality and the occurrence of multiple pregnancies. Fertil Steril 1992; 57:626–630.
69. Hsu M-I, Mayer J, Aronshon M, Lanzendorf S, Muasher S, Kolm P, Oehninger S. Embryo implantation in in vitro fertilization and intracytoplasmic sperm injection: impact of cleavage status, morphology grade, and number of embryos transferred. Fertil Steril 1999;72:679–685.
70. Shapiro BS, Harris DC, Richter KS. Predictive value of 72-hour blastomere cell number on blastocyst development and success of subsequent transfer based on the degree of blastocyst development. Fertil Steril 2000;73: 582–586.
71. Martin PM, Welch HG. Probabilities for singleton and multiple pregnancies after in vitro fertilization. Fertil Steril 1998;70:478–481.
72. Trimarchi JR. A mathematical model for predicting which embryos to transfer – an illusion of control or a powerful tool? Fertil Steril 2001;76:1286–1288.
73. Staessen C, Janssenswillen C, Van Den Abbeel E, Devroey P, Van Steirteghem A. Avoidance of triplet pregnancies by elective transfer of two good quality embryos. Hum Reprod 1993;8:1650–1653.
74. Templeton A, Morris JK. Reducing the risk of multiple birth by transfer of two embryos after in vitro fertilization. N Engl J Med 1998;339:573–577.
75. Milki AA, Fisch JD, Behr B. Two-blastocyst transfer has similar pregnancy rates and a decreased multiple gestation rate compared with three-blastocyst transfer. Fertil Steril 1999;72:225–228.

76. Dean NL, Philips SJ, Buckett WM, Biljan MM, Lin Tan S. Impact of reducing the number of embryos transferred from three to two in women under the age of 35 who produced three or more high-quality embryos. Fertil Steril 2000;74: 820–823.
77. Ozturk O, Bhattacharya S, Templeton A. Avoiding multiple pregnancies in ART. Evaluation and implementation of new strategies. Hum Reprod 2001;16:1319–1321.
78. Strandell A, Bergh C, Lundin K. Selection of patients suitable for one-embryo transfer may reduce the rate of multiple births by half without impairment of overall birth rates. Hum Reprod 2000;15:2520–2525.
79. Croucher CA, Lass A, Margara R, Winston RM. Predictive value of the results of a first in-vitro fertilization cycle on the outcome of subsequent cycles. Hum Reprod 1998;13: 403–408.
80. Bates GW, Ginsburg ES. Early pregnancy loss in in vitro fertilization (IVF) is a positive predictor of subsequent IVF success. Fertil Steril 2002;77:337–341.
81. Pickering BJ, Taylor A, Johnson MH, Braude PR. An analysis of multinucleated blastomere formation in human embryos. Mol Hum Reprod 1995;10:1912–1922.
82. Kligman I, Benadiva C, Alikani M, Munné S. The presence of multinucleated blastomeres in human embryos is correlated with chromosomal abnormalities. Hum Reprod 1996;11:1492–1498.
83. Jackson KV, Ginsburg ES, Hornstein MD, Rein MS, Clarke RN. Multinucleation in normally fertilized embryos is associated with an accelerated ovulation induction response and lower implantation and pregnancy rates in in vitro fertilization-embryo transfer cycles. Fertil Steril 1998;70:60–66.
84. Palmstierna M, Murkes D, Cseminczky, Andersson O, Wramby H. Zona pellucida thickness variation and occurrence of visible mononucleated blastomeres in preembryos are associated with a high pregnancy rate in IVF treatment. J Ass Reprod Genet 1998;15:70–74.
85. Pelinck MJ, De Vos M, Dekens M, Van der Elst J, De Sutter P, Dhont M. Embryos cultured in vitro with multinucleated blastomeres have poor implantation potential in human in-vitro fertilization and intracytoplasmic sperm injection. Hum Reprod 1998;13:960–963.
86. Van Royen E, Mangelschots K, Vercruyssen M, De Neubourg D, Valkenburg M, Ryckaert G, Gerris J. Multinucleation in cleavage stage embryos. Hum Reprod 2003;18:1062–1069.
87. Papanikolaou EG, D'haeseleer E, Verheyen G, Van de Velde H, Camus M, Van Steirteghem A, Devroey P, Tournaye H. Live birth rate is significantly higher after blastocyst transfer than after cleavage-stage embryo transfer when at least four embryos are available on day 3 of embryo culture. A randomized prospective study. Hum Reprod 2005;20: 3198–3203.
88. Coskun S, Hollanders J, Al-Hassan S, Al-Sufyan H, Al-Mayman H, Jaroudi K. Day 5 versus day 3 embryo transfer: a controlled randomized trial. Hum Reprod 2000;15:1947–1952.
89. Rienzi L, Ubaldi F, Iacobelli M, Ferrero S, Minasi MG, Martinez F, Tesarik J, Greco E. Day 3 embryo transfer with combined evaluation at the pronuclear and cleavage stages compares favourably with day 5 blastocyst transfer. Hum Reprod 2002;17:1852–1855.
90. Bungum M, Bungum L, Humaidan P, Yding Andersen C. Day 3 versus day 5 embryo transfer: a prospective randomized study. RBM Online 2003;7:98–104.
91. Kolibianakis EM, Devroey P. Blastocyst culture: facts and fiction. RBM Online 2002;5:285–293.
92. Utsunomiya T, Ito H, Nagaki M, Sato J. A prospective, randomized study: day 3 versus hatching blastocyst stage. Hum Reprod 2004;19:1598–1603.
93. Kolibianakis EM, Zikopoulos K, Verpoest W, Joris H, Van Steirteghem AC, Devroey P. Should we advise patients undergoing IVF to start a cycle leading to a day 3 or a day 5 transfer? Hum Reprod 2004;19:2550–2554.
94. Blake D, Proctor M, Johnson N, Olive D. The merits of blastocyst versus cleavage stage embryo transfer: a Cochrane Review. Hum Reprod 2004;19:795–807.
95. Gerris J, De Neubourg D, De Sutter P, Van Royen E, Mangelschots K, Vercruyssen M. Cryopreservation as a tool to reduce multiple birth. RBM Online 2003;7: 286–294.
96. Catt J, Wood T, Henman M, Jansen R. Single embryo transfer in IVF to prevent multiple pregnancies. Twin Res 2003;6:536–539.
97. Uchiyama K, Aono F, Kuwayama M, Osada H, Kato O. The efficacy of single embryo transfer with vitrification. Hum Reprod 2004;19(suppl 1):i135.
98. Jackson RA, Gibson KA, Wu YW, Croughan MS. Perinatal outcome in singletons following in vitro fertilization: a meta-analysis. Obstet Gynecol 2004;103:551–563.
99. De Sutter P, Bontinck J, Schutysers V, Van der Elst J, Gerris J, Dhont M. First-trimester bleeding and pregnancy outcome in singletons after assisted reproduction. Hum Reprod 2006;21:1907–1911.
100. De Sutter P, Delbaere I, Gerris J, Verstraelen H, Goetgeluk S, Van der Elst J, Temmerman M, Dhont M. Birthweight of singletons in ART is higher after single than after double embryo transfer. Hum Reprod 2006;21: 2633–2537.
101. Pinborg A, Lidegaard Ø, la Cour Freiesleben N, Andersen AN. Consequences of vanishing twins in IVF/ICSI pregnancies. Hum Reprod 2005;20:2821–2829.
103. Collins JA. An international survey of the health economics of IVF and ICSI. Hum Reprod Update 2002;8:265–277.
104. Jain T, Harlow BL, Horstein MD. Insurance coverage and outcomes of in vitro fertilization. N Engl J Med 2002;347:661–666.
105. Reynolds MA, Schieve L, Jeng G, Peterson HB. Does insurance coverage decrease the risk for multiple births associated with assisted reproductive technology? Fertil Steril 2003;80:16–22.
106. Buckett W, Tan SL. What is the most relevant standard of success in assisted reproduction? The importance of informed choice. Hum Reprod 2004;19:1043–1045.
107. D'Alton M. Infertility and the desire for multiple births. Fertil Steril 2004;81:523–525.
108. Hartshorne GM, Lilford RJ. Different perspectives of patients and health care professionals on the potential benefits and risks of blastocyst culture and multiple embryo transfer. Hum Reprod 2002;17:1023–1030.

109. Ryan GL, Van Voorhis BJ. The desire of infertile patients for multiple gestations – do they know the risks. Fertil Steril 2004;81:526.
110. Murray S, Shetty A, Rattray A, Taylor V, Bhattacharya S. A randomized comparison of alternative methods of information provision on the acceptability of elective single embryo transfer. Hum Reprod 2004;19:911–916.
111. Pinborg A, Loft A, Schmidt L, Andersen NA. Attitudes of IVF/ICSI-twin mothers towards twins and single embryo transfer. Hum Reprod 2003;18:621–627.

# Obesity and In Vitro Fertilization (IVF) Outcomes

Anuja Dokras

**Abstract** Obesity in reproductive age women is common and associated with various serious comorbidities. In women attempting pregnancy, obesity portends an independent risk factor for maternal complications such as preeclampsia and gestational diabetes, each of which carries its own set of comorbidities. Obesity in in vitro fertilization (IVF) patients has been associated with increased cycle cancellation rates, reduced live birth rates, and increased risk of mis-carriage. Additionally, obese and morbidly obese women are more likely to encounter delivery complications including preterm delivery, fetal macrosomia, increased need for induction of labor, greater utilization of instrumental delivery and a higher risk for emergency cesarean section. We recommend that obese and morbidly obese women should be strongly counseled regarding the importance of weight reduction and offered effective strategies during preconception visits and prior to initiation of infertility workup.

**Keywords** Obesity • Polycystic ovarian disease • PCOS • IVF outcome • Anovulation • Hyperinsulinemia

## 1 Introduction

Recent estimates suggest that approximately 60% of U.S. women are overweight, nearly one-third are obese and 6% are morbidly obese (1, 2). Obesity in women is characterized by similar comorbidities as in men, namely, increased risk of type II diabetes, coronary artery disease, gall bladder disease, osteoporosis, and certain cancers including breast and uterine cancer. The relative risk of mortality in the reproductive age group from obesity-associated complications in the U.S. is annually 1.83 (CI 1.27–2.62) (3). Unfortunately, over the past decade population-based trends show a 40% increase in prepregnancy with overweight and obesity and a two-fold increase in prepregnancy with morbid obesity in women (4). This increase in obesity has several health implications during pregnancy. Obesity is an independent risk factor for maternal complications such as preeclampsia and gestational diabetes, each of which carries its own set of comorbidities (5–7). Additionally, obese and morbidly obese women are more likely to encounter delivery complications including preterm delivery, fetal macrosomia, increased need for induction of labor, greater utilization of instrumental delivery and a higher risk for emergency cesarean section (5, 7, 8) In each case, the magnitude of risk increases with increasing maternal body mass index (BMI). Furthermore, adverse neonatal outcomes such as CNS abnormalities, shoulder dystocia, stillbirth, and death have been associated with maternal obesity, though obesity was not an independent risk factor in all studies (6, 7, 9, 10).

## 2 Links Between Obesity and Reproductive Outcomes

Recently, in a study of over 7,000 women fecundity was found to be significantly reduced in obese women (OR = 0.82, 95% CI 0.72–0.95) compared to normal-weight

A. Dokras
Department of Obstetrics and Gynecology,
University of Pennsylvania, 3701 Market St,
Philadelphia, PA 19104, USA
e-mail: adokras@obgyn.upenn.edu

D.T. Carrell et al. (eds.), *Biennial Review of Infertility*, DOI: 10.1007/978-1-60327-392-3_12

women and this was more evident in obese primiparous women (OR = 0.66, 95% CI 0.49–0.89) (11). Importantly, these findings persisted even in the subset of women with regular menstrual cycles. In a large British study, obesity at age 7 and obesity at age 23 independently increased the risk of menstrual problems at age 33 (OR = 1.59, 1.75, respectively, $n$ = 5,799) (12). Consistent with these findings, obese women at age 23 years were less likely to conceive within 12 months of unprotected intercourse (RR = 0.69) compared to normal-weight woman. A cohort study of 53,910 couples enrolled in the Danish National Birth Cohort found a dose-response relationship between increasing female-BMI category and subfecundity (time to pregnancy >12 months; OR = 1.32, 95% CI 1.26–1.37) (13). These studies collectively indicate that obese women are at a higher risk of infertility; however, the underlying mechanisms are unclear. Many obese women are hyperinsulinemic and therefore have endocrine profiles similar to women with polycystic ovary syndrome (PCOS). Serum hormone profiles are characterized by elevated insulin and LH levels, an elevated LH–FSH ratio and low mid-luteal progesterone levels. This profile reflects anovulation and has been referred to as "relative functional hyperandrogenism" to distinguish from PCOS (14). The ability of metformin, an insulin sensitizing agent, to restore ovulation further emphasizes the role of insulin in oocyte development and release in obese individuals. In addition, the endocrine changes seen after bariatric surgery provide evidence that weight loss helps correct the abnormal hormonal milieu that is associated with obesity and anovulation (15). In this study by Teitelman et al., the mean menstrual cycle length preoperatively among those women categorized as ovulatory and anovulatory was 27.3 and 127.5 days, respectively. Of the 98 patients who were anovulatory preoperatively, 70 patients (71.4%) regained normal menstrual cycles after surgery. The women who regained ovulation had greater weight loss than those who remained anovulatory (61.4 vs. 49.9 kg, $p = 0.02$) supporting the association between obesity and anovulation.

## 3 IVF Outcomes and Obesity

With the increasing prevalence of obesity worldwide, more women seeking in vitro fertilization (IVF) as a treatment for infertility are obese. The data regarding the impact of obesity on pregnancy rates after IVF are conflicting. This can be partly explained by the lack of uniformity in the definition of obesity and different end points (clinical pregnancy, live birth rate) used in these studies. Further, the high proportion of women with PCOS among the obese population may also influence some of the outcomes associated with IVF (16).

Given the impact of obesity on obstetric outcomes, the end point of IVF treatment in this population should be the live birth rate. Live birth, as an outcome measure, has been reported by a small number of studies. A few studies have shown no effect of increasing BMI on IVF success rates after controlling for patients age and dose of gonadotropins administered (17–19). In a large Dutch study, BMI > 27 was associated with no significant difference when live birth rate per oocyte retrieval was compared with the normal-weight group (20). Other groups have reported decreased cumulative live birth rates after IVF with increasing BMI (21–23). In a study from Norway ($n$ = 5,019) the cumulative live birth rates showed a negative trend with increase in BMI (21). BMI ≥ 30 had a cumulative live birth rate of 41.4% after three IVF cycles compared to 50.3% in normal-weight women. Similarly, in an Australian study ($n$ = 3,586) the likelihood of achieving at least one pregnancy after assisted reproductive treatment in obese women [BMI ≥ 30, OR = 0.73 (0.57–0.95)] and very obese women [BMI > 35, OR = 0.5 (0.32–0.77)] was significantly reduced (23).

We reported live birth rates after IVF in 1,293 patients (<38 years) undergoing their first fresh IVF or IVF with ICSI cycle (24). Women were divided into BMI groups, as determined by weight and height measured at the initial IVF consultation [weight (kg)/height (meters)$^2$] based on the World Health Organization (WHO) and National Institute of Health (NIH) definitions: normal weight (BMI < 25), overweight (BMI 25–29.9), obese (BMI 30–39.9) and morbidly obese (BMI ≥ 40) (1, 25). The study population's clinical pregnancy rate per cycle start was 47.6% with no significant difference among the four BMI groups with regard to clinical pregnancy (presence of fetal heart beat). After adjusting for the year of study, diagnosis of PCOS and age with multifactorial logistic regression analysis, we did not detect a significant difference in clinical pregnancy rate with increasing BMI. The overall delivery or live birth rate was 41.6%. We also did not find a difference in live birth rate with BMI. This is the only study to include women with BMI > 40. Although the morbidly obese women ($n$ = 79) had a slightly lower clinical pregnancy (41.7 vs. 46.8%) and delivery rate (36.7, 41.5%) compared to normal-weight women these were not statistically significant.

Recently, a meta-analysis reported the odds of live birth rate after IVF in women with BMI < 25 as 1.08 (95% CI 0.92–1.26) compared to BMI ≥ 25 (total number of studies = 3) (26). In women with BMI < 30 the OR for live birth was 1.12 (95% CI 0.91–1.37) when compared to BMI ≥ 30.In the same analysis, women with BMI ≥ 25 had a lower chance of pregnancy (biochemical, clinical, ongoing) following IVF (OR = 0.71, 95% CI 0.62, 0.81) compared with women having a BMI < 25 (total number of studies = 6). In women with a BMI of < 30, the odds of pregnancy was 1.16 (95%: CI 0.95, 1.43) when compared with women having a BMI of ≥ 30. Taken together, data from these few studies suggest that obese women may have lower clinical pregnancy rates after IVF. Future studies examining the effects of obesity on IVF outcomes should include live birth as the end point.

## 4 Increased IVF Cancellation Rates

Several studies have demonstrated higher rates of IVF cycle cancellation prior to oocyte retrieval in overweight and obese women (19, 21, 27). We found a significantly higher cancellation rate of 25.3% in the morbidly obese group ($n$ = 79) compared to 10.8% in the normal-weight and overweight women ($n$ = 978, $p < 0.004$) (24). After adjusting for the year of treatment, age and diagnosis of PCOS, the OR for cancellation in women with BMI ≥ 40 compared to normal-weight women was 2.73 (95% CI 1.49–5.0). In our study, obese women had a cancellation rate comparable to overweight and normal-weight women. For the patients who did undergo oocyte retrieval, there was a significant trend towards increasing length of gonadotropin stimulation days with increasing BMI ($p < 0.001$). Despite the longer stimulation for women with increased BMI, the peak estradiol levels showed a significant linear reduction across the BMI groups ($p < 0.001$). All women included in our study were administered gonadotropins intramuscularly and for women >91 kgs 2 in. needles were used instead of 1 and ½ in. needles. One study has demonstrated lower absorption of recombinant FSH in obese women with both the intramuscular and subcutaneous routes of administration (28). We examined the second cycles of morbidly obese women who were cancelled in our study and found a similar high cancellation rate despite an increase in gonadotropin dose (24). Other studies have also reported increased gonadotropin use in obese subjects undergoing IVF (21, 29). In a retrospective study of 5,019 IVF or IVF/ICSI treatments in 2,660 couples, a positive correlation was reported between BMI and gonadotropin requirement during stimulation and a negative correlation between BMI and the number of oocytes collected (21). A recent meta-analysis showed that BMI ≥ 30 was associated with a higher odds of cancellation 1.35 (95% CI 0.99, 1.84) compared to those with BMI < 30. Similarly, women with BMI ≥ 30 required higher dose of gonadotropins (weighed mean differences 361.9, 95% CI: 156.4, 567.4) compared to women with BMI < 30. The precise mechanisms for increased gonadotropin requirements and higher cancellation rate in obese women undergoing IVF remain unclear. Although it is possible that obesity may be associated with decreased absorption of gonadotropins, it has also been suggested that the FSH threshold maybe increased resulting in impaired ovarian response in this population.

## 5 Miscarriage Rates After IVF in Obese Women

The data regarding the effects of obesity on miscarriage rates after IVF are controversial (18, 21, 22, 24, 29–31). One of the reasons for this discrepancy maybe the varying definition of miscarriage used in the above studies (less than 6 weeks, up to 20 weeks gestation). We detected a higher spontaneous miscarriage rate in obese women after IVF as compared to normal-weight women (24). Increased risk of miscarriage in women with PCOS has not been shown to be independent of obesity (16). In a large study from Norway after adjusting for diagnosis of infertility, the OR for early miscarriage was 1.69 (1.1.3–2.51, $p$ = 0.003) in obese women (BMI ≥ 30) compared to normal-weight women (21). Recently, there have been two meta-analysis examining the risk of miscarriage after IVF. Maheshwari et al. reported an increased risk of miscarriage (6–20 weeks) in women with BMI ≥ 25 OR = 1.33 (1.06–1.68) compared to BMI < 25, and in women with BMI ≥ 30 an increased risk of 1.53 (1.27–1.84) compared to women with BMI < 30 (number of studies = 10) (29). Interestingly, in another meta-analysis ($n$ = 16 studies) patients with a BMI ≥ 25 had significantly higher odds of miscarriage, regardless of the method of conception (odds ratio, 1.67; 95% CI, 1.25–2.25). This study showed that both oocyte donor recipients with BMI ≥ 25 have significantly higher odds of miscarriage (OR = 1.52; 95% CI 1.10–2.09) and women treated with ovulation induction medications (OR = 5.11; 95% CI 1.76–14.83) (32). These findings suggest that the increased risk of miscarriage was related to obesity rather than the type of infertility treatment.

The studies that report an increased risk of miscarriage in obese subjects are not specifically designed to determine the cause of this association. In a retrospective study of 712 ovum donation cycles, the rate of miscarriage was 13.3% in normal-weight patients, 15.5% in overweight patients, and 38.1% in obese patients (BMI ≥ 30) (1, 33). This model suggests that altered endometrial receptivity may contribute to the increased miscarriage rate observed in obese women. More studies are needed especially in the infertility population to clearly determine the risk of miscarriage with obesity and the potential contribution of prediabetes/insulin resistance.

## 6 Independent Effect of PCOS on IVF Outcomes

Although a large number of women with PCOS are obese in the US, it is not clear whether the above reported effects of obesity on IVF outcomes were entirely independent of the effects of PCOS. The data on pregnancy outcomes in women with PCOS are controversial and IVF studies comparing PCOS women to weight-matched controls are limited (16). A meta-analysis (nine studies) demonstrated that the cycle cancellation rate was significantly increased (12.8 vs. 4.1%; OR = 0.5, 95% CI 0.2–1.0), duration of gonadotropin stimulation was significantly longer (1.2 days, 95% CI: 0.9–1.5) and more cumulus–oocyte complexes (2.9, 95% CI: 2.2–3.6) were retrieved in women with PCOS as compared with women without PCOS (16). The high cancellation rate may be secondary to hyperstimulation indicating that these findings are not entirely similar to those summarized for obese women in this chapter. We examined the independent effects of PCOS and obesity in women undergoing IVF treatment (24). We reported the overall cancellation rate in the non-PCOS morbidly obese women was almost three times higher compared to the PCOS women (33.3 vs.12.9%). These findings underscore the observed association between obesity and decreased ovarian response to exogenous gonadotropins. Overall, there was no significant difference in clinical pregnancy rates, miscarriage rates and live birth rates in women with or without PCOS when matched for obesity and morbidly obesity. In a large Australian study discussed above, the likelihood of achieving a pregnancy in very obese women (BMI > 35) was half that of the normal-weight group after controlling for the cause of infertility (23). The same study reported PCOS to have an independent effect on fecundity. Another study has reported the OR for live birth rate after IVF as 0.75 (0.57–0.98, $p$ = 0.05) in obese women after adjusting for diagnosis of infertility (21).

## 7 Effect of Obesity on Obstetric Outcomes After IVF

As mentioned in the Introduction, prepregnancy obesity is associated with significant obstetric and neonatal complications. Our data confirm previously reported associations between obesity and obstetric complications in the infertility population (6–8, 24). We have reported that women with a BMI ≥ 40 undergoing IVF were almost twice as likely to have a Cesarean section (68.9%) than women with a BMI < 25 (36%, $p < 0.002$). Also, there was a significant trend towards increased risk of gestational diabetes ($p < 0.01$) and preeclampsia ($p < 0.001$) with increasing BMI and after adjusting for multiple gestation. Morbidly obese patients were also more likely than women with a BMI < 25 to develop preeclampsia (21 vs. 7%; $p < 0.001$) and gestational diabetes (10.3 vs. 3.1%; $p = 0.03$). The risk of preterm delivery and multiple births was similar among BMI groups. Further, the morbidly obese group had significantly higher risk for singleton fetal birth weight >4,000 g compared to the normal-weight group (23.5 vs. 9.7%, $p < 0.05$).

Analysis of a large multicenter database in the US showed that obesity and morbid obesity had a statistically significant association with preeclampsia (OR =

1.6 and 3.3), gestational diabetes (OR = 2.6 and 4.0) and fetal birth weight >4,000 g (OR = 1.7 and 1.9) (34). The association between maternal BMI and cesarean delivery has been shown to be independent of fetal macrosomia (4). The same authors reported that one in seven cesarean deliveries of singleton infants were attributable to overweight and obesity. Operative and postoperative complications in these BMI groups include increased blood loss, increased operative time, wound infections and endometritis (35).

## 8 Pathophysiology of the Effects of Obesity on IVF Outcomes

Both ovarian and endometrial mechanisms may contribute to the outcomes of IVF in obese patients. It is likely that the impact of obesity on IVF pregnancy rates may be secondary to reduced ovarian response as reflected by the high cancellation rate and increased requirement for gonadotropins. In addition, we reported fewer mature oocytes in women with a BMI $\geq 40$ compared to normal-weight women ($p < 0.02$) (24). Other authors have examined the role of the endometrium on IVF outcomes in obese patients. In oocyte donation cycles, ongoing pregnancy rates per cycle were lower (38.3%) in the overweight ($n = 450$) and obese recipient groups ($n = 122$) compared to the underweight ($n = 471$) and normal groups ($n = 1,613$, 45.5%) (36). Recently, BMI was reported as an independent risk factor for the development of endometrial polyps in patients undergoing IVF (37). Although the precise effect of endometrial polyps on IVF outcomes is unclear, this study showed a positive correlation between obesity and occurrence of polyps, size of the polyps, and occurrence of multiple polyps. A combination of higher miscarriage and lower clinical pregnancy rates in overweight and obese women after IVF could also account for the observed reduced live birth rate in some studies.

## 9 Discussion

This chapter highlights the increased obstetric risks in a population that has undergone a planned intervention to achieve pregnancy and warrants urgent attention. This is a target group that may benefit from counseling regarding the complications of obesity in early and late pregnancy and perhaps delaying ART treatment to allow for weight loss. In 2006, the British Fertility Society, which represents professionals working with assisted conception, issued recommendations on eligibility for IVF in the National Health System (NHS). They suggested that woman who are obese or severely overweight (BMI $\geq$ 36) should not get IVF treatment until they have lost weight (38). The American Society for Reproductive Medicine does not recommend an upper limit for BMI prior to IVF. The American Society for Obstetrics and Gynecology (ACOG) recommends that obstetricians provide preconception counseling and education about the specific maternal and fetal risks of obesity in pregnancy (5). Setting an initial goal of losing 5–10% of body weight over a 6-month period is realistic and achievable. The target population should include obese women seen at annual examinations and also children and adolescents as childhood onset of obesity contributes to 25% of adult obesity (39). ACOG further recommends that referral for further evaluation and treatment should be considered when resources of the clinician are insufficient to meet the needs of obese women (40). For women with morbid obesity, a combination of medications and group lifestyle modifications results in greater weight loss than medication or lifestyle modifications alone (41). Not surprisingly, the epidemic of obesity seen in the pregnant population will have significant public health implications. It is therefore not surprising that countries offering universal health care wish to implement upper limits of weight for infertility treatment. There are currently no estimates on the economic impact of obesity on pregnancy. We recommend that obese and morbidly obese women should be strongly counseled regarding the importance of weight reduction and offered effective strategies during preconception visits and prior to initiation of infertility workup. Once patients are referred for IVF treatment, acceptance of weight loss therapies that require delay in child bearing is difficult. Obese women who do not have PCOS should also be counseled regarding their significantly increased risk of IVF cycle cancellation. However, the obstetrics risk in the obese and morbidly obese women who successfully complete an IVF cycle, underscores the importance of early initiation of weight loss therapies.

## References


1. World Health Organization. Obesity: preventing and managing the global epidemic, WHO technical report series 894. Geneva, Switzerland: World Health Organization, 2000.
2. Hedley AA, Ogden CL, Johnson CL, Carroll MD, Curtin LR, Flegal KM. Prevalence of overweight and obesity among US children, adolescents and adults, 1999–2002. JAMA 2004;291:2847–50.
3. Flegal KA, Graubard BI, Williamson DF, Gail MH. Excess deaths associated with underweight, overweight, and obesity. JAMA 2005;293:1861–7.
4. LaCoursiere DY, Bloebaum L, Duncan JD, Varner MW. Population-based trends and correlates of maternal overweight and obesity, Utah 1991–2001. Am J Obstet Gynecol 2005;192:832–9.
5. American College of Obstetrics and Gynecology Committee on Obstetric Practice. Obesity in pregnancy: Committee opinion number 315. Obstet Gynecol 2005;106:671–5.
6. Cedergren MI. Maternal morbid obesity and the risk of adverse pregnancy outcome. Obstet Gynecol 2004;103:219–24.
7. Sebire NJ, Jolly M, Harris JP, et al. Maternal obesity and pregnancy outcome: a study of 287,213 pregnancies in London. Int J Obes 2001;25:1175–82.
8. Ehrenberg HM, Mercer BM, Catalano PM. The influence of obesity and diabetes on the prevalence of macrosomia. Am J Obstet Gynecol 2004;191:964–8.
9. Anderson JL, Walter K, Canfield MA, Shaw GM, Watkins ML, Werler MM. Maternal obesity, gestational diabetes, and central nervous system birth defects. Epidemiology 2005;16:87–92.
10. Kristensen J, Vestergaard M, Wisborg K, Kesmodel U, Secher NJ. Pre-pregnancy weight and the risk of stillbirth and neonatal death. Br J Obstet Gynaecol 2005;112:403–8.
11. Gesink Law DC, Maclehose RF, Longnecker MP, Obesity and timeto pregnancy. Hum Reprod 2007;22(2):414–20.
12. Lake JK, Power C, Cole TJ. Child to adult body mass index in the1958 British birth cohort: associations with parental obesity. Arch Dis Child 1997;77(5):376–81.
13. Ramlau-Hansen CH, Thulstrup AM, Nohr EA, Bonde JP, Sorensen TIA, Olsen J. Subfecundity in overweight and obese couples. Hum Reprod 2007;22:1634–7.
14. Pasquali R, Gambineri A, Pagotto U. The impact of obesity on reproduction in women with polycystic ovary syndrome. BJOG 2006;113:1148–59.
15. Teitelman M, Grotegut CA, Williams NN, Lewis JD. The impact of bariatric surgery on menstrual patterns. Obes Surg 2006;16(11):1457–63.
16. Heijnen EM, Eijkemans MJ, Hughes EG, Laven JS, Macklon, NS, Fauser, BC. A meta-analysis of outcomes of conventional IVF in women with polycystic ovary syndrome. Hum Reprod Update 2006;12(1):13–21.
17. Lewis CG, Warnes GM, Wang KJ, Matthews CD. Failure of body mass index or body weight to influence markedly the response to ovarian hyperstimulation in normal cycling women. Fertil Steril 1990;53:1097–9.
18. Lashen H, Ledger W, Bernal AL, Barlow D. Extremes of body mass do not adversely affect the outcome of superovulation and in-vitro fertilization. Hum Reprod 1999;14:712–5.
19. Spandorfer SD, Kump L, Goldschlag D, et al. Obesity and in vitro fertilization: negative influences on outcome. J Reprod Med 2004;49:973–7.
20. Lintsen AME, Pasker-de Jong PCM, de Boer EJ, et al. Effects of subfertility cause, smoking and body weight on the success rate of IVF. Hum Reprod 2005;20:1867–75.
21. Fedorcsak P, Dale PO, Storeng R, et al. Impact of overweight and underweight on assisted reproduction treatment. Hum Reprod 2004;19:2523–8.
22. Nichols JE, Crane MM, Higdon HL, Miller PB, Boone WR. Extremes of body mass index reduce in vitro fertilization pregnancy rates. Fertil Steril 2003;79(3):645–7.
23. Wang JX, Davies M, Norman RJ. Body mass and the probability of pregnancy during assisted reproduction treatment: retrospective study. BMJ 2000;321:1320–1.
24. Dokras A, Baredziak L, Blaine J, Syrop C, VanVoorhis BJ, Sparks A. Obstetric outcomes after in vitro fertilization in obese and morbidly obese women. Obstet Gynecol 2006;108(1):61–9.
25. National Heart, Lung, and Blood Institute (NHLBI) and National Institute for Diabetes and Digestive and Kidney Diseases (NIDDK). Clinical guidelines on the identification, evaluation, and treatment of overweight and obesity in adults. The evidence report. Obes Res 1998;6(suppl 2):51S–210S.
26. Maheshwari A, Stofberg, L, Bhattacharya S. Effect of overweight and obesity on assisted reproductive technology – a systematic review. Hum Reprod Update 2007;13(5):433–44.
27. Mulders AG, Laven JS, Imani B, Eijkemans MJ, Fauser BC. IVF outcome in anovulatory infertility (WHO group 2) including PCOS-following previous unsuccessful ovulation induction. Reprod Biomed Online 2003;7(1):50–8.
28. Steinkampf MP, Hammond KR, Nichols JE, Slayden SH. Effect of obesity on recombinant follicle stimulating hormone absorption: subcutaneous versus imtramuscular administration. Fertil Steril 2003;80(1):99–102.
29. Dechaud H, Anahory T, Reyftmann L, Loup V, Hamamah S, Hedon B. Obesity does not adversely affect results in patients who are undergoing in vitro fertilization and embryo transfer. Eur J Obstet Gynecol Reprod Biol 2006; 127(1):88–93.
30. Wang JX, Davies MJ, Norman RJ. Obesity increases the risk of spontaneous abortion during infertility treatment. Obes Res 2002;10:551–4.
31. Metwally M, Ong KJ, Ledger WL, Li TC. Does high body mass index increase the risk of miscarriage after spontaneous and assisted conception? A meta-analysis of the evidence. Fertil Steril 2007;90(3):714–26.
32. Bellver J, Rossal LP, Bosch E, et al. Obesity and the risk of spontaneous abortion after oocyte donation. Fertil Steril 2003;79:1136–40.
33. Winter E, Wang J, Davies MJ, Norman R. Early pregnancy loss following assisted reproductive technology treatment. Hum Reprod 2002;17(12):3220–23.
34. Weiss JL, Malone FD, Emig D, et al. Obesity, obstetric complication and cesarean delivery rate – a population-based screening study. Am J Obstet Gynecol 2004; 190:1091–7.
35. Kabiru W, Raynor BD. Obstetric outcomes associated with increase in BMI category during pregnancy. Am J Obstet Gynecol 2004;191:928–32.

36. Bellver J, Melo MA, Bosch E, Serra V, Remohí J, Pellicer A. Obesity and poor reproductive outcome: the potential role of the endometrium. Fertil Steril 2007;88(2):446–51.
37. Onalan R, Onalan G, Tonguc E, Ozdener T, Dogan M, Mollamahmutoglu L. Body mass index is an independent risk factor for the development of endometrial polypsin patients undergoing in vitro fertilization. Fertil Steril 2008 Mar 4 [Epub ahead of print].
38. O'Dowd A. Society issues guidance on IVF. BMJ 2006;333:517.
39. Dietz WH, Robinson TN. Clinical practice. Overweight children and adolescents. N Engl J Med 2005;352(20):2100–9.
40. ACOG Committee Opinion, Management of obesity. Obstet Gynecol 2005;106(4):895–9.
41. Wadden TA, Berkowitz RI, Womble LG, et al. Randomized trial of lifestyle modification and pharmacotherapy for obesity. N Engl J Med 2005;353(20):2111–20.

# Human Oocyte Abnormalities: Basic Analyses and Clinical Applications

Vanessa Y. Rawe and Catherine M. H. Combelles

**Abstract** Oocyte quality impacts early embryonic survival and the establishment and maintenance of pregnancy. Although meiosis may be completed successfully, there are a variety of other processes occurring within the cytoplasm of the oocyte that are required for complete developmental competence following fertilization. Morphological criteria are insufficient to give information on the oocyte's developmental ability, so it is of importance to understand the cellular and molecular basis of the oocyte pathology and determine the classification criteria for the selection of oocytes with superior developmental ability. In the absence of a comprehensive oocyte grading scheme, the power of morphological observations to aid oocyte/embryo selection is reduced. Until the mechanisms underlying oocyte quality are elucidated, efforts to apply assisted reproductive technologies in the treatment of human infertility will not be maximized. Exciting new technologies and data on oocyte biology have emerged in the last few years. In the present review, we briefly consider morphological characteristics with regard to oocyte developmental competency and then summarize key cellular and molecular findings as related to the pathophysiology of human oocytes. Finally, we consider some possible clinical predictors for assessing oocyte quality in ART.

**Keywords** Oocyte quality • Oocyte morphology • Female gamete • Assisted reproduction techniques • *In vitro* fertilization • Intracytoplasmic sperm injection

V.Y. Rawe (✉) and C.M.H. Combelles
Centro de Estudios en Ginecología y Reproducción (CEGyR), Buenos Aires, Argentina
e-mail: vrawe@cegyr.com

## 1 Introduction

Oocytes play a central role in the establishment of embryonic fate. Cellular and molecular events progressively provide the oocyte with the ability to complete meiosis (1), to ensure normal fertilization (2) and to undergo embryo development (3). Any dysfunction or dislocation of oocyte components will decrease oocyte competence with subsequent detrimental effects on embryo quality (4, 5). Of the oocytes retrieved after ovarian stimulation, only a minority (5–10%) can generate embryos with full developmental potential (6). Furthermore, only a small percentage of morphologically normal oocytes give rise to pregnancies, suggesting that most of the problems leading to poor embryonic development and implantation failure cannot be detected using standard microscopic evaluation. While morphological abnormalities appear to be associated with compromised oocyte quality, their precise identification and impact on embryo development is currently lacking. Characterization of the structural and functional deficiencies will help design strategies to improve fertilization and embryo development.

In the following review, we provide a summary of (1) morphological characteristics as related to oocyte developmental competence, (2) cellular and molecular findings for understanding the pathophysiology of human oocytes, and (3) possible clinical predictors for the evaluation of oocyte quality in ART.

## 2 Morphological Characteristics of Oocytes

When considering oocyte morphology, focus should not only include the oocyte, but also its extracellular

D.T. Carrell et al. (eds.), *Biennial Review of Infertility*, DOI: 10.1007/978-1-60327-392-3_13

accompanying compartments and cells, namely the cumulus cells, zona pellucida, and perivitelline space.

## 2.1 Extracytoplasmic

### 2.1.1 Cumulus Cells

The cumulus cells are the specialized granulosa cells that directly surround the oocyte during antral follicular development. Importantly, these cells accompany the oocyte throughout the development from an immature to a fully mature ovulated gamete, as well as beyond, as it awaits fertilization in the fallopian tube. Not surprisingly, cumulus cells thus serve a pivotal role in supporting the oocyte, whether *in vivo* or *in vitro*. Considerable evidence buttresses the interdependence between cumulus cells and the oocyte, including compromised oocyte quality when completing its developmental program and maturation in the absence of cumulus cells. Functionally, the oocyte is known to depend on its surrounding somatic cells for a myriad of activities, ranging from sources of signaling molecules to metabolites (7–9). Interestingly, the interdependence between the two cell compartments of the cumulus–oocyte complex (COC) is reciprocal. Indeed, the cumulus cells also depend on the oocyte for their normal differentiation, regulation, and functions (10–12).

Mechanistically, the development of cumulus cells and oocyte appear coordinated through a complex and regulated set of intercellular interactions, including direct cell–cell contacts, gap junctional communications, and paracrine signaling (11, 13, 14). Specialized cellular projections (from the cumulus cells to the oocyte surface) permit a physical and close link with the oocyte. These transzonal projections exist in COCs of all mammalian systems described to date; they are rich in either microtubules or microfilaments, and are reminiscent of cell processes in neurons, themselves examples of another cell type that rely extensively on cell communication and support from other cells. Gap junctions exist between cumulus cells and oocytes, and their functional roles are supported by genetic programming and several *in vitro* lines of evidence (13–15). Furthermore, communication between cumulus cells and oocytes appear to rely on several members of the transforming growth factor-β superfamily (11, 16). On the basis of the pivotal roles and influences of cumulus cells and oocytes on each other, clinical efforts should also focus on identifying cumulus abnormalities. Another essential component of the COC is the extracellular matrix (ECM) within which cumulus cells are embedded. Studies using animal models support the roles of adequate COC matrix in not only ovulation but also fertilization (17, 18). Ovulation is a complex event that entails the upregulation and secretion of ECM molecules leading to cumulus expansion, itself a process believed to provide the necessary environment and cues for sperm penetration and eventual fertilization.

In the clinic, COCs may be routinely graded based on gross evaluations under light microscopy. Upon retrieval, COCs vary considerably in their appearance; early attempts at classifying morphologies of the cumulus mass described the number of cell layers vesting the oocyte, the visibility of the oocyte, as well as the tightness of cell interactions in contrast to an expanded disposition of the cumulus–corona complex. Upon receiving the ovulatory signal, COCs are stimulated to mature and normally respond with the expansion and mucification of their cumulus masses (18). So, it was initially proposed that oocytes from a COC with a dense compact cumulus represent a state of maturity less advanced than those from COCs with expanded radial arrays of cells (19). However, the predictive value of variations in COC morphologies has largely fallen by the wayside (20). Previous studies evaluated COC grading in relation to nuclear maturity of the oocyte and/or subsequent embryo and pregnancy outcomes. Rattanachaiyanont et al. (21) reported a decrease in the proportion of mature oocytes in COCs with a dense layer of coronal cells although over 60% of oocytes were still meiotically mature in this group; none of the other COC grades appeared to relate to the maturity state of the oocyte on the day of retrieval. There were also no detectable links among COC grades, fertilization rates, and embryo cleavages; however, ICSI was employed and thus the potential influences of varying cumulus morphologies on normal routes of fertilization could not be determined (21). In contrast, another study documented improved fertilization rates and chances of pregnancy for expanded COCs in conventional IVF cycles (22). Overall, it remains uncertain whether COC grading could reliably pinpoint the deviant oocytes that are destined for fertilization; perhaps, the use of COC grading remains most relevant to applications aimed at maturing oocytes *in vitro* as opposed to mature eggs obtained after ovarian stimulation. In addition, many issues in COC grading remain, including a certain level of subjectivity, an inability to identify a morphological scheme with actual predictive value, and the superimposed confounding influences of hormone stimulation on the organization of the COC. However, on the basis of the biological underpinnings of the COC and cooperation between the oocyte and cumulus cells, it remains likely that features of the COC (if assessed adequately) may detect oocyte abnormalities. Only new approaches and future research will unravel this interesting possibility.

Another point of clinical relevance to cumulus cells that merits mention is the routine removal of these cells for intracytoplasmic sperm injection (ICSI) within a 2–4 h window post-retrieval. Given the known influences of cumulus cells on oocyte maturation and fertilization, it is not unreasonable that a premature removal of cumulus cells may compromise the last steps of oocyte development and competence acquisition. For instance, oocytes that progressed from metaphase-I to metaphase-II shortly after retrieval exhibit compromised fertilization rates when compared to oocytes already in metaphase-II (23). Extending the time of culture prior to ICSI may permit some of the oocytes to complete their developmental programs, a situation particularly relevant to those remaining slightly immature at the time of retrieval. For this subset of oocytes, studies tested the effects of delayed sperm injection on oocyte maturation and fertilization rates; the use of such a rescue maturation step was shown to provide an increased number of available embryos, albeit of compromised quality (24–26). However, rescued M-I oocytes have only been cultured thus far in the absence of cumulus cells. Future studies, therefore, should not ignore the seminal roles of cumulus cells, with efforts aiming to ensure that any oocytes remaining to complete their maturation programs *in vitro* can do so under the most optimal and efficient of culture conditions.

### 2.1.2 Zona Pellucida

The zona pellucida (ZP) is the specialized ECM layer that directly surrounds the oocyte. As such, the ZP represents the interface between the oocyte and its enclosing cumulus cells. The normal development of follicles, and thus the oocytes, depends on the presence and integrity of the ZP (13, 27, 28). Beyond an involvement in oocyte–somatic cell interactions, the ZP also plays essential roles at fertilization permitting sperm–egg interactions, the acrosome reaction, and an adequate block to polyspermy. The clinical introduction of ICSI has permitted not only the treatment of male factor infertility and the ability to circumvent many cases of fertilization failures, but also the identification of variants in ZP morphology. In contrast to IVF, the removal of cumulus cells before ICSI allows the visualization of the ZP shortly after retrieval and prior to fertilization. A large number of ZP variants (appearance, thickness, irregularities, composition, and organization) have been described with the advent of ICSI (Fig. 1). Thicker ZPs are associated with decreased fertilization rates, implantation, and pregnancy rates (29, 30). The dynamic features of the ZP were also later evaluated, with thickness variation (ZPTV) measured along the circumference of the zona; the more variable the ZP thickness, the better the quality of the embryos (31), and the higher the implantation and pregnancy rates (32). Extending these retrospective analyses, a randomized controlled trial showed the significant value of using ZPTV measurements to select embryos, although only among a cohort of poor quality ones; no benefits were apparent in other instances (33), thereby arguing for the need to combine and tailor the use of various morphological markers.

Recent studies have taken advantage of polarized microscopy (described in technical details in Sect. 3.1.2) to detect noninvasively variations in ZP organization and relate these to embryonic and clinical outcomes (34–36). The use of the Polscope™ has permitted the identification of three ZP layers, each with different light-retardance properties and thicknesses, in turn reflecting the various orientations of filaments (34). These zona properties differ within and across the maturation states (34). ZP evaluations performed on the day of retrieval indicate a positive relationship between increased retardance and thickness of the inner layer, and embryo cohorts of good quality (36), and elevated pregnancy rates (35). Together, these more recent studies highlight the advantages of examining the ZP layers both qualitatively and quantitatively by polarized microscopy and the potential weaknesses of measuring total ZP thickness alone.

Taken together, available studies reveal significant variances in ZP organization which, in turn, reflect heterogeneity in oocyte quality within a retrieved cohort. Indeed, during oogenesis, the ZP is laid down in a very

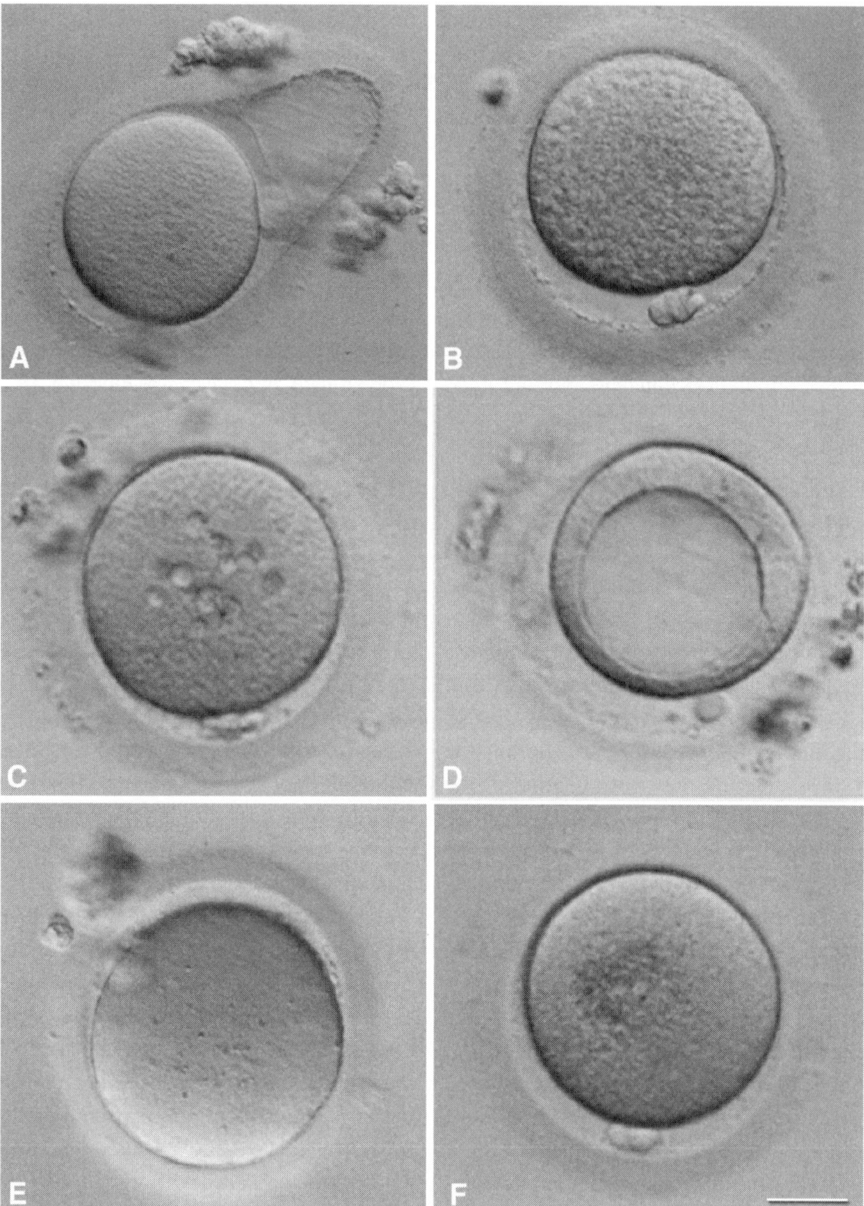


**Fig. 1** Light microscopy of MII human oocyte abnormalities. (**a**) Large perivitelline space (PVS). (**b**) Extremely granulated oocyte. Note the presence of debris in the PVS, a dark and thick zona pellucida and a fragmented polar body. (**c**) Presence of small vacuoles within the ooplasm. (**d**) Large vacuole. (**e**) Presence of cytoplasmic inclusions. (**f**) Excessive centrally located granularity and dark cytoplasm. Images were kindly donated by Dr. Mariana Hernández and Dr. Andrea De Matteis (CIGOR, Córdoba, Argentina). *Scale bar* represents 50 mm

orderly fashion (in both time and space) and given its critical roles during oocyte and embryo development, the zona is likely a good predictor of oocyte quality. The ZP has been imaged at different time points, on the day of retrieval or postembryo culture. While ZP thickness varies and becomes thinner postfertilization, there is still a clear value to examining the zona on the day of retrieval, that is after it has reached its maximal thickness post oocyte maturation and before later remodeling events. Interestingly, in the clinic the organization of the ZP appears influenced by intrinsic factors in the oocyte from the time of retrieval, hormonal stimulation

(37), and subsequent ZP thickening and hardening during culture (discussed below). Albeit invasive in nature, Familiari et al. (38) undertook an ultrastructural study of human ZPs using electron microscopy; spongy, mesh-like vs. compact ZP filaments were characteristic of mature vs. immature or atretic oocytes, respectively. These observations further support the relevance of ZP organization in predicting oocyte quality. Mechanistically, the biological significance of the ZP ultrastructure remains uncertain, but it may relate to differences in chemical permeability. In theory, a spongy ZP network may facilitate sperm binding and digestion through the zona at fertilization (38).

The ZP also plays a pivotal role in preimplantation embryos; for instance, abnormalities in oocyte (and thus ZP) shape are associated with irregular cleavage patterns, compromised cell–cell contacts, and subsequent difficulties in developmental progression (39). The importance of the ZP continues until the blastocyst stage, a time when the embryo needs to hatch out of the zona prior to implanting into the uterine epithelium. Interestingly, the zona pellucida thickness marker discussed above may reflect a subsequent ability of the embryo to hatch and implant successfully (32). Although still contentious, there may be a causal relationship between recurrent implantation failure and an inability of embryos to escape normally from the ZP (40). In the clinic, assisted hatching of the ZP is sometimes used to facilitate the release of the embryo from its ZP. Randomized controlled trials do not support a beneficial use of AH in all patients but rather in specific circumstances such as in cases of recurrent pregnancy losses (41, 42). However, other than targeting a particular patient population, no useful morphological predictors of the zona (not even its thickness) yet exist to identify embryos that could benefit from AH. A need for AH may relate to intrinsic aberrations (due to advanced maternal age, infertility diagnosis, hormones) (40, 42) and/or culture-induced changes in zona properties. For instance, prolonged and nonphysiological culture conditions may lead to irreversible chemical modifications or zona hardening (41). With much of the focus placed on evaluations of the ZP at the embryonic stage, there is a need to ascertain whether ZP morphological features or abnormalities in the oocyte may predict any potential benefits of circumventing these with the use of AH prior to embryo transfer. In addition, AH may also only be beneficial for a subset of embryos within a cohort. Clearly, we need to augment our knowledge regarding abnormalities in zona morphology and their potential clinical significance.

### 2.1.3 Perivitelline Space

The perivitelline space (PVS) represents the acellular compartment in between the plasma membrane of the oocyte and its ZP. It becomes clearly visible in a mature oocyte with the extruded polar body located in its most prominent portion (Fig. 1). There is a gradient of possible PVS arrangements: from directly apposed to the membrane, to separate and distinguishable, to be exaggerated. These variants may exist within the circumference of a single female gamete or across a cohort of oocytes. A challenge still resides in unequivocally assigning a PVS arrangement with what may be typical or deviant from normal. An indistinguishable PVS typically corresponds to immature oocytes while a distinct space to mature oocytes (43). In contrast, the exact significance of an exaggerated PVS remains uncertain even though it is typically described as aberrant in spite of equivocal evidence. One retrospective study demonstrated a correlation between a large PVS and a decline in both fertilization and embryo quality (44), while others reported a lack of any such relationships (45–47). Recently, Ten et al. (48) reported no influence of PVS size on fertilization, but improved embryo quality in oocytes with large PVS. When examining oocyte cohorts, the incidence of large PVS is rather common, in 23% of retrieved oocytes (46), 11% of donor oocytes (48), and 50% of fertilized zygotes (47). However, there is still no consensus as to whether PVS assessment alone may predict oocyte quality.

Given the paucity of knowledge, one can only speculate on the relevance of a minimal as opposed to large PVS. On one hand, a large PVS may result in disrupted or compromised communication between the cumulus cells and the oocyte, particularly via gap junctions and transzonal projections. On another hand, it may be advantageous to interrupt certain modes of cell communication at the right time, and there may be a mechanism by which the PVS influences oocyte development, a possibility that merits experimental consideration. It may be hypothesized that the PVS contains and houses molecules essential to oocyte and/or cumulus cell development. Conversely, secreted molecules may become inadequately trapped in the PVS, thereby hindering their availability to the oocyte and/or cumulus cells. Interestingly, at least in the mouse, there is selectivity with respect to the entrance and retention of certain molecules in the PVS (49). Besides the speculations on potential developmental implications, the reasons for an exaggerated PVS also remain unknown.

Relatively little attention has focused on the composition of the PVS, although it does contain a matrix of proteins and hyaluronic acid organized as granules and filaments (50). The exact origin of the PVS chemicals remains unknown with the cumulus cells and oocyte representing likely candidates. Indeed, there is some support for the presence of cortical granule material in the PVS, as well as the formation of a cortical granule envelope within the PVS (43, 50). In this vein, the PVS may influence sperm penetration, fertilization, and a proper block to polyspermy. Early work also reported the accumulation of other materials in the PVS, including secreted glycoproteins of oviductal origin (49, 51). However, these factors are only present in naturally ovulated oocytes and not in gametes obtained and manipulated for ART. Future studies should explore the possibility that deficiencies in PVS content may reside in *in vitro* fertilized oocytes with no exposure to the natural oviductal milieu.

Another measurable morphological feature of the PVS is the presence or absence of debris, with about 40% of donor oocyte (48) and 50% of zygote cohorts (47) displaying PVS debris. The origin of such debris, as observed in the clinic, remains unknown; Xia (44) proposed that it might arise from premature exocytosis of cortical granules (see Sect. 3.1.3). Future work will also be needed to distinguish normal changes in PVS content from abnormalities. A retrospective analysis in donor oocytes showed no correlations between the presence of debris, fertilization rates, and embryo quality (48). Although grossly understudied to date, future oocyte studies cannot afford to ignore the PVS, its exact and dynamic content, as well as its morphological and clinical significance.

Taken together, morphological evaluations of the three extracellular components of the oocyte provide a certain measure of oocyte assessment while not independently providing predictors of oocyte quality. Current modes of assessment likely merit further refinements and evaluations in combination, with the acceptance that their potential utility may ultimately be limited in scope. Indeed, it is conceivable that morphology of the cumulus cells, ZP, and PVS may distinguish inherently compromised oocytes within a heterogeneous cohort, while never enabling distinction among the top quality gametes. Furthermore, issues pertaining to inter- and intra-observer variability will likely exist. Given the complexity in morphological variants, much work remains in accurately detecting and assessing these characteristics, and then in establishing their clinical significance. Randomized controlled trials may then test the value of using any single extracytoplasmic assessment, or combination of features on pregnancy outcomes.

## 2.2 Intracytoplasmic

### 2.2.1 Polar Body

The mammalian oocyte is arrested in diakinesis of prophase I at birth. It retains an intact nucleus (the germinal vesicle, GV) until ovulation at which time exposure to luteinizing hormone (LH) triggers meiotic resumption. After germinal vesicle breakdown (GVBD), a short anaphase I (A-I) and telophase I (T-I) take place and the first polar body (PB) is extruded. Finally, the oocyte becomes arrested at the metaphase-II (MII) stage until fertilization. In 1995, Eichenlaub-Ritter et al. (52) postulated that morphology of the first PB reflected the postovulatory age of the oocyte. At present, some data support the conclusion that PB shape, size, surface and integrity can predict oocyte quality (44, 53–55), but other studies show no correlation between PB characteristics and oocyte developmental competence (46, 56, 57) or genetic constitution of the embryo (58). Polar bodies contain a redundant set of cytoplasm, organelles, and chromosomes/chromatids and they can provide useful information about the genetics of the oocyte without potentially jeopardizing it. Cytogenetic analysis of both PBs using fluorescent in situ hybridization (FISH) and chromosomal painting allows the prediction of the partial or total chromosome status of the oocyte. PBs can also be used to screen for mitochondrial mutations and deletions. Thus, the study of PBs may serve as a powerful genetic diagnostic tool during prefertilization screening without the need for embryo biopsy (59). Although a clear advantage of PB biopsy vs. embryo PGD is that the information can be obtained earlier in the culture process, some limitations should be considered (60). First, only the maternal genetic contribution can be studied. Second, potential nonseparation of sister chromatids during meiosis II can occur, requiring PB2 analysis. Third, polar body chromosomes are shorter, which makes the technique more difficult. Technical problems such as lack of metaphase preparation, loss of chromosomes, signal overlap, and hybridization failure should also be taken into account when considering PBs analysis.

### 2.2.2 Ooplasm

In order to guarantee adequate oocyte quality, nuclear and cytoplasmic maturation must take place in a synchronized manner. In this context, nuclear maturity refers to the resumption of meiosis and the progression to metaphase II, the arrested stage at the time of ovulation. The metaphase promoting factor (MPF) formed by cyclin B and p34cdc2 supports the transition from $G_2$ to M phase. Active MPF in turn permits the initiation of nuclear maturation (e.g., germinal vesicle breakdown) and condensation of metaphase I (MI) chromosomes, then a decrease in MPF leads to entry into anaphase I and a second peak in MPF activity drives the oocyte to metaphase II (61).

Even if oocytes possess nuclear competence, they still may be deficient in cytoplasmic maturation, which refers to all processes preparing the oocytes for activation, fertilization, and embryo development. Completion of both types of maturation are highly susceptible to abnormalities in follicular hormonal milieu and/or *in vitro* culture conditions (e.g., pH, temperature, oxygen) that may cause alterations in oocyte morphology (Fig. 1), with some of these anomalies being visible at the light-microscopic level (62, 63).

With the advent of ICSI, removal of cumulus cells has allowed direct observation of oocyte morphological characteristics under light microscopy. Several ooplasmic features such as the presence or absence of granularity (Fig. 1b), coloration, presence of vacuoles (Fig. 1c, d), inclusion, and organelles clustering are typically observed (Fig. 1e, f) (44, 64, 65). Indeed, more than 50% of human oocytes show at least one of these morphological abnormalities (66). In contrast, a "good looking" MII oocyte typically shows a clear cytoplasm with moderate granulation and no inclusions, while an oocyte with a dark ooplasm decreases by 83% the likelihood of obtaining good quality embryos (48).

Vacuoles and aggregations of smooth endoplasmic reticulum (sER) were found to be the most apparent cytoplasmic feature that impairs developmental capacity. Vacuoles arise spontaneously (67) by fusion of preexisting vesicles derived from the sER or Golgi apparatus (68). Very few reports studied the effect of vacuoles on oocyte competence in humans (67, 69–71), but the majority of them established a negative impact on fertilization rates and development to blastocyst stage. Otsuki et al. (72) reported that the presence of smooth Endoplasmic Reticulum Clusters (sERCs) is associated with reduced chances of successful pregnancy, even in sERC-negative oocytes from the same cohort that are transferred along with the sERC-positive oocytes.

Treatment of human infertility typically involves the administration of exogenous gonadotropins to stimulate aggressively the ovaries to produce the maximal number of mature oocytes. Ovarian stimulation in mice causes delayed embryonic development, increased abnormal blastocyst formation, fetal growth retardation, and increased fetal loss (73). Similar detrimental effects of superovulation on oocyte quality may occur in human-assisted reproduction. In fact, in the study by Otsuki et al. (72) a correlation between the level of estradiol on the day of HCG administration and the presence of sERC was found.

Despite these broad associations among oocyte morphology, embryo quality, and ovarian stimulation, it is clear that microscopic visualization of morphology is not sufficient to understand the basis of an underlying pathology, or its relative impact in assisted reproduction technologies. Researching these events is a major challenge, which will be undoubtedly rewarded by new knowledge and, in the long term, by the improved treatments of infertility.

### 2.2.3 Meiotic Spindle

The defining feature of meiosis is that chromosome replication in S-phase is followed by two consecutive cell divisions to produce haploid gametes. Aneuploidy is a major obstacle in achieving reproductive success. About 20% of all human oocytes are regarded as aneuploid although this figure can vary widely, from 10% to as high as 40–60% (74–76). The incidence of aneuploidy increases with advanced maternal age (77). These aneuploidies are believed to result primarily from errors in maternal meiosis I (78, 79). The nondisjunction of bivalent chromosomes appears as a key mechanism for age-related aneuploidy (80). Aberrant spindle assembly (81) or other meiotic errors (79) may also be partly to blame. The vast majority of embryos formed from aneuploid oocytes are nonviable and lost at some point before term. Unfortunately, standard morphological evaluation cannot detect chromosomal anomalies and thus cannot guide the decision of which embryo(s) to transfer.

The structure and function of the meiotic spindle is fundamental to ensuring correct chromosome segregation at MI and MII. Characteristics of the spindle such as its presence, location, and length, are often used to evaluate oocyte quality. In somatic cells, the spindle is under the control of backup mechanisms, ensuring that each phase of chromosome segregation is not triggered unless the previous phase is correctly completed (82). In contrast, in mammalian oocytes these checkpoints are not strictly implemented during the meiotic process (83, 84) which, in turn, may result in chromosome missegregation occurring under conditions of spindle disorganization. Furthermore, oocytes from older women (81), either grown under suboptimal conditions or exposed to environmental chemicals (85, 86), are particularly susceptible to the consequences of such a "leaky" control mechanism of chromosome segregation. For these reasons, it has been suggested (87–89) that analysis of the spindle may be a valuable criterion for assessing oocyte quality. Indeed, while no relationship was found between the relative position of the meiotic spindle (with respect to the PB) and oocyte developmental competence, spindle length has been reported to correlate with oocyte quality (4, 87).

There are two approaches to studying the meiotic spindle: noninvasive method, using an optical system termed "polarization light microscopy" (Polscope™, Fig. 2a, b) and a second, invasive method using fluorescence (conventional or confocal) immunostaining microscopy (Fig. 3, see Sect. 3.1.2).

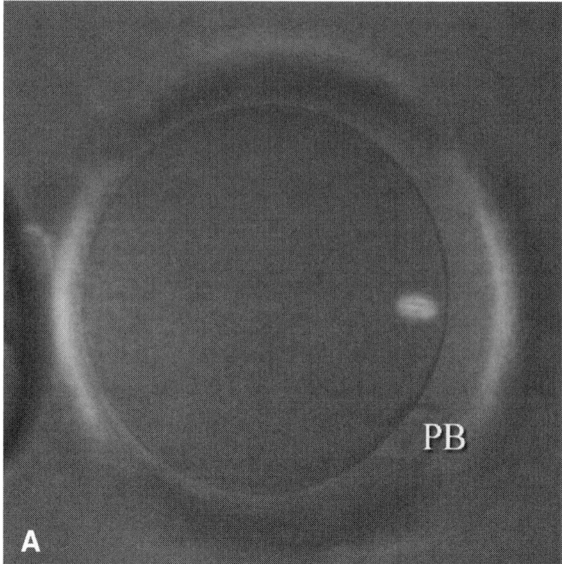


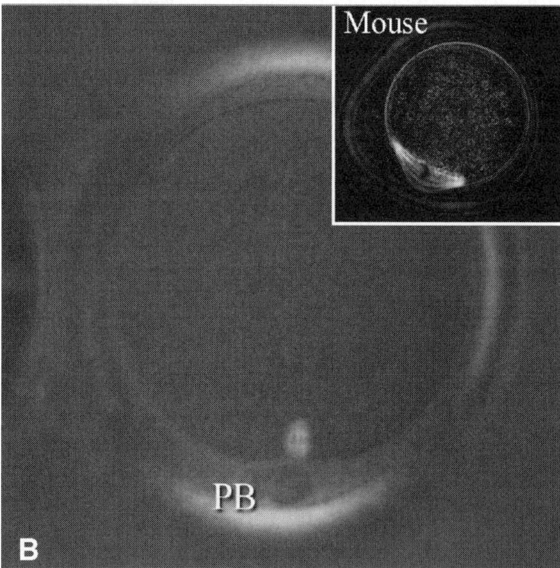


**Fig. 2** Polarization microscopy of MII human oocytes. (**a**) Living human oocyte with a spindle rotated approximately 30° from the polar body (PB). (**b**) Oocyte with the spindle located near the PB. The inset in B shows a polarization image of a mouse oocyte. Note the difference in the length and position of the meiotic spindle. Images A and B were generously donated by Dr. Ariel Ahumada (Procrearte, Buenos Aires, Argentina). *Scale bar* represents 50 μm

Polarized light is the light in which all the rays vibrate in one plane. A polarizing microscope has two disk accessories. They are made up of polarizing plastic that allows light to pass that is only vibrating in one plane. One of the discs is called a polarizer (placed below the condenser). Another similar disc is placed in the top part of the microscope and cuts off all the light vibrating in a perpendicular plane. This disc is called analyzer. The placement of the discs is such that they allow light vibrating in planes perpendicular to each other. Hence, when both the disks are in place, no light can pass to the eyepieces and the field of view is dark unless a doubly refractile object like polymerized microtubules is placed in the path of polarized light. In this instance, microtubules of the meiotic spindle,

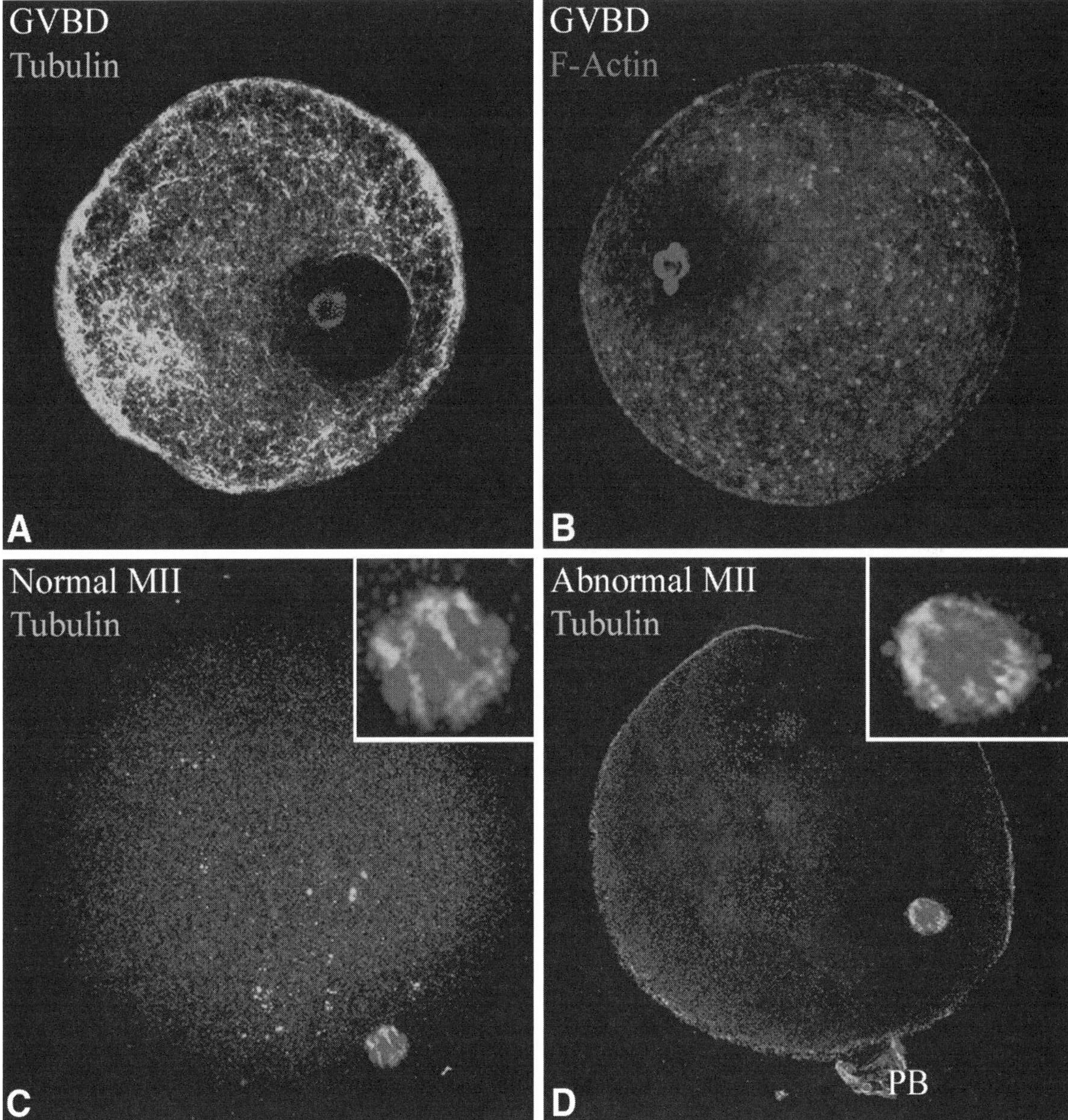


**Fig. 3** Confocal microscopy of human oocytes at different maturational stages: cytoskeleton markers. (**a**) During Germinal Vesicle Breakdown (GVBD stage), oocytes show a network of tubulin (*green*) organized throughout the ooplasm and surrounding the germinal vesicle where the chromatin (*blue*) is tightly associated with the nucleolus. (**b**) Filamentous actin (F-actin) is visualized using 568-Phalloidin (*red*) in GVBD human oocytes. Microfilaments are distributed in the ooplasm and enriched at the oocyte cortex. Note the different distribution of microfilaments around the human GV when compared with microtubules (**a** vs. **b**), suggesting that the migration of the nucleus during meiosis I in humans is a microtubule (and not microfilament) dependent event. (**c** and **d**) MII oocytes show microtubules polymerized in the meiotic spindle (*green*). In **c**, a normal morphology of the spindle and an organized metaphase plate are observed (inset) in contraposition to **d**, where chromosomes are not well aligned and the meiotic spindle is rotated with respect to the polar body (PB). (**e**) Profilin (an actin-related protein) distributes to specific foci inside the GVBD nucleus and throughout the ooplasm. It promotes the incorporation of actin monomers into filaments and the nucleation of them is catalyzed by the Arp 2/3 complex. (**f**) Wiskott-Aldrich syndrome protein family verprolin-homologous protein (WAVE1) regulates the actin cytoskeleton and is observed associated with Golgi apparatus in human GV oocytes (unpublished observations). Images were obtained using an Olympus spectral confocal microscope, with laser lines at 488-, 568-, and 633-nm wavelengths (University of Buenos Aires, Faculty of Exact and Natural Sciences) and then processed by Adobe Photoshop 7.0. *Scale bar* represents 20 μm (*see Color Plates*)

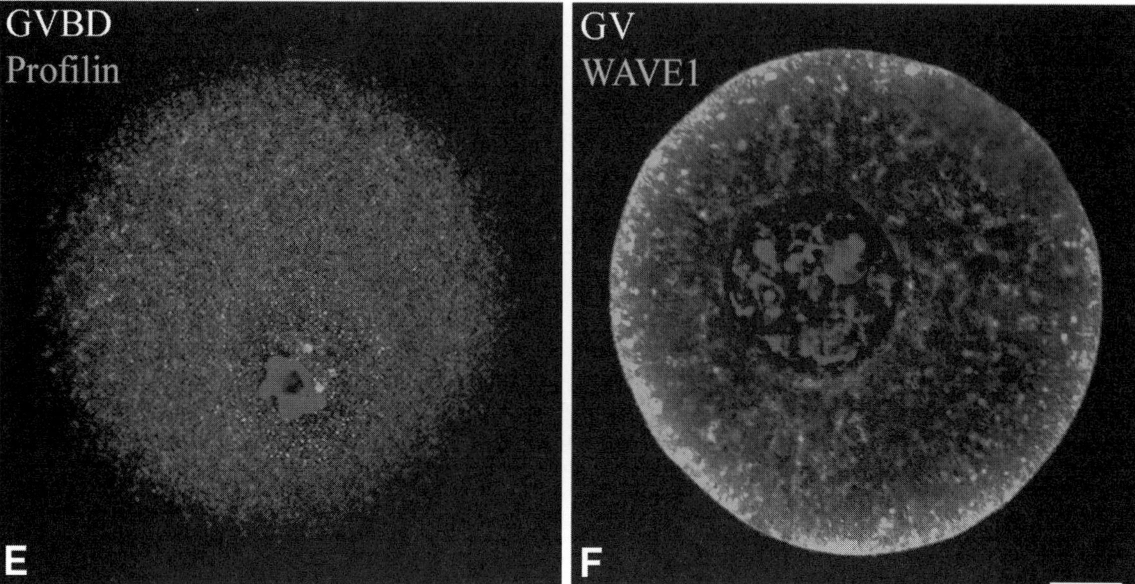


**Fig. 3** (continued)

for example, appear illuminated against the ooplasm that appears as a dark background.

Compared with immunostaining or other microscopy methods, the Polscope™ offers the unique advantage of being totally noninvasive, preserving oocyte viability, and allowing repeated observations to be performed (Fig. 2) (87, 90, 91). Using this approach, numerous studies have assessed the relationship between spindle appearance and/or position and oocyte developmental competency. Wang et al. (87) suggested that more oocytes with birefringent spindles than oocytes without spindles fertilized normally after ICSI (61.8 vs. 44.2%). Oocytes in which the spindle is shifted more than 90° relative to the position of the first polar body also display reduced fertilization rates. Confocal studies confirmed that spindles structures were almost identical to Polscope™ images of spindle birefringence.

Rienzi et al. (89) have shown that the absence of the MII spindle is associated with reduced rates of fertilization and blastocyst formation. Interestingly, a percentage of oocytes showing a first polar body may not have completed nuclear maturation. Eichenlaub-Ritter et al. (92) and De Santis et al. (57) have found that human oocytes without birefringent spindles may still be at the telophase or prometaphase I stage, and as a consequence, have worse prognosis after IVF/ICSI.

## 3 Cellular/Molecular Parameters of Oocytes

### 3.1 *Invasive Analysis*

#### 3.1.1 Mitochondria

The distribution of mitochondria is a highly dynamic process during oocyte maturation, fertilization, and early embryonic development (93, 94). Mitochondria are the main energy producers in oocytes, using the oxidative phosphorylation pathway to supply ATP for all cellular activities requiring energy. The abnormal redistribution of mitochondria throughout the ooplasm is a marker of cytoplasm immaturity and is strongly linked to low developmental ability (93–96). Santos et al. (97) demonstrated that the average mtDNA copy number was significantly lower in cohorts of human unfertilized oocytes than cohorts with normal fertilization. Furthermore, mtDNA deletions have been associated with impaired oocyte quality and insufficient embryonic development (98, 99). Consistent with these observations, variations in ATP levels significantly affect oocyte quality and embryonic development (100, 101).

The regulation of spindle formation, as well as progression of meiotic maturation, necessitates the interaction of mitochondria and the activity of microtubule motor proteins (see Sect. 3.1.2). Mitochondria translocate to the perinuclear region during formation of the first metaphase spindle and subsequently disperse during extrusion of the first polar body (102). Recently, Zeng et al. (103) applied the Polscope™ to assess the presence of the meiotic spindle and for the quantification of mtDNA and ATP content to *in vitro* matured human oocytes. Interestingly, they found a significant positive relationship between elevated mtDNA, ATP content and detectable meiotic spindles.

Taken together, mitochondrial distribution as well as cytoplasmic mtDNA and ATP content may be regarded as potential predictors of oocyte developmental competence. However, these methods are invasive and therefore have no value as prediction tools in the clinical IVF laboratory.

### 3.1.2 Cytoskeleton Structure (Epifluorescence and Confocal Microscopy)

Confocal microscopy offers the most detailed and informative data on spindle structure and the cytoskeleton components in general (**Fig. 3**). It allows the analysis of fluorescently labeled thick specimens without physical sectioning. Optical sections are generated by eliminating out-of-focus fluorescence and displayed as digitalized images. It allows 3-dimensional reconstruction (XYZ) and time analysis (XYT), thus providing a unique chance to link morphology with cell function. Since images are obtained by scanning, excess illumination of the specimen and quick decrease of the fluorescent signal are avoided. Nevertheless, this technique unfortunately requires a fixation step that causes loss of oocyte viability and thereby is unpractical for application with oocytes destined for clinical use. However, the identification of factors responsible for the developmental competency within the oocyte is essential not only to establish objective criteria of oocyte quality, but also to aid in improving methods for gamete selection.

Published protocols detail how to perform parallel, multichannel immunodetection and imaging of human oocyte, zygote, and embryo components by epifluorescence or confocal microscopy (104). As far as the oocyte cytoskeleton is concerned, the plasticity of rodent and nonrodent mammals is different. Therefore, some differences between mouse and human oocytes have to be considered before generalizations and extrapolations are made among mammalian species. Mouse oocytes exhibit a polarized distribution of actin filaments, cortical granules, and microvilli, prior to fertilization. Human oocytes, on the contrary, show no polarization of these components (Fig. 3b). The meiotic spindle in rodent oocytes is arranged tangentially to the plasma membrane (see inset Fig. 2b), while in human oocytes it is smaller and arranged radially (Figs. 2a, b and 3c, d). Numerous cytoplasmic microtubule asters are found in the unfertilized mouse oocyte. After fertilization, they elongate and, together with actin filaments, form the scaffolding necessary for pronuclear migration and apposition. By contrast, in nonrodent species the centrosome degenerates in the oocyte and is retained in the sperm during the maturation process. Human spermatozoa contribute the centrosome during fertilization, which serves as the dominant microtubule-organizing center in the zygote, and nucleates microtubules from a central structure known as the γ-tubulin ring complex. Also, during fertilization in nonrodent mammals the microtubules, but not the actin filaments, are required for pronuclear migration and apposition (105).

Meiotic spindles in mammalian oocytes lack centrioles, which are present only up to the pachytene stage during oogenesis (106). Contrarily to rodents where several pericentriolar material (PCM) foci including γ-tubulin have been found at the acentriolar meiotic spindle poles and in the cytoplasm (107), metaphase II arrested oocytes from pig (108), sheep (109), and cow (110) do not have cytoplasmic microtubule organizing centers (MTOC). Different pathways of spindle formation have been described for several species but in the majority of them, common components are used (111). Microtubule-associated molecular motors such as DYNC1I1 (cytoplasmic dynein 1 intermediate chain), and its cofactor DCTN1 (dynactin p150$^{Glued}$) are critically involved in the transport of vesicles and formation of the meiotic spindle (112). The role of microtubule-associated molecular motors like HSET, Eg5 and the mitotic antigen NuMA have been observed in nonhuman primates oocytes (113, 114) and just recently identified in human oocytes (115, 116). The identification of HSET, Eg5 and NuMA in human oocytes suggests that their presence may be necessary for controlled microtubule dynamics. As stated before (see Sect. 2.2.3), approximately 20% of all human oocytes are considered aneuploid, and it is thus of particular interest to understand the establishment of a normal bipolar spindle and the respective roles of microtubules and motor proteins in chromosomal segregation. According to Blake et al. (117), approximately 35% of transferred human embryos/blastocysts derived from *in vivo* maturation develop to term. In contrast, when meiotically immature oocytes are recovered from stimulated ovaries and matured *in vitro* (IVM), only 12% of the resulting zygotes progress to the blastocyst stage (24) and only a mere 14% of transferred embryos develop to term (118, 119). It is clear, therefore, that even if oocytes are meiotically mature, they still may be deficient in cytoplasmic maturation.

Comprehending the events responsible for a balanced coordination of nuclear and cytoplasmic maturation is of clinical relevance since there are sporadic, yet accumulating, instances of meiotic arrests in ART. Controlled ovarian stimulation typically results in maturation rates of about 90%, with the remaining oocytes either meiotically incompetent or only able to resume meiosis upon *in vitro* maturation (IVM) (120). However, there are unusual clinical patient cases when IVM fails to rescue oocytes that are immature across an entire cohort. These oocytes appear irreversibly, uniformly, and repeatedly arrested in defined phases of meiosis, including cases in prophase-I or metaphase-I (121–125). Given the tight cell cycle controls that preside over meiotic resumption and progression, it is not surprising that errors may arise. For instance, deficiencies in the cell cycle regulator CDC25B may preclude oocytes from exiting prophase-I arrest (126). Metaphase-I arrest may result from aberrant meiotic recombination events, defects in MPF or PKC regulation, or spindle malfunctions (127). It is important to acknowledge that even oocytes that are mature at the time of retrieval may fail to fertilize, predominantly because of defects in oocyte activation (128). Etiologies may include spindle abnormalities and/or defects in the normal dynamics of cell cycle molecules. To date, much of the evaluation of these arrested oocytes has relied on endpoint nuclear and cytoskeletal evaluations using the aforementioned immunofluorescence approaches. Although these techniques are invasive, they enable the systematic detection of oocytes possessing aberrant nuclear and/or cytoplasmic maturation (notably chromosomal and cytoskeletal defects), together with the identification of relevant underpinnings. Such knowledge may then allow improved management along with targeted treatment strategies in patients afflicted by meiotic arrest.

### 3.1.3 Calcium and Cortical Granules

Beyond the evaluation of the cytoskeleton, cellular mediators of oocyte activation ought to be considered. A central middleman is calcium with its well-described oscillations downstream of sperm entry and upstream of cell cycle regulators (129). Future studies should assess whether the processing of sperm factors, calcium stores, oscillations, and/or calcium response elements are compromised in human oocytes that fail to exit metaphase-II arrest and activate. The ability of an oocyte to mount and sustain calcium oscillations is relevant to any effort aimed at identifying human oocyte abnormalities. Indeed, previous animal studies demonstrated that calcium-signaling activity is acquired during follicular and oocyte development (130), and it is further influenced by many factors pertinent to clinical ART (including age, hormonal stimulation, and *in vitro* culture) (131). Now that the early embryonic events are also known to depend on calcium oscillations in the oocyte (132), it is all the more paramount to understand and identify any interruptions in egg activation and calcium-signaling pathways of the human oocyte.

Cortical granules (CGs) constitute a complement of organelles essential to egg activation and fertilization (133). CGs are Golgi-derived, specialized secretory vesicles of the oocyte; they accumulate during oogenesis with a final location in the microfilament-rich cortex of the oocyte. CGs are filled with mucopolysaccharides, peroxidases, and proteolytic enzymes; upon exocytosis into the PVS for eventual transport through the ZP, CG enzymes mediate irreversible changes in the ZP, resulting in zona hardening. Zona hardening, characterized by an increased resistance to denaturing agents, prevents polyspermy and provides protection to the embryo (133). CGs are normally found in very high density and docked at the oolemma, awaiting a cue prior to their fusion and release of contents. CG exocytosis (i.e., the cortical reaction) takes place in response to the calcium rises at oocyte activation (2). Given the importance of calcium signaling and secretory pathways in oocytes (134), it is not surprising that CG abnormalities arise in ART. Van Blerkom (67) documented that about 15% of mature human oocytes exhibit premature CG exocytosis, thereby interrupting the normal sequence of egg activation events. The demonstration that failed to fertilize human eggs may experience precocious CG release (135) corroborates the importance of these organelles in identifying and managing oocyte abnormalities. The cortical reaction may not always be premature; for instance, the extended culture of mature mouse oocytes actually interferes with normal CG exocytosis (136). CGs thus serve as a marker of cytoplasmic maturation, and their total complements as well as localization merit analysis in human oocytes; this can be done using routine fluorescence microscopy and simultaneously with nuclear and cytoskeletal parameters (137). Microfilaments also play a role in CG migration and cortical positioning (138), and ovarian stimulation with large quantities of gonadotropins negatively influence microfilament and CG distribution in hamster oocytes (139). Lastly, it is important to note that not all oocytes are competent to undergo CG exocytosis in response to calcium increases; indeed, immature mouse oocytes are not able to do so even downstream of intracellular calcium rises (140). Abnormalities in both CG translocation to the plasma membrane and calcium-dependent signaling molecules characterize immature mouse oocytes (141). In this vein, organelle and/or CG-related molecular defects merit further consideration in human oocytes.

### 3.1.4 Ubiquitin-Proteasome System

In eukaryotes, proteasomes are ubiquitous and essential for cellular viability; they represent the major site of proteolytic activity in mammalian cells and constitute up to 1% of cellular proteins (142, 143). Over the past few years, intensive research has focused on the 20S proteasome and its molecular structure and function. It is present in the cytoplasm and nucleus of eukaryotic cells and when associated with regulatory particles, it forms the 26S proteasome with a catalytic core. The 26S proteasome is an essential component of ubiquitin-dependent proteolysis, a process by which most proteins become degraded. Besides the tightly controlled degradation of regulatory proteins (cyclins, transcription factors, etc.), proteasomes degrade the bulk of proteins as part of a quality control process. They have recently been described in gametes, with specific roles during fertilization in different species (144–147).

While the importance of the proteasome system to degrade cell cycle regulatory proteins is well established during mammalian preimplantation embryonic development, its role in regulating oocyte quality is much less understood. Nevertheless, in the last few years, studies have explored the distribution of proteasomes during various stages of mammalian oocyte maturation together with the effects of proteasome inhibitors on oocyte quality. Preliminary results suggest that the differential presence of proteasomes may play an important role in remodeling cytoplasmic and nuclear events during human oocyte maturation, fertilization, and early embryonic development (148, 149). Failure of proteasome-mediated quality control may be a hidden cause for poor oocyte and embryo quality observed during assisted reproduction techniques.

## 3.2 Non-Invasive

### 3.2.1 Proteome, Secretome, and Metabolome

While considerable knowledge can be gained from invasive evaluations, a critical impetus prevails to identify predictors of oocyte quality in a noninvasive manner. Other requirements pertaining to oocyte assessment include the need for accuracy, high-throughput analysis, and rapid turnaround with results available prior to the time of embryo transfer. These are some of the constraints within which approaches are explored, and despite the significant efforts that remain, this is a booming and exciting time in the field of noninvasive oocyte assessment.

Much attention has been placed on the complementary assessment of all available sample types in the clinic. These samples (both cellular and noncellular) are routinely discarded and they will presumably reflect the developmental competence of the corresponding oocyte. To date, studies have investigated the potential use of serum, follicular fluid, follicular cells (both granulosa and cumulus cells), and the spent culture medium. Analyses have detected the presence and/or activity of a wide set of molecules. A focus on molecular parameters would conceivably provide more precise markers of cellular functions; an important premise of such analysis is that the presence and/or regulated expression of a gene product would reflect its physiological or pathophysiological roles. For instance, if the culture medium within which an oocyte is held were to contain a high level of stress-related proteins, this may indicate a compromised quality of the gamete. It may conversely be envisaged that elevated levels of stress proteins may indicate an oocyte's ability to respond to stressful culture conditions, thereby potentially reflecting its superior quality and developmental competencies. Therefore, only longitudinal studies that unequivocally correlate levels of a protein to clinical outcome are of ultimate value.

Proteomics or the profiling of expressed proteins with high-throughput analysis is an emerging and invaluable approach to detect the protein signatures of clinical samples. For instance, serum proteomics can allow the identification of biomarkers in patients at elevated risks of certain diseases (150). Similarly, proteomics may be applied to serum or other fluids of infertility patients for subsequent correlations with the quality of their embryo cohorts. With respect to serum, one of the limitations is that it is too dynamic and non-specific of a sample type. Thus, serum does not necessarily reflect the microenvironment of the developing oocyte with any accuracy. Analyses of follicular fluid address this deficiency of serum since this is the very milieu within which the COC completes its development *in vivo*. Indeed, many studies have focused on measuring the levels of pertinent molecules (namely a myriad of hormones, paracrine factors, and cytokines), and some of these factors have showed correlations with oocyte quality (151–153). However, while follicular fluid remains an invaluable resource (readily available and likely to reflect the developmental potential of an oocyte), its testing as a predictor of oocyte quality is fraught by many limitations. Issues include the lack of sample representation across a patient's cohort, confounding variables not systematically controlled for, and the use of outcome measures not always proven to relate to live birth (such as oocyte/embryo morphological grading). More generally, there is a limited ability to correlate directly follicular fluid content with the fate of a given oocyte or embryo. Taken together, follicular fluid studies provide an invaluable glimpse into potential markers of oocyte health, but its clinical and irrefutable use in selecting the golden oocyte is not yet ready for primetime. Perhaps, novel markers of oocyte health or aberrations should be considered; along these lines, more recent analyses of follicular fluids using proteomic approaches may permit the detection of new factors for future validation (154–157).

The follicular cells retrieved at the time of follicular aspiration constitute another sample type readily available for analysis without any detriment to the oocytes. The two follicular cell types obtained are the membrana granulosa cells and the cumulus cells. Of the two, membrana granulosa cells are the most immediately available for analysis, since they are routinely discarded upon removal of the COC from the follicular aspirates. As one potential biomarker of oocyte health, several studies have focused on the luteinized status of the membrana granulosa cell population with, for example, apoptosis of luteinized granulosa cells serving as an indicator of fertilization outcome (158). However, many factors confound most membrana granulosa cell studies, including cell pooling across follicular aspirates, contaminants, and differentiation states that have already become modified by the hormone stimulation treatments. Indeed, membrana granulosa cells are known to respond to exogenous hormone regimens, thereby artificially affecting a physiological balance of cell proliferation and differentiation. More precisely, granulosa cells typically become luteinized in response to ovarian stimulation (159), and thus true biomarkers of the follicular environment within which an oocyte developed *in vivo* may no longer be represented accurately by the analysis of granulosa cells during IVF. Nonetheless, one must acknowledge that granulosa cell studies may provide invaluable clues into their roles and potential regulation of oocyte quality.

The cumulus cells are the second type of somatic cell having potential use as biomarkers of oocyte quality. These cells are typically left intact during conventional insemination cycles, but undergo dispersal during overnight incubation with sperm, after which they are mechanically removed. There are two occasions when studies collect and analyze cumulus cells: postinsemination or pre-ICSI following the enzymatic and mechanical removal of cumulus cells. In the first case, the cumulus cells are alas not pristine since they may be contaminated by sperm cells. Their assessment may also be confounded by a superimposed period of *in vitro* culture for up to 24 h, thereby no longer accurately representing the developmental potential of the oocyte. Also, a large number of embryology laboratories do not inseminate COCs singly but rather in groups of 2–4, thereby eliminating any possibility of direct correlation of a cumulus cell biomarker from a given COC with the quality of its associated oocyte. In contrast, cumulus cells obtained prior to ICSI can be obtained within a few hours of retrieval, washed free of contaminants, and readily tracked to the fate of a single oocyte, early embryo, and fetus. As to the types of evaluations, these include gene expression patterns in cumulus cells (see Sect. 3.2.2). The growth patterns of cultured cumulus cells have also been considered, with the analysis of their cell proliferation and death properties (19, 31, 160, 161). For instance, Host et al. (31) put forth an association between more apoptosis in cumulus cells and subsequent quality of the associated oocyte, based on compromised clinical outcomes. Unfortunately, these studies remain extremely preliminary and of weak predictive value. This is despite the indisputable influences of cumulus cells on the oocyte as evidenced by animal studies (see Sect. 2.1.1); also of importance may be the consideration that not all cumulus cells within a COC are created equal, as documented by the detection of gradients of apoptotic activities in the various cumulus layers of bovine COCs (162).

A last set of samples that is routinely discarded in the clinic are all of the culture media, which were "conditioned" or "spent" by eggs or embryos. It is important to note that, to date, testing has focused on insemination and embryo culture media in an attempt to relate biomarkers to embryo, and thus, by inference, oocyte quality. Directly analyzing the conditioned media of unfertilized oocytes presents additional challenges because the cells are cultured for a relatively short time before insemination or injection. The minute amount of products that may be detectable is a likely limitation, but the additional time that can be allotted for analysis (that is prior to embryo transfer) is a definite advantage of oocyte analyses. Nevertheless, the evaluation of embryo conditioned media is a reasonable approach given that the health of the embryo ultimately depends on the initial quality of the oocyte, thereby underlying the future development of the resulting fetus. Analyses of embryo conditioned media range from assessment of specific potential candidates to profiling using high-throughput mass spectrometry.

Initial studies on soluble human leukocyte antigen G (HLA-G) pinpointed the likely need to examine more than one predicting factor out of the embryo secretome (163). The use of high-throughput mass spectrometry methodologies was reported in embryo spent media for the initial detection of novel protein candidates (164), all of which necessitate later confirmation with other more specific technologies (e.g., immunoassays). The results to date are still preliminary and illustrate a need for further validation of the employed methodologies, successful and independent use by multiple laboratories, and demonstration of powerful predictor values (165, 166).

Regarding the direct analysis of conditioned media from cultured COCs on the day of retrieval, Cecconi et al. (20) tested its use in conjunction with COC grading and evaluation of cell morphology. The presence of a 31-kDa band correlated with conception cycles, thereby suggesting that analyzing the secretome of cumulus cells may prove of superior predictive value when compared to mere morphological assessment. Animal studies also support the relevance of measuring molecules secreted by the oocyte as predictors of oocyte quality (11, 167). Given the known influence of cumulus cell- and oocyte-secreted factors on the normal function of the COC (11), studies targeting the secretome of cumulus cells and/or the oocyte should come as no surprise.

When it comes to monitoring the oocyte noninvasively and safely, techniques are still limited and our incomplete understanding of oocyte biology still precludes the development and implementation of novel assays. That acknowledged, efforts are already under way to assess the physiology of the oocyte using technologies that, for instance, permit the output of certain metabolites in the surrounding milieu or, conversely, their depletion. To date, studies focused on cultured mouse embryos and their oxygen/glucose consumption, lactate production, and amino acid turnover (168, 169). Together, these markers indicate that a "quieter" rather than a more "active" metabolism is associated with improved embryo viability (170). The noninvasive measurements of respiration rates also permit the identification of embryos of good quality (171). Technologies for the characterization of oocyte physiology at the single-cell level are still highly complex, require a certain level of expertise, and are neither available nor yet validated for routine use in the ART laboratory. Clearly, these are exciting and innovative areas of future product development and testing. Previous studies point towards the relevance of evaluating the metabolic states of oocytes following retrieval (172). While current efforts focus on profiling the metabolomes of human embryos, such knowledge and technological developments will surely impact oocyte studies, particularly ones that will rely on oocyte spent media samples.

In summary, noninvasive assessments will permit the identification of abnormalities and the preselection of the best quality oocytes. Despite the many potential directions explored to date, there still remain technological advances to apply, improve on, and test through large cohort randomized controlled studies that will compare clinical outcomes with or without the use of noninvasive predictors.

### 3.2.2 Gene Expression and Microarray Studies

Despite all of the undeniable and practical advantages of noninvasive oocyte assessment, including analyses of secretomes and metabolomes, invaluable information may be gained from invasive, yet complementary, gene expression studies. Indeed, only when relevant molecular pathways and players are identified, may future efforts zero in on their noninvasive evaluations. In the meantime, gene expression and microarray studies are also being applied to oocytes and cumulus cells, with the latter sample type analyzed without compromising current laboratory practices.

Initial reports performed gene microarray analyses of human oocytes that vary in their meiotic and/or developmental competences. Although these studies are preliminary and notes of caution remain as to the origin and thus informative nature of the human oocytes, there is support for significant variation in gene expression levels. For instance, *in vitro* and *in vivo* matured human oocytes (known to diverge in their developmental competencies) display differences in the groups of genes that they express (173, 174). Instances of differentially expressed gene families include ones involved in gene expression, cell cycle regulation, transport, cell organization, metabolism, and signaling. Gene profiling of human and animal oocytes also identified new cumulus- and oocyte-specific genes that may prove of developmental relevance (175, 176). Oocytes from older women represent another example of gametes that harbor compromised quality in conjunction with significant changes in gene expression profiles (177). Taken together, all of the emerging microarray studies have identified relevant and new targets to the evaluation and management of oocyte health.

As in the case of oocytes, microarray studies in cumulus cells promise to complement hypothesis-driven efforts; many of these have already identified a growing list of gene markers that may relate to the quality of oocytes. To date, recurring cumulus cell gene groups with potential predictive value include ones related to paracrine signaling, the cumulus matrix, and hypoxia (178–181). A microarray analysis of human granulosa cells also identified a subset of genes (mostly involved in steroidogenesis) with differential expressions depending on the pregnancy outcome (182).

Extending and often confirmatory of microarray profiles are reports that carefully analyze candidate genes (in oocytes and/or cumulus cells), their dynamic expression, and potential prognostic value in terms of oocyte competence. Some of these studies have already undergone testing in an ART setting and in relation to embryo outcomes (178, 181, 183). To date, most studies focus on analysis at the mRNA transcript level, largely because of available technologies and the ability to amplify the very little amount of samples available. However, there are clear benefits to profiling the proteome of oocytes and cumulus cells (184), particularly since the final gene products are the ones that carry out cellular functions, and posttranscriptional regulation is a common process in female gametes. Proteomic findings are currently preliminary and seriously limited by sensitivity, quantification, and sample needs. Lastly, future studies must focus on not only the assessment of individual gene marker or gene families, but also the use of a systems biology approach in order to avoid any bias and unwanted omissions in our quest for oocyte quality predictors.

## 4 Conclusions

The central role of oocyte competence in determining embryo developmental fate has spurred an extensive search for reliable predictors of oocyte quality. Attempts to characterize morphological attributes associated with oocyte quality have achieved very limited success. Among all of the morphological, cellular, and molecular parameters presented above, a pivotal overarching theme is our need to characterize a "normal" oocyte. From this platform, we will then be positioned to develop diagnostic methodologies to detect oocyte abnormalities. Insight into the subcellular nature of oocyte abnormalities and into the mechanisms that lead to aberrant oocyte maturation has only recently began to unfold. The understanding of cellular and molecular basis of morphological characteristics will allow the identification of reliable predictors of oocyte quality. In the absence of a comprehensive oocyte grading scheme, the power of morphological observations to aid oocyte/embryo selection is reduced.

Technologies should be tailored towards detecting the abnormal. Many challenges remain ahead but excitingly, several paths have now been paved towards much-awaited breakthroughs in the detection of oocytes exhibiting compromised quality.

## References


1. Sorensen RA, Wassarman PM. Relationship between growth and meiotic maturation of the mouse oocyte. Dev Biol 1976; 50(2):531–6.
2. Abbott AL, Ducibella T. Calcium and the control of mammalian cortical granule exocytosis. Front Biosci 2001;6: D792–806.
3. Schroeder AC, Eppig JJ. The developmental capacity of mouse oocytes that matured spontaneously in vitro is normal. Dev Biol 1984;102(2):493–7.
4. Coticchio G, Sereni E, Serrao L, Mazzone S, Iadarola I, Borini A. What criteria for the definition of oocyte quality? Ann N Y Acad Sci 2004;1034:132–44.
5. Combelles CM, Racowsky C. Assessment and optimization of oocyte quality during assisted reproductive technology treatment. Semin Reprod Med 2005;23(3):277–84.
6. Patrizio P, Bianchi V, Lalioti MD, Gerasimova T, Sakkas D. High rate of biological loss in assisted reproduction: it is in the seed, not in the soil. Reprod Biomed Online 2007;14(1): 92–5.
7. Sugiura K, Pendola FL, Eppig JJ. Oocyte control of metabolic cooperativity between oocytes and companion granulosa cells: energy metabolism. Dev Biol 2005;279(1):20–30.
8. Hussein TS, Thompson JG, Gilchrist RB. Oocyte-secreted factors enhance oocyte developmental competence. Dev Biol 2006;296(2):514–21.
9. Su YQ, Sugiura K, Wigglesworth K, et al. Oocyte regulation of metabolic cooperativity between mouse cumulus cells and oocytes: BMP15 and GDF9 control cholesterol biosynthesis in cumulus cells. Development 2008;135(1):111–21.
10. Matzuk MM, Burns KH, Viveiros MM, Eppig JJ. Intercellular communication in the mammalian ovary: oocytes carry the conversation. Science 2002;296(5576):2178–80.
11. Gilchrist RB, Lane M, Thompson JG. Oocyte-secreted factors: regulators of cumulus cell function and oocyte quality. Hum Reprod Update 2008;14(2):159–77.
12. Gilchrist RB, Ritter LJ, Armstrong DT. Oocyte-somatic cell interactions during follicle development in mammals. Anim Reprod Sci 2004;82–83:431–46.
13. Albertini DF, Combelles CM, Benecchi E, Carabatsos MJ. Cellular basis for paracrine regulation of ovarian follicle development. Reproduction 2001;121(5):647–53.
14. Kidder GM, Mhawi AA. Gap junctions and ovarian folliculogenesis. Reproduction 2002;123(5):613–20.
15. Simon AM, Goodenough DA, Li E, Paul DL. Female infertility in mice lacking connexin 37. Nature 1997;385(6616): 525–9.
16. Knight PG, Glister C. TGF-beta superfamily members and ovarian follicle development. Reproduction 2006;132(2): 191–206.
17. Zhuo L, Kimata K. Cumulus oophorus extracellular matrix: its construction and regulation. Cell Struct Funct 2001; 26(4):189–96.
18. Russell DL, Salustri A. Extracellular matrix of the cumulus-oocyte complex. Semin Reprod Med 2006;24(4):217–27.
19. Gregory L, Booth AD, Wells C, Walker SM. A study of the cumulus-corona cell complex in in-vitro fertilization and embryo transfer; a prognostic indicator of the failure of implantation. Hum Reprod 1994;9(7):1308–17.
20. Cecconi S, Rossi G, Gualtieri R, Talevi R. Presence of a 31-kD protein band in human cumulus – corona radiata – conditioned media and pregnancy outcome. Fertil Steril 2001;75(5):966–72.
21. Rattanachaiyanont M, Leader A, Leveille MC. Lack of correlation between oocyte-corona-cumulus complex morphology and nuclear maturity of oocytes collected in stimulated cycles for intracytoplasmic sperm injection. Fertil Steril 1999;71(5):937–40.
22. Ng ST, Chang TH, Wu TC. Prediction of the rates of fertilization, cleavage, and pregnancy success by cumulus-coronal morphology in an in vitro fertilization program. Fertil Steril 1999;72(3):412–7.
23. De Vos A, Van de Velde H, Joris H, Van Steirteghem A. In-vitro matured metaphase-I oocytes have a lower fertilization rate but similar embryo quality as mature metaphase-II oocytes after intracytoplasmic sperm injection. Hum Reprod 1999;14(7):1859–63.
24. Chen SU, Chen HF, Lien YR, Ho HN, Chang HC, Yang YS. Schedule to inject in vitro matured oocytes may increase pregnancy after intracytoplasmic sperm injection. Arch Androl 2000;44(3):197–205.
25. Strassburger D, Friedler S, Raziel A, Kasterstein E, Schachter M, Ron-El R. The outcome of ICSI of immature MI oocytes and rescued in vitro matured MII oocytes. Hum Reprod 2004;19(7):1587–90.
26. Vanhoutte L, De Sutter P, Van der Elst J, Dhont M. Clinical benefit of metaphase I oocytes. Reprod Biol Endocrinol 2005;3:71.
27. Rankin T, Soyal S, Dean J. The mouse zona pellucida: folliculogenesis, fertility and pre-implantation development. Mol Cell Endocrinol 2000;163(1–2):21–5.
28. Rankin TL, O'Brien M, Lee E, Wigglesworth K, Eppig J, Dean J. Defective zonae pellucidae in Zp2-null mice disrupt folliculogenesis, fertility and development. Development 2001;128(7):1119–26.
29. Cohen J, Inge KL, Suzman M, Wiker SR, Wright G. Videocinematography of fresh and cryopreserved embryos: a retrospective analysis of embryonic morphology and implantation. Fertil Steril 1989;51(5):820–7.
30. Bertrand E, Van den Bergh M, Englert Y. Does zona pellucida thickness influence the fertilization rate? Hum Reprod 1995;10(5):1189–93.
31. Host E, Gabrielsen A, Lindenberg S, Smidt-Jensen S. Apoptosis in human cumulus cells in relation to zona pellucida thickness variation, maturation stage, and cleavage of the corresponding oocyte after intracytoplasmic sperm injection. Fertil Steril 2002;77(3):511–5.
32. Gabrielsen A, Bhatnager PR, Petersen K, Lindenberg S. Influence of zona pellucida thickness of human embryos on clinical pregnancy outcome following in vitro fertilization treatment. J Assist Reprod Genet 2000;17(6):323–8.

33. Gabrielsen A, Lindenberg S, Petersen K. The impact of the zona pellucida thickness variation of human embryos on pregnancy outcome in relation to suboptimal embryo development. A prospective randomized controlled study. Hum Reprod 2001;16(10):2166–70.
34. Pelletier C, Keefe DL, Trimarchi JR. Noninvasive polarized light microscopy quantitatively distinguishes the multilaminar structure of the zona pellucida of living human eggs and embryos. Fertil Steril 2004;81 Suppl 1:850–6.
35. Shen Y, Stalf T, Mehnert C, Eichenlaub-Ritter U, Tinneberg HR. High magnitude of light retardation by the zona pellucida is associated with conception cycles. Hum Reprod 2005;20(6):1596–606.
36. Rama Raju GA, Prakash GJ, Krishna KM, Madan K. Meiotic spindle and zona pellucida characteristics as predictors of embryonic development: a preliminary study using Polscope imaging. Reprod Biomed Online 2007;14(2): 166–74.
37. Bertrand E, Van den Bergh M, Englert Y. Clinical parameters influencing human zona pellucida thickness. Fertil Steril 1996;66(3):408–11.
38. Familiari G, Relucenti M, Heyn R, Micara G, Correr S. Three-dimensional structure of the zona pellucida at ovulation. Microsc Res Tech 2006;69(6):415–26.
39. Ebner T, Shebl O, Moser M, Sommergruber M, Tews G. Developmental fate of ovoid oocytes. Hum Reprod 2008; 23(1):62–6.
40. Edi-Osagie E, Hooper L, Seif MW. The impact of assisted hatching on live birth rates and outcomes of assisted conception: a systematic review. Hum Reprod 2003;18(9): 1828–35.
41. De Vos A, Van Steirteghem A. Zona hardening, zona drilling and assisted hatching: new achievements in assisted reproduction. Cells Tissues Organs 2000;166(2):220–7.
42. Germond M, Primi MP, Senn A. Hatching: how to select the clinical indications. Ann N Y Acad Sci 2004;1034:145–51.
43. Talbot P, Dandekar P. Perivitelline space: does it play a role in blocking polyspermy in mammals? Microsc Res Tech 2003;61(4):349–57.
44. Xia P. Intracytoplasmic sperm injection: correlation of oocyte grade based on polar body, perivitelline space and cytoplasmic inclusions with fertilization rate and embryo quality. Hum Reprod 1997;12(8):1750–5.
45. De Sutter P, Dozortsev D, Qian C, Dhont M. Oocyte morphology does not correlate with fertilization rate and embryo quality after intracytoplasmic sperm injection. Hum Reprod 1996;11(3):595–7.
46. Balaban B, Urman B, Sertac A, Alatas C, Aksoy S, Mercan R. Oocyte morphology does not affect fertilization rate, embryo quality and implantation rate after intracytoplasmic sperm injection. Hum Reprod 1998;13(12):3431–3.
47. Plachot M, Selva J, Wolf JP, Bastit P, de Mouzon J. [Consequences of oocyte dysmorphy on the fertilization rate and embryo development after intracytoplasmic sperm injection. A prospective multicenter study]. Gynecol Obstet Fertil 2002;30(10):772–9.
48. Ten J, Mendiola J, Vioque J, de Juan J, Bernabeu R. Donor oocyte dysmorphisms and their influence on fertilization and embryo quality. Reprod Biomed Online 2007;14(1):40–8.
49. Kapur RP, Johnson LV. Selective sequestration of an oviductal fluid glycoprotein in the perivitelline space of mouse oocytes and embryos. J Exp Zool 1986;238(2):249–60.
50. Dandekar P, Talbot P. Perivitelline space of mammalian oocytes: extracellular matrix of unfertilized oocytes and formation of a cortical granule envelope following fertilization. Mol Reprod Dev 1992;31(2):135–43.
51. Buhi WC. Characterization and biological roles of oviduct-specific, oestrogen-dependent glycoprotein. Reproduction 2002;123(3):355–62.
52. Eichenlaub-Ritter U, Schmiady H, Kentenich H, Soewarto D. Recurrent failure in polar body formation and premature chromosome condensation in oocytes from a human patient: indicators of asynchrony in nuclear and cytoplasmic maturation. Hum Reprod 1995;10(9):2343–9.
53. Ebner T, Moser M, Sommergruber M, Yaman C, Pfleger U, Tews G. First polar body morphology and blastocyst formation rate in ICSI patients. Hum Reprod 2002;17(9):2415–8.
54. Ebner T, Moser M, Yaman C, Feichtinger O, Hartl J, Tews G. Elective transfer of embryos selected on the basis of first polar body morphology is associated with increased rates of implantation and pregnancy. Fertil Steril 1999;72(4):599–603.
55. Ebner T, Yaman C, Moser M, Sommergruber M, Feichtinger O, Tews G. Prognostic value of first polar body morphology on fertilization rate and embryo quality in intracytoplasmic sperm injection. Hum Reprod 2000;15(2):427–30.
56. Ciotti PM, Notarangelo L, Morselli-Labate AM, Felletti V, Porcu E, Venturoli S. First polar body morphology before ICSI is not related to embryo quality or pregnancy rate. Hum Reprod 2004;19(10):2334–9.
57. De Santis L, Cino I, Rabellotti E, et al. Polar body morphology and spindle imaging as predictors of oocyte quality. Reprod Biomed Online 2005;11(1):36–42.
58. Verlinsky Y, Lerner S, Illkevitch N, et al. Is there any predictive value of first polar body morphology for embryo genotype or developmental potential? Reprod Biomed Online 2003;7(3):336–41.
59. Gitlin SA, Gibbons WE, Gosden RG. Oocyte biology and genetics revelations from polar bodies. Reprod Biomed Online 2003;6(4):403–9.
60. Munne S. Preimplantation genetic diagnosis of structural abnormalities. Mol Cell Endocrinol 2001;183 Suppl 1:S55–8.
61. Eppig JJ. Coordination of nuclear and cytoplasmic oocyte maturation in eutherian mammals. Reprod Fertil Dev 1996;8(4):485–9.
62. Hu Y, Betzendahl I, Cortvrindt R, Smitz J, Eichenlaub-Ritter U. Effects of low O2 and ageing on spindles and chromosomes in mouse oocytes from pre-antral follicle culture. Hum Reprod 2001;16(4):737–48.
63. Van Blerkom J, Antczak M, Schrader R. The developmental potential of the human oocyte is related to the dissolved oxygen content of follicular fluid: association with vascular endothelial growth factor levels and perifollicular blood flow characteristics. Hum Reprod 1997;12(5):1047–55.
64. Van Blerkom J, Henry G. Oocyte dysmorphism and aneuploidy in meiotically mature human oocytes after ovarian stimulation. Hum Reprod 1992;7(3):379–90.
65. Kahraman S, Yakin K, Donmez E, et al. Relationship between granular cytoplasm of oocytes and pregnancy outcome following intracytoplasmic sperm injection. Hum Reprod 2000;15(11):2390–3.
66. Ebner T, Moser M, Sommergruber M, Tews G. Selection based on morphological assessment of oocytes and embryos at different stages of preimplantation development: a review. Hum Reprod Update 2003;9(3):251–62.

67. Van Blerkom J. Occurrence and developmental consequences of aberrant cellular organization in meiotically mature human oocytes after exogenous ovarian hyperstimulation. J Electron Microsc Tech 1990;16(4):324–46.
68. El Shafie M, Sousa M, Windt ML, Kruger TF. Ultrastructure of human oocytes: a transmission electron microscopic view. In: El Shafie M, Sousa M, Windt ML, Kruger TF, eds. An Atlas of the Ultrastructure of Human Oocytes: A Guide for Assisted Reproduction. New York, London: Parthenon; 2000:151–71.
69. Nayudu PL, Lopata A, Jones GM, et al. An analysis of human oocytes and follicles from stimulated cycles: oocyte morphology and associated follicular fluid characteristics. Hum Reprod 1989;4(5):558–67.
70. Alikani M, Palermo G, Adler A, Bertoli M, Blake M, Cohen J. Intracytoplasmic sperm injection in dysmorphic human oocytes. Zygote 1995;3(4):283–8.
71. Loutradis D, Drakakis P, Kallianidis K, Milingos S, Dendrinos S, Michalas S. Oocyte morphology correlates with embryo quality and pregnancy rate after intracytoplasmic sperm injection. Fertil Steril 1999;72(2):240–4.
72. Otsuki J, Okada A, Morimoto K, Nagai Y, Kubo H. The relationship between pregnancy outcome and smooth endoplasmic reticulum clusters in MII human oocytes. Hum Reprod 2004;19(7):1591–7.
73. Van der Auwera I, D'Hooghe T. Superovulation of female mice delays embryonic and fetal development. Hum Reprod 2001;16(6):1237–43.
74. Kuliev A, Cieslak J, Verlinsky Y. Frequency and distribution of chromosome abnormalities in human oocytes. Cytogenet Genome Res 2005;111(3–4):193–8.
75. Rosenbusch BE, Schneider M. Cytogenetic analysis of human oocytes remaining unfertilized after intracytoplasmic sperm injection. Fertil Steril 2006;85(2):302–7.
76. Pacchierotti F, Adler ID, Eichenlaub-Ritter U, Mailhes JB. Gender effects on the incidence of aneuploidy in mammalian germ cells. Environ Res 2007;104(1):46–69.
77. Munne S. Chromosome abnormalities and their relationship to morphology and development of human embryos. Reprod Biomed Online 2006;12(2):234–53.
78. Hassold T, Jacobs PA, Leppert M, Sheldon M. Cytogenetic and molecular studies of trisomy 13. J Med Genet 1987; 24(12):725–32.
79. Angell R. First-meiotic-division nondisjunction in human oocytes. Am J Hum Genet 1997;61(1):23–32.
80. Dailey T, Dale B, Cohen J, Munne S. Association between nondisjunction and maternal age in meiosis-II human oocytes. Am J Hum Genet 1996;59(1):176–84.
81. Battaglia DE, Goodwin P, Klein NA, Soules MR. Influence of maternal age on meiotic spindle assembly in oocytes from naturally cycling women. Hum Reprod 1996;11(10):2217–22.
82. Gardner RD, Burke DJ. The spindle checkpoint: two transitions, two pathways. Trends Cell Biol 2000;10(4):154–8.
83. Hodges CA, Ilagan A, Jennings D, Keri R, Nilson J, Hunt PA. Experimental evidence that changes in oocyte growth influence meiotic chromosome segregation. Hum Reprod 2002;17(5):1171–80.
84. Jones KT. Meiosis in oocytes: predisposition to aneuploidy and its increased incidence with age. Hum Reprod Update 2008;14(2):143–58.
85. Yin H, Baart E, Betzendahl I, Eichenlaub-Ritter U. Diazepam induces meiotic delay, aneuploidy and predivision of homologues and chromatids in mammalian oocytes. Mutagenesis 1998;13(6):567–80.
86. Yin H, Cukurcam S, Betzendahl I, Adler ID, Eichenlaub-Ritter U. Trichlorfon exposure, spindle aberrations and nondisjunction in mammalian oocytes. Chromosoma 1998;107(6–7):514–22.
87. Wang WH, Meng L, Hackett RJ, Keefe DL. Developmental ability of human oocytes with or without birefringent spindles imaged by Polscope before insemination. Hum Reprod 2001;16(7):1464–8.
88. Moon JH, Hyun CS, Lee SW, Son WY, Yoon SH, Lim JH. Visualization of the metaphase II meiotic spindle in living human oocytes using the Polscope enables the prediction of embryonic developmental competence after ICSI. Hum Reprod 2003;18(4):817–20.
89. Rienzi L, Ubaldi F, Martinez F, et al. Relationship between meiotic spindle location with regard to the polar body position and oocyte developmental potential after ICSI. Hum Reprod 2003;18(6):1289–93.
90. Navarro PA, Liu L, Trimarchi JR, Ferriani RA, Keefe DL. Noninvasive imaging of spindle dynamics during mammalian oocyte activation. Fertil Steril 2005;83 Suppl 1:1197–205.
91. Keefe D, Liu L, Wang W, Silva C. Imaging meiotic spindles by polarization light microscopy: principles and applications to IVF. Reprod Biomed Online 2003;7(1):24–9.
92. Eichenlaub-Ritter U, Shen Y, Tinneberg HR. Manipulation of the oocyte: possible damage to the spindle apparatus. Reprod Biomed Online 2002;5(2):117–24.
93. Bavister BD, Squirrell JM. Mitochondrial distribution and function in oocytes and early embryos. Hum Reprod 2000;15 Suppl 2:189–98.
94. Sun QY, Wu GM, Lai L, et al. Translocation of active mitochondria during pig oocyte maturation, fertilization and early embryo development in vitro. Reproduction 2001; 122(1):155–63.
95. Brevini TA, Vassena R, Francisci C, Gandolfi F. Role of adenosine triphosphate, active mitochondria, and microtubules in the acquisition of developmental competence of parthenogenetically activated pig oocytes. Biol Reprod 2005;72(5):1218–23.
96. Au HK, Yeh TS, Kao SH, Tzeng CR, Hsieh RH. Abnormal mitochondrial structure in human unfertilized oocytes and arrested embryos. Ann N Y Acad Sci 2005;1042:177–85.
97. Santos TA, El Shourbagy S, St John JC. Mitochondrial content reflects oocyte variability and fertilization outcome. Fertil Steril 2006;85(3):584–91.
98. Hsieh RH, Tsai NM, Au HK, Chang SJ, Wei YH, Tzeng CR. Multiple rearrangements of mitochondrial DNA in unfertilized human oocytes. Fertil Steril 2002;77(5):1012–7.
99. Gibson TC, Kubisch HM, Brenner CA. Mitochondrial DNA deletions in rhesus macaque oocytes and embryos. Mol Hum Reprod 2005;11(11):785–9.
100. Slotte H, Gustafson O, Nylund L, Pousette A. ATP and ADP in human pre-embryos. Hum Reprod 1990;5(3):319–22.
101. Van Blerkom J, Davis PW, Lee J. ATP content of human oocytes and developmental potential and outcome after in-vitro fertilization and embryo transfer. Hum Reprod 1995;10(2):415–24.
102. Wilding M, Dale B, Marino M, et al. Mitochondrial aggregation patterns and activity in human oocytes and preimplantation embryos. Hum Reprod 2001;16(5):909–17.

103. Zeng HT, Ren Z, Yeung WS, et al. Low mitochondrial DNA and ATP contents contribute to the absence of birefringent spindle imaged with Polscope in in vitro matured human oocytes. Hum Reprod 2007;22(6):1681–6.
104 Rawe VY, Chemes HE. Exploring the cytoskeleton after intracytoplasmic sperm injection in humans. Methods Mol Biol 2009;518:1–18.
105. Navara CS, Wu GJ, Simerly C, Schatten G. Mammalian model systems for exploring cytoskeletal dynamics during fertilization. Curr Top Dev Biol 1995;31:321–42.
106. Szollosi D, Calarco P, Donahue RP. Absence of centrioles in the first and second meiotic spindles of mouse oocytes. J Cell Sci 1972;11(2):521–41.
107. Maro B, Howlett SK, Webb M. Non-spindle microtubule organizing centers in metaphase II-arrested mouse oocytes. J Cell Biol 1985;101(5 Pt 1):1665–72.
108. Kim NH, Funahashi H, Prather RS, Schatten G, Day BN. Microtubule and microfilament dynamics in porcine oocytes during meiotic maturation. Mol Reprod Dev 1996;43(2):248–55.
109. Le Guen P, Crozet N. Microtubule and centrosome distribution during sheep fertilization. Eur J Cell Biol 1989;48(2):239–49.
110. Long CR, Pinto-Correia C, Duby RT, et al. Chromatin and microtubule morphology during the first cell cycle in bovine zygotes. Mol Reprod Dev 1993;36(1):23–32.
111. Merdes A, Cleveland DW. Pathways of spindle pole formation: different mechanisms; conserved components. J Cell Biol 1997;138(5):953–6.
112. Barton NR, Goldstein LS. Going mobile: microtubule motors and chromosome segregation. Proc Natl Acad Sci U S A 1996;93(5):1735–42.
113. Simerly C, Dominko T, Navara C, et al. Molecular correlates of primate nuclear transfer failures. Science 2003;300(5617):297.
114. Simerly C, Navara C, Hyun SH, et al. Embryogenesis and blastocyst development after somatic cell nuclear transfer in nonhuman primates: overcoming defects caused by meiotic spindle extraction. Dev Biol 2004;276(2):237–52.
115. Hall VJ, Compton D, Stojkovic P, et al. Developmental competence of human in vitro aged oocytes as host cells for nuclear transfer. Hum Reprod 2007;22(1):52–62.
116. Rawe VY, Espanol AJ, Nodar F, Brugo-Olmedo S. Mammalian oocyte maturation and microtubule-associated proteins dynamics. Fert Ster Suppl 2005;84 Suppl 1:S143.
117. Blake D, Proctor M, Johnson N, Olive D. Cleavage stage versus blastocyst stage embryo transfer in assisted conception. Cochrane Database Syst Rev 2005;(4):CD002118.
118. Veeck LL, Wortham JW, Jr., Witmyer J, et al. Maturation and fertilization of morphologically immature human oocytes in a program of in vitro fertilization. Fertil Steril 1983;39(5):594–602.
119. Nagy ZP, Cecile J, Liu J, Loccufier A, Devroey P, Van Steirteghem A. Pregnancy and birth after intracytoplasmic sperm injection of in vitro matured germinal-vesicle stage oocytes: case report. Fertil Steril 1996;65(5):1047–50.
120. Combelles CM, Cekleniak NA, Racowsky C, Albertini DF. Assessment of nuclear and cytoplasmic maturation in in-vitro matured human oocytes. Hum Reprod 2002;17(4): 1006–16.
121. Bergere M, Lombroso R, Gombault M, Wainer R, Selva J. An idiopathic infertility with oocytes metaphase I maturation block: case report. Hum Reprod 2001;16(10):2136–8.
122. Levran D, Farhi J, Nahum H, Glezerman M, Weissman A. Maturation arrest of human oocytes as a cause of infertility: case report. Hum Reprod 2002;17(6):1604–9.
123. Neal MS, Cowan L, Louis JP, Hughes E, King WA, Basrur PK. Cytogenetic evaluation of human oocytes that failed to complete meiotic maturation in vitro. Fertil Steril 2002; 77(4):844–5.
124. Schmiady H, Neitzel H. Arrest of human oocytes during meiosis I in two sisters of consanguineous parents: first evidence for an autosomal recessive trait in human infertility: case report. Hum Reprod 2002;17(10):2556–9.
125. Combelles CM, Albertini DF, Racowsky C. Distinct microtubule and chromatin characteristics of human oocytes after failed in-vivo and in-vitro meiotic maturation. Hum Reprod 2003;18(10):2124–30.
126. Lincoln AJ, Wickramasinghe D, Stein P, et al. Cdc25b phosphatase is required for resumption of meiosis during oocyte maturation. Nat Genet 2002;30(4):446–9.
127. Mrazek M, Fulka Jr J, Jr. Failure of oocyte maturation: possible mechanisms for oocyte maturation arrest. Hum Reprod 2003;18(11):2249–52.
128. Ben-Yosef D, Shalgi R. Oocyte activation: lessons from human infertility. Trends Mol Med 2001;7(4):163–9.
129. Ducibella T, Fissore R. The roles of Ca2+, downstream protein kinases, and oscillatory signaling in regulating fertilization and the activation of development. Dev Biol 2008;315(2):257–79.
130. Cheung A, Swann K, Carroll J. The ability to generate normal Ca(2+) transients in response to spermatozoa develops during the final stages of oocyte growth and maturation. Hum Reprod 2000;15(6):1389–95.
131. Martins OG, Pesty A, Gouveia-Oliveira A, Cidadao AJ, Plancha CE, Lefevre B. Oocyte Ca2+ spike acquisition during in vitro development of early preantral follicles: influence of age and hormonal supplementation. Zygote 2002;10(1):59–64.
132. Ducibella T, Schultz RM, Ozil JP. Role of calcium signals in early development. Semin Cell Dev Biol 2006;17(2): 324–32.
133. Ducibella T. The cortical reaction and development of activation competence in mammalian oocytes. Hum Reprod Update 1996;2(1):29–42.
134. Ducibella T, Matson S. Secretory mechanisms and ca(2+) signaling in gametes: similarities to regulated neuroendocrine secretion in somatic cells and involvement in emerging pathologies. Endocr Pathol 2007;18(4):191–203.
135. Ducibella T, Dubey A, Gross V, et al. A zona biochemical change and spontaneous cortical granule loss in eggs that fail to fertilize in in vitro fertilization. Fertil Steril 1995;64(6):1154–61.
136. Abbott AL, Xu Z, Kopf GS, Ducibella T, Schultz RM. In vitro culture retards spontaneous activation of cell cycle progression and cortical granule exocytosis that normally occur in in vivo unfertilized mouse eggs. Biol Reprod 1998;59(6):1515–21.
137. Miyara F, Aubriot FX, Glissant A, et al. Multiparameter analysis of human oocytes at metaphase II stage after IVF

failure in non-male infertility. Hum Reprod 2003;18(7): 1494–503.

138. Sun QY, Schatten H. Regulation of dynamic events by microfilaments during oocyte maturation and fertilization. Reproduction 2006;131(2):193–205.
139. Lee ST, Han HJ, Oh SJ, Lee EJ, Han JY, Lim JM. Influence of ovarian hyperstimulation and ovulation induction on the cytoskeletal dynamics and developmental competence of oocytes. Mol Reprod Dev 2006;73(8):1022–33.
140. Abbott AL, Fissore RA, Ducibella T. Incompetence of preovulatory mouse oocytes to undergo cortical granule exocytosis following induced calcium oscillations. Dev Biol 1999;207(1):38–48.
141. Abbott AL, Fissore RA, Ducibella T. Identification of a translocation deficiency in cortical granule secretion in preovulatory mouse oocytes. Biol Reprod 2001;65(6):1640–7.
142. Tanaka K. Molecular biology of proteasomes. Mol Biol Rep 1995;21(1):21–6.
143. Tanaka K, Yoshimura T, Ichihara A, Kameyama K, Takagi T. A high molecular weight protease in the cytosol of rat liver. II. Properties of the purified enzyme. J Biol Chem 1986;261(32):15204–7.
144. Wojcik C, Benchaib M, Lornage J, Czyba JC, Guerin JF. Proteasomes in human spermatozoa. Int J Androl 2000; 23(3):169–77.
145. Sutovsky P, Manandhar G, McCauley TC, et al. Proteasomal interference prevents zona pellucida penetration and fertilization in mammals. Biol Reprod 2004;71(5):1625–37.
146. Sutovsky P, McCauley TC, Sutovsky M, Day BN. Early degradation of paternal mitochondria in domestic pig (Sus scrofa) is prevented by selective proteasomal inhibitors lactacystin and MG132. Biol Reprod 2003;68(5):1793–800.
147. Rawe VY, Diaz ES, Abdelmassih R, et al. The role of sperm proteasomes during sperm aster formation and early zygote development: implications for fertilization failure in humans. Hum Reprod 2008;23(3):573–80.
148 Branzini C, Perez Tito L, Maggiotto G, Abdelmassih R, Wojcik C, Rawe VY. Proteasome dynamics during maturation and fertilization of human oocytes. Fert Ster Suppl 2007;Suppl 1:S297.
149 Etcheverry M, Wojcik C, Branzini MC, Abdelmassih S, Reis A, Rawe VY. Oocyte quality control and proteasomes in human oocytes, fertilization, and early embryo development. Fert Ster Suppl 2006;Suppl 2:S39.
150. Hanash S. Disease proteomics. Nature 2003;422(6928): 226–32.
151. Mendoza C, Ruiz-Requena E, Ortega E, et al. Follicular fluid markers of oocyte developmental potential. Hum Reprod 2002;17(4):1017–22.
152. Xia P, Younglai EV. Relationship between steroid concentrations in ovarian follicular fluid and oocyte morphology in patients undergoing intracytoplasmic sperm injection (ICSI) treatment. J Reprod Fertil 2000;118(2):229–33.
153. Wu YT, Tang L, Cai J, et al. High bone morphogenetic protein-15 level in follicular fluid is associated with high quality oocyte and subsequent embryonic development. Hum Reprod 2007;22(6):1526–31.
154. Thomas N, Goodacre R, Timmins EM, Gaudoin M, Fleming R. Fourier transform infrared spectroscopy of follicular fluids from large and small antral follicles. Hum Reprod 2000;15(8):1667–71.
155. Kim YS, Kim MS, Lee SH, et al. Proteomic analysis of recurrent spontaneous abortion: identification of an inadequately expressed set of proteins in human follicular fluid. Proteomics 2006;6(11):3445–54.
156. Schweigert FJ, Gericke B, Wolfram W, Kaisers U, Dudenhausen JW. Peptide and protein profiles in serum and follicular fluid of women undergoing IVF. Hum Reprod 2006;21(11):2960–8.
157. Hanrieder J, Nyakas A, Naessen T, Bergquist J. Proteomic analysis of human follicular fluid using an alternative bottom-up approach. J Proteome Res 2008;7(1):443–9.
158. Oosterhuis GJ, Michgelsen HW, Lambalk CB, Schoemaker J, Vermes I. Apoptotic cell death in human granulosa-lutein cells: a possible indicator of in vitro fertilization outcome. Fertil Steril 1998;70(4):747–9.
159. Murphy BD. Models of luteinization. Biol Reprod 2000; 63(1):2–11.
160. Lee KS, Joo BS, Na YJ, Yoon MS, Choi OH, Kim WW. Cumulus cells apoptosis as an indicator to predict the quality of oocytes and the outcome of IVF-ET. J Assist Reprod Genet 2001;18(9):490–8.
161. Moffatt O, Drury S, Tomlinson M, Afnan M, Sakkas D. The apoptotic profile of human cumulus cells changes with patient age and after exposure to sperm but not in relation to oocyte maturity. Fertil Steril 2002;77(5):1006–11.
162. Hussein TS, Froiland DA, Amato F, Thompson JG, Gilchrist RB. Oocytes prevent cumulus cell apoptosis by maintaining a morphogenic paracrine gradient of bone morphogenetic proteins. J Cell Sci 2005;118(Pt 22):5257–68.
163. Katz-Jaffe MG, Gardner DK. Embryology in the era of proteomics. Theriogenology 2007;68 Suppl 1:S125–30.
164. Katz-Jaffe MG, Schoolcraft WB, Gardner DK. Analysis of protein expression (secretome) by human and mouse preimplantation embryos. Fertil Steril 2006;86(3):678–85.
165. Combelles CM, Racowsky C. Protein expression profiles of early embryos – an important step in the right direction: just not quite ready for prime time. Fertil Steril 2006;86(2):493; author reply.
166. Sargent I, Swales A, Ledee N, Kozma N, Tabiasco J, Le Bouteiller P. sHLA-G production by human IVF embryos: can it be measured reliably? J Reprod Immunol 2007;75(2): 128–32.
167. Vanderhyden BC, Caron PJ, Buccione R, Eppig JJ. Developmental pattern of the secretion of cumulus expansion-enabling factor by mouse oocytes and the role of oocytes in promoting granulosa cell differentiation. Dev Biol 1990;140(2):307–17.
168. Sturmey RG, Leese HJ. Energy metabolism in pig oocytes and early embryos. Reproduction 2003;126(2): 197–204.
169. Houghton FD, Leese HJ. Metabolism and developmental competence of the preimplantation embryo. Eur J Obstet Gynecol Reprod Biol 2004;115 Suppl 1:S92–6.
170. Leese HJ, Sturmey RG, Baumann CG, McEvoy TG. Embryo viability and metabolism: obeying the quiet rules. Hum Reprod 2007;22(12):3047–50.
171. Lopes AS, Greve T, Callesen H. Quantification of embryo quality by respirometry. Theriogenology 2007;67(1):21–31.
172. Singh R, Sinclair KD. Metabolomics: approaches to assessing oocyte and embryo quality. Theriogenology 2007;68 Suppl 1:S56–62.

173. Jones GM, Cram DS, Song B, et al. Gene expression profiling of human oocytes following in vivo or in vitro maturation. Hum Reprod 2008;23(5):1138–44.
174. Wells D, Patrizio P. Gene expression profiling of human oocytes at different maturational stages and after in vitro maturation. Am J Obstet Gynecol 2008;198(4):455 e1–9; discussion e9–11.
175. Yao J, Ren X, Ireland JJ, Coussens PM, Smith TP, Smith GW. Generation of a bovine oocyte cDNA library and microarray: resources for identification of genes important for follicular development and early embryogenesis. Physiol Genomics 2004;19(1):84–92.
176. Gasca S, Pellestor F, Assou S, et al. Identifying new human oocyte marker genes: a microarray approach. Reprod Biomed Online 2007;14(2):175–83.
177. Steuerwald NM, Bermudez MG, Wells D, Munne S, Cohen J. Maternal age-related differential global expression profiles observed in human oocytes. Reprod Biomed Online 2007;14(6):700–8.
178. Zhang X, Jafari N, Barnes RB, Confino E, Milad M, Kazer RR. Studies of gene expression in human cumulus cells indicate pentraxin 3 as a possible marker for oocyte quality. Fertil Steril 2005;83 Suppl 1:1169–79.
179. Cillo F, Brevini TA, Antonini S, Paffoni A, Ragni G, Gandolfi F. Association between human oocyte developmental competence and expression levels of some cumulus genes. Reproduction 2007;134(5):645–50.
180. Assidi M, Dufort I, Ali A, et al. Identification of potential markers of oocyte competence expressed in bovine cumulus cells matured with follicle-stimulating hormone and/or phorbol myristate acetate in vitro. Biol Reprod 2008;79(2):209–22.
181. van Montfoort AP, Geraedts JP, Dumoulin JC, Stassen AP, Evers JL, Ayoubi TA. Differential gene expression in cumulus cells as a prognostic indicator of embryo viability: a microarray analysis. Mol Hum Reprod 2008;14(3):157–68.
182. Hamel M, Dufort I, Robert C, et al. Identification of differentially expressed markers in human follicular cells associated with competent oocytes. Hum Reprod 2008; 23(5):1118–27.
183. McKenzie LJ, Pangas SA, Carson SA, et al. Human cumulus granulosa cell gene expression: a predictor of fertilization and embryo selection in women undergoing IVF. Hum Reprod 2004;19(12):2869–74.
184. Memili E, Peddinti D, Shack LA, et al. Bovine germinal vesicle oocyte and cumulus cell proteomics. Reproduction 2007;133(6):1107–20.

# In Vitro Maturation of Mammalian Oocytes

John J. Bromfield, Katie L. Jones, and David F. Albertini

**Abstract** Efforts to optimize oocyte quality as a result of *in vitro* maturation (IVM) are critical to achieving patient-specific success in assisted reproductive techniques. Traditional approaches to human IVM have been replaced by methodologies aimed at recapitulating the changing milieu of the ovulatory follicle following reception of signals initiated by LH. These include the deployment of sequential media changes that more accurately reflect the temporal shift in balance between biosynthetic and metabolic alterations that occur within the cumulus cells and their enclosed oocytes. Distinctions in cumulus cell physiology and gene expression in an *in vivo* and *in vitro* context are likely to serve as useful noninvasive biomarkers for the developmental potential of human oocytes that complete nuclear and cytoplasmic maturation under ex vivo conditions.

**Keywords** Oocyte • Germinal vesicle • Metabolic cooperation • Junctions • Cumulus oocyte complex cytoskeleton • Meiotic spindle • Chromosomes • Cell cycle

## 1 Introduction

The link between oocyte quality and the developmental capability of an embryo has long been appreciated. But exactly what properties in the oocyte, both prior to and following maturation, confer developmental competence to the conceptus has evaded rigorous definition until recently. What has become clear is that a protracted series of molecular and cellular modifications must occur during both the growth and maturation stages of oogenesis in mammals to realize successful preimplantation embryogenesis (1). While achieving ex vivo oogenesis is a novel and much sought after paradigm within emerging assisted reproductive techniques (ART), manipulating the final stages of oocyte maturation for purposes of embryo production has been at the heart of contemporary ART, originating with the classical studies of Edwards (2, 3). His work foresaw the need to develop and optimize cell culture techniques that would sustain oocyte maturation, and heralded 40 years of active research in animal and human systems. As the clinical application of *in vitro* maturation in human oocytes has entered the mainstream of ART, so too has the need to better understand the *in vivo* conditions that stimulate oocyte maturation during ovulation. Thus the purpose of this review is to outline recent evidence based on the physiology of ovulation and pose a series of questions that would allow for comparison of the quality of oocytes produced under *in vivo* and *in vitro* conditions. It is hoped that the concepts put forth here will stimulate further research designed to improve *in vitro* maturation for clinical applications.

### 1.1 Historical Considerations

Even before the classical studies of Edwards (2), there was ample evidence demonstrating the feasibility of *in vitro* maturation in mammalian oocytes based on the pioneering efforts of Pincus and his colleagues (4) (Table 1). Pincus' success in documenting the spontaneous maturation of rabbit oocytes from the germinal vesicle to metaphase-II stage of meiosis in culture

J.J. Bromfield, K.L. Jones, and D.F. Albertini (✉)
Center for Reproductive Sciences, Kansas University Medical Center, 3901 Rainbow Boulevard, Kansas City, KS, USA
e-mail: dalbertini@kumc.edu

D.T. Carrell et al. (eds.), *Biennial Review of Infertility*, DOI: 10.1007/978-1-60327-392-3_14

**Table 1** Historical milestones in development of IVM

| Author/Year | Observation | Ref. |
|---|---|---|
| Pincus and Enzmann, 1935 | Spontaneous maturation of rabbit oocytes | (4) |
| Rock and Menkin, 1944 | Spontaneous maturation of human oocytes | (5) |
| Edwards, 1965 | Spontaneous maturation is common amongst mammals | (3) |
| Biggers et al., 1967 | Oocyte metabolism depends on follicle cells | (6) |
| Cho et al., 1974 | cAMP blocks meiotic resumption | (7) |
| Anderson and Albertini, 1976 | Gap junctions connect oocyte and granulose cells in mammals | (8) |
| Schroeder and Eppig, 1984 | IVM in mice allows birth of live young | (9) |
| Downs et al. 1988 | Oocyte maturation can be induced by FSH and EGF | (10) |

prompted one of the first documented efforts to achieve IVM in the human. In 1944, Menkin and Rock (5) published what was debated to be the first "successful" IVF study in humans using aspirated follicular oocytes from the ovaries of women judged to be peri-ovulatory. They reported that in excess of 800 human oocytes were retrieved between 1938 and 1944 and were "bathed in Locke's solution and incubated in the patient's blood serum for 24 h to bring them to maturity." While many of these oocytes were observed to have matured based on the extrusion of a first polar body, it remains speculation as to whether or not any of these patients would have undergone an endogenous gonadotropin surge to influence these earliest results. Nevertheless, the concept that human oocytes could undergo spontaneous IVM was established.

From the outset, there was little doubt that traditional culture conditions would support at least nuclear maturation but short of carrying out IVF and embryo culture, evidence was lacking to support the idea that IVM oocytes from any animal species had acquired the necessary cytoplasmic properties that would support embryonic development. This barrier to further advances was in part dictated by the lack of information on the basic metabolism of the mammalian oocyte. Biggers et al. (6) were the first to study this problem and in the mouse, showed that metabolism of the mouse embryo was comparable to that of the oocytes in terms of using pyruvate as a preferred energy substrate, and more importantly, identified the source of this substrate as the follicle cells attached to the oocyte. This fundamental observation has withstood the test of time and laid the foundation for appreciating the extreme dependence of the embryo's metabolism upon energy resources derived from the companion cells of the cumulus oophorus. Following this work, a series of discoveries was made over the next 20 years in animal models that would set the stage for using human IVM (Table 1). These included identification of cAMP as a meiosis arresting agent (7), the discovery of gap junctions between oocytes and granulosa cells (8), the demonstration that mouse oocytes matured *in vitro* could develop to blastocysts and yield live young after IVF and embryo transfer (9), and the finding that even under conditions of meiotic arrest, FSH or EGF could promote IVM in mice with the resulting oocytes exhibiting higher developmental potential than oocytes matured in the absence of cumulus cells or hormonal supplements (10). Collectively, this body of knowledge established the notion that factors within the ovarian follicle suppressed spontaneous maturation using metabolic cooperation between the oocyte and granulosa cells, and that hormonal signals relieved this inhibition, supporting IVM in a fashion consistent with achieving conceptus developmental competence.

Concurrent with these substantive advances were initial (11, 12) and then later (13–15) attempts to undertake human IVM using explanted follicular oocytes cultured in a single medium for variable amounts of time. In 1997, Bavister and Boatman working with the rhesus monkey introduced the notion of deploying a sequential medium postulating that the needs and requirements for the oocyte and cumulus cells changed at successive stages of the maturation process (16). As will be discussed further, new information on the cascade of signals generated during ovulation suggests that indeed the microenvironment in which the oocyte undergoes final maturation is a changing one and will need to be tightly regulated under *in vitro* conditions to consistently and efficiently achieve full nuclear and cytoplasmic maturation (Fig. 1).

## 2 In Vivo Vs. In Vitro Maturation of Oocytes

### *2.1 A Revised Physiological Perspective of the Follicular Milieu*

Over the past 10 years, collective evidence from primarily rodent model systems has added complexity to our understanding of the intrafollicular sequence of

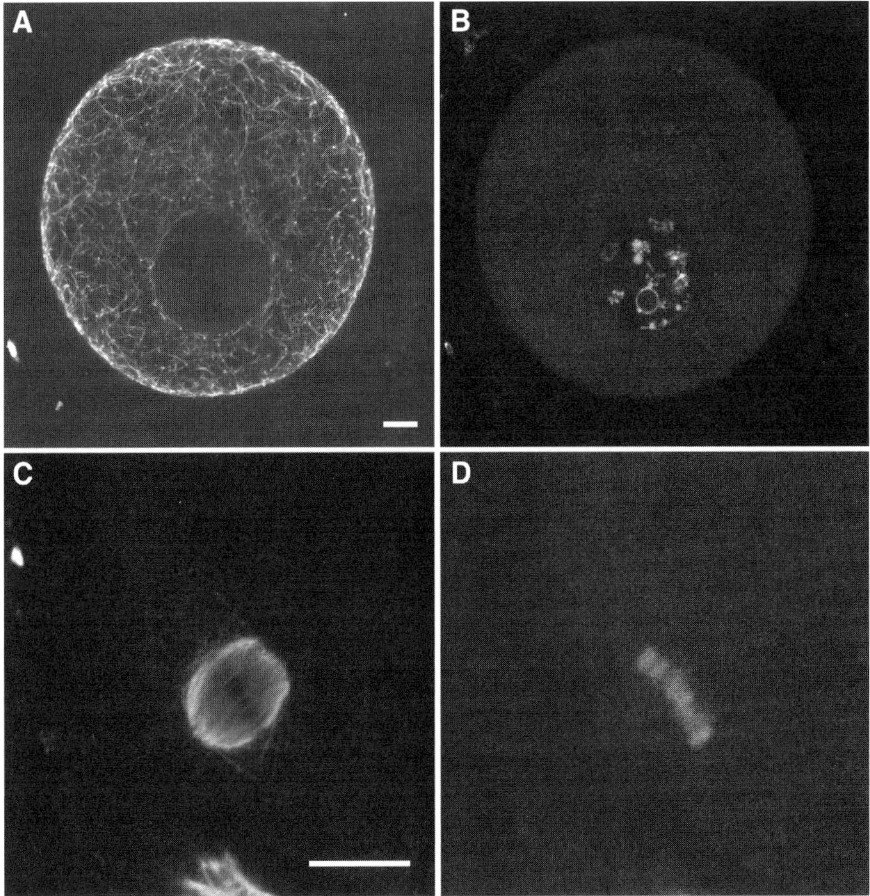


**Fig. 1 Configuration of immature germinal vesicle and MII stage human oocytes.** Confocal scanning microscopy of human oocytes at the germinal vesicle (A, B) and MII (C, D) stage. Germinal vesicle oocytes show an extensive tubulin network throughout the entire oocyte (**A**) and condensed chromatin within the germinal vesicle with a distinctive ring surrounding the nucleolus (**B**). MII stage oocytes display a well organized meiotic spindle with microtubules meeting at flattened poles adjacent to the oocyte cortex (**C**) with aligned chromatids along an equatorial plate (**D**). *Scale bars* represent 10 μm

events that are elicited by the LH surge during ovulation. Central to this new paradigm is the notion that a cascade of signaling steps brings about significant changes in the transcriptional activity of granulosa cells resulting in the synthesis and secretion of EGF-like molecules whose primary target is the cumulus oophorus (17, 18). Buttressed by the long-standing idea that the cumulus–oocyte complex is a highly integrated heterocellular syncytium, two key questions have remained that would mechanistically contribute to the problem of oocyte *in vitro* maturation. First, how is the switch from diplotene arrest into meiotic maturation triggered at the level of the oocyte? Second, how do cumulus cells participate in the resumption of meiosis and what role does this level of communication have in conferring cytoplasmic competency to the mature oocyte? These two questions lie at the heart of the technical and conceptual problems presently impeding optimization of IVM for human ARTs.

By tradition, and for lack of better alternatives, the inclusion of gonadotropins, steroids, growth factors, serum, and antioxidants has been used in the design of culture media to mimic what has been postulated to be an ex vivo environment within which immature oocytes could proceed through meiosis-I and progress through to metaphase of meiosis-II. However, it is not clear that persistent exposure to gonadotropins is beneficial in the context of cumulus–oocyte interactions during meiotic resumption or at later transition stages of oocyte maturation. In fact, many of the genes that direct the pathway of luteinization become transcriptionally activated within hours of LH treatment in mice and these seem sufficient to direct terminal differentiation of the mural cell compartment. Although we know little about the lifespan of ligand–receptor activation and stability during ovulation, persistent exposure in a culture setting is likely to bring about inappropriate signaling of a prolonged duration that interferes with the maintenance of structural integrity within the cumulus oophorus. In animal models, this condition directly impacts cell cycle progression during IVM and further results in a failure to maintain meiotic arrest at metaphase-II (19). Moreover, both clinical and research programs have now reached a consensus that excess gonadotropin brings about a reduction in oocyte quality further emphasizing the need to use hormone supplements judiciously in designing IVM protocols that would better mimic follicular physiology in the context of ovulation.

Thus, mapping of the transcriptional requirements for oocyte and follicular maturation *in vivo* has already identified a triggering rather than constitutive role for the peri-ovulatory gonadotropin and pinpointed as an intermediary in this process, the generation of EGF-like molecules as pertinent to the microenvironment that sustains oocyte maturation (17, 18). It follows then that temporally limiting exposure to gonadotropins in combination with supplements conducive to both cumulus expansion and oocyte maturation provide logical first steps in the development of efficacious IVM protocols.

## 2.2 Signaling Meiotic Resumption

It has long been appreciated that coordination of nuclear maturation with that of the cytoplasm leads to oocytes exhibiting good developmental potential. How such coordination is achieved is a more perplexing problem but in general, the assumption that these events are temporally, if not spatially, synergized has provided a backdrop for studies on oocyte IVM. With respect to nuclear maturation, the first overt sign that diplotene arrest has been overcome and that there is a commitment to proceed through meiosis-I, is the process of germinal vesicle breakdown. While commitment to engage in M-phase progression is tantamount to the activation of the cdk/cyclin/kinase complex, an upstream signal releasing a state of cell cycle arrest is pivotal to initiating meiotic maturation. Recent evidence has shed important new light on how this critical early step is regulated in the rodent.

Within 1–3 h of receptor activation by LH in mural granulosa cells, EGF-like proteins including amphiregulin and epiregulin are synthesized from newly transcribed mRNAs (17, 18). These factors can elicit oocyte maturation as long as granulosa cells are present, again indicating that the signal to commence maturation is transduced through the cumulus oophorus and is not the direct result of LH per se. As discussed earlier, cAMP is believed to be a central regulator of meiotic resumption due to the ability of oocytes to generate this factor which exerts a direct PKA-mediated negative effect on the MPF activator CDC25 (20). What therefore regulates cAMP levels in the oocyte? In the mouse, this pivotal function appears to rely upon a Gs-coupled receptor (GPR3) located in the oocyte plasma membrane. Studies by Mehlmann et al. (21) have shown that when GPR3 is genetically depleted from mice, oocytes undergo precocious maturation in the follicle, and meiotic arrest can be restored by replenishing the mRNA for GPR3 in oocytes from the mutant mice. Thus the long-standing model invoking cAMP metabolism in maintenance of meiotic arrest finds support from these recent studies and has been used clinically to synchronize immature human oocytes prior to IVM (22).

Clearly, the ability to regulate the onset and progression of meiotic maturation in mammalian oocytes are important factors to consider in designing clinically appropriate protocols for human oocyte IVM. At least in the case of releasing meiotic arrest, pharmacological agents such as phosphodiesterase inhibitors have been used to block the precocious advancement of the oocyte cell cycle (22). It will be necessary to identify agents that delay or impede cumulus cell responses to EGF to synchronize the metabolism of the cumulus with that of the oocyte upon release from meiotic arrest. The more pressing challenge will be to determine the causes of cytoplasmic maturation and the role of cumulus cell integrity on this developmentally relevant aspect of oocyte quality (Table 2).

## 2.3 Linking Cumulus Oocyte Integrity to Cytoplasmic Maturation

The most obvious changes that distinguish oocyte maturation *in vivo* from those which occur *in vitro* relate to the state of cell interactions within the cumulus–oocyte complex (Table 2). Specifically, little is known about the short or long term effects of follicular disruption

**Table 2** Mechanisms integrating COC metabolism

| Interface | Transfer mode | Substrate or signal propagated |
|---|---|---|
| Granulosa-Granulosa | Gap junction | ATP, GSH, cAMP, Ca |
| | Adhesion junctions | Receptor tyrosine kinases |
| Granulosa-Zona pellucida | Integrins, proteases, crosslinkers, hyaluronic acid matrix binding | EGF, IL-6, GDF-9, BMP-15 |
| Granulosa-Oocyte | Gap junction | ATP, GSH, cAMP, Ca |
| | Adherens junctions | RTKs, scaffold proteins |
| | Lipid exchange | Cholesterol, phosphoinositides |
| | Local endocytosis and exocytosis | Proteolytic cleavage products |

induced during the process of ovum retrieval. For achieving IVM, it is known that the presence of cumulus cells provides a physical basis for integrating both nutrient supply and signal conveyance if the contacts between the oocyte and cumulus cells are retained. But again, the dynamics of the cumulus–oocyte-complex (COC) are subject to progressive change due to the process of cumulus expansion and the resulting subdivision of labor between those cumulus cells that retain adhesive contacts with the zona pellucida and those that assume more distal locations as cumulus expansion progresses. Models of these interactions have been proposed but most tend to ignore the consequences of diluting COCs into relatively large volumes of medium that would irreversibly modify both the structure and contents of the extracellular matrix enveloping the oocyte (23). The importance of this interaction, and a major reason to think that it must be sustained throughout the course of meiotic maturation, is that after signaling to resume meiosis, major changes in oocyte structure and metabolism occur that are linked to cytoplasmic maturation (Table 2).

Amongst the more recent principles governing cellular regulation in many systems is the notion that mRNAs are localized within the cytoplasm to perform site specific functions, once activated for translation to occur. Thus, both maintenance of appropriate levels of mRNAs by establishing a means for preventing degradation, and assignment to correct locations, synergize to produce robust responses controlling cell cycle progression and timing, and organelle positioning and activation (24). These processes are hallmarks of oocyte maturation. Correct readout of stored maternal mRNAs, positioning of mitochondria and the meiotic spindle, and timely initiation of anaphase onset at both meiosis-1 and 2 are vital to ensure the synchronous maturation of the nucleus and cytoplasm. Notably, none of these processes would involve transcription, thereby emphasizing the need to focus on posttranslational dynamics in the case of the oocyte itself.

In contrast, transcriptional regulation at the level of the cumulus cells is characteristic of their function both prior to and following the LH surge, as noted above. Here, several aspects of cumulus cell function are subject to regulation not only via the activation of LH or FSH receptors but also by the system of TGF beta molecules derived from the oocyte itself (1). For example, the inability of the oocyte to undergo glycolysis and derive energy substrates like pyruvate is compensated for by the metabolism of the granulosa cells to which it is attached. Recent evidence in the mouse now shows that BMP-15 and FGF-8 are made in the oocyte, and their secreted products stimulate glycolysis in the cumulus cells (25). Moreover, in the mouse, GDF-9 and BMP-15 also seem to influence the delivery of cholesterol to the oocyte after it is synthesized in the cumulus cells (26). There is then precedence for so-called metabolic cooperation at many stages in the process that regulates meiotic maturation beginning with energy substrate provision, and ending with the loading of important molecules like glutathione and ATP. The common feature that links cumulus integrity with achieving cytoplasmic maturation appears then, to be based in an architecture that satisfies a symbiotic relationship between oocyte and cumulus cell, as summarized in Table 2. Defining this architecture and understanding how it changes in space and time during ovulation will set the stage for improvements in human IVM.

The metabolic demands during meiotic maturation are formidable (27). A constant energy supply is required to sustain ATP-consuming kinases that, in turn, drive entry into metaphase-I and maintain metaphase-II arrest. The intrinsic lack of a glutathione generating capacity in the oocyte means that the only source of this essential redox regulator is from the surrounding cumulus cells (28). Stored maternal proteins are needed to generate the meiotic spindle and, in murine models, this has been shown to be directly influenced by IVM conditions. Specifically, the localization and assembly of the meiotic spindle *in vivo* involves a spatial restriction that limits the amount of tubulin that is effectively integrated during progression of meiosis (29); *in vitro* maturation under conditions that compromise cumulus cell attachment leads to excess tubulin recruitment into spindles and a loss of this maternal protein into the polar bodies. It was recently shown that spindle enlargement is due to the failure to retain gamma-tubulin containing organizing centers in the oocyte cortex, again due to a loss in cumulus cell contact (30). Similar forces acting to stabilize the oocyte cortex during maturation are likely to influence the location and integrity of other organelles required during preimplantation development. This aspect of IVM needs to be better characterized in human oocytes especially with reference to the nature of oocyte granulosa cell interactions (31).

## 3 Lessons Learned

Optimizing conditions for human IVM has, under certain circumstances, drawn upon discoveries made with animal models. These animal systems offer abundant material, the ability to manipulate gene and protein actions, and more importantly, in the case of the mouse and cow, the ability to translate IVM conditions to a clinical outcome measure whether it be pregnancy establishment or term birth. On the other hand, without a clear picture of normo-ovulatory processes in humans and nonhuman primates there are likely to be additional or different factors that are called into play to achieve oocyte maturation *in vivo* or *in vitro*. While this is an unrealistic research scenario for studies on humans, future work in this area can be guided by the principles of ovulatory physiology gleaned from animal studies and suggest that the lessons learned in these models will find application in the clinic (Table 3).

One set of lessons can be viewed from the perspective of oversimplification. Just as the facility to study gene transcription set the stage for deducing many of the gene networks involved in murine ovulation, so too will the need to map the spatial and temporal aspects of oocyte proteins that underlie developmental competencies. Given the oocyte's transcriptionally dormant state and its reliance on the cumulus cells for fundamental aspects of metabolism, it will be essential to achieve effective support of mRNA processing and the lifetimes for specific proteins in cell cycle control. This will ultimately require definition of the protein factors that drive chromosome alignment and segregation at both meiotic anaphases, and those maternally inherited proteins that support the fidelity of cell division in the early conceptus. What sets the primate oocyte apart from other mammals in this regard remains a perplexing problem, given the high incidence of aneuploidy that is known to compromise human oocyte health.

Another example of oversimplification derives from the microenvironment that the oocyte finds itself in both prior to, and following, cumulus expansion. Viscous hyaluronate-rich gels provide physical rigidity and biochemical accessibility for growth factors in many developmental systems and this should not be overlooked in the case of the COC. If nothing else, mounting evidence for the dualistic functions of both granulosa and oocyte secreted proteins argues strongly that any enzymatic or dilution effect imposed on the COC is likely to alter the immediate interfaces being used to initiate or sustain signaling cascades as oocyte maturation progresses. Likewise the basic culture conditions now employed are also apt to generate stress responses in both cumulus cells and oocytes due to the heightened metabolism of the former, and the protracted dependence of the latter, on the energy requirements for both the oocyte and zygote. Addressing both the sources of and ways to micromanage reactive oxygen species will measurably

**Table 3** Physicochemical factors required for IVM optimization

| Factors | Consequence | Remediation prospect |
|---|---|---|
| Matrix stability | Loss of growth factors | Substitution of enriched artificial matrices |
| Diffusion | Reversal of local metabolite and protein gradients | Limit vessel volume and number of medium exchanges |
| Culture stress | ROS generation, metabolic diversion | Medium quenching, directed metabolism |
| Enhanced catabolism | Precocious depletion of maternal mRNAs, proteins | Medium conditioners to adjust protein phosphatase, proteosome, and RNA degrading machinery |
| Cell contact interactions | Loss of metabolic cooperation | Identify and overexpress/stabilize junctional complexes |
| Oolemma stability | Modification of oocyte domain structure and linkage to cytoskeleton initiates macromolecular turnover | Identify cumulus/zona (extrinsic) and oocyte (intrinsic) molecules that regulate membrane stability using pharmacological agents |

serve to protect both long lived and rapidly turning over proteins that determine oocyte quality. And finally, taking the dimensions of time and space and putting them into the context of the changing demands on the oocyte while cumulus expansion proceeds, will necessitate the adoption of microfluidic technology to effect the *in vivo* situation. While some of these modifications from existing clinical approaches are underway and promising, the majority of clinics retain standards for IVM that require updating in an effort to improve the efficiency and safety of this form of ART.

## 4 Clinical Applications Summary

Human oocyte IVM will continue to be used for clinical embryo production. This need will be driven by benefits to patients that include lessening the risk of ovarian hyperstimulation syndrome (OHSS), especially in cases of polycystic ovary syndrome (PCOS), minimizing both costs and adverse oocyte quality derivative from excessive follicular stimulation, and offering in general a more patient-friendly experience. This potentially major role that human IVM may play in current ART practices is likely to grow as more suitable conditions are defined for manipulating both oocyte and cumulus cell physiology with respect to the array of factors yet to be discovered that contribute to establishing consistent and high levels of oocyte quality. One of the more relevant questions at this point then pertains to identifying biomarkers that directly or indirectly reflect cytoplasmic maturation without compromising the functionality of the cumulus–oocyte complex. New assays are under development that will allow for rapid detection of mRNAs from cumulus cells that might have biomarker potential for assessing oocyte quality. Alternatively, using microassays and sensitive detection strategies to monitor COC metabolism based on catabolism and metabolite secretion might afford the opportunity to profile a given COCs metabolome that could in practice serve as a quality indicator. While all of these approaches offer some merit for clinical application, predictors of oocyte quality will ultimately depend on demonstration of the features of oocytes that best dictate the initiation and persistence of an otherwise error-prone program for pre and post implantation development. Thus, any summary of the state of human IVM must look beyond currently accepted practices, such as whether to use hCG priming or not, and introduce practical modifications in technology that are based on our best guess, drawn from results with animal models such as nonhuman primates.

An impending opportunity for carrying out studies on human IVM should derive from the introduction of fertility preservation programs. Specifically, the use of oocytes isolated from grafted pieces of ovarian cortex and grown to maturity will expand research-oriented clinical programs to analyze the developmental program for human oogenesis at a level of detail not previously appreciated. Moreover, the growth of cryopreservation options for both immature and mature human oocytes will similarly stimulate more study into the staging of oocyte maturation in a context that will bear fruits consistent with improved clinical outcome. As always, the burden of proof in any new procedure will be enhancement of pregnancy rates and birth of healthy offspring in large numbers; data we await from the initial phase of human IVM.

## References


1. Rodrigues P, Limback D, McGinnis LK, Plancha CE, Albertini DF. Oogenesis: prospects and challenges for the future. J Cell Physiol 2008;216(2):355–65.
2. Edwards RG. Maturation in vitro of mouse, sheep, cow, pig, rhesus monkey and human ovarian oocytes. Nature 1965; 208(5008):349–51.
3. Edwards RG. Maturation in vitro of human ovarian oocytes. Lancet 1965;2(7419):926–9.
4. Pincus G, Enzmann E. The comparative behavior of mammalian eggs in vivo and in vitro. 1. The activation of ovarian eggs. J Exp Med 1935;62:665–75.
5. Rock J, Menkin MF. In vitro fertilization and cleavage of human ovarian eggs. Science 1944;100(2588):105–7.
6. Biggers JD, Whittingham DG, Donahue RP. The pattern of energy metabolism in the mouse oocyte and zygote. Proc Natl Acad Sci 1967;58(2):560–7.
7. Cho WK, Stern S, Biggers JD. Inhibitory effect of dibutyryl cAMP on mouse oocyte maturation in vitro. J Exp Zool 1974; 187(3):383–6.
8. Anderson E, Albertini DF. Gap junctions between the oocyte and companion follicle cells in the mammalian ovary. J Cell Biol 1976;71(2):680–6.
9. Schroeder AC, Eppig JJ. The developmental capacity of mouse oocytes that matured spontaneously in vitro is normal. Dev Biol 1984;102(2):493–7.
10. Downs SM, Daniel SA, Eppig JJ. Induction of maturation in cumulus cell-enclosed mouse oocytes by follicle-stimulating hormone and epidermal growth factor: evidence for a positive

stimulus of somatic cell origin. J Exp Zool 1988;245(1): 86–96.
11. Veeck LL, Wortham JW, Jr., Witmyer J, et al. Maturation and fertilization of morphologically immature human oocytes in a program of in vitro fertilization. Fertil Steril 1983;39(5):594–602.
12. Cha KY, Koo JJ, Ko JJ, Choi DH, Han SY, Yoon TK. Pregnancy after in vitro fertilization of human follicular oocytes collected from nonstimulated cycles, their culture in vitro and their transfer in a donor oocyte program. Fertil Steril 1991;55(1):109–13.
13. Trounson A, Wood C, Kausche A. In vitro maturation and the fertilization and developmental competence of oocytes recovered from untreated polycystic ovarian patients. Fertil Steril 1994;62(2):353–62.
14. Cha KY, Chian RC. Maturation in vitro of immature human oocytes for clinical use. Hum Reprod Update 1998; 4(2):103–20.
15. Smith SD, Mikkelsen A, Lindenberg S. Development of human oocytes matured in vitro for 28 or 36 hours. Fertil Steril 2000;73(3):541–4.
16. Bavister BD, Boatman DE. The neglected human blastocyst revisited. Hum Reprod 1997;12(8):1607–10.
17. Ashkenazi H, Cao X, Motola S, Popliker M, Conti M, Tsafriri A. Epidermal growth factor family members: endogenous mediators of the ovulatory response. Endocrinology 2005;146(1):77–84.
18. Park JY, Su YQ, Ariga M, Law E, Jin SL, Conti M. EGF-like growth factors as mediators of LH action in the ovulatory follicle. Science 2004;303(5658):682–4.
19. Plancha CE, Albertini DF. Protein synthesis requirements during resumption of meiosis in the hamster oocyte: early nuclear and microtubule configurations. Mol Reprod Dev 1992; 33(3):324–32.
20. Lincoln AJ, Wickramasinghe D, Stein P, et al. Cdc25b phosphatase is required for resumption of meiosis during oocyte maturation. Nat Genet 2002;30(4):446–9.
21. Mehlmann LM, Saeki Y, Tanaka S, et al. The Gs-linked receptor GPR3 maintains meiotic arrest in mammalian oocytes. Science 2004;306(5703):1947–50.
22. Nogueira D, Ron-El R, Friedler S, et al. Meiotic arrest in vitro by phosphodiesterase 3-inhibitor enhances maturation capacity of human oocytes and allows subsequent embryonic development. Biol Reprod 2006;74(1):177–84.
23. Albertini DF. Oocyte-granulosa cell interactions. In: Blerkom JV, Gregory L, eds. Essential IVF: Reviews of Topical Issues in Clinical In Vitro Fertilization. Boston: Kluwer; 2002:43–58.
24. Bromfield J, Messamore W, Albertini DF. Epigenetic regulation during mammalian oogenesis. Reprod Fertil Dev 2008;20(1):74–80.
25. Sugiura K, Su Y-Q, Diaz FJ, et al. Oocyte-derived BMP15 and FGFs cooperate to promote glycolysis in cumulus cells. Development 2007;134(14):2593–603.
26. Su YQ, Sugiura K, Wigglesworth K, et al. Oocyte regulation of metabolic cooperativity between mouse cumulus cells and oocytes: BMP15 and GDF9 control cholesterol biosynthesis in cumulus cells. Development 2008;135(1):111–21.
27. Thompson JG, Lane M, Gilchrist RB. Metabolism of the bovine cumulus-oocyte complex and influence on subsequent developmental competence. Soc Reprod Fertil Supplil 2007;64:179–90.
28. Combelles CM, Cekleniak NA, Racowsky C, Albertini DF. Assessment of nuclear and cytoplasmic maturation in in-vitro matured human oocytes. Hum Reprod 2002;17(4):1006–16.
29. Sanfins A, Lee GY, Plancha CE, Overstrom EW, Albertini DF. Distinctions in meiotic spindle structure and assembly during in vitro and in vivo maturation of mouse oocytes. Biol Reprod 2003;69(6):2059–67.
30. Barrett SL, Albertini DF. Allocation of gamma-tubulin between oocyte cortex and meiotic spindle influences asymmetric cytokinesis in the mouse oocyte. Biol Reprod 2007;76(6):949–57.
31. Cekleniak NA, Combelles CM, Ganz DA, Fung J, Albertini DF, Racowsky C. A novel system for in vitro maturation of human oocytes. Fertil Steril 2001;75(6):1185–93.

# The Use of Oocyte and Embryo Vitrification in Assisted Reproductive Technology

Tetsunori Mukaida

**Abstract** Refined slow freezing and new vitrification methods have significantly improved cryopreservation of human oocytes and embryos. Slow freezing techniques using a programmed cryo-machine have been traditionally employed, but usually take several hours to complete and involve ice-crystal formation during freezing. Vitrification has become a reliable strategy, not only because it is very simple but also because it can lead to high survival rates and viability. The underlying concept of vitrification is to transform the cells into an amorphous glassy state inside and outside the vitrified cell, instead of ice crystal formation. This requires high concentrations of cryoprotectancts (CPAs) and rapid cooling and warming steps. Conventional vitrification, using cryostraws with relatively high concentration of CPAs was not clinically effective compared with slow freezing, especially in oocyte and blastocyst. However, ultra-rapid vitrification, using a minimized volume of vitrification solution, has been adopted and could dramatically improve survival rate and viability. In order to vitrify the cells in liquid nitrogen, sufficient dehydration and permeation of the CPA are necessary, in any stage of gametes and embryos, although this ultra-rapid vitrification does not require full equilibration of CPAs because of its extremely high cooling rate. This is why this approach could decrease the concentration of CPAs to reach the vitrified state during the cooling and warming steps that could reduce the toxicity of CPA without forming ice-crystals inside the cell. Recently cryoloop, cryotop, hemistraw, open pulled straw (OPS), and EM grid were introduced as tools to minimize the vitrification solution at the final steps. In this chapter, the basic concepts and methodologies of both conventional vitrification and ultra-rapid vitrification will be discussed.

**Keywords** Vitrification • Cryotop • Cryoloop • Cryopreservation • Cryoprotectant • Embryo • Blastocyst • Oocyte

## 1 Introduction

In assisted reproductive technology (ART), cryopreservation of embryos has proven important for the best use of supernumerary embryos. In the cryopreservation of embryos, there is a risk of various types of injury (1, 2). Among them, the formation of intracellular ice appears to be the most damaging. The first strategy to prevent intracellular ice from forming was to adopt a lower concentration of cryoprotectant and a long slow-cooling stage. This slow freezing method has proven effective for embryos of a wide range of mammalian species. Unlike embryos of laboratory animals and domestic animals, in which dimethylsulphoxide (DMSO), glycerol or ethylene glycol (EG) are commonly used as the cryoprotectant (Cryoprotective agent: CPA), human embryos at early cleavage stages have most often been frozen in a solution of propanediol supplemented with sucrose (3), although those at the blastocyst stage have more frequently been frozen with glycerol and sucrose (4–6). With slow freezing, however, it is difficult to completely eliminate injuries occurring from ice formation. Furthermore, the slow freezing method requires a long period of time before embryos are stored in liquid nitrogen ($LN_2$).

T. Mukaida
Hiroshima HART Clinic, 5-7-10 Ohtemachi, Naka-ku, Hiroshima 730-0051, Japan
e-mail: info@hiroshima-hart.jp

D.T. Carrell et al. (eds.), *Biennial Review of Infertility*, DOI: 10.1007/978-1-60327-392-3_15

In 1985, Rall and Fahy reported (7) an innovative approach called "vitrification," in which injuries related to ice crystal are minimized by using very high concentrations of CPAs. Vitrification is the solidification of a solution at a low temperature without the formation of ice crystals, by increasing the viscosity using high cooling rates (1). The rapid cooling process can minimize chilling injury and osmotic shock to the embryos. Vitrification, with recent improvements, has become a reliable strategy, not only because it is very simple but also because it can lead to high survival rates. To induce vitrification in $LN_2$, the solution must contain a high concentration of CPAs (2). This approach simplifies the cooling process, because embryos can be rapidly cooled directly in $LN_2$. Although embryos subjected to vitrification are more liable to be injured by the toxicity of the high concentration of CPAs, the method has been refined and proven to be effective for the cryopreservation of embryos at various stages of development in laboratory and domestic species. In 1998, we showed that vitrification using an EG-based vitrification solution (8) (EFS40) with conventional cryostraws was effective for human embryos at the 4–8 cell stage (9). The effectiveness of vitrification was confirmed for human embryos at the 8–16 cell stage (10) and the morula stage (11), using EG-based solutions.

The basic procedure for vitrification is simple. Embryos are suspended in a vitrification solution and then plunged in $LN_2$. Embryos are warmed rapidly and diluted quickly with a sucrose solution. The most important stage is the exposure of embryos to the vitrification solution before cooling. To prevent intracellular ice from forming, a longer period of exposure is desirable. However, if the exposure is too long, cells suffer from the toxicity of the solution. Therefore, the optimal exposure time for successful vitrification must be a compromise between preventing the formation of intracellular ice and preventing toxic injury. Actually, however, embryos may be injured by the toxicity of the cryoprotectant before enough cryoprotectant can permeate the cells. Therefore, a two-step procedure is commonly adopted in which embryos are first equilibrated in a dilute (e.g., 10%) CPA solution, followed by a brief (30–60 s) exposure to a vitrification solution before the cells is cooled with liquid nitrogen. The optimal exposure time in the vitrification solution depends not only on the CPA solution but also on the temperature, since both the permeability of embryos and the toxicity of the CPA are largely influenced by temperature (6, 7).

In vitrification, the selection of CPAs requires extreme care because their concentration can be as high as 6 M, which can make the toxicity of these compounds a key limiting factor in cryobiology. The most appropriate characteristics of a penetrating CPA are low toxicity and high permeability. For cryopreservation of human embryos, PROH and DMSO have been used as the dominant CPAs, although glycerol is used when embryos are frozen at the blastocyst stage (6). As a less toxic CPA, ethylene glycol is commonly and widely used (2). However, few comparative studies have examined the effect of the CPA on the survival of vitrified embryos.

## 2 Day 2–3 Embryo Vitrification

In 1998, we performed an investigation to find a suitable CPA and suitable conditions for exposing embryos to a vitrification solution using 8-cell mouse embryos (9). The survival rates of 8-cell embryos vitrified in various solutions after exposure to the solutions for 0.5 and 2 min at 20 and 25°C are summarized in Fig. 1. The highest rates of survival were obtained, regardless of the time and temperature, with ethylene glycol-based solutions. Although none of the vitrified embryos were morphologically normal when embryos were vitrified after 0.5 min exposure to any mixture of 30% CPA, the survival rate was over 90% when embryos were treated for a longer time (2 min) at a higher temperature (25°C), or when embryos were treated with a higher concentration of ethylene glycol (EFS40) at a higher temperature (25°C).

In addition, a small saccharide (e.g., sucrose) and a macromolecule (e.g., Ficoll 70, BSA or PVP) are frequently included in vitrification solutions. These non-permeating agents are much less toxic, and are known to promote vitrification of the solution (8). Therefore, their inclusion can reduce the toxicity of the solution by decreasing the concentration of the permeating agent required for vitrification. In addition, inclusion of a saccharide promotes shrinkage of embryos, and thus reduces the amount of intracellular cryoprotectant, which will also reduce the toxic effect of the permeating CPA (8). At the same time, the osmotic action of saccharide plays an important role in minimizing the

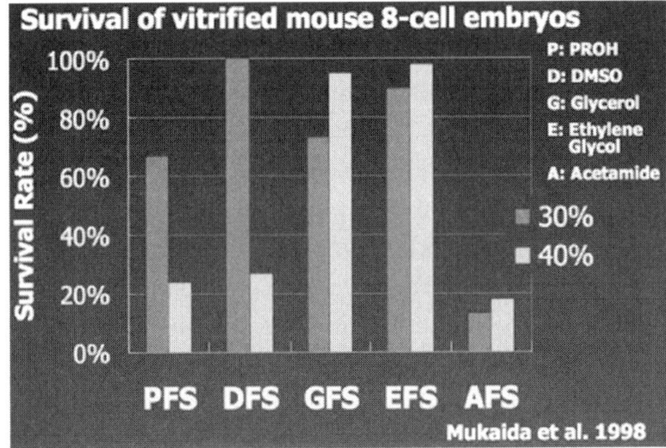


**Fig. 1** Survival of vitrified 8-cell mouse embryos, assessed by their ability to develop into expanded blastocysts, expressed as the percentage of morphologically normal embryos at recovery for each vitrification solution, regardless of the time and temperature of exposure. Vitrification solutions contain 30% (*closed bar*) or 40% (*hatched bar*) permeating cryoprotectant. All the concentrations were diluted with FS solution (PB1 medium containing 30% Ficoll + 0.5 M sucrose). $^{**}p < 0.01$, $^{*}p < 0.05$; significantly different within solutions containing the same permeating cryoprotectant. *AFS* acetamide-based solution; *PFS* propanediol-based solution; *DFS* dimethylsulphoxide-based solution; *GFS* glycerol-based solution; *EFS* ethylene glycol-based solution

swelling of embryos during dilution, since a quick dilution is necessary to prevent the toxic effect of the solution.

## 3 Protocols and Clinical Results of Day 2–3 Vitrification

### *3.1 Vitrification Using Conventional Cryostraws for Day 2–3 Embryos*

A two-step protocol for straw vitrification using ethylene glycol-based solutions, EFS20 and EFS40, has been described (1, 12). This method has been proven suitable for human embryos on day 2–3 (9, Mukaida et al., unpublished data). The two solutions (EFS20 and EFS40) are used for pretreatment and vitrification, respectively. The base medium used for vitrification of embryos is modified phosphate-buffered saline (PB1), in which BSA is replaced with human serum albumin (HSA). Ethylene glycol is diluted to 20 or 40% (v/v) with Ficoll-sucrose (FS) solution; the components of the FS solution are 30% (w/v) Ficoll 70 (average molecular weight 70,000, Amersham Pharmacia Biotech, Buckinghamshire, England), and 0.5 M sucrose in PB1 medium. The respective vitrification solutions are designated EFS20 and EFS40. The final concentrations of Ficoll 70 and sucrose are 24% (w/v) and 0.4 M, respectively, in EFS20, and 18% (w/v) and 0.3 M, respectively, in EFS40. For dilution, PB1 medium containing 0.5 M sucrose (S-PB1) is prepared.

All the solutions are placed in a room at 25–27°C, at which temperature embryos are manipulated. A 0.25 ml plastic straw (~132 mm including the cotton plug) is prepared for embryo loading by drawing S-PB1 medium up to a depth of ~60 mm, followed by air (~25–30 mm), EFS40 (~5 mm), another volume of air (~5 mm) and finally more EFS40 (~12 mm). First, embryos are pretreated by being suspended in a drop of EFS20 in the lid of a culture dish (or a dish) for 2 min. Then, embryos are transferred into the larger column of FES40 near the mouth of the straw. The contents of the straw are aspirated until the first column of S-PB1 medium is in contact with the cotton plug, and the straw is sealed with the heat-sealer. After exposure of embryos to EFS40 for ~30 s, the straw is positioned in the $LN_2$ vapor phase by placing it horizontally on a ~1 cm thick Styrofoam boat floating on the surface of the $LN_2$ in a Dewar vessel (inner diameter, 140 mm). After 3 min or more, the straw is placed in a canister and stored in $LN_2$. EFS40 and EFS20 are prepared in 1 ml syringes equipped with 18-G needles, and new small drops are placed on the lid of a dish just before use for each sample, to prevent concentration of the solution by evaporation.

For embryo recovery, the straw is kept in air for 10 s and then immersed in water at 25–28°C. When the crystallized S-PB1 medium in the straw begins to melt (after about 7 s), the straw is removed from the water, quickly wiped dry, and cut at both ends. The contents of the straw are expelled into a culture dish by flushing the straw with 0.8 ml of S-PB1 medium using a 1 ml syringe attached with an 18-G needle. After gently agitating the culture dish to promote mixing of the contents, the embryos are pipetted into fresh S-PB1 medium. About 5 min after being flushed out, the embryos are transferred to fresh PB1 medium. Embryos are further washed with fresh PB1 medium, and are transferred to a culture medium for culture until transfer.

In 1998, we reported (9) the effectiveness of this vitrification method for day 2–3 human embryos, more trials on this straw vitrification were performed in the HART Clinic group (Hiroshima HART Clinic, Osaka HART Clinic, and Tokyo HART Clinic), and its effectiveness was confirmed. In our unpublished data for day 2–3 embryos, a total of 661 embryos were vitrified, and 486 (74%) of them had 50% or more morphologically intact blastomeres after warming, confirmed by further development of these vitrified embryos on the day after warming. A total of 335 vitrified embryos were transferred in 127 cycles at one or two days after warming, 34 (26.8%) women became pregnant and 22 women (17%) delivered babies.

### 3.2 Vitrification Using Cryoloops for Day 2–3 Embryos

Here we describe an ultra-rapid vitrification approach using the cryoloop (13–16). This method is available not only for embryos on day 2–3, but also for blastocysts, for which conventional vitrification using a straw was found to be less effective. The protocol for vitrification using the cryoloop can be found in the following section on vitrification of blastocysts, which is basically the same technique.

At the HART Clinic group, cryoloop vitrification is adopted for cryopreservation of supernumerary human embryos on day 2–3 for a short period of time, and mainly blastocysts on day 5–6 after oocytes pick-up that were obtained from culture in sequential media. Available data are as follows: For embryos on day 2–3, a total of 269 embryos have been vitrified, and 188 (70%) of them had 50% or more morphologically intact blastomeres, confirmed by further development on the day after warming. A total of 112 vitrified embryos were transferred into 44 patients, and 14 (32%) of these women conceived (Mukaida et al., unpublished data).

In 2007, Desai et al. (17) reported the postvitrification development, pregnancy outcomes and live births for cryoloop vitrification of human day 3 cleavage-stage embryos. Tables 1 and 2 include their protocol and results, which presented consecutive vitrification-warming cycles performed over a 2.5-year interval. A total of 236 embryos were warmed, and the average number of embryos transferred per patient was 2.66 ± 0.86. They reported that the clinical pregnancy rate was 44% (34/77), and the implantation rate was 20% (40/201). The postwarming survival rate was 85% (201/236). They also reported that 78% (184/236) of warmed embryos showed signs of embryonic compaction and/or blastulation by the time of transfer. That means those surviving embryos were confirmed as potentially viable. Theoretically, vitrification does not involve ice crystal formation, and survival judged by the morphological appearance may not always be related to their viability. Therefore, confirmation of further development is necessary and one of the important factors to evaluate after warming.

In 2005, Raju et al. (18) reported a modified protocol for vitrification of human 8-cell embryos using the cryoloop technique. They reported using 10% ethylene glycol (EG) for 5 min at 37°C as a equilibration phase, and 40% EG in 0.6 mol/l sucrose for 30 s as a vitrification phase. Human 8-cell embryos were loaded onto a nylon loop made in their biomechanical Department at the Krishna IVF Clinic. Also, the nylon loop with a thin filmy layer of vitrification solution and vitrified embryos was directly placed into a cryovial containing liquid nitrogen. Loading and storage steps were similar to our cryoloop protocol described above, however, the protocol including the type of cryoprotectant and duration of exposure was different. Initially, embryos were suspended in a 10% ethylene glycol solution for 5 min at 37°C, and transferred to a 40% ethylene glycol in 0.6 mol/l sucrose solution for 30 s. For warming, vitrified embryos were passed through four different concentrations of sucrose solution i.e., 1, 0.5, 0.25, and 0.125 mol/l for 2.5 min at each step at 37°C (Table 1). Table 2 includes their results. Mean age of patients was 31.3 ± 4.5 years. The post-thaw survival rate of embryos was 95.3%. The clinical pregnancy rate and implantation rates were 35.0 and 14.9%, respectively.

### 3.3 Vitrification Using Cryotops

Since in our center (Hiroshima HART clinic) the cryoloop system has only been applied for the cryopreservation of embryos at the blastocyst stage, the protocol and data of vitrification using cryotops in this chapter were adopted from the study carried out at the IVF Nagata Clinic, Hakata, Japan. Their protocol and data of vitrification were described briefly as follows: 346

# Color Plates

CGH Array (Female Patient: Male Reference) Shows

Principles of Analysis:

- Examines the genome at a resolution of 1 Mb intervals (or less)
- Detects abnormalities at a rate: ~12%
- Detects 99% of clinically significant abnormalities detected by karyotype
  - XX Female shows X gain and absence of Y when tested against male reference DNA
- High-throughput analysis using minimal amounts of DNA

Limitation

Unable to detect balanced translocations

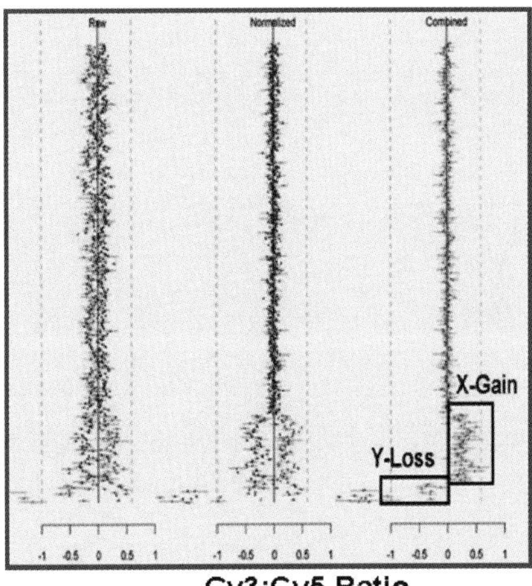


**Chapter 8, Fig. 3** The *lower panel* shows an actual analysis of gender mismatched DNA to show the principles of the assay. In this study a BAC array was illustrate and female DNA patient DNA competed with male reference DNA and then hybridized to the CGH array. The array shows the loss of the entire Y chromosome in the XX female and the gain of an extra X chromosome

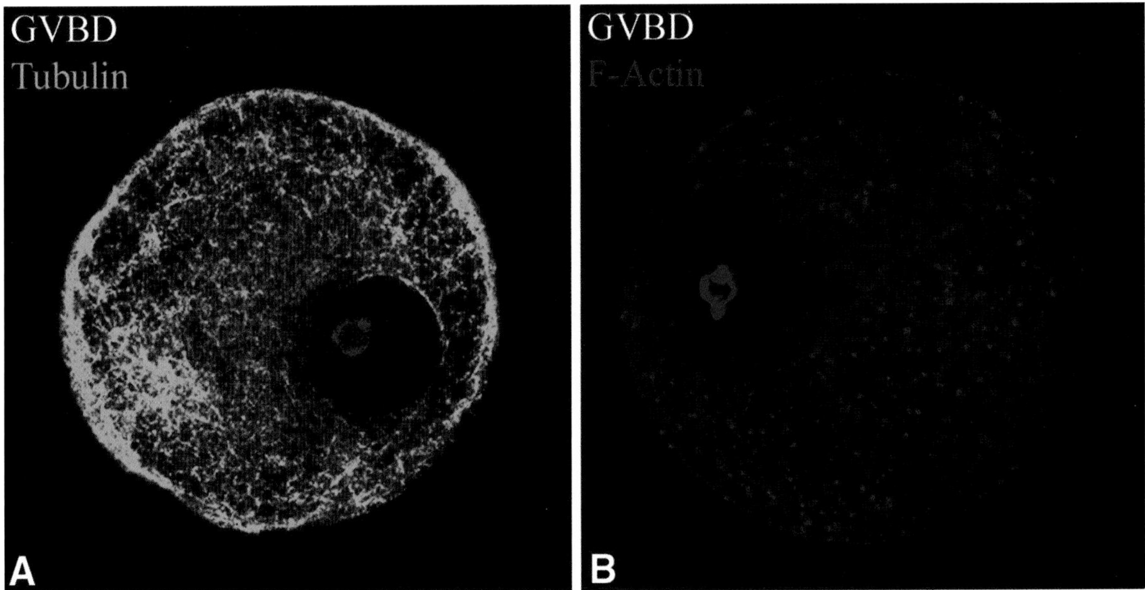


**Chapter 13, Fig. 3** (continued)

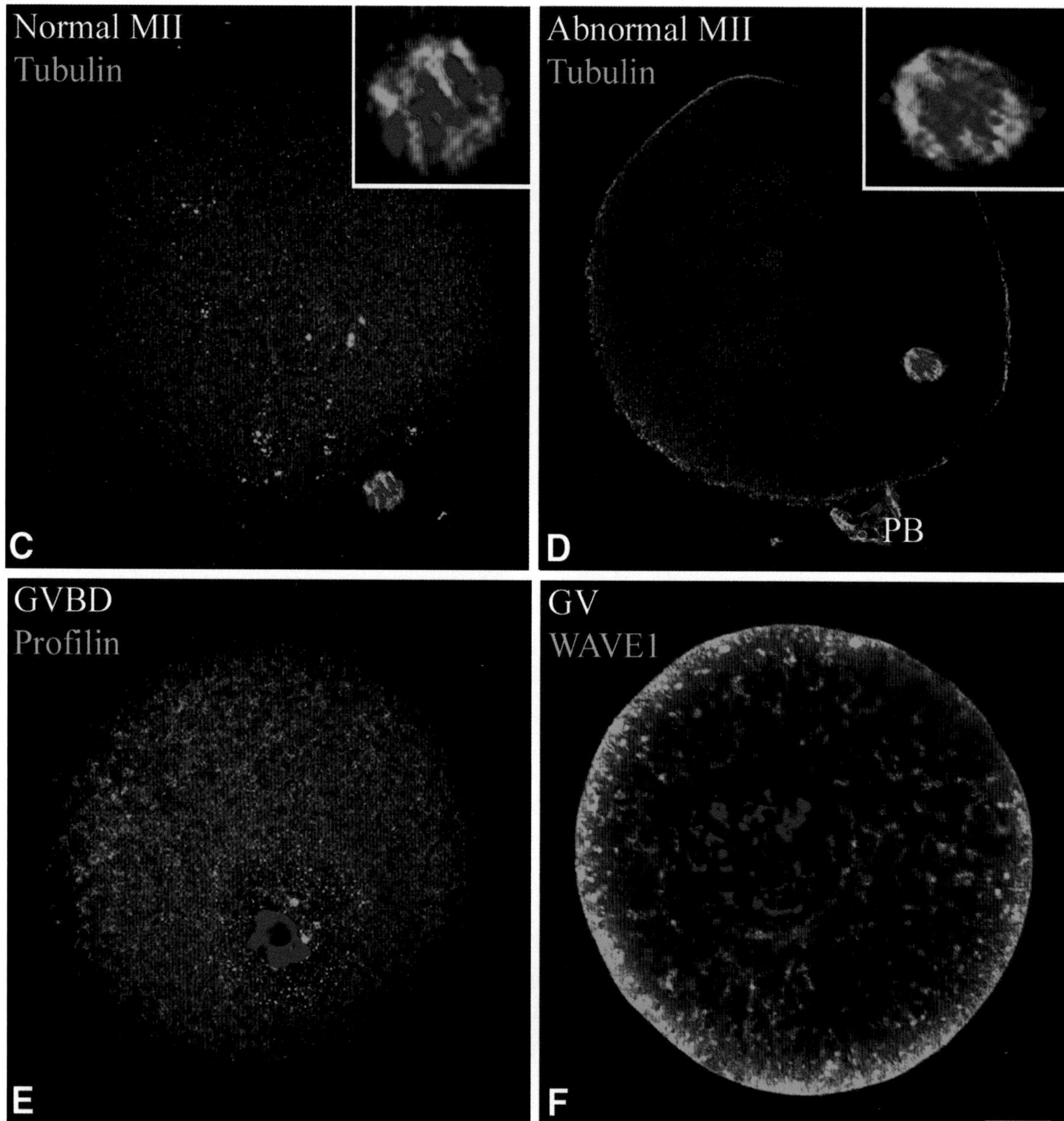


**Chapter 13, Fig. 3** Confocal microscopy of human oocytes at different maturational stages: cytoskeleton markers. (**a**) During Germinal Vesicle Breakdown (GVBD stage), oocytes show a network of tubulin (*green*) organized throughout the ooplasm and surrounding the germinal vesicle where the chromatin (*blue*) is tightly associated with the nucleolus. (**b**) Filamentous actin (F-actin) is visualized using 568-Phalloidin (*red*) in GVBD human oocytes. Microfilaments are distributed in the ooplasm and enriched at the oocyte cortex. Note the different distribution of microfilaments around the human GV when compared with microtubules (**a** vs. **b**), suggesting that the migration of the nucleus during meiosis I in humans is a microtubule (and not microfilament) dependent event. (**c** and **d**) MII oocytes show microtubules polymerized in the meiotic spindle (*green*). In **c**, a normal morphology of the spindle and an organized metaphase plate are observed (inset) in contraposition to **d**, where chromosomes are not well aligned and the meiotic spindle is rotated with respect to the polar body (PB). (**e**) Profilin (an actin-related protein) distributes to specific foci inside the GVBD nucleus and throughout the ooplasm. It promotes the incorporation of actin monomers into filaments and the nucleation of them is catalyzed by the Arp 2/3 complex. (**f**) Wiskott-Aldrich syndrome protein family verprolin-homologous protein (WAVE1) regulates the actin cytoskeleton and is observed associated with Golgi apparatus in human GV oocytes (unpublished observations). Images were obtained using an Olympus spectral confocal microscope, with laser lines at 488-, 568-, and 633-nm wavelengths (University of Buenos Aires, Faculty of Exact and Natural Sciences) and then processed by Adobe Photoshop 7.0. *Scale bar* represents 20 μm

patients who needed to have their embryos cryopreserved on day 2 of development to avoid either OHSS or as supernumerary embryos for subsequent transfer attempts, agreed to cryopreservation of the embryos by vitrification. A total of 1,774 day 2 embryos were vitrified with equilibration solution, an equal mixture of 7.5% DMSO and 7.5% ethylene glycol (EG) in HTF supplemented with 20% HSA and a vitrification solution, using a mixture of 15% DMSO, 15% EG and 0.5 M sucrose in HTF/HSA. Initially, embryos were exposed to the equilibration solution for 5–10 min, and to the vitrification solution for 1 min at room temperature (25–27°C). The duration of the equilibration time was adjusted by morphological changes that indicated shrinkage for dehydration and reexpansion for cryoprotectant (CPA) permeation, and was individually recorded for further analysis. Embryos were then loaded onto a minute nylon sheet (cryotop), and plunged into $LN_2$ immediately. For warming, vitrified embryos on the tip of a cryotop were dipped and kept in 1 M of sucrose solution for 1 min. and then diluted in 0.5 M of sucrose solution for 3 min. Embryos with 70% or more intact blastomeres were considered as indicative of survival and kept in culture until transfer on the following day (Table 1).

Table 2 includes the results from the use of the Cryotops at Nagata Clinic. Briefly, 346 patients with day 2 embryos that were to be cryopreserved to avoid either OHSS or as supernumerary embryos for subsequent transfer attempts were entered in this investigation.

**Table 1** Summary of each vitrification protocol with respect to the concentration, time and properties of vitrification solution for day 2–3 human embryo cryopreservation

| | Cryostraw | Cryoloop (1) | Cryoloop (2) | Cryotop |
|---|---|---|---|---|
| Temperature | Room (25–27°C) | Warm stage (37°C) | Warm stage (37°C) | Room (25–27°C) |
| Equilibration step | EG.F.S. 20:20%EG (2 min) | 7.5%EG + 7.5%DMSO (2 min) | 10%EG (5 min) | 7.5%EG + 7.5%DMSO (5–10 min[a]) |
| Vitrification step | EG.F.S. 40 :40%EG (1 min) | 15%EG + 15%DMSO + F + S (35 s) | 40%EG + S (30 s) | 15%EG + 15%DMSO + S (1 min) |
| Cooling system | Vapor phase $LN_2$ (3 min), then plunged into $LN_2$ | Plunged into $LN_2$ directly (Ultra-rapid cooling) | Plunged into $LN_2$ directly (Ultra-rapid cooling) | Plunged into $LN_2$ directly (Ultra-rapid cooling) |
| Warming step | One step<br>0.5 M S (5 min) | Two steps<br>0.25 M S (2 min)<br>0.125 M S (3 min) | Four Steps<br>1 M S (2.5 min)<br>0.5 M S (2.5 min)<br>0.25 M S (2.5 min)<br>0.125 M S (2.5 min) | Two Steps<br>1 M S (1 min)<br>0.5 M S (3 min) |

*EG* ethylene glycol; *F* ficoll; *S* sucrose
Cryoloop (1): Reported by Desai (17). Cryoloop (2): Reported by Raju (18)
[a] The duration of equilibration is adjusted according to the time needed for reexpansion of the vitrified embryos

**Table 2** Summary of the clinical results in each vitrification approach for day 2–3 embryos. Results in each vitrification protocol for human day 2–3 vitrified embryos

| Age | Cryostraw | Cryoloop (1) 34.1±4.5 | Cryoloop (2) 31.3±4.5 | Cryotop 35.0±4.5 |
|---|---|---|---|---|
| No. of cycles | 127 | 77 | 40 | 604 (346 patients) |
| Survival rate | | 201/236 (85) | 121/127 (95) | 1,701/1,774 (95.9) |
| Cleavage rate[a] | 486/661 (76) | 184/236 (78) | | 1,289/1,774 (72.7) |
| Pregnancy rate | 34/127 (26.8) | 34/77 (44.2) | 14/40 (35.0) | 164/604 (27.2) |
| Implantation rate | | 40/201 (19.9) | 18/121 (14.9) | 192/1,442 (13.3) |
| Delivery rate[b] | 22/127 (17) | | 13/40 (32.5) | 118/604 (19.5) |

Cryoloop (1): Reported by Desai (17). Cryoloop (2): Reported by Raju (18)
Values in parentheses indicates percentage
[a] Including survival and further cleavage rate
[b] Including on-going pregnancy

A total of 1,774 day 2 embryos were warmed in 604 transfer cycles. One thousand, seven hundred and one of the vitrified embryos survived and 1,442 of them were transferred. Pregnancy was confirmed in one hundred sixty four cycles, and 192 of them were implanted as confirmed by the presence of a gestational sac. Forty six cycles were ended in miscarriage, and 67 deliveries were achieved. Others are ongoing pregnancies.

Total survival and cleavage rates were 95.9% (1,701/1,774) and 75.8% (1,289/1,701), respectively. The mean number of embryos transferred was 2.4 ± 0.7, the pregnancy rate was 27.2% (164/604), the implantation rate was 13.3% (192/1,442), and the abortion rate was 28.0% (46/164). Ninety nine healthy babies were born from 84 deliveries (boys: 49, girls: 50).

## 4 Blastocyst Vitrification

Recent advances in culture systems with sequential media have made it possible to develop human IVF embryos to the blastocyst stage quite easily. Because the blastocyst is better suited to the uterine environment and blastocyst formation is a form of selection for more viable embryos, blastocyst transfer has become a promising option to raise the overall pregnancy rate (19, 20). Accordingly, the need to cryopreserve human blastocysts is increasing. Menezo et al. (3) cryopreserved human cocultured blastocysts using the slow freezing method with glycerol and obtained reasonable clinical results (27% pregnancy rate, 17% implantation rate). However results reported by other clinics have not been consistent (21–23). Menezo et al. (3) speculated that the cryopreservation outcome is influenced by the culture conditions, such as a coculture system.

Recently, human blastocysts were successfully vitrified in straws (24). However, our own attempts to vitrify human blastocysts using straws resulted in only 45% survival (39/86) (unpublished data). Vanderzwalmen et al. (25) also reported a low pregnancy rate with human blastocysts vitrified in straws. This is probably because human blastocysts are much less permeable to CPA and water, since we have observed that they shrink more slowly than mouse and bovine blastocysts in the CPA solution. This suggests that human blastocysts are more likely to be injured by intracellular ice crystal formation.

Increased rates of cooling and warming can help circumvent the problem of intracellular ice formation in less permeable embryos. Faster rates of cooling and warming can be achieved by minimizing the volume of the solution with which embryos are vitrified, i.e., by using minute tools such as electron microscopic(EM) grids (26), open pulled straws (27) or cryoloops (2, 28). We showed that transfers of human blastocysts vitrified with cryoloops led to the first successful birth of a baby (13). Since our original report, we have continued to use this vitrification approach in our group of three clinics (Tokyo, Osaka, Hiroshima HART clinic) for the cryopreservation of blastocysts on day 5 and day 6. This chapter includes our summary of the clinical outcomes from our blastocyst vitrification program for the last 8 years, which confirms the effectiveness of the cryoloop technique for the cryopreservation of human blastocysts.

## 5 Protocol for Blastocysts Vitrification

The protocol for the cryoloop vitrification of blastocysts was adopted from a previous report (16), albeit with slight modifications, and has been described previously (13–15). The cryoloop consisted of a nylon loop (20 mm wide; 0.5–0.7 mm in diameter) mounted on a stainless steel pipe inserted into the lid of a cryovial (Hampton Research, Laguna Niguel., CA, USA) (Fig 2). A metal insert on the lid enables the use of a stainless steel handling rod with a small magnet (Crystalwand, Hampton Research) for manipulation of the loop at low temperature.

One or two blastocysts were vitrified in one cryoloop after a two-step procedure to load the blastocysts with CPAs at ~37°C. As the base medium, HEPES-buffered modified hTF medium supplemented with 10% (v/v) synthetic serum substitute (SSS) was used. Initially, blastocysts were placed in the base medium containing 7.5% (v/v) DMSO and 7.5% (v/v) EG (CPA solution I). After 2 min, the blastocysts were transferred into CPA solution II, which is the base medium containing 15% (v/v) DMSO, 15% (v/v) EG, 10 mg/ml of Ficoll 70 (average molecular weight 70,000; Pharmacia Biotech, Uppsala, Sweden) and 0.65 mol/l sucrose (CPA solution II). Both CPA solutions had

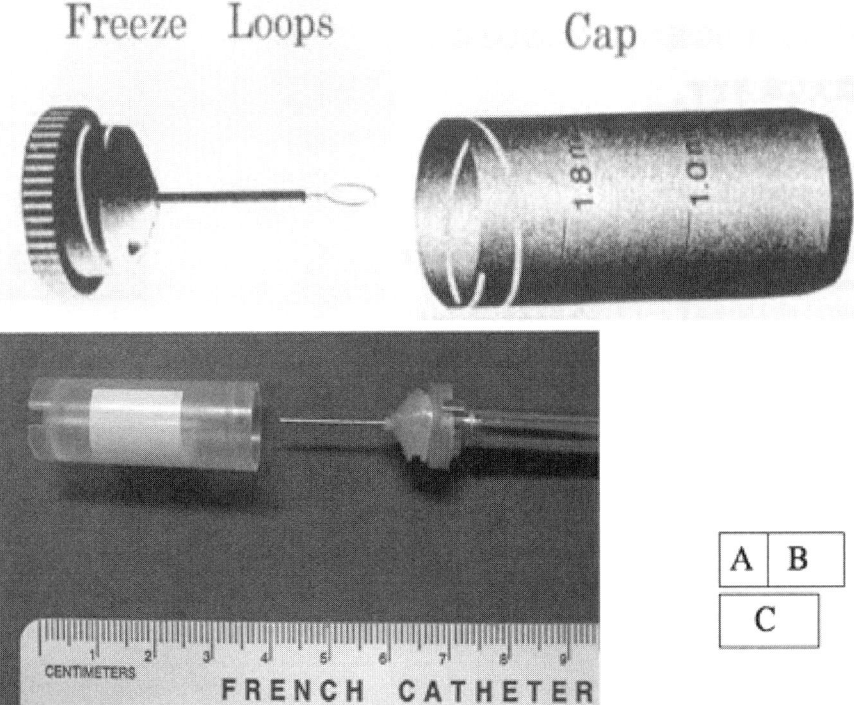


**Fig. 2** (**a**) Capping portion of the cryovial, which consists of a minute nylon loop (20 µm wide, 0.5–0.7 mm in diameter) mounted on a stainless steel tube inserted into the lid of a cryovial. (**b**) Container part of the cryovial. The shape and the size are similar to those of Nunc Cryovials used for semen cryopreservation. (**c**) The capping portion attached to a stainless steel handling rod with a small magnet for manipulation of the loop at low temperature

been warmed briefly in an incubator at 37°C and blastocysts were handled on the stage warmer of a dissecting microscope at 37°C.

While the blastocysts were suspended in CPA solution II, a cryoloop was dipped into CPA solution II in order to create a thin, filmy layer of solution, by surface tension, on the nylon loop. The blastocysts were then washed quickly in solution II and transferred onto the filmy layer on the nylon loop using a micropipette. Immediately after the loading of blastocysts, the cryoloop was plunged into $LN_2$. The time blastocysts were exposed to solution II before cooling was limited to 25–30 s. Using a stainless steel rod, the loop containing the blastocysts was sealed in a cryovial, which was previously submerged in $LN_2$. The vials were attached to standard canes and stored in $LN_2$. The entire procedure was completed within 5 min. Vitrified blastocysts were kept in the $LN_2$ tank for one month to 6 years depending on the patients' background.

## 6 Warming of Blastocysts, Assisted Hatching and Assessment of Survival

In a four-well multi-dish, ~1 ml of base medium containing 0.5 mol/l sucrose in no.1 well, base medium containing 0.25 mol/l sucrose in no. 2 well, and base medium in no. 3 well were warmed briefly in an incubator at 37°C and then placed on the stage warmer of a dissecting microscope. With the cryovial submerged in liquid nitrogen, the vial was opened with the aid of the stainless steel rod, and the loop containing blastocysts was removed from the liquid nitrogen and placed directly and quickly into the well containing the 0.5 mol/l sucrose solution (no.1) well. Blastocysts immediately fell from the loop into the solution. Thus blastocysts were warmed and diluted instantly at around 37°C adjusted by the stage warmer. After 2 min, the blastocysts were transferred to the 0.25 mol/l

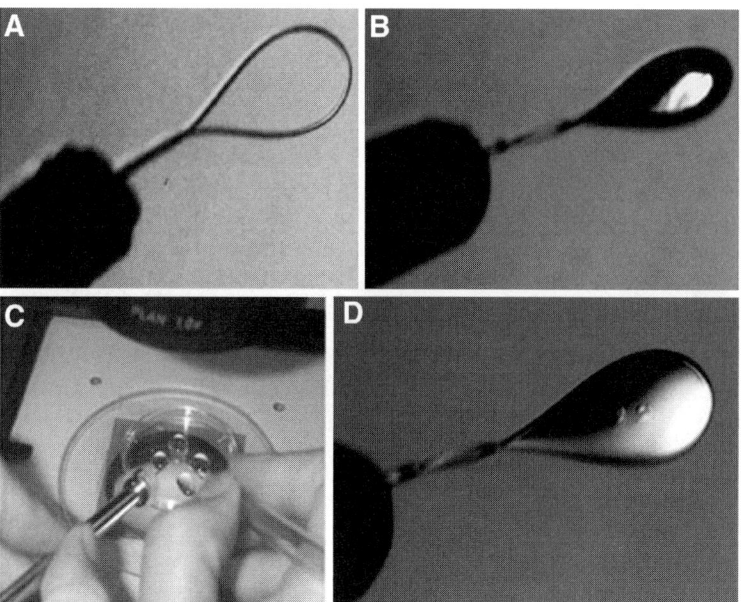


**Fig. 3** (**a**) A minute nylon loop (20 mm wide, 0.5–0.7 mm in diameter) mounted on a stainless steel pipe under 100× magnification. (**b**) A thin layer of the vitrification solution on the nylon loop after dipping the loop into the solution. (**c**) Under a dissecting microscope, the capping portion of cryovial with the cryoloop attached with a stainless steel handling rod for manipulation is held by left hand, and a pulled Pasteur pipette with blastocysts is held by the right hand. Prior to loading, blastocysts are rinsed several times in small drops of final vitrification solution (solution II) on the lid of a culture dish. (**d**) Blastocysts on the loop with thin layer of vitrification solution

sucrose solution in no. 2 well. After an additional 3 min, blastocysts were washed and kept in the base medium in no. 3 well for 5 min. During this 5 min. assisted zona hatching was always performed on warmed blastocysts with either acidic tyrode as previously described (29, 30) or Laser pulse on warmed blastocysts (Fig. 3). Then blastocysts were returned to Blast Assist Medium 2 (Medicult) medium or Global (Life Global) medium for further culture until transfer.

About 2–3 h after warming, the appearance of the blastocysts was examined on an inverted microscope at 400× magnification, and survival was assessed based on the morphological integrity of the blastomeres, inner cell mass and trophectoderm, and reexpansion of the blastocoele. The surviving blastocysts were scored as to developmental stage and were graded according to quality as described in the section on grading of blastocysts.

## 7 Patients and Grading of Blastocysts

We perform blastocyst transfer programs on patients who have had previous multiple failures of conventional day 2 or day 3 embryo transfer and who have agreed to use of the cryoloop vitrification method to cryopreserve their supernumerary blastocysts obtained 5 or 6 days after oocyte retrieval.

On day 5 after the oocyte pick up, blastocyst development was examined. Only on day 5, each embryo developed to the blastocyst stage was scored depending on the developmental stage, and graded according to quality criteria 32 with slight modifications (31).

Briefly, blastocysts were first given a numerical score from 1 to 6 on the basis of their degree of development. Secondly, the blastocysts were graded in three ranks based on morphological appearance. For example, the inner cell mass (ICM) was graded as A (many tightly packed cells), B (several loosely grouped cells), or C (few cells) and the trophectoderm was graded as A (many cells forming a cohesive epithelium), B (fewer cells forming a loose epithelium) or C (very few large cells).

When patients had their fresh embryos transferred on day 2–3, all the remaining embryos were cultured to allow those that developed into blastocysts to be vitrified. Patients who received transfers of fresh blastocysts had all their remaining supernumerary blastocysts vitrified. On day 5, if at least one supernumerary blastocyst was graded as A or B, all the blastocysts of the patient were vitrified regardless of the developmental stage and the grading. In a few cases, compacted morulae forming the cavity were also vitrified with the blastocysts. If all the blastocysts of the patient were graded C, they were not cryopreserved. On day 6, if at least one blastocyst had a large blastocoele (i.e., scored as 3–6) and was graded as A or B, all the developed blastocysts scored as 3–6 were vitrified.

## 8 Artificial Shrinkage (AS) of Expanded Blastocyst (Figs. 4, 5)

As previously mentioned, the first successful outcome of blastocyst vitrification using a cryoloop was originally reported in 2001(13), and in 2003, the summary of the clinical results with 223 warming cycles confirmed the effectiveness of the cryoloop technique for the cryopreservation of human blastocysts (14). However, this previous report in 2003 revealed that the survival rates were dependent on the developmental stage of blastocysts and were negatively correlated with the expansion of the blastocoele (32). The survival rate of early blastocysts with a smaller blastocoelic cavity, which was scored 1 and 2 according to Gardner's criteria (33), were 87% (48/55) and 97% (62/64) respectively. Also, full blastocysts lacking an expanded blastoceolic cavity, which were scored 3, had a survival rate of 89% (99/111). The total survival rate of blastocysts scored 1–3 together was 91% (209/230). However, the survival rate of both expanded and hatching blastocysts, scored 4 and 5 respectively was 85.0% (288/339), which was significantly lower than that of the score 1–3 group ($p < 0.05$). We therefore postulated that a large blastocoele might lessen cryopreservative potential due to ice crystal formation during the rapid cooling phase of vitrification. In order to overcome this problem, shrinkage of the blastoceole was thought to be the appropriate approach. Several studies reported an increase in the survival rate of blastocysts when the volume of the blastocoele was artificially reduced with glass microneedle (32), 29-gauge needle (34), or micropipetting with a hand-drawn Pasteur pipette (35).

Since 2003, therefore, we added artificial shrinkage (AS) after puncturing the blastocoele with a microneedle or laser pulse using a cryoloop technique prior to vitrification to improve the survival rate and clinical outcome of vitrified blastocyst transfer programs. In 2006, we reported the effectiveness of AS prior to vitrification, including the confirmation of the safety of this procedure (31).

The technique of shrinkage using microneedle puncture has been described previously (32). Briefly, about ten minutes before the vitrification, the expanded blastocysts were placed in 50 μl drops of preequilibrated Blast Assist Medium 2 (Medicult) or Global (Life Global) medium. The expanded blastocyst was held with a holding pipette connected to the micromanipulator, and the ICM was placed at the 6 or 12 o'clock position, a glass microneedle was pushed through the cellular junction of the trophectoderm into the blastocoele cavity until it shrank (Fig. 4). After removing the microneedle, contraction of the blastocoele was observed within a few minutes. After complete shrinkage of the blastocoele, the blastocyst was vitrified and stored in a $LN_2$ tank.

Since September of 2004, a laser pulse generated by laser system ZILOS-tkTM (Hamilton Thorn Bioscience Inc., Beverly, MA., USA) has been introduced to perform the artificial shrinkage, instead of microneedle puncture. The inner cell mass should be located away from the targeted point of the laser pulse. One single laser pulse (200 ms) targeted at the cellular junction of the trophectoderm creates a hole to induce collapsing of the blastocoelic cavity. The blastocoele of the expanded blastocyst shrank immediately (Fig. 5). With the use of this laser system, it is not necessary to hold and locate the expanded blastocyst with a holding pipette connected to the micromanipulator. The laser technique makes the procedures simple and convenient (31).

## 9 Clinical Results of Vitrified Blastocysts Transfer

At the HART clinic, a vitrified blastocysts transfer program using a cryoloop between November 1999 and December 2007 was analyzed (Fig. 6). A total of 5,412 blastocysts originating from 2,670 cycles were vitrified and warmed. Mean age was 36.2 years. Vitrified blastocysts were generated in three categories of patient groups. Group.1: Patients who had their fresh embryos transferred on day 2–3, and all the remaining embryos were cultured to allow those which developed into blastocysts to be vitrified. Group.2: Patients who received transfers of fresh blastocysts and had all their

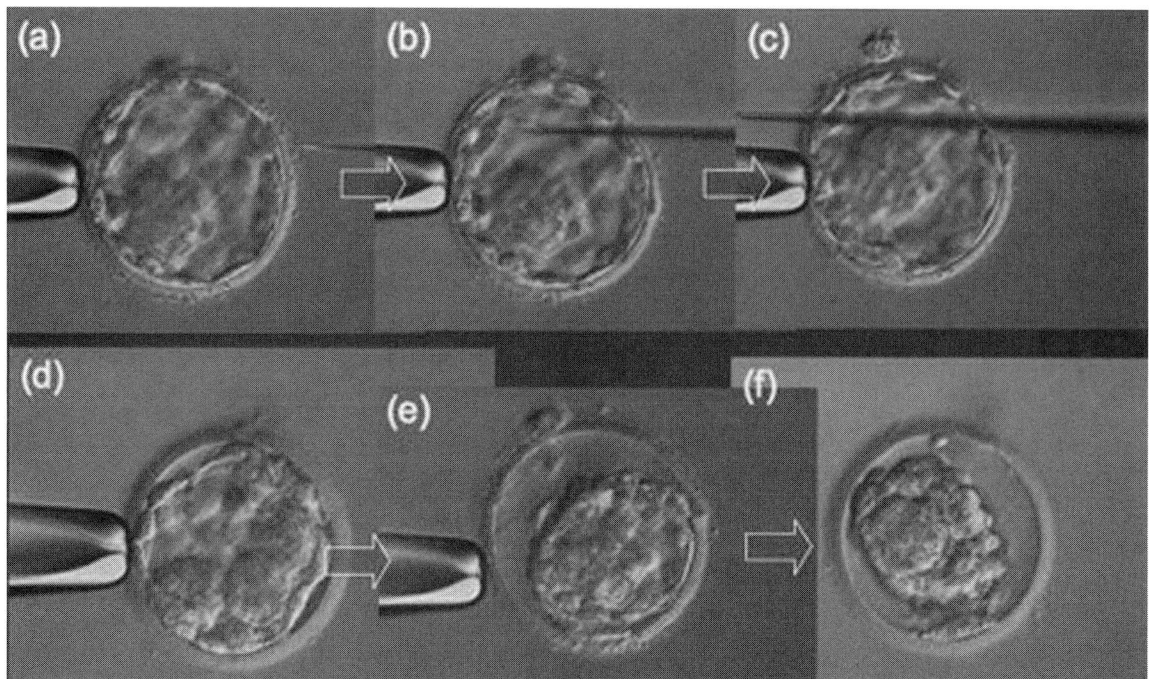


**Fig. 4** Artificial shrinkage of expanded blastocyst with the microneedle. (**a**) Holding the expanded blastocyst with holding micropipette connected to micromanipulation, (**b**) insertion of the microneedle inside the blastocoele at a point away from the inner cell mass, (**c**) Puncture through the blastocoele and removing the microneedle gradually, (**d**) beginning of shrinkage 10 s after puncture, (**e**) partial shrinkage 30 s after puncture, (**f**) complete shrinkage 1 min after puncture

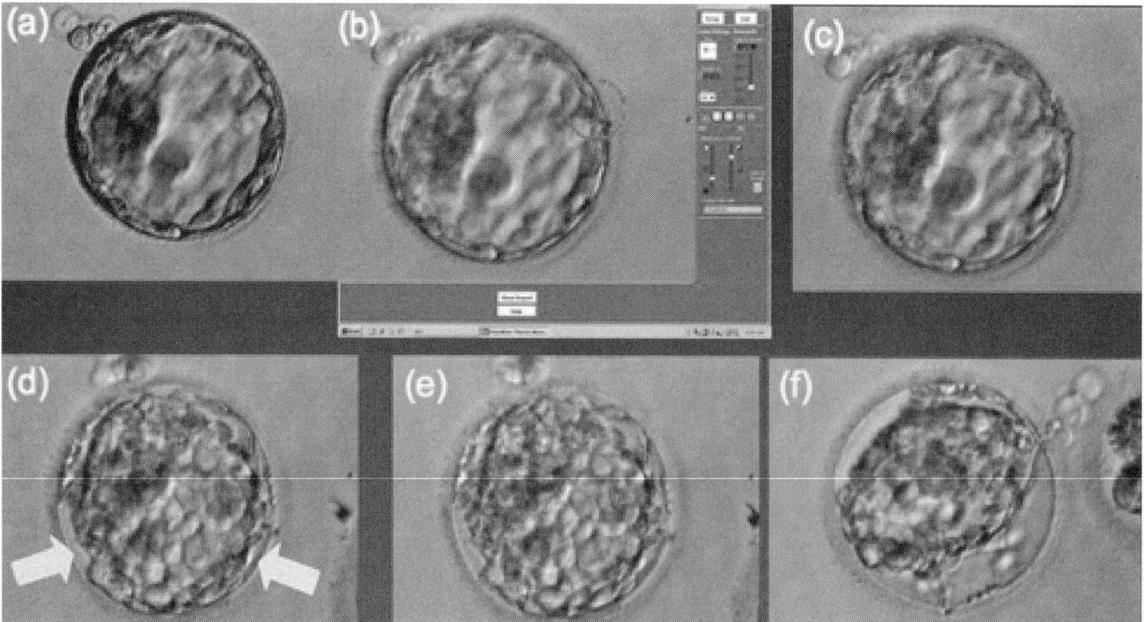


**Fig. 5** Artificial shrinkage of expanded blastocyst with a single laser pulse. (**a**) Prior to the artificial shrinkage, (**b**) a single laser pulse at the point of the cellular junction of trophectoderm cell at a point away from the inner cell mass (*circle* indicated), (**c**) beginning of shrinkage 5 s after laser shooting and arrows indicated formation of perivitelline space because of contraction, (**d**) shrinkage 10 s after laser shooting, (**e**) shrinkage 20 s after laser shooting, (**f**) almost complete shrinkage 30 s after laser shooting

| Clinical outcome of vitrification | |
|---|---|
| HART Clinics | 1999-2007 |
| Total No. of attempted cycles | 2670 |
| Total No. of warmed vitrified Bl. | 5412 |
| Total No. of survived Bl. | 4984 |
| Survival rate | 92.1% |
| No. of transferred cycles | 2599 |
| Mean No. of BL transferred | 1.65 |
| No. of clinical pregnancies(%/BT) | 1281 (49.3%) |
| No. of Implantation (%) | 1538 (35.9%) |
| No. of birth (babies; boy : girl) | 572 (706;351:355) |
| No. of Miscarriage (%) | 336 (26.2%) |

**Fig. 6** Clinical outcome data following blastocyst vitrification at the HART clinic

remaining supernumerary blastocysts vitrified. Group.3: Patients who had no fresh embryo transfer due to either OHSS symptom or attempting only vitrified blastocyst transfer intentionally, along with controlled endometrial cycle supplemented by exogenous female hormones in order to overcome multiple implantation failures, because uterine receptivity under controlled endometrial cycles was indicated as better than that under stimulated cycles. In HART clinics, fresh blastocyst transfer is intentionally avoided after two or three failures of fresh transfer. One of the reasons why fresh transfer is intentionally avoided is that ovarian hyperstimulation does not always create a suitable uterine receptivity and environment for implantation compared with controlled endometrial preparation using exogenous hormone.

After warming of vitrified blastocysts for transfer, 4,984 (92.1%) of the embryos survived. In 61 cycles, no blastocysts survived and embryo transfer was not conducted. In ten cycles, viable blastocysts were obtained but embryo transfer was cancelled because the number of cells that survived and the quality of the embryos were low. A total of 4,289 blastocysts were transferred in 2,599 cycles. The mean number of blastocysts transferred per cycle was 1.65. Of 2,599 transfers, 1,281 resulted in clinical pregnancy (confirmed by gestational sac in the uterus); the pregnancy rate was 48.0% per warming cycle, and 49.3% per transfer. The implantation rate was 35.9% (1,538/4,289). Seven hundred and six healthy babies were born in 572 deliveries, and 373 pregnancies are ongoing or have not been followed up. No bias in the sex ratio was observed since 351 babies were boys and 355 were girls. Three hundred thirty six pregnant cycles ended in miscarriage (26.2%). In comparison of 1,187 pregnancies established from fresh blastocyst transfers in our group of clinics during the same period, 249 (21.1%) resulted in miscarriages, and no difference was observed between them.

## 10 Clinical Results of Artificial Shrinkage (AS) Procedures

As we described (31), when we cryopreserve human blastocysts using the above vitrification technique at full, or more advanced, stages including expanded and hatching blastocysts, the AS procedure is always necessary prior to vitrification.

In order to show the effectiveness of AS, 270 cycles with 245 patients who had only expanded and/or hatching blastocysts vitrified were retrospectively evaluated. The average age of the patients was 35.6 years (27–41). Two hundred and sixty-six cycles had vitrified blastocyst transfer with artificial shrinkage. In four cycles, no blastocysts survived and embryo transfer was cancelled. Five hundred and two vitrified blastocysts were warmed for transfer, and 488 survived. Survival rate was 97.2%. Four hundred and forty-eight vitrified blastocysts were transferred, and the mean number of blastocysts transferred per cycle was 1.7. Of 266 transfers, 160 resulted in clinical pregnancy; the pregnancy rate was 59.3% per warming cycle (160/270), and 60.2% per transfer (160/266).

Results of vitrified expanded and hatching blastocysts in our previous study reported in 2003 served as a control group. Survival rate of both expanded and hatching blastocysts, scored 4 and 5 respectively was 85.0% (288/339). A statistical difference was noted between the study and the control groups ($p < 0.05$). When the pregnancy rate of the study group was compared with the control group, a statistically significant improvement was noticed in the AS group (60.2 vs. 34.1%; $p < 0.01$).

Also we performed preliminary comparisons between the results achieved by using microneedle or laser pulse for blasocoele shrinkage, to show the difference of methodologies for AS. AS using a microneedle was performed in 240 cycles with 462 blastocysts, and AS using a laser pulse was performed in 26 cycles with 40 blastocysts. The survival rates achieved with

**Table 3** Artificial Shrinkage using either microneedle or laser pulse

| | Microneedle | Laser pulse |
|---|---|---|
| No. of cycles with vitrified blastocyst transfer | 240 | 26 |
| No. of blastocysts vitrified | 462 | 40 |
| No. of vitrified blastocysts that survived | 449 | 39 |
| Survival rate (%) | 97.2 | 97.5 |
| Mean no. of blastocysts transferred | 1.6 | 1.4 |
| Clinical pregnancies | 144 | 16 |
| Percentage (%) | 60.0 | 61.5 |
| No. of implantation | 191 | 18 |
| Implantation rate (%) | 46.5 | 48.6 |
| No. of cycles miscarried | 32 | 3 |
| Percentage (%) | 22.2 | 18.8 |

the two methods were similar (microneedle: 97.2% vs. laser pulse: 97.5%). The mean number of survived blastocysts transferred was also similar. Clinical pregnancy, implantation and miscarriage rates were also similar. No statistical difference was observed in the results achieved with the two methods (31, Table 3). We reported the perinatal outcome (36) of our vitrified blastocyst transfer program in 2004.

## 11 Discussion

Numerous protocols for the cryopreservation of mammalian embryos have been reported. The protocols can be classified into four methods, original slow freezing, conventional slow freezing, conventional vitrification using the conventional cryo-straw and ultra-rapid vitrification using a minute tool. Although strategies to circumvent various injuries (especially from the formation of intracellular ice) are different, the principle of cryopreservation is the same. The most suitable protocol should be adopted for each case. For certain types of embryos such as human blastocysts and bovine embryos at earlier stages, ultra-rapid vitrification will be the preferred choice, because the survival rates of embryos cryopreserved by other methods have been low. For other embryos, e.g., mouse embryos, bovine blastocysts and human embryos at 2–8 cell stages, both slow freezing and conventional vitrification have proven effective. However, vitrification has a potential advantage in that higher survival rates can be obtained if conditions, such as temperature and duration of exposure of embryos to the CPA, as well as the skill of pipetting, are optimized. Therefore, vitrification would be a preferred method of cryopreservation to the slow-cooling method because of both the lack of ice crystal formation and its greater convenience.

We have already reported (9) a simple vitrification method using an ethylene glycol-based solution for 4–8 cell human embryos frozen in conventional cryo-straws. Moreover, the success of vitrification procedures has recently been increased by techniques that substantially reduce the volume of the vitrification solution. Among such techniques, the Cryoloop and Cryotops are the most refined strategy. A major difference between the Cryoloop, the Cryotop, and the conventional cryo-straw for vitrification is the cooling and warming rate. The Cryoloop and the Cryotop enable ultra-rapid cooling and warming, and this may have prevented intracellular ice formation, more consistently since we have observed that human embryos are dehydrated and concentrated more slowly than other types of embryos, suggesting that intracellular ice is more likely to form. The difference between the Cryoloop and the Cryotop is only in the way vitrified embryos are held. In the Cryoloop system, the vitrified embryo is almost floating in the thin filmy layer of the droplet on the nylon loop, and heat conduction to the embryos becomes homogenous. In the Cryotop, the vitrified embryo is placed on the surface of nylon sheet, and heat conduction might not be homogenous especially from the sides of the plastic tip. For the cryopreservation of multiple cells or a small amount of tissue, this may create uneven heat conduction; however, for a smaller number of eggs or embryos, it does not seem to make any difference.

In conclusion, for day 2–3 human embryos, vitrification through ultra-rapid cooling achieved by direct contact with $LN_2$ seems preferable, and either EG only or EG + DMSO as CPAs are acceptable. For equilibration prior to vitrification, a two step approach is enough to obtain acceptable clinical results. Moreover, individual adjustment of cryoprotectant exposure times depending on the morphological change is always better for equilibration compared with the fixed duration protocol. Theoretically, the Rama Raju et al. (18) protocol for equilibration and warming adding individual adjustments in each step will be the most appropriate approach based on our review. Finally, maximizing the cooling rate and minimizing the concentration of croprotectants is critical to establish the protocol for vitrification with any stage of embryo, and vitrification of day 2–3 human embryos is more effective than using the slow cooling approach.

With the development of sequential culture media, based upon the physiology of the human reproductive tract and the changing physiology of the developing embryos, it is possible to grow viable blastocysts easily in vitro. And because of the resulting high implantation rates, blastocyst transfer will necessarily be a good approach in ART. Accordingly, the need to cryopreserve human blastocysts is increasing.

The cryoloop enables ultra-rapid cooling and warming, and this may consistently prevent intracellular ice formation, since we have observed that human blastocysts are dehydrated and concentrated more slowly than in earlier stage embryos, suggesting that intracellular ice is more likely to form in blastocysts. Furthermore the technique using the cryoloop is easier and simpler than that using the cryo-straw.

## 12 Oocyte Vitrification

Cryopreservation of human oocytes has been significantly improved by the refined slow-freezing methods and new vitrification techniques. The establishment of oocyte cryopreservation techniques would provide a number of benefits. First it could prevent ethical and legal problems associated with embryo freezing, particularly in certain countries where embryo freezing is banned or limited by law. Second, the age at which people marry is rising, resulting in infertility issues, and an egg bank would create an option for older women to have children later in life. Third, it would allow enough time for genetic and infectious screening in donor oocyte programs. It would also provide the convenience for synchronization of procedures and utilize precious donor oocytes efficiently thereby avoiding the unnecessary use of fertilization by the recipient's husband's sperm. Finally oocyte freezing gives the option of fertility preservation for patients who receive anticancer treatment or oophorectomy.

Although cryopreservation has a lot of advantages as above, clinical outcomes remain unsatisfactory due to lower pregnancy and implantation rate resulting from decrease in survival rates and poor embryo development.

There are many reasons to be listed as to why cryopreservation of oocytes does not achieve satisfactory results. The size and shape of the oocyte are quite obvious reasons. Cryobiologically, those reasons are quite important to achieve acceptable permeation of CPA, dehydration and rehydration. Moreover, another reason is that the oocyte itself is single cell. Survival can be judged as all or nothing. Multicellular embryos can survive and compensate for as much as half of the loss of their cells, as demonstrated by biopsy and further development after cryosurvival.

Apart from the factors mentioned above, there are many other factors that influence the sensitivity of oocytes to cryobiological damages. In terms of CPA permeability, the plasma membrane is extremely sensitive and rapidly undergoes a transition from the liquid state to the gel state, an irreversible process that is detrimental for further development. For some reasons including the releasing of cortical granules, after fertilization, the plasma membrane of the zygote is much less sensitive to this type of injury. Chilling injury that occurs at relatively high temperatures induces irreversible damage of cytoplasmic lipid droplets, lipid-rich plasma membranes, and microtubules (37). The osmotic shock at equilibration may result in shrinking and deformity of oocytes, supposedly damaging the cytoskeleton. On the other hand, osmotic swelling shock that can occur during the dilution (rehydration) steps may results in extensive swelling, rupture of the membrane, lysis, and immediate death of the oocyte. These damages might relate the depolymerization of microtubules, misalignment of chromosomes, and the possible increased risk of aneuploidy. However, similar to somatic cell nuclear transfer, in human oocyte, spindle reorganization (38) may occur surprisingly efficiently, and the number of chromosomal abnormalities in children born after oocyte vitrification does not seem to find a significant increase.

Based on the factors listed above, principles of a successful cryopreservation strategy can be found in an ultra-rapid vitrification system for the following reasons. The large cell and spherical shape of the oocyte necessitate the use of high permeable cryoprotectants with low toxicity. According to earlier investigations in rabbits (39), the permeability of ethylene glycol is facilitated by dimethylsulphoxide (DMSO). A possible way to minimize toxic and osmotic effects of CPA is to decrease the required concentration of CPA while maintaining the ice-free solidification pattern. The only practical way to achieve above circumstances is to induce extreme increase in cooling rates. For this purpose, electron microscope(EM) grids (26), cryoloops (28), and cryotops (40) seems to be the most appropriate tools as well as containers. And the problem of zona hardening and subsequent low level of fertilization has been eliminated entirely with the discovery and subsequent widespread application of ICSI.

Since vitrification was introduced as an alternative approach for cryopreservation of human gametes and embryos, vitrification, with recent improvements, has become a more reliable strategy, not only because it is very simple but also because it can lead to high clinical efficiency along with better clinical outcome. In particular, ultra-rapid vitrification opens a new era for oocyte and blastocyst cryopreservation as described by the author in this chapter. Classically, enough equilibration of CPA and dehydration are necessary to cryopreserve gametes and embryos. However, extremely high cooling rates achieved by direct plunging into $LN_2$ with minimal volume (≤0.5 ml) of final vitrification solution including vitrified cells, could obtain high survival rate and better viability and help us to escape ice crystal formation even with the lower concentration of CPA, that could cause devitrification (ice crystal formation) if conventional cooling was applied. Recently this ultra-rapid vitrification approach was applied for ovarian tissue cryopreservation and stem cell cryopreservation. With the proper preparation of ovarian tissue such as 1 cm square shape and less than 1 mm thickness with properly designed container, high survival and better postwarming viability can be expected in this vitrification approach. In future, vitrification will become the most suitable method for cryopreservation of any cells and tissues.

## 12.1 Materials and Methods of Oocyte Vitirifcation

Recently, many reports related to oocyte vitrification have been coming out with ultra-rapid vitrification technique, especially cryotop (40) method. That was why I chose cryotop technique to describe the clinical usefulness of oocyte vitrification in this chapter.

The cryotop that was originally introduced (40) by Kuwayama is now used in an increasing number of laboratories worldwide for oocyte vitrification as well as embryo cryopreservation. The technique of the cryotop vitrification for oocyte was reported in number of scientific papers (41, 42) and cryotop vitrification kit (Kitazato, Tokyo, Japan) has been commercially available for the last 4 years. The kit contains the cryotop device, a filmstrip attached to a plastic handle also equipped with a cap to cover the filmstrip for safe handling and storage, and all media required for washing, equilibration, vitrification, warming, and dilution. These solutions are based on TCM199 medium supplemented with synthetic serum substitute (SSS), and containing ethylene glycol, DMSO, as permeable CPA and sucrose as non permeable CPA. Concept and concentration of these solutions are quite similar to cryoloop vitrification described preciously. However, no Ficoll is added in the vitrification solution for cryotop technique.

All media and manipulations should be performed at 25–27°C, except for thawing where the medium should be warmed to 37°C. Oocytes can be vitrified 2–6 h after the ovum pick-up, immediately after denudation. A stepwise, very mild initial equilibration procedure can be carried out by making 20 µL droplets of washing and equilibration solutions (one and two droplets, respectively) close to each other, and unifying droplets when oocytes seem to have completely recovered from the osmotic effect (a total of approximately 6 min). Finally, oocytes should be placed into an equilibration drop and incubated until they are completely recovered (approximately in an additional 9 min). Subsequently, one oocyte should be placed into a large volume of vitrification solution, mixed well, and after 60 s loaded on the film strip of the cryotop. All excess media should be removed leaving only the oocyte covered with a thin layer of vitrification solution. Then the film part should be submerged into liquid nitrogen with a quick and continuous vertical movement to ensure the maximum cooling rate (23,000°C/min). Finally, under the liquid nitrogen, the cap should be fixed on the cryotop with forceps to protect the film part from mechanical damage during transfer to the container and storage. At warming, the film part of the cryotop should be submerged quickly into the 37°C warming solution to reach extremely high warming rate (42,000°C/min). After 10 s, the oocyte can be gently removed from the surface of the cryotop and kept submerged in the warming solution. After 1 min, the dilution should be continued in the dilution and washing solutions for 3, 5 min, respectively. Oocytes should be kept for an additional 2 h before the ICSI.

### 12.2 Results of Oocyte Vitrification with Cryotop Technique

The cryotop is now used in an increasing number of laboratories world wide for oocyte vitrification. Luccena et al. (41) reported 89.2% survival rates after cryotop vitrification and a total pregnancy rate of 56.5% (13 of 23 patients) with and average of 4.63 embryos transferred to each patient. Ruvalcava et al. (42) from Mexico have reported 401/445 (90.1%) survival and 34.1% pregnancy rates. In Valencia, Spian, Cobo et al., (submitted) have vitrified a total of 225 MII oocytes. Of which 217 (96.5%) survived, and 165(76.0%) were normally fertilized after ICSI, which was not different from the controls. Of zygotes 93.9% underwent cleavage on day 2 and 22.4% of them reached blastocyst stage. Twenty-one cycles of embryo transfer were performed and resulted in 13 pregnancies (61.9% pregnancy and 37.2% implantation rates). Kato Ladies Clinic, where Dr. Kuwayama belongs, also reported more than 90% of survival and cleavage rate, resulting in around 40–50% pregnancy rates (personal communication). They concluded that cryotop vitrification of oocytes may soon exceed the total numbers of babies born after other cryopreservation methods worldwide with high survival and implantation potential.

## 13 Conclusions

For embryo cryopreservation, the vitrification method has many advantages over the slow freezing method: (1) injuries related to ice are less likely to occur (2) survival of embryos can be maintained at a higher level if conditions for embryo treatment are optimized and (3) embryos can be cryopreserved by a simple method in a short period without a programmable freezer. Therefore, vitrification is suitable for human embryos, in which a small number of embryos are cryopreserved frequently. Human embryos at early cleavage stages can be cryopreserved by conventional vitrification using cryostraws or by ultrarapid vitrification using cryoloops. Human blastocysts are more efficiently cryopreserved by the ultra-rapid approach. Our clinical outcome shows that vitrification of blastocysts using the cryoloop technique results in high survival and high pregnancy rates, and confirms the safety of this procedure as seen in our perinatal evaluation.

## References


1. Kasai M. Simple and efficient methods for vitrification of mammalian embryos. Anim Reprod Sci 1996;42: 67–75.
2. Kasai M. Advances in the cryopreservation of mammalian oocytes and embryos: development of ultrarapid vitrification. Reprod Med Biol 2002;1: 1–9.
3. Lassalle B, Testart J, and Renard JP. Human embryo features that influence the success of cryopreservation with the use of 1,2 propanediol. Fertil Steril 1985;44: 645–651.
4. Fehilly CB, Cohen J, Edwards RG, et al. Cryopreservation of cleaving embryos and expanded blastocysts in the human: a comparative study. Fertil Steril 1985;44: 638–644.
5. Hartshorne GM, Elder K, Edwards RG, et al. The influence of in-vitro development upon post-thaw survival and implantation of cryopreserved human blastocysts. Hum Reprod 1991;6: 136–141.
6. Menezo Y, Nicollet B, Andre D, et al. Freezing cocultured human blastocysts. Fertil Steril 1992;58: 977–980.
7. Rall WF, Fahy GM. Ice-free cryopreservation of mouse embryos at −196°C by vitrification. Nature 1985;313: 573–575.
8. Kasai M, Komi JH, Machida T, et al. A simple method for mouse embryo cryopreservation in a low toxicity vitrification solution, without appreciable loss of viability. J Reprod Fertil 1990;89: 91–97.
9. Mukaida T, Takahashi K, Kasai M, et al. Vitrification of human embryos based on the assessment of suitable conditions for 8-cell mouse embryos. Hum Reprod 1998;13: 2874–2879.
10. Saito H, Kaneko T, Hiroi M, et al. Application of vitrification to human embryo freezing. Gynecol Obstet Invest 2000;49: 145–149.
11. Yokota Y, Yokota H, Araki Y, et al. Birth of healthy twins from in vitro development of human refrozen embryos. Fertil Steril 2001;76: 1063–1065.
12. Kasai M. Vitrification: refined strategy for the cryopreservation of mammalian embryos. J Mamm Ova Res 1997;14: 17–28.
13. Mukaida T, Kasai M, Takahashi K, et al. Successful birth after transfer of vitrified human blastocysts with use of a cryoloop containerless technique. Fertil Steril 2001;76: 618–620.
14. Mukaida T, Oka C, Takahashi K, et al. Vitrification of human blastocysts using cryoloops: clinical outcome of 223 cycles. Hum Reprod 2003;18: 384–391.
15. Mukaida T, Takahashi K, Kasai M, et al. Blastocyst cryopreservation: ultrarapid Vitrification using cryoloop technique. Reprod BioMed Online 2003;6: 221–225.
16. Lane M, Schoolcraft WB, and Gardner DK. Vitrification of mouse and human blastocysts using a novel cryoloop container-less technique. Fertil Steril 1999;72: 1073–1078.

17. Desai N, Blackmon H, Goldfarb J, et al. Cryoloop vitrification of human day 3 cleavage-stage embryos: post-vitrification development, pregnancy outcomes and live births. Reprod BioMed Online 2007;14: 208–213.
18. Rama Raju GA, Haranath GB, Madan K, et al. Vitrification of human 8-cell embryos, a modified protocol for better pregnancy rates. Reprod BioMed Online 2005;11: 434–437.
19. Gardner DK, Schoolcraft WB, Stevens J, et al. A prospective randomized trial of blastocyst culture and transfer in in vitro fertilization. Hum Reprod 1998;13: 3434–3440.
20. Cruz JR, Dubey AK, Gindoff PR, et al. Is blastocyst transfer useful as an alternative treatment for patients with multiple in vitro fertilization failures? Fertil Steril 1999;72: 218–220.
21. Troup SA, Matson PL, Lieberman BA, et al. Cryopreservation of human embryos at the pronucleate, early cleavage, or expanded blastocyst stages. Eur J Obstet Gynecol Reprod Biol 1990;38: 133–139.
22. Nakayama T, Goto Y, Noda Y, et al. Developmental potential of frozen-thawed human blastocysts. J Assist Reprod Genet 1995;12: 239–243.
23. Ludwig M, Al-Hasani S, Diedrich K, et al. New aspects of cryopreservation of oocytes and embryos in assisted reproduction and future perspectives. Hum Reprod 1999;14:Suppl 1: 162–185.
24. Yokota Y, Sato S, Araki Y, et al. Birth of a healthy baby following vitrification of human blastocysts. Fertil Steril 2001;75: 1027–1029.
25. Vanderzwalmen P, Zech H, Van Roosendaal E, et al. Pregnancy and implantation rates after transfers of fresh and vitrified embryos on day 4 or 5. J Assist Reprod Genet 1999;16: 147.26.
26. Martino A, Songsasen N, and Leibo SP. Development into blastocysts of bovine oocytes cryopreserved by ultra-rapid cooling. Biol Reprod 1996;54: 1059–1069.
27. Vajta G, Kuwayama M, Callesen H, et al. Open Pulled Straw (OPS) vitrification: a new way to reduce cryoinjuries of bovine ova and embryos. Mol Reprod Dev 1998;51: 53–58.
28. Lane M, Bavister BD, Forest KT, et al. Containerless vitrification of mammalian oocytes and embryos. Nat Biotechnol 1999;17: 1234–1236.
29. Cohen J, Alikani M, Rosenwaks Z, et al. Implantation enhancement by selective assisted hatching using zona drilling of human embryos with poor prognosis. Hum Reprod 1992;7: 685–691.
30. Obruca A, Strohmer H, Sakkas D. Use of lasers in assisted fertilization and hatching. Hum Reprod 1994;9: 1723–1726.
31. Mukaida T, Takahashi K, Oka C, et al. Artificial Shrinkage of blastocoele using either micro-needle or laser pulse prior to the cooling steps of vitrification improves survival rate and pregnancy outcome of vitrified human blastocysts. Hum Reprod 2006;21: 3246–3252.
32. Vanderzwalmen, P, Mukaida, T, Schoysman, R, et al. Births after vitrification at morula and blastocyst stages: effect of artificial reduction of the blastocoelic cavity before vitrification. Hum Reprod 2002;17: 744–751.
33. Gardner DK, and Schoolcraft WB. In-vitro culture of human blastocyst. In Jansen, R. Mortimer, D, eds, Towards Reproductive Certainty: Infertility and Genetics Beyond 1999. Carnforth: Parthenon Press, 1999: 378–388.
34. Son WY, Yoon SH, Lim JH, et al. Pregnancy outcome following transfer of human blastocysts vitrified on electron microscopy grids after induced collapse of the blastocoele. Hum Reprod 2003;18: 137–139.
35. Hiraoka K, Hiraoka K, Kinutani K, et al. Blastocoele collapse by micropipetting prior to vitrification gives excellent survival and pregnancy outcomes for human day 5 and 6 expanded blastocysts. Hum Reprod 2004;19: 2884–2888.
36. Takahashi K, Mukaida T, Oka C, et al. Perinatal outcome of blastocyst transfer with vitrification using cryoloop: A 4 year follow-up study. Fertil Steril 2005;84: 88–92.
37. Ghetler Y, Yavin S, Shalgi R, et al. The effect of chilling on membrane lipid phase transition in human oocytes and zygotes. Hum Reprod 2005;20: 3385–3389.
38. Santhananthan AH, Ng SC, Trounson A, et al. The effects of ultrarapid freezing on mitotic spindles of oocytes and embryos. Gamete Res 1998;21: 385–401.
39. Vicente JS, Garicia-Ximenez F. Osmotic and cryoprotecitve effects of a mixture of DMSO and ethylene glycol on rabbit morulae. Theriogenology 1994;42: 1205–15.
40. Kuwayama M, Vajta G, Kato O, et al. Highly efficient vitrification method for cryopreservation of human oocytes. Reprod BioMed Online 2005;11: 300–308.
41. Lucena E, Bernal DP, Lucena A, et al. Successful ongoing pregnancies after vitrification of oocytes. Fertil Steril 2006;85: 108–111.
42. Ruvalcaba L, Garcfa M, Martinez R, et al. Oocyte vitrification success: first ongoing pregnancy in Mexico. Reprod Hum 2005;3: 7–10.

# Imprinting Errors and IVF

Victoria K. Cortessis

**Abstract** Imprinting disorders have been reported in children conceived by IVF. There is concern that procedures of IVF may interfere with epigenetic processes responsible for setting imprint marks during gametogenesis. This possibility seems plausible in light of the rarity of these conditions and results of experiments examining imprint marks in model organisms subjected to *in vitro* manipulations. We quantitatively summarized published human data on this question by meta-analysis, relating IVF to the risk of four model imprinting disorders. Estimates of summary relative risk were 3.7 (95% confidence interval (CI) = 1.7–7.8) for Angelman syndrome, 6.1 (95% CI = 3.8–11) for Beckwith-Wiedemann syndrome, and 5.7 (95% CI = 1.4–22) for Prader-Willi syndrome. Published data were insufficient to conduct meaningful analyses of risk of Silver-Russel syndrome. These results are consistent with the elevated risk of imprinting disorders following IVF, although absolute risk of these outcomes remains low. Elevated risk could in theory arise from either detrimental effects of IVF procedures or increased occurrence of aberrant methylation of imprinted genes in gametes of subfertile parents.

**Keywords** Imprinted gene • Angelman syndrome (AS) • Beckwith-Wiedemann syndrome (BWS) • Prader-Willi syndrome (PWS) • Silver-Russel syndrome (SRS) • *In vitro* fertilization • (IVF) Assisted reproductive technology (ART)

V.K. Cortessis
Department of Preventive Medicine, Keck School of Medicine, Norris Comprehensive Cancer Center, University of Southern California, Los Angeles, CA, USA
e-mail: cortessi@usc.edu

## 1 Introduction

### 1.1 Imprinted Genes

In diploid organisms including humans, autosomal genes are present in two copies or alleles. Most autosomal genes are expressed from both the maternal and the paternal alleles (gene copies inherited from the mother and the father, respectively). However, in placental mammals, a small subset of autosomal genes, the "imprinted genes," are expressed from only one allele, determined by the parent of origin. Imprinted genes are characterized by the allele that is not expressed. Thus, under normal circumstances "paternally imprinted genes" are expressed from the maternal allele, and "maternally imprinted genes" from the paternal allele. To date, nearly 50 imprinted genes have been identified in the human genome (1, 2), although several times this number are postulated to exist.

Parent-of-origin expression of imprinted genes appears to be controlled largely by epigenetic mechanisms of gene regulation. These mechanisms do not rely on DNA sequence differences of expressed versus unexpressed alleles. Instead, alleles inherited from each parent are differentially packaged in other molecules. At imprinting control regions, often in the vicinity of imprinted genes, proteins and covalently bound molecules are arranged in distinct patterns – termed "imprints" – on the maternal versus paternal alleles. Methyl groups bound to DNA are the imprint marks that have been most thoroughly characterized to date. The imprints are reset in each generation, in a multi-staged process that includes several key events: protection of imprint marks in the preimplantation embryo, erasure of imprint marks during migration of primordial germ cells to the genital ridges, and resetting imprint marks

D.T. Carrell et al. (eds.), *Biennial Review of Infertility,* DOI: 10.1007/978-1-60327-392-3_16

in gender-specific patterns at various stages of gametogenesis.

## 1.2 Functional Haploidy of Imprinted Genes

Genes that are expressed from both alleles have functional redundancy: even if one allele does not encode functional RNA or protein, it is very likely that the other one does. The advantage of such redundancy is apparent in numerous X-linked recessive disorders, such as some forms of muscular dystrophy and color blindness. Among females who carry two copies of each X chromosome gene, these conditions are far rarer than among males with a single copy of each. Haploid males develop these conditions after inheriting a single allele with significant functional deficits, whereas females who inherit such an allele are generally protected by functional RNA or protein encoded by a second, intact allele.

A similar situation exists at imprinted loci: although two copies of each imprinted gene are present, only one is expressed. Imprinted genes are therefore functionally haploid. As a consequence, they can convey vulnerabilities associated with functional deficits of the expressed allele, even in the presence of a second allele. Unlike X chromosome genes, however, imprinted genes impart haploid vulnerability to both sexes.

## 1.3 Origin of Imprinted Genes

It is widely accepted that the biological benefits of sexual reproduction outweigh disease risk arising from the haploid state of the male X chromosome. What biological benefit could balance the consequences to both sexes of the functional haploidy of imprinted genes? One hypothesis postulates that patterns of expression of imprinted genes have resulted from differing selective pressures on maternal versus paternal alleles (3). Based on the premise that maternal strategies for promoting offspring survival would distribute resources among all of a female's pregnancies, whereas paternal strategies would concentrate resources on each ongoing pregnancy, one prediction of the hypothesis relates to growth control by imprinted genes. Specifically, paternally expressed genes were predicted to promote fetal growth, while maternally expressed genes were predicted to restrict it. Aspects of these predictions have been borne out in subsequent research on the function of molecules encoded by imprinted genes, the majority of which influence embryonic development and fetal growth (4, 5).

## 1.4 Consequences of Improper Parental Contributions of Imprinted Genes

The phenotypic consequences of uniparental gestation – in which a conceptus receives the usual number of chromosomes from a single parent – have been demonstrated both experimentally and clinically. In an elegant set of experiments conducted in the 1980s, fertilized mouse eggs were manipulated to contain two pronuclei of uniparental origin. Although each conceptus had a full set of genetic material, development was very abnormal: bi-paternal conceptuses experienced minimal embryonic development but had overgrown extra-embryonic tissue, whereas bi-maternal embryos developed to early somite stage but had very little extra-embryonic tissue (6). These experiments provided dramatic evidence of the nonequivalence of maternal and paternal DNA, a phenomenon now attributed to genetic imprinting. In the clinical setting, two gynecologic tumor types originate from uniparental gestation: the DNA of ovarian mature teratomas is of solely maternal origin whereas that of complete hydatidiform moles is of solely paternal origin (7).

Dramatic phenotypes can also result from improper complements of far smaller subsets of the genome containing imprinted genes. Uniparental disomy is the rare state in which an individual has received both copies of an autosomal gene or chromosome from the same parent. A number of dramatic developmental phenotypes result from uniparental disomy involving chromosomal regions containing imprinted genes. Many of the same disorders can occur in the absence of disomy, resulting instead from either genetic errors, such as deletion or mutation of an imprinted gene, or from improperly set imprint marks, also called imprinting defects. The anticipated molecular consequence of each of these etiologies is the improper expression of one or more imprinted genes. The resulting sets of conditions are called "model imprinting disorders."

## 2 Imprinting Disorders Following In Vitro Fertilization (IVF)

Model imprinting disorders are individually and collectively extremely rare. Reports that one of these disorders, Angelman syndrome, was diagnosed in several children conceived by IVF, was therefore interpreted as a possible indication that assisted reproductive technology may have the potential to cause improper imprinting (6, 7). Occurrence of a second model imprinting disorder, Beckwith-Wiedeman syndrome, was subsequently reported among children conceived by IVF. Similarities between the overgrowth phenotype observed in this syndrome and the veterinary condition large offspring syndrome intensified concerns about a possible role of IVF, since large offspring syndrome appeared to be induced by conditions of embryo culture (10). Very recent experiments conducted on the laboratory mouse demonstrated the plausibility of a causal role of IVF, reporting aberrant imprints in embryo DNA, (11) and abnormal placental expression of imprinted genes (12) following superovulation, as well as aberrant embryonic expression of imprinted genes following IVF, (13) and manipulation of embryos (14).

### 2.1 Body of Review

To examine published human data on associations between IVF and imprinting disorders, we conducted an extensive literature review on associations between a history of IVF conception and occurrence of each of four imprinting disorders: Angelman syndrome and Beckwith-Wiedemann syndrome (Table 1) had been postulated previously to have IVF as a possible etiology, and both conditions are associated with disrupted imprinting of maternal origin. Prader-Willi syndrome and Silver-Russel (Table 1) are regarded as reciprocal conditions to Angelman syndrome and Beckwith-Wiedemann syndrome, respectively, because they are associated with disrupted paternal imprinting of the same chromosomal regions. These latter conditions were addressed in this review in order to examine the possible role of paternal imprinting in the IVF setting.

### 2.2 Methods

MEDLINE and PubMed were searched for all articles published in English through April 2008 describing

**Table 1** Population frequencies and proportionate contributions of described etiologies of four imprinting disorders

| Disorder | Population frequency | Described etiologies and approximate proportion attributed to each |
|---|---|---|
| Syndromes associated with imprinting defects of maternal origin | | |
| Angelman syndrome MIM#105830 | 1/15,000 | 80% genetic (70% deletion maternal 15q11–q13; 10% *UBE3A* mutation) (29)<br>0% unknown (29)<br>5% paternal UPD (29)<br>5% maternal ID (29) |
| Beckwith-Wiedemann syndrome MIM#130650 | 1/14,5000 | 45% maternal ID chromosome 11 (40% hypomethylated ICR2; 5% hypermethylated ICR1) (30)<br>22–27% unknown (30)<br>20% paternal UPD chromosome 11 (30)<br>7% genetic (2% paternal deletion or maternal rearrangement chromosome 11p15.5; 5% *CDKN1C* mutation; 5% ICR1 or ICR2 deletion) (30) |
| Syndromes associated with imprinting defects of paternal origin | | |
| Prader-Willi syndrome MIM#176270 | 1/10,000–1/15,000 | 80% genetic (75% deletion paternal 15q11–q13; 5% balanced translocation or other) (31)<br>20% maternal UPD (31)<br>1% paternal ID (31) |
| Silver-Russell syndrome MIM%180860 | 1/3,000–1/100,000 | 50% maternal UPD chromosome 7 (32)<br>40% unknown (32)<br>10% paternal ID (hypomethylation) chromosome 11 (32) |

*ICR* imprinting control region; *UPD* uniparental disomy; *ID* imprinting defect

associations between conception by ART and occurrence of imprinting disorders. Publications were reviewed in detail and selected for inclusion in the meta-analysis if they met two criteria: (1) specifically reported on occurrence of one or more imprinting disorders in a defined series of children conceived following ART, and (2) reported on occurrence of the same set of disorders in a comparable population conceived without ART. A single reviewer extracted data from each of the reports found to meet these criteria. Data were extracted directly from the articles as numbers of affected and unaffected children among ART and comparison groups, or as point and interval estimates of relative risk provided in the original article.

Cells with zero counts were included in the analysis by imputation of 0.5 cases. Meta-analyses were implemented separately for each disorder using Stata statistical software (Stata/SE 9.0, College Station, TX) and specifying a random effects model. We graphically displayed the point and 95% confidence interval for each contributing study in a Forrest plot (Figs.1a, 2a and 3a) and assessed the possibility of publication bias

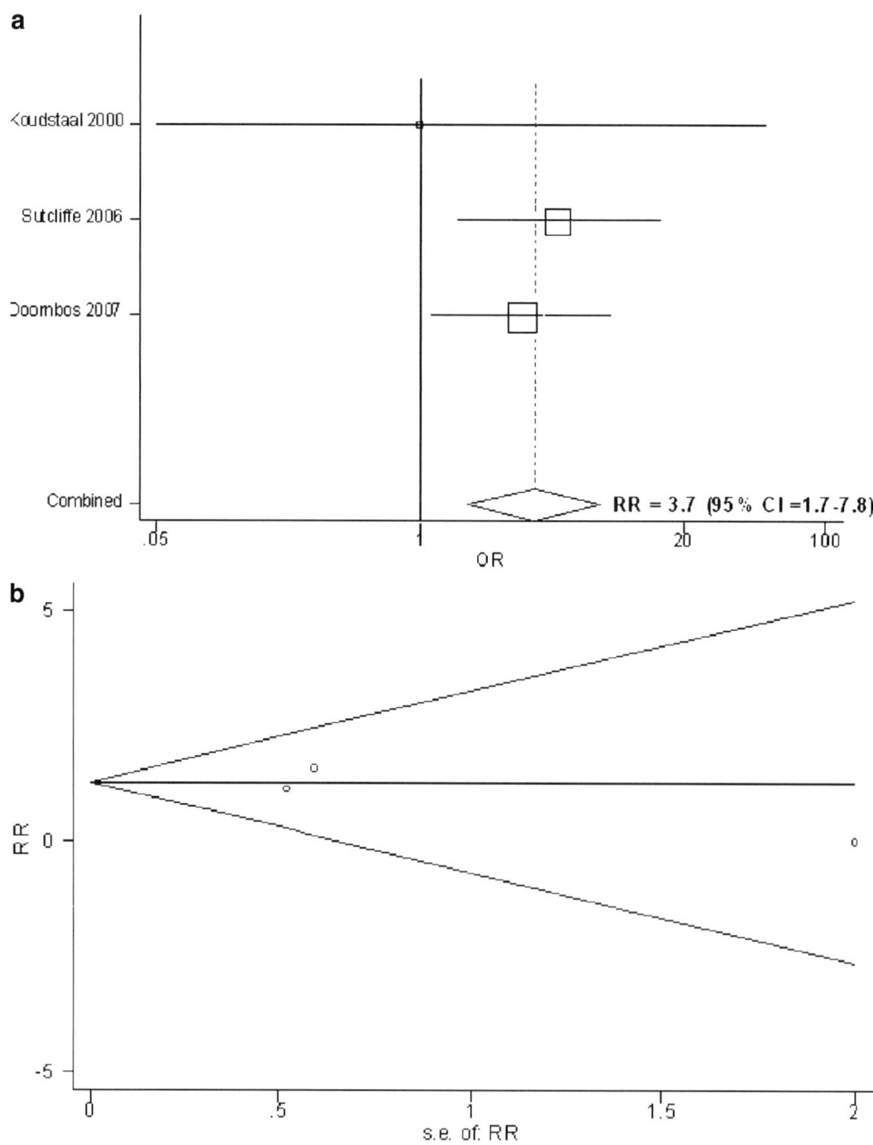


**Fig. 1** Results of meta-analysis estimating summary relative risk of Angelman syndrome following IVF (**a**) Forest plot, (**b**) Funnel plot

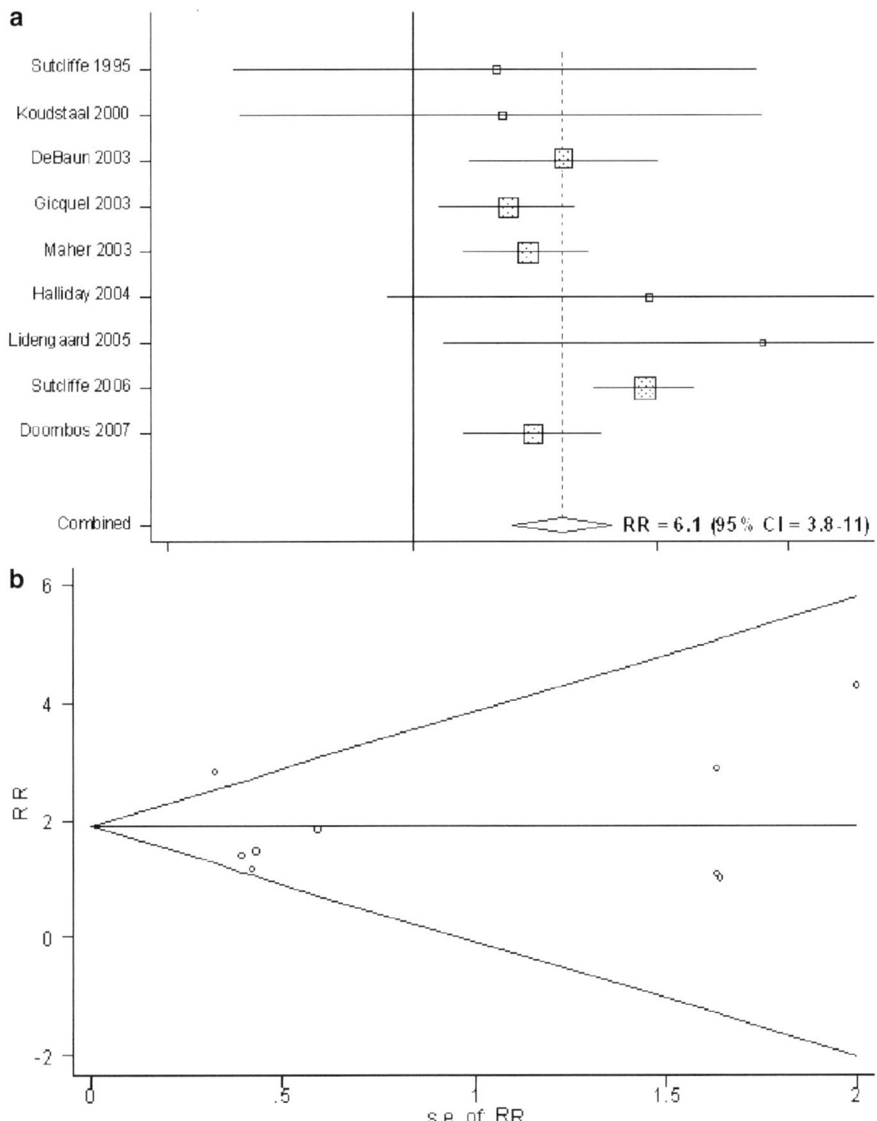


**Fig. 2** Results of meta-analysis estimating summary relative risk of Beckwith-Wiedemann syndrome following IVF (**a**) Forest plot, (**b**) Funnel plot

using Egger's unweighed regression asymmetry test (15). To examine dispersion of the data, we created Begg's funnel plots (Figs. 1b, 2b and 3b), which display for each study the risk ratio versus its standard error. Results distributed within the "funnel" defined by 95% confidence limits can be interpreted as variation due to sampling error. Variation due to differences in design and conduct of the studies is termed statistical heterogeneity, and may result in over-dispersion of results (e.g., outside the confidence limits).

## 2.3 Results

The literature search identified three articles providing association data on ART and AS (16–18), nine providing data on BWS (16–24), four providing data on PWS (16–18, 24), and one providing data on RSS (17). Specific etiology was not provided for most cases, so effects of imprinting defects versus other etiologies could not be addressed. Meta-analysis of data on AS,

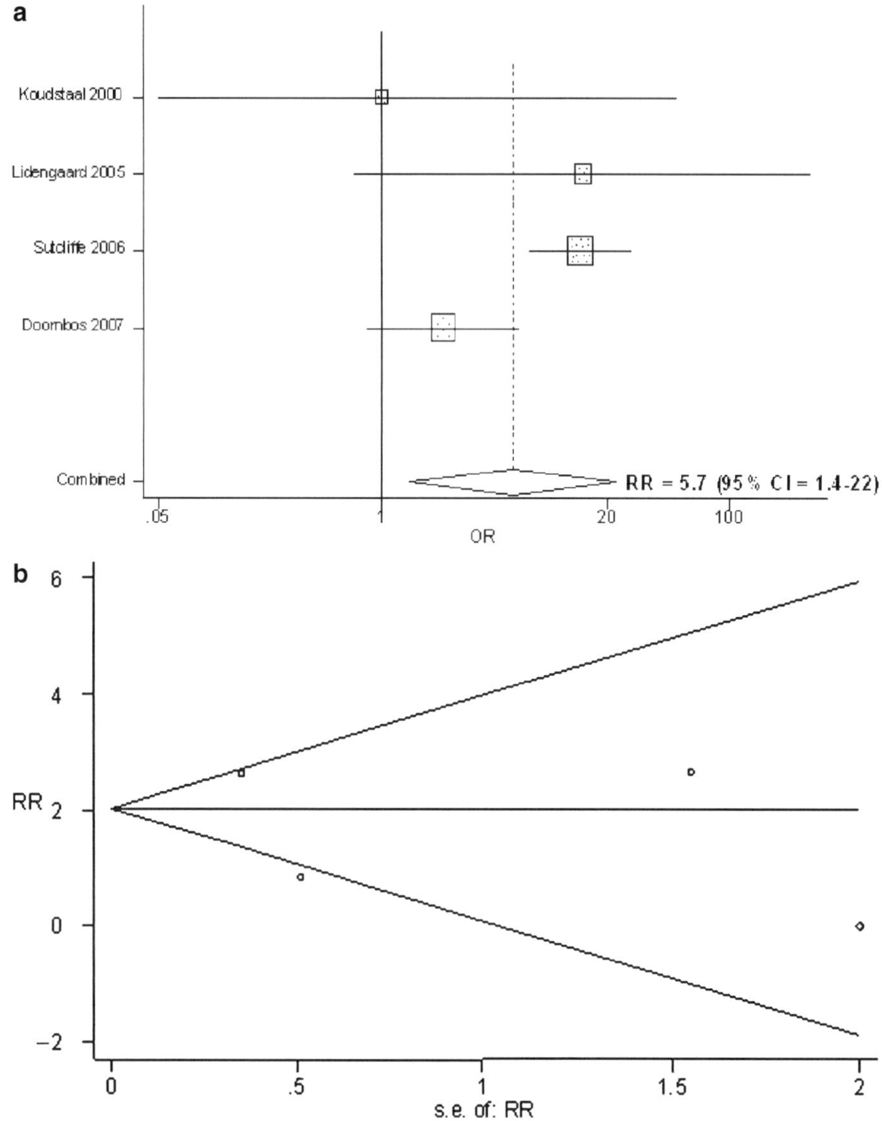


**Fig. 3** Results of meta-analysis estimating summary relative risk of Prader-Willi syndrome following IVF (**a**) Forest plot, (**b**) Funnel plot

BWS and PWS provided statistically significant summary relative risk ratio estimates consistent with increased risk of each of these conditions following IVF conception. The estimates were 3.7 (95% confidence interval (CI) = 1.7–7.8) for AS (Fig. 1a), 6.1 (95% CI = 3.8–11) for BWS (Fig. 2a), and 5.7 (95% CI = 1.4–22) for PWS (Fig. 3a). The single data set on RSS following ART revealed a statistically nonsignificant relative risk estimate of 14.6 (95% CI = 0.70–304).

Egger's test statistics were 0.519 for AS, 0.928 for BWS and 0.629 for PWS, providing no indication of publication bias for any of the disorders (i.e., smaller studies did not systematically estimate stronger associations than larger studies). Moreover, funnel plots (Figs. 1b, 2b and 3b) provide little evidence of statistical heterogeneity since results of all (AS) or most contributing studies (BWS, PWS) are distributed within the 95% confidence limits.

## 3 Discussion

Results of the meta-analysis suggest that there may be increased risk of imprinting disorders following IVF. This is the first comprehensive meta-analysis relating published data on IVF to these imprinting disorders, and results must be interpreted with caution for both statistical and logical reasons. Studies contributing to the analysis were few in number and reported small numbers of cases from a variety of settings, such that unidentified sources of bias may have influenced the summary risk ratio estimates to some extent. More importantly, even truly increased risk of imprinting disorders following IVF does not necessarily indicate a causal relationship between procedures of IVF and these conditions. Several alternate explanations cannot be ruled out on the basis of purely observational data. First, sub-fertile parents electing for IVF may produce gametes with improper imprints at an elevated frequency. This possibility is consistent with recent reports of elevated rates of aberrant methylation of imprinted genes among men with poor semen parameters (25–28). Moreover, couples undergoing IVF are quite unlike the general populations in which they reside with respect to age and income, two factors associated with numerous environmental exposures and physiologic process that may have unrecognized roles in the etiology of these disorders. Thus, confounding of the results by indication for IVF remains a real possibility. Perhaps the greatest value of these results is the early indication that epigenetic processes may be important in either the etiology of subfertility or as a complication of IVF.

## 4 Conclusions

Couples considering IVF may be counseled that according to preliminary data the risk of the birth of a child with a rare imprinting disorder may be increased several-fold following IVF, although absolute risk remains very low. The substantial magnitudes of the associations reported here indicate that further investigation of both possible explanations for these results is warranted, in the light of the high prevalence of idiopathic infertility as well as societal patterns of increasing use of assisted reproductive techniques.

**Acknowledgments** Southern California Environmental Health Sciences Center (grant # 5P30ES007048) funded by the National Institute of Environmental Health Sciences. The author thanks Carol Davis-Dao and Peter George Cortessis the younger for technical assistance.

## References

1. http://www.geneimprint.com/site/genes-by-species, 2008.
2. Maeda N, Hayashizaki Y. Genome-wide survey of imprinted genes. *Cytogenet Genome Res* 2006;113(1–4):144–52.
3. Wilkins J. Genomic imprinting and methylation: epigenetic canalization and conflict. *Trends Genet* 2005;21(6):356–65.
4. Abu-Amero S, Monk D, Apostolidou S, Stanier P, Moore G. Imprinted genes and their role in human fetal growth. *Cytogenet Genome Res* 2006;113(1–4):262–70.
5. Tycko B, Morison I. Physiological functions of imprinted genes. *J Cell Physiol* 2002;192(3):245–58.
6. Surani M, Barton S, Norris M. Development of reconstituted mouse eggs suggests imprinting of the genome during gametogenesis. *Nature* 1984;308(5959):548–50.
7. Mutter G. Role of imprinting in abnormal human development. *Mutat Res* 1997;396(1–2):141–7.
8. Cox G, Bürger J, Lip V, Mau U, Sperling K, Wu B, et al. Intracytoplasmic sperm injection may increase the risk of imprinting defects. *Am J Hum Genet* 2002;71(1):162–4.
9. Ørstavik K, Eiklid K, van der Hagen C, Spetalen S, Kierulf K, Skjeldal O, et al. Another case of imprinting defect in a girl with Angelman syndrome who was conceived by intracytoplasmic semen injection. *Am J Hum Genet* 2003;72(1):218–9.
10. Sinclair K. Assisted reproductive technologies and pregnancy outcomes: mechanistic insights from animal studies. *Semin Reprod Med* 2008;26(2):153–61.
11. Sato A, Otsu E, Negishi H, Utsunomiya T, Arima T. Aberrant DNA methylation of imprinted loci in superovulated oocytes. *Hum Reprod* 2007;22(1):26–35.
12. Fortier A, Lopes F, Darricarrère N, Martel J, Trasler J. Superovulation alters the expression of imprinted genes in the midgestation mouse placenta. *Hum Mol Genet* 2008;17(11):1653–65.
13. Li T, Vu T, Ulaner G, Littman E, Ling J, Chen H, et al. IVF results in de novo DNA methylation and histone methylation at an Igf2-H19 imprinting epigenetic switch. *Mol Hum Reprod* 2005;11(9):631–40.
14. Rivera R, Stein P, Weaver J, Mager J, Schultz R, Bartolomei M. Manipulations of mouse embryos prior to implantation result in aberrant expression of imprinted genes on day 9.5 of development. *Hum Mol Genet* 2008;17(1):1–14.
15. Egger M, Davey Smith G, Schneider M, Minder C. Bias in meta-analysis detected by a simple, graphical test. [see comment]. *BMJ* 1997;315(7109):629–34.
16. Koudstaal J, Braat D, Bruinse H, Naaktgeboren N, Vermeiden J, Visser G. Obstetric outcome of singleton pregnancies after IVF: a matched control study in four Dutch university hospitals. *Hum Reprod* 2000;15(8):1819–25.

17. Sutcliffe A, Peters C, Bowdin S, Temple K, Reardon W, Wilson L, et al. Assisted reproductive therapies and imprinting disorders – a preliminary British survey. *Hum Reprod* 2006;21(4):1009–11.
18. Doornbos M, Maas S, McDonnell J, Vermeiden J, Hennekam R. Infertility, assisted reproduction technologies and imprinting disturbances: a Dutch study. *Hum Reprod* 2007;22(9):2476–80.
19. DeBaun M, Niemitz E, Feinberg A. Association of in vitro fertilization with Beckwith-Wiedemann syndrome and epigenetic alterations of LIT1 and H19. *Am J Hum Genet* 2003;72(1):156–60.
20. Gicquel C, Gaston V, Mandelbaum J, Siffroi J, Flahault A, Le Bouc Y. In vitro fertilization may increase the risk of Beckwith-Wiedemann syndrome related to the abnormal imprinting of the KCN1OT gene. *Am J Hum Genet* 2003;72(5):1338–41.
21. Maher E, Afnan M, Barratt C. Epigenetic risks related to assisted reproductive technologies: epigenetics, imprinting, ART and icebergs? *Hum Reprod* 2003;18(12):2508–11.
22. Sutcliffe A, D'Souza S, Cadman J, Richards B, McKinlay I, Lieberman B. Minor congenital anomalies, major congenital malformations and development in children conceived from cryopreserved embryos. *Hum Reprod* 1995;10(12):3332–7.
23. Halliday J, Oke K, Breheny S, Algar E, J Amor D. Beckwith-Wiedemann syndrome and IVF: a case-control study. *Am J Hum Genet* 2004;75(3):526–8.
24. Lidegaard O, Pinborg A, Andersen A. Imprinting diseases and IVF: Danish National IVF cohort study. *Hum Reprod* 2005;20(4):950–4.
25. Hartmann S, Bergmann M, Bohle R, Weidner W, Steger K. Genetic imprinting during impaired spermatogenesis. *Mol Hum Reprod* 2006;12(6):407–11.
26. Marques C, Carvalho F, Sousa M, Barros A. Genomic imprinting in disruptive spermatogenesis. *Lancet* 2004;363(9422): 1700–2.
27. Manning M, Lissens W, Liebaers I, Van Steirteghem A, Weidner W. Imprinting analysis in spermatozoa prepared for intracytoplasmic sperm injection (ICSI). *Int J Androl* 2001;24(2):87–94.
28. Houshdaran S, Cortessis V, Siegmund K, Yang A, Laird P, Sokol R. Widespread epigenetic abnormalities suggest a broad DNA methylation erasure defect in abnormal human sperm. *PLoS ONE* 2007;2(12):e1289.
29. Lalande M, Calciano M. Molecular epigenetics of Angelman syndrome. *Cell Mol Life Sci* 2007;64(7–8):947–60.
30. Maher E. Imprinting and assisted reproductive technology. *Hum Mol Genet* 2005;14 Spec No 1:R133–8.
31. Chen C, Visootsak J, Do;;s S. Graham JM. Proader-Willi Syndrome: an update and review for the primary pediatrician. *Clin Pediatr (Phila)* 2007;46(7):580–591.
32. Abu-Amero S, Monk D, Frost J, Preece M, Stanier P, Moore G. The genetic aetiology of Silver-Russell syndrome. *J Med Genet* 2008;45(4):193–9.

# Section IV
# Evolving Controversies in Contemporary Reproductive Medicine

## Varicocelectomy or ART for Male Factor Infertility Due to A Varicocele?

# Discriminate Use of Varicocelectomy in Light of Advances in Assisted Reproductive Technologies

John M. Csokmay and Alan H. DeCherney

**Abstract** Varicoceles are common in the population and pose a challenge to infertility providers. The data to support varicocelectomy in infertile males is limited and controversial. Varicocelectomy does demonstrate improvement in semen parameters and may be considered the sole infertility management in only a limited subset of the infertile population. Current advances in assisted reproductive technologies (ART) have demonstrated superior success rates and shorter time to pregnancy compared to surgical repair of varicocele in the sub-fertile male and should be considered the primary treatment.

**Keywords** Varicocele • Varicocelectomy • Infertility • Male factor • Assisted reproductive technologies (ART) • In vitro fertilization (IVF) • Intra-cytoplasmic sperm injection (ICSI) • Semen analysis; Oligospermia; Anti-sperm antibodies

## 1 Introduction

A varicocele is an enlarged, tortuous spermatic vein above the testis that almost always occurs on the left side (1). The left-sided predominance is probably reflective in the venous drainage of the right (into inferior vena cava) and left (into left renal vein) testicular veins. This usual presentation includes a soft mass or swelling above the testis noted when the male patient stands or with valsalva. It has commonly been referred to as a "bag of worms" on physical examination (Fig. 1).

Varicoceles are prevalent in the population and occur in approximately 15% of normal males. The prevalence may be as high as 40% in males presenting with infertilitly (2). A varicocele is the most common surgically correctable abnormality found in infertile men and the available clinical and animal model data on varicoceles indicate an adverse effect of spermatogenesis (1). It has been assumed, therefore, that correction of a varicocele would improve fertility. For many years, varicocelectomy has remained a standard treatment of infertile males with varicoceles despite a paucity of evidence. The purpose of this review is to evaluate the current literature and knowledge of varicocelectomy and its utility in the sub-fertile patient in light of advances in assisted reproductive technologies (ART).

## 2 Pathophysiology of Varicoceles

The proposal that varicoceles are associated with male sub-fertility is widely accepted, but the pathophysiology and mechanisms by which fertility is affected are not completely understood. Based upon the available literature, varicocele effects on spermatogenesis appear to be multifactorial (Fig. 2).

Alterations in spermatogenesis may be explained by the increased scrotal temperature which results from impaired blood drainage from the testes (3, 4). Yamaguchi et al. demonstrated that intra-testicular temperatures increased by 0.78°C in men with varicoceles when moving from a supine to standing position. This is in contrast to men without varicoceles in whom a 0.5°C decrease in scrotal temperature was observed (5). Other studies have supported the presence of higher intra-scrotal temperatures in males with varicoceles (6–8). Interestingly, increases in bilateral testicular

J.M. Csokmay and A.H. DeCherney (✉)
National Institute of Child Health and Human Development, National Institutes of Health, Bethesda, MD 20892, USA
e-mail: decherna@mail.nih.gov

D.T. Carrell et al. (eds.), *Biennial Review of Infertility,* DOI: 10.1007/978-1-60327-392-3_17

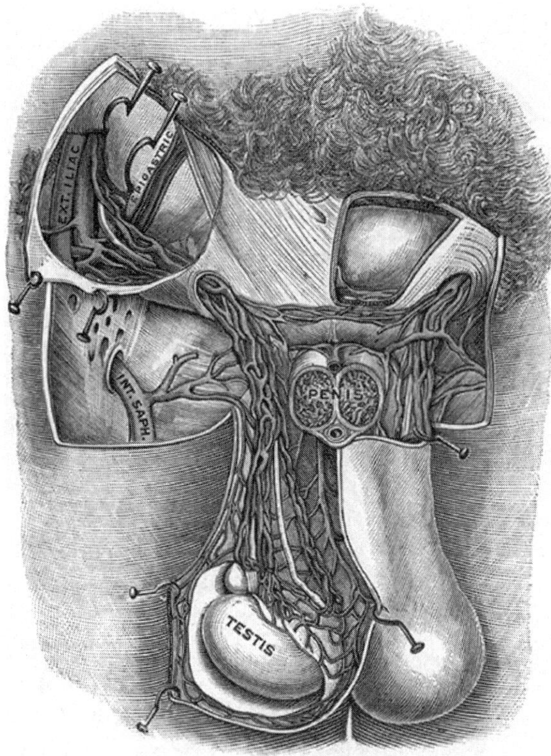


**Fig. 1** Demonstrating the abnormal dilation of spermatic vein found in varicocele (Figure originally from *Gray's Anatomy*, now in public domain.)

temperature occur in the setting of unilateral varicoceles. This bilateral effect was established in animal models in which the production of unilateral varicoceles resulted in bilateral increases in testicular blood flow and temperature (9).

Other mechanisms by which varicoceles may adversely affect spermatogenesis include hypoxia (10, 11), the reflux of adrenal and renal metabolites from the renal vein (12–14), the presence of reactive oxygen species (15), and the presence of anti-sperm antibodies (16, 17). The association of varicoceles and anti-sperm antibodies remains controversial (18).

## 3 Varicocelectomy and the Semen Analysis

The strongest argument for the routine use of varicocelectomy in the sub-fertile male has arisen from the literature showing that these men frequently have semen parameters that improve following surgical correction. A recent meta-analysis of seventeen studies in 2007 demonstrated a positive effect of varicocelectomy on semen parameters. The population studied included infertile men with a clinically palpable varicocele who had undergone varicocelectomy., and with at least one abnormal semen parameter, The analysis demonstrated an overall statistically significant increase in sperm concentration by 9.7–12.0 × 10(6)/mL$^{-1}$ and an increase in motility by 9.9–11.7% after microsurgical and high ligation varicocelectomies, respectively. It also demonstrated a 3.16% improvement of sperm morphology as per the World Health Organization sperm morphology (19).

Improvement in semen parameters following varicocelectomy would intuitively imply improved fertility; however, trials have not consistently demonstrated

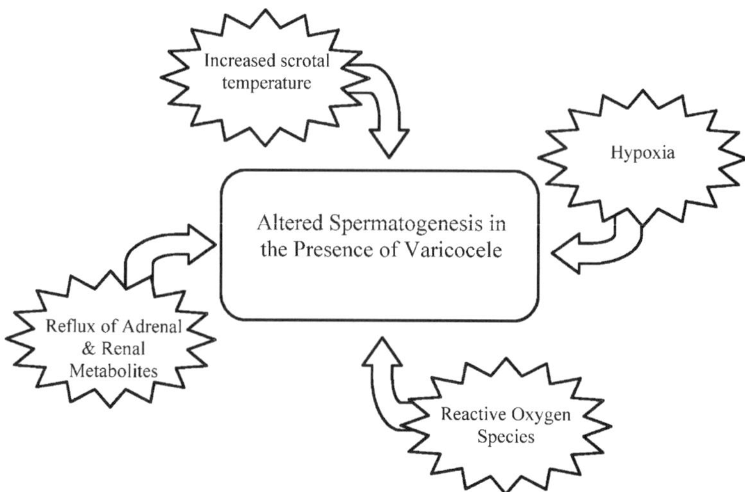


**Fig. 2** The factors implicated in altered spermatogenesis as found in varicocele

an improvement in pregnancy rates compared to no treatment.

## 4 Varicoceles in the Adolescent

The presence of varicocele in the adolescent poses a unique dilemma. There is sufficient data to support that varicocele has a progressive and deleterious effect in the adolescent patient. Varicoceles in the pubertal male either decrease or prevent an increase in testicular volume (20, 21). When examining treatment of varicoceles in adolescents, randomized prospective trials have demonstrated "catch-up" growth after repair (22–25). There is also evidence to suggest that semen analysis parameters are improved with treatment (22, 24). Based upon these data, it is the recommendation of the American Society of Reproductive Medicine (ASRM) that "adolescents who have a varicocele and objective evidence of reduced ipsilateral testicular size should be offered varicocele repair" (26). The question of whether this progressive effect (and improvement with repair) exists in adulthood is an area of debate. At the present time, the treatment of varicocele in the adolescent should be considered a special entity, different from that of adults.

## 5 Varicoceles and Fertility

Past data have brought into question the relationship of varicocele to infertility. Indeed, it is the most commonly identified abnormality in sub-fertile males, but this does not necessarily translate into a causal relationship of varicocele and infertility. Reported in 1968, Uehling described examining 776 men during routine military physical. Within this group 440 (57%) were married and a varicocele was present in 25% of married men. There was no difference in the percentage of childless couples between married men with and without varicocele (31% and 32%, respectively) (27). Similarly, Thomason et al. examined over 900 men for routine physical examinations and noted the prevalence of varicocele was not different between the whole group (31%) and the subgroup of men ($n = 299$, 33%) who reported fathering a child (29%) (28).

The wide variation in reported prevalence rates of varicocele may be influenced by examiner bias in the detection of varicocele in infertile males as suggested by Redmon (29). Within this review, the authors cite varicocele prevalence rates ranging from 4 to 47% depending on the source of the information. In an effort to describe this observation, it is stated that the "data raise the possibility that reported prevalence rates of varicocele from examination of men attending infertility clinics may be subject to examiner bias. Men referred for infertility evaluation almost universally have had one or more abnormal semen analyses prompting a referral. In most cases there is no obvious factor found. In a search for an explanation for the abnormal semen analyses, examiners may be unconsciously biased to detect a varicocele" (29).

## 6 Controversies of Varicocelectomy: Review of the Literature

In 1995, Nieschlag stated that "therapeutic recommendations in male infertility, as in other fields of medicine, should be based exclusively on properly controlled clinical trials" (30). Indeed, in an age of evidence based medicine one cannot rely upon anecdotal or inadequate information. Considering this thought, many practitioners have based their treatment recommendations of varicoceles on "less than optimal" data. A review of the literature reveals many conflicting opinions on the use of varicocelectomy in the treatment of the sub-fertile male.

There has not yet been a definitive randomized controlled trial of varicocele treatment versus expectant management in the sub-fertile male that effectively resolves the controversy. Two of the most thorough randomized controlled trials of sub-fertile males with varicoceles have shown dramatically different outcomes (31, 32). The most convincing data in support of surgical varicocelectomy is demonstrated by Madgar et al. with a remarkable pregnancy rate of 60% in the treated group versus 10% in the untreated group ($p < 0.001$) at 12 months (31). This is in contrast to the larger study by Neischlag (30, 32) which concluded no improvement in varicocele treatment (surgical varicocelectomy and embolization) compared to counseling alone, with pregnancy rates of 29 and 25%, respectively (NS) (32). Both of these studies included only couples in which the female infertility factor had been excluded.

Careful examination of both of these studies reveals several limitations. These studies suffered a large drop-out rate of patients. The Madgar study considered 210 patients initially, but ultimately only 45 patients were randomized (25 to treatment and 20 to no treatment). Within this relatively small group was a significant difference in pregnancy rates between treated/untreated males that has not been reproduced in later trials. The mean age of the male partner was 28-years old within this group (31). While the Nieschlag study was larger, it too suffered from large drop-out rate. Of the initial 226 patients who fulfilled the entry criteria, 203 were randomized but 78 couples subsequently dropped out leaving 125 patients for analysis (63 received counseling versus 62 with varicocele treatment). The mean age of the males in this study was 32 (32). Both of these studies included men only from couples with sub-fertility, although the Madgar study did exclude men with severe oligospermia (<5 million $mL^{-1}$).

Many criticisms have been made of both of these landmark trials in addition to the limitations already discussed. One such criticism of the Nieschlag trial was that varicocelectomy repair included both surgical as well as embolization treatment. Subsequent trials have demonstrated embolization therapy to be inferior to surgical correction; a potential reason for a non-significant difference in pregnancy rates when compared to no treatment (counseling alone). The Nieschlag trial described a strategy for concealment that was not reported by Madgar. The study by Madgar et al. did not include men with severe oligospermia. Both studies reported a follow-up time of 12 months. Neither study was blinded.

Numerous other investigations within the literature are equally divided in the use of varicocelectomy. Table 1 represents a partial list of the published evaluations of varicocelectomy in treating the infertile male demonstrating the disparity of data that exists.v

**Table 1** Summary of trials/analyses which have addressed the utility of varicocelectomy in the infertile male

| For varicocelectomy | Against varicocelectomy |
|---|---|
| Madgar 1995 (31) | Neischlag 1995/98 (30, 32) |
| Schlesinger 1994 (42) | Krause 2002 (47) |
| Onozawa 2002 (43) | Grasso 2000 (48) |
| Marmar 1994 (44) | Bresnik 1993 (49) |
| Sayfan 1992 (45) | Nilsson 1979 (50) |
| Cayan 2000 (46) | Rageth 1992 (51) |
| Marmar 2007 (34) | Evers 2004 (33) |

## 6.1 Meta-analyses and Varicocelectomy

Because of the limited and conflicting data, several meta-analyses have attempted to pool the data and make more solid conclusions. In 2004, Evers and Collins conducted an analysis of eight studies (607 participants) that met their inclusion criteria. Randomized clinical trials were included if they reported pregnancy rates and compared treated and untreated groups. The combined Peto odds ratio of the eight studies was 1.10 (95% CI, 0.73–1.68) which indicated "no benefit of varicocele treatment over expectant management in sub-fertility couples in whom varicocele in the man is the only abnormal finding" (33) (Table 2).

In contrast to the analysis by Evers and Collins, a more recent meta-analysis conducted by Marmar et al. concluded a benefit of varicocelectomy. This analysis included only studies that involved infertile males with clinical varicocele and abnormal semen analysis, treated with surgical varicocelectomy. Five studies were included in the analysis (570 participants) and the pooled odds ratio was 2.87 (95% CI, 1.33–6.20), demonstrating an improvement in the odds of spontaneous pregnancy following varicocelectomy (34) (Table 3).

Just as the individual trials have received criticism and have been deemed "poor studies," the meta-analyses have also been met with hesitation. The analysis by Evers and Collins included a study in which embolization for treatment of varicocele was included, three studies evaluating men with subclinical varicoceles, and one study involved clinical varicocele but normal semen analysis. Together, some suggest that these studies favor "no difference" with treatment. Similarly, criticisms of the analysis by Marmar are present. The main criticism surrounds the inclusion of observational studies (three out of the five studies) in the analysis. In addition, it excluded the large randomized controlled trial by Nieschlag due to its use of embolization in the treatment arm. The potential inclusion bias in this meta-analysis may imply a difference with treatment that does not really exist.

Meta-analytical studies are only as good as the studies included therein; they cannot overcome flaws in the design or implementation of the individual studies. They are also subject to risks such as publication bias (negative studies are less likely to be published)

**Table 2** Evers and Collins meta-analysis summary

| Study | Treatment n/N | Control n/N | Weight (%) | Peto Odds Ratio 95% CI |
|---|---|---|---|---|
| Breznik 1993 | 18/43 | 17/36 | 22.4 | 0.81 [0.33, 1.96] |
| Grasso 2000 | 1/34 | 2/34 | 3.3 | 0.50 [0.05, 5.01] |
| Krause 2002 | 5/33 | 6/34 | 10.7 | 0.84 [0.23, 3.02] |
| Madgar 1995 | 15/25 | 2/20 | 12.2 | 8.00 [2.41, 26.55] |
| Nieschlag 1995/1998 | 18/62 | 16/63 | 28.6 | 1.20 [0.55, 2.63] |
| Nilsson 1979 | 4/51 | 8/45 | 12.1 | 0.41 [0.12, 1.36] |
| Unal 2001 | 2/21 | 1/21 | 3.3 | 2.02 [0.20, 20.52] |
| Yamamoto 1996 | 3/45 | 4/40 | 7.4 | 0.65 [0.14, 3.02] |
| Total (95% CI) | 314 | 293 | 100.0 | 1.10 [0.73, 1.68] |

Total events: 66 (Treatment), 56 (Control)
Test for heterogeneity chi-square=14.99 df=7 p=0.04 I² =53.3%
Test for overall effect z=0.46 p=0.6

Peto Odds Ratio 95% CI: 0.1 0.2 0.5 1 2 5 10 — Favours Treatment / Favours Control

**Table 3** Marmar et al. meta-analysis summary

| Study | Varicocelectomy n/N | Control n/N | OR (random) 95% CI |
|---|---|---|---|
| Grasso et al 2000 | 1 / 34 | 2 / 34 | 0.48 [0.04, 5.61] |
| Madgar et al 1995 | 16 / 25 | 2 / 20 | 13.50 [2.55, 71.40] |
| Marmar et al 1994 | 66 / 186 | 3 / 19 | 2.93 [0.82, 10.44] |
| Okuyama et al 1988 | 43 / 141 | 15 / 83 | 1.99 [1.02, 3.86] |
| Onozawa et al 2002 | 6 / 10 | 5 / 18 | 3.90 [0.76, 19.95] |
| Total (95% CI) | 396 | 174 | 2.87 [1.33, 6.20] |

Total events: 131 (Varicocelectomy), 27 (Control)
Test for heterogeneity: Chi² = 8.47, df = 4 (P= 0.17), r = 38.1%
Test for overall effect Z = 2.68 (P < 0.00001)

OR (random) 95% CI: 0.01 0.1 1 10 100 — Favors control / Favors surgery

and selection/inclusion bias. As such, the ideal study to derive solid evidence would consist of a prospective, blinded, randomized control trial. Blinding is not reasonable as a surgical treatment consists of one arm of the study and a study volunteer would be unlikely to agree to the idea of sham surgery. In regards to the need for a properly constructed RCT, Evers and Collins state that "it will become increasingly difficult to conduct such a study, since the introduction of IVF/ICSI in the fertility clinic will make many men reluctant to take the risk of being allocated to the no-treatment arm of such a study, when at the same time a treatment of proven effectiveness is readily available in the form of IVF/ICSI" (33).

## 7 Varicocele in Light of Advances in Assisted Reproductive Technologies

All of the studies listed thus far have examined a subfertile couple population that was designated as pure male factor. These studies all claim to have excluded female infertility factors. Epidemiologic data suggests that 20% of infertility couples are due to solely to male factor, but combined male and female factors contribute to an additional 30–40% of infertility (35).

Given the prevalence of combined male and female infertility and the advances made in the field of ART, recent analyses have begun to examine the natural history of varicocele and its relationship with ART, with or without varicocelectomy. In 2004, O'Brien et al. conducted a retrospective cohort analysis with couples with advanced female age comparing microsurgical varicocelectomy versus no treatment; both groups were free to undergo ART (36). Within the 202 couples identified, 108 males chose to have microsurgical varicocelectomy and 94 elected to no surgery. At a mean of 30 months follow up, 41% of couples from both groups had achieved pregnancy. Within the surgically treated group 35% obtained spontaneous pregnancy and an additional 6% from the use of ART. Within the non-surgical group, 25% achieved spontaneous pregnancy and an additional 16% through ART (all non-significant differences). The authors conclude that the natural history of infertile men with varicocele (with the option of ART) demonstrated similar pregnancy rates between surgical and non-surgical arms (36) (Table 4).

A larger retrospective study has recently been reported by Zini et al. which confirms these conclusions (37). This retrospective cohort of six hundred and ten (610) couples demonstrated overall comparable rates of pregnancy (spontaneous and assisted pregnancies) between the observational and surgical groups. They conclude that the surgical group had statistically lower sperm concentration and motility while the observation group was more likely to utilize ART (37) (Table 5).

**Table 4** Summary of results from O'Brien et al. (36)

| | Surgery | No surgery | *p* |
|---|---|---|---|
| *n* | 108 | 94 | |
| Follow up time (months) | 30.1 | 32.9 | NS |
| Female age | 37.4 | 38.5 | 0.01 |
| Spontaneous pregnancy rate (%) | 35 | 25 | NS |
| Overall pregnancy rate (%) | 41 | 41 | NS |
| ART use (%) | 20 | 45 | NS |
| Time to pregnancy (months) | 16 | 11 | NS |

**Table 5** Summary of results from Zini et al. (37)

| | Surgery | No surgery | *p* |
|---|---|---|---|
| *n* | 363 | 247 | |
| Follow up time (months) | 36 | 40 | NS |
| Spontaneous pregnancy rate (%) | 39 | 32 | NS |
| Overall pregnancy rate (%)[a] | 53 | 56 | NS |
| ART use (%) | 38 | 54 | 0.002 |

[a] Overall pregnancy rate (spontaneous + ART pregnancies)

## 8 Advantages of Assisted Reproductive Technologies

Before the advent of intra-cytoplasmic sperm injection (ICSI) in 1992, males with varicoceles and severe male factor infertility had no reasonable treatment alternatives to surgical repair. With ICSI, the effect of male factor infertility on pregnancy rates became less pronounced. The 1997 American Society for Reproductive Medicine (ASRM) report stated that "clinics with proficiency in ICSI may be able to mitigate the effects of male factor infertility. When all IVF cycles were classified by male factor and other diagnoses, patients with male factor infertility experienced a higher delivery rate per retrieval (25.5%) than those with other diagnoses (23.4%)" (38).

In vitro fertilization with ICSI now allows for successful fertilization of the human oocyte despite severe oligozoospermia, asthenozoospermia (low sperm motility), and teratozoospermia (higher rate of abnormal sperm morphology). With advances in surgical techniques, even males without sperms in the ejaculate may be candidates for ICSI procedures. Spermatozoa now may be obtained through testicular biopsy or fine needle aspirates with good success (39, 40). Important to the discussion of ART is that infertility due to female factors (tubal obstruction, anovulation, etc.) are addressed simultaneously.

The success rates and efficacy of assisted reproductive technologies are well documented. All clinics performing in vitro fertilization are required to report their statistics to the Society for Assisted Reproductive Technology (SART). Figure 3 demonstrates the success rates of fresh, non-donor oocyte cycles as stratified by female age. The overall success is greatest in the <35 year old age group and live birth rates per transfer have risen from 33.6% in 1996, to 43.3% in 2005 (41). Male factor infertility accounts for approximate 17% of all IVF cycles. When evaluating cycles of IVF/ICSI for male factor infertility, approximately 85% utilize ICSI and the success rates are at an impressive 42.6% in 2006 (41). The use of ICSI has increased significantly due to its proven success. The American Society for Reproductive Medicine (ASRM) report of 1997 documented that 35.7% of all IVF cycles used ICSI (38). This has increased to approximately 62% by the year 2006. Table 6 summarizes the trend in ART in couples with only a male factor diagnosis (41).

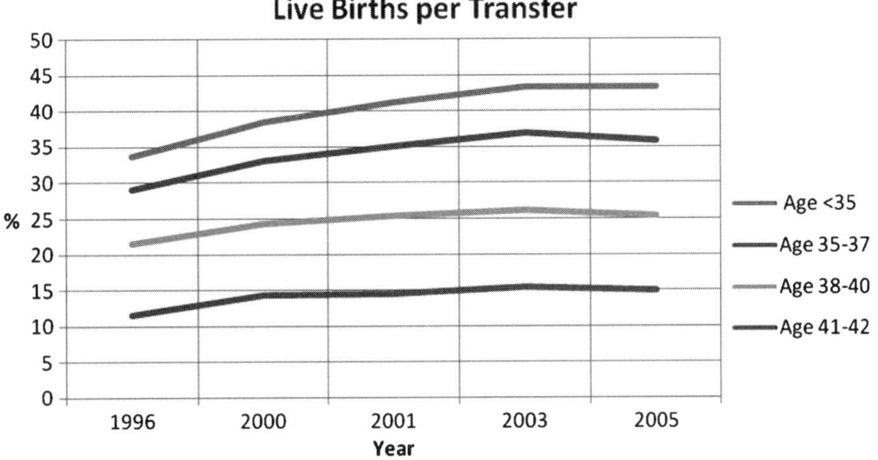


**Fig. 3** In vitro fertilization success rates as reported by Society for Assisted Reproductive Technology. Based upon fresh, nondonor oocytes cycles and stratified by female age

**Table 6** SART/CDC published data on all reported assisted reproductive technology cycles per year. Cycle specific data limited to cycles performed for male factor only. Data limited to fresh nondonor oocyte cycles with female age < 35 years

| | 2004 | 2005 | 2006 |
|---|---|---|---|
| Total ART cycles per year | 119,461 | 123,200 | 126,706 |
| All ART cycles done for male factor only (%) | 17 | 17 | 17 |
| All ART cycles utilizing ICSI (%) | 57 | 59 | 62 |
| *Male Factor Only ART Data* | | | |
| Number of ART cycles for male factor | 8,899 | 9,051 | 9,023 |
| Male factor cycles utilizing ICSI (%) | 85 | 85 | 86 |
| Cycles resulting in pregnancies (%) | 44.6 | 44.7 | 48.8 |
| Cycles resulting in live births (%) | 38.8 | 39.2 | 42.6 |
| Cancellations (%) | 6.9 | 6.3 | 5.9 |
| Implantation rate (%) | 28.4 | 29.3 | 33.1 |

In addition to superior pregnancy rates, ART offers the additional advantage of a decreased time to pregnancy. As demonstrated in Table 6, the pregnancy rate per IVF cycle in 2006 was 48.8% (41). In contrast, the time to pregnancy for the varicocelectomy group (with the option of ART) as documented in the O'Brien analysis was 16 ± 5 months (36). Clearly, ART offers an abbreviated interval to pregnancy while maintaining better success rates. To further support the use of ART, Zini et al. reported that 38% of men who chose primary surgical management (varicocelectomy) ultimately did utilize ART. This is in contrast to the group who chose the observation arm in which 54% underwent some form of ART; no difference was noted in the pregnancy rates between these two groups.

The data support that ART offers excellent pregnancy rates of the infertile couple and it is able to treat both male and female factor infertility. The advances in ART (with ICSI) have been significant over the past 10 years and there is clear and reproducible published data to support its efficacy.

## 9 Conclusions

Varicoceles are prevalent in the infertile male population and the detrimental effect on spermatogenesis is well documented. Varicocelectomy may prove to be the treatment of choice in the adolescent to prevent progressive testicular damage. However, the association of varicoceles and infertility does not prove causality. Despite evidence that shows improvement in semen parameters following surgery, varicocelectomy has not been clearly proven to improve pregnancy rates. Furthermore, many sub-fertile couples exhibit a concurrent female abnormality contributing to the problem, which obviously is not addressed by varicocelectomy. At this time ART has superior success rates and shorter time to pregnancy compared to surgical repair of varicocele. Varicocelectomy may have a role in a limited subset of patients, but the data supporting its use are controversial and do not demonstrate it to be superior to ART.

## References


1. Wein AJ, Kavoussi LR, Novick AC, Partin AW, Peters CA, editors. Campbell-Walsh Urology. 9th ed: W.B. Saunders, Philadelphia; 2007.
2. Sharlip ID, Jarow JP, Belker AM, et al. Best practice policies for male infertility. Fertility and Sterility 2002;77(5):873–882.
3. Pryor JL, Howards SS. Varicocele. The Urologic clinics of North America 1987;14(3):499–513.
4. Zorgniotti AW. Testis temperature, infertility, and the varicocele paradox. Urology 1980;16(1):7–10.
5. Yamaguchi M, Sakatoku J, Takihara H. The application of intrascrotal deep body temperature measurement for the noninvasive diagnosis of varicoceles. Fertility and Sterility 1989;52(2):295–301.
6. Ali JI, Weaver DJ, Weinstein SH, Grimes EM. Scrotal temperature and semen quality in men with and without varicocele. Archives of Andrology 1990;24(2):215–219.
7. Lerchl A, Keck C, Spiteri-Grech J, Nieschlag E. Diurnal variations in scrotal temperature of normal men and patients with varicocele before and after treatment. International Journal of Andrology 1993;16(3):195–200.
8. Zorgniotti AW, Macleod J. Studies in temperature, human semen quality, and varicocele. Fertility and Sterility 1973;24(11):854–863.
9. Saypol DC, Howards SS, Turner TT, Miller ED. Influence of surgically induced varicocele on testicular blood flow, temperature, and histology in adult rats and dogs. The Journal of Clinical Investigation 1981;68(1):39–45.
10. Chakraborty J, Hikim AP, Jhunjhunwala JS. Stagnation of blood in the microcirculatory vessels in the testes of men with varicocele. Journal of Andrology 1985;6(2):117–126.
11. Gat Y, Zukerman Z, Chakraborty J, Gornish M. Varicocele, hypoxia and male infertility. Fluid mechanics analysis of the impaired testicular venous drainage system. Human Reproduction (Oxford, England) 2005;20(9):2614–2619.
12. Comhaire F, Vermeulen A. Varicocele sterility: cortisol and catecholamines. Fertility and Sterility 1974;25(1):88–95.
13. Cohen MS, Plaine L, Brown JS. The role of internal spermatic vein plasma catecholamine determinations in subfertile men with varicoceles. Fertility and Sterility 1975;26(12):1243–1249.
14. Camoglio FS, Zampieri N, Corroppolo M, et al. Varicocele and retrograde adrenal metabolites flow. An experimental study on rats. Urologia Internationalis 2004;73(4):337–342.
15. Koksal IT, Usta M, Orhan I, Abbasoglu S, Kadioglu A. Potential role of reactive oxygen species on testicular pathology associated with infertility. Asian Journal of Andrology 2003;5(2):95–99.
16. Golomb J, Vardinon N, Homonnai ZT, Braf Z, Yust I. Demonstration of antispermatozoal antibodies in varicocele-related infertility with an enzyme-linked immunosorbent assay (ELISA). Fertility and sterility 1986;45(3):397–402.
17. Knudson G, Ross L, Stuhldreher D, Houlihan D, Bruns E, Prins G. Prevalence of sperm bound antibodies in infertile men with varicocele: the effect of varicocele ligation on antibody levels and semen response. The Journal of Urology 1994;151(5):1260–1262.
18. Oshinsky GS, Rodriguez MV, Mellinger BC. Varicocele-related infertility is not associated with increased sperm-bound antibody. The Journal of Urology 1993;150(3): 871–873.
19. Agarwal A, Deepinder F, Cocuzza M, et al. Efficacy of varicocelectomy in improving semen parameters: new meta-analytical approach. Urology 2007;70(3):532–538.
20. Haans LC, Laven JS, Mali WP, te Velde ER, Wensing CJ. Testis volumes, semen quality, and hormonal patterns in adolescents with and without a varicocele. Fertility and Sterility 1991;56(4):731–736.
21. Sayfan J, Siplovich L, Koltun L, Benyamin N. Varicocele treatment in pubertal boys prevents testicular growth arrest. The Journal of Urology 1997;157(4):1456–1457.
22. Okuyama A, Nakamura M, Namiki M, et al. Surgical repair of varicocele at puberty: preventive treatment for fertility improvement. The Journal of Urology 1988;139(3):562–564.
23. Paduch DA, Niedzielski J. Repair versus observation in adolescent varicocele: a prospective study. The Journal of Urology 1997;158(3 Pt 2):1128–1132.
24. Yamamoto M, Hibi H, Katsuno S, Miyake K. Effects of varicocelectomy on testis volume and semen parameters in adolescents: a randomized prospective study. Nagoya Journal of Medical Science 1995;58(3–4):127–132.
25. Laven JS, Haans LC, Mali WP, te Velde ER, Wensing CJ, Eimers JM. Effects of varicocele treatment in adolescents: a randomized study. Fertility and Sterility 1992;58(4): 756–762.
26. Report on varicocele and infertility. Fertility and Sterility 2006;86(5 Suppl):S93–S95.
27. Uehling DT. Fertility in men with varicocele. International Journal of Fertility 1968;13(1):58–60.
28. Thomason AM, Fariss BL. The prevalence of varicoceles in a group of healthy young men. Military Medicine 1979;144(3):181–182.
29. Redmon JB, Carey P, Pryor JL. Varicocele–the most common cause of male factor infertility? Human Reproduction Update 2002;8(1):53–58.
30. Nieschlag E, Hertle L, Fischedick A, Behre HM. Treatment of varicocele: counselling as effective as occlusion of the vena spermatica. Human Reproduction (Oxford, England) 1995;10(2):347–53.
31. Madgar I, Weissenberg R, Lunenfeld B, Karasik A, Goldwasser B. Controlled trial of high spermatic vein ligation for varicocele in infertile men. Fertility and Sterility 1995;63(1):120–124.
32. Nieschlag E, Hertle L, Fischedick A, Abshagen K, Behre HM. Update on treatment of varicocele: counselling as effective as occlusion of the vena spermatica. Human Reproduction (Oxford, England) 1998;13(8):2147–2150.
33. Evers JL, Collins JA. Surgery or embolisation for varicocele in subfertile men. Cochrane Database of Systematic Reviews (Online) 2004(3):CD000479.

34. Marmar JL, Agarwal A, Prabakaran S, Agarwal R, Short RA, Benoff S, et al. Reassessing the value of varicocelectomy as a treatment for male subfertility with a new meta-analysis. Fertility and Sterility 2007;88(3): 639–648.
35. Thonneau P, Marchand S, Tallec A, et al. Incidence and main causes of infertility in a resident population (1,850,000) of three French regions (1988–1989). Human Reproduction (Oxford, England) 1991;6(6):811–816.
36. O'Brien JH, Bowles B, Kamal KM, Jarvi K, Zini A. Microsurgical varicocelectomy for infertile couples with advanced female age: natural history in the era of ART. Journal of Andrology 2004;25(6):939–943.
37. Zini A, Boman J, Baazeem A, Jarvi K, Libman J. Natural history of varicocele management in the era of intracytoplasmic sperm injection. Fertility and Sterility 2008; 90(6):2251–2256.
38. [No Authors Listed]Assisted reproductive technology in the United States: 1997 results generated from the American Society for Reproductive Medicine/Society for Assisted Reproductive Technology Registry. Fertility and Sterility 2000;74(4):641–653; discussion 53–54.
39. Schlegel PN, Palermo GD, Goldstein M, Menendez S, Zaninovic N, Veeck LL, et al. Testicular sperm extraction with intracytoplasmic sperm injection for nonobstructive azoospermia. Urology 1997;49(3):435–440.
40. Tournaye H, Camus M, Goossens A, Liu J, Nagy P, Silber S, et al. Recent concepts in the management of infertility because of non-obstructive azoospermia. Human Reproduction (Oxford, England) 1995;10 Suppl 1:115–119.
41. Society For Assisted Reproductive Technology. SART National Summary. 1209 Montgomery Highway, Birmingham, AL 35216 2008 (Online).
42. Schlesinger MH, Wilets IF, Nagler HM. Treatment outcome after varicocelectomy. A critical analysis. Urologic Clinics of North America 1994;21(3):517–529.
43. Onozawa M, Endo F, Suetomi T, Takeshima H, Akaza H. Clinical study of varicocele: statistical analysis and the results of long-term follow-up. Internation Journal of Urology 2002;9(8):455–61.
44. Marmar JL, Kim Y. Subinguinal microsurgical varicocelectomy: a technical critique and statistical analysis of semen and pregnancy data. Journal of Urology 1994;152(4): 1127–1132.
45. Sayfan J, Soffer Y, Orda R. Varicocele treatment: prospective randomized trial of 3 methods. Journal of Urology. 1992;148(5):1447–1449.
46. Cayan S, Kadioglu TC, Tefekli A, Kadioglu A, Tellaloglu S. Comparison of results and complications of high ligation surgery and microsurgical high inguinal varicocelectomy in the treatment of varicocele. Urology 2000;55(5):750–754.
47. Krause W, Müller HH, Schäfer H, Weidner W. Does treatment of varicocele improve male fertility? results of the 'Deutsche Varikozelenstudie', a multicentre study of 14 collaborating centres. Andrologia 2002;34(3):164–171.
48. Grasso M, Lania C, Castelli M, Galli L, Franzoso F, Rigatti P. Low-grade left varicocele in patients over 30 years old: the effect of spermatic vein ligation on fertility. BJU International 2000;85(3):305–307.
49. Breznik R, Vlaisavljevic V, Borko E. Treatment of varicocele and male fertility. Archives of Andrology 1993;30:157–160.
50. Nilsson S, Edvinsson A, Nilsson B. Improvement of semen and pregnancy rate after ligation and division of the internal spermatic vein: fact or fiction? British Journal of Urology 1979;51(6):591–596.
51. Rageth JC, Unger C, DaRugna D, Steffen R, Stucki D, Barone C, et al. Long-term results of varicocelectomy. Urology International 1992;48(3):327–331.
52. Unal D, Yeni E, Verit A, Karatas OF. Clomiphene citrate versus varicocelectomy in treatment of subclinical varicocele: a prospective randomized study. International Journal of Urology 2001;8(5):227–230.
53. Yamamoto M, Hibi H, Hirata Y, Miyake K, Ishigaki T. Effect of varicocelectomy on sperm parameters and pregnancy rate in patients with subclinical varicocele: a randomized prospective controlled study. Journal of Urology 1996;155(5):1636–8.

# The Use of Varicocelectomy Surgery in the Treatment of the Infertile Male

Joel L. Marmar

**Abstract** Varicoceles are diagnosed in about 15% of men in the general population, but these lesions are seen in 40% of male infertility patients. For decades, urologists have considered these lesions as a possible cause of male infertility, and they have performed varicocelectomies on infertile men with palpable varicoceles and at least one persistently abnormal semen parameter. With the advancements in IVF/ICSI, reproductive endocrinologists (REs) have taken a different approach and they usually recommend some form of ART instead of the surgical alternative. In recent years, the debate has intensified because of conflicting publications and subsequent commentaries on the subject of varicoceles and pregnancy. There have been limited prospective randomized trials (PRTs), and many uncontrolled studies. Nevertheless, urologists generally contend that there is sufficient experimental and clinical evidence to support the surgical correction of these lesions, whereas the REs usually minimize the role of varicoceles as a cause of infertility. The conflicting opinions reached new heights recently, when two meta-analyses on varicoceles and fertility appeared in prominent peer review journals with completely opposite results. One meta-analysis was written by two REs, whereas the other was written by a team of urologists, basic scientists and statisticians. In this chapter, the differences between these meta-analyses will be explored, current concepts related to the pathophysiology of varicoceles will be presented, different methods for the correction of varicoceles will be considered and new protocols will be analyzed that combine surgery and ART. The intent of the chapter will be to enlighten both urologists and REs with current information related to varicoceles, varicocelectomies and ART.

**Keywords** Varicocele • Varicocelectomy • Male infertility • Meta-analysis • Apoptosis • Oxidative stress • IUI • IVF/ICSI

## 1 Introduction

When urologists examine infertile men, they usually search for a varicocele because they are taught that this lesion may be a possible cause of infertility. In fact, most urologists utilize specific clinical routines to search for these lesions that are consistent with the recommendations of the Best Policy Practice Committees of both the American Urologic Association (AUA) and the American Society of Reproductive Medicine (ASRM) (1, 2). These include examinations of the patient in both the recumbent and upright positions, an examination during valsalva maneuver, and a Doppler examination for clarification of inconclusive cases. This diagnosis seems important because the committees have stated "correction of varicoceles is indicated for infertile men with palpable lesions and one or more abnormal semen parameters or an abnormal sperm function test." Furthermore, in the urologic literature, there have been numerous reports of benefits following varicocele surgery (3–11).

When Reproductive Endocrinologists (REs) counsel infertile couples, their opinions often differ from those of urologists regarding the diagnosis and treatment of varicoceles. RE's often take the position proposed by

J.L. Marmar
Robert Wood Johnson School of Medicine at Camden, Cooper University Hospital, 3 Cooper Plaza – Suite 411, Camden, NJ 08103, USA
e-mail: marmar-joel@cooperhealth.edu

D.T. Carrell et al. (eds.), *Biennial Review of Infertility*, DOI: 10.1007/978-1-60327-392-3_18

the National Collaborating Centre for Women's and Children's Health, 2005 (12) that "men should not be offered surgery for varicoceles as a form of fertility treatment because it does not improve pregnancy rates." Furthermore, RE's often cite other studies, usually not done by urologists, that suggest no benefit from surgery (13–18). As an alternative, these specialists often recommend IVF/ICSI.

Recently, these opposing positions were clearly represented in two meta-analyses. The first report was written by two gynecologists and the authors concluded that varicocele repair does not seem to be an effective treatment for male infertility or unexplained subfertility (19). The second meta-analysis was written by a collaboration of urologists, basic scientists and statisticians and demonstrated improved pregnancy rates after surgery (20). Both of these publications have been widely critiqued, but even the commentaries appear to be quite partisan. The commentaries written by REs supported the data presented by Evers and Collins (19) whereas the commentaries by urologists supported Marmar et al. (20).

Clearly, these positions represent clinical polarization by specialty, and they beg the question, where do we go from here? If selected infertile men may benefit from a simple outpatient surgical procedure, then as scientists and clinicians, it seems important for all of the specialists involved in these cases to gain a greater understanding of the issues. If young couples want more than one child and a varicocelectomy enables them to accomplish their goal, then a carefully planned procedure should be carried out to avoid repetitive cycles of IVF/ICSI. On the other hand, if there is no valid reason to recommend a varicocelectomy, then the unbiased facts should be known.

The purpose of this chapter will be to review information related to varicoceles in several ways. First, the differences between these two meta-analyses will be highlighted. Second, there will be an explanation of the clinical diversity among men with varicoceles, and aspects of the pathophysiology of varicoceles will be discussed in the light of current molecular and genetic studies. Third, the chapter will present the pros and cons of specific varicocelectomy procedures. Lastly, the outcomes and costs will be reviewed for protocols that include both varicocele surgery and ART (IUI and IVF/ICSI). It is hoped that this chapter will offer new ideas about varicoceles for both REs and urologists.

## 2 The Differences Between Recent Meta-analyses on Varicocelectomy and Pregnancy

### 2.1 The First Meta-analysis

The first meta-analysis (19) included only Level I evidence from a group of prospective randomized trials (PRTs). The study concluded that varicocele surgery did not improve fertility. However, this meta-analysis was reviewed by several critics and they cited methodological flaws that may have introduced bias. Specifically, the National Collaborating Centre for Women's and Children's health (12) offered criticisms for several reasons: the selected studies included in the meta-analysis had clinical heterogeneity among the subjects, differences in the mean ages, differences in the duration of infertility and high dropout rates after randomization. The editorial comment that immediately followed the meta-analysis (21) raised the question of "publication bias" because Evers and Collins exclude data from a large WHO study that was presented in the abstract form. The multicenter WHO report concluded that varicocele surgery may improve pregnancy rates and the exclusion of these data may have made a difference. Other critics pointed out that this meta-analysis included data from men with subclinical varicoceles and men with normal semen parameters (22). In a separate analysis (23), several studies were eliminated from the Evers and Collins meta-analysis that included subjects with subclinical varicoceles and normal semen analyses. Recomputation of the data was limited to three studies, and these results changed the conclusions because these data did not allow the reader to draw any favorable or adverse conclusions about the treatment of varicoceles in infertile couples. Furthermore, two of these three studies showed significant improvement in semen parameters which was consistent with the findings of another recent meta-analysis that reported improved semen findings following varicocele surgery on infertile men with palpable lesions and at least one abnormal preoperative semen parameter (24). The data in this study were collected and analyzed by the same team involved with the study of Marmar et al. and they used similar scoring systems to evaluate bias when selecting studies for their meta-analysis (20).

Although some published literature has been critical of the fact that most varicocele studies were uncontrolled and not PRTs (25), others pointed out potential problems associated with PRTs. The studies may be costly and difficult to complete without high drop out rates after randomization (26–28). Still others have cited potential ethical issues with some PRTs because the randomization and informed consent may not reach international standards, and in most cases they are done without peer review (29). Lastly, some critics of the PRTs considered them unfair to the infertile couples because they offered no treatment in one arm of the trial, when alternative treatment was available such as IVF/ICSI (21). In these instances, treatment delays may expose these couples to the disadvantage of advancing age on pregnancy outcome. The question that remained was whether other data from existing PRTs and observational studies could be used together to evaluate the relationship between varicocelectomies and pregnancies?

### 2.2 The Second Meta-analysis

The second meta-analysis by Marmar et al. (20) used data from both PRTs and observational studies. The authors followed the guidelines established by the Potsdam Coalition (30). This approach may be controversial to some, but the Potsdam Coalition suggested that observational studies should not be abandoned, especially when there is a lack of data from PRTs (30). Others noted that observational studies may be included in a meta-analysis after critical appraisal and methodological evaluation (27), and a combination of data from several smaller observational studies may be an efficient, effective and perhaps the only means of reaching a conclusion about a clinical topic (31). Still others commented that decisions about clinical practices should be based on the combined weight of the evidence from available reports, but the challenge to develop a methodology for evaluating observational studies and deciding which to include in a particular meta-analysis remained (28).

Marmar et al. addressed the challenge of study design in several ways. Initially, all of the articles for this meta-analysis were blinded for the reviewers and then specifically scored for four types of bias – selection, confounding, informational and "other." A scoring system was developed related to each type of bias. A higher score indicated that the study met most of the criteria required to avoid bias, but an article was eliminated whenever it failed to reach the threshold score in more than one category of bias. If only one category scored below the threshold range, then the study was reexamined for inclusion in the meta-analysis. The articles for inclusion contained only infertile men with palpable varicoceles and at least one abnormal semen parameter on at least three semen analyses. The treatment included only men with surgical repairs because this approach minimized heterogeneity and addressed the difference of opinion regarding outcomes with surgery compared to embolization (32, 33). Lastly, Marmar et al. selected articles that included data on "spontaneous or natural" pregnancy rates, and excluded men who had undergone IVF/ICSI.

There were 101 articles retrieved from the search, but most were eliminated because of the study design. A total of 15 studies were blinded for the reviewers, but after scoring for bias, five articles (two RCTs and three observational studies) were included in the final meta-analysis. The results suggest that after varicocelectomy, compared to no treatment, the odds of a spontaneous pregnancy was 2.87 (95% CI, 1.33–6.20, $p = 0.007$). Within the five studies, there were 131 pregnancies among 396 couples where the husband had surgery (33.0%) vs. 27 pregnancies among 174 controls (15.5%). The number needed to treat was 5.7 (95% CI, 4.1–9.5). Based on these data, the authors concluded that a surgical varicocelectomy was an effective treatment for improving the spontaneous pregnancy rate for couples with an infertile male partner who had at least one low semen parameter and a palpable varicocele.

## 3 The Need for Specific Entry Criteria in Varicocelectomy Studies

Clinicians in the field of infertility realize that questions related to varicocelectomies and pregnancy rates have not been settled, but why are the opinions on these matters so different and so polarized? How could experienced clinicians and scientists reach such different conclusions about the role of varicocelectomy and fertility? One explanation may relate to diversity among the patients, which in turn may necessitate careful consideration of the entry criteria and study designs. For example, PRTs have been considered to be the highest level of evidence for medical research, but some investigators have noted that there maybe significant heterogeneity among the PRT study groups with a level of variability that may produce contradictory results between studies. Other investigators have been concerned about observational studies because they may over state the benefit of a specific procedure or treatment. Both of these concerns were addressed in a review that evaluated the outcomes of both observational studies and PRTs on similar topics (34). The results proved to be similar so long as the entry criteria were the same for the patients in these studies. Therefore, the next sections will address specific factors that may influence entry criteria, such as: the clinical diversity among varicocele patients, the molecular differences among the patients and the differences among varicocelectomy procedures.

## 3.1 Understanding Clinical Diversity

As a practical matter, men with varicoceles demonstrate considerable clinical diversity (35). Some men with these lesions are fertile and have normal semen parameters (36, 37). Others are infertile, and show a variety of semen findings (5). Some men have left sided lesions alone, but many are bilateral. Some men seem to improve after varicocelectomy, but others show no benefit following this surgery. Bilateral varicocelectomies may lead to significantly better pregnancy rates vs. unilateral repairs (38). These differences demonstrate the need for strict entry criteria to accommodate for the diversity.

One entry criterion to consider is the size of the varicocele and methods used for testing the size. The size of the lesions may vary considerably, and the effect of varicocele size on semen parameters may be used to illustrate the complexity of the varicocelectomy debate. A study reported maximum benefit from varicocelectomies among men with large lesions and lower sperm densities (38, 39). Others demonstrated improvement mostly among men with large varicoceles so long as the sperm densities were <40 million sperm/ml (40). They suggested a "ceiling effect" or no improvement when the initial sperm densities were >40 million sperm/ml. In contrast to these reports, other studies have shown improvement with varicocelectomies among selected men with small or subclinical varicoceles diagnosed by ultrasound (41–43). Others have suggested that repair of small varicoceles offers no benefit to the patient (1, 2). These conflicting findings may depend on the method used for diagnosis and for classification.

An early classification of varicoceles included four categories: Grade 3 – large and visible, Grade 2 – palpable, Grade 1 – only palpable with a valsalva maneuver and Grade 0 – nonpalpable or subclinical (43). This classification has been used for years and predates the use of clinical venography and ultrasound. Presently, the "gold standard" for the diagnosis of varicoceles has been venography, but it is an invasive procedure and is not practical for routine use. More recently, ultrasound studies have been used for the diagnoses, and these protocols include measurable and reproducible parameters that provide a high degree of sensitivity and specificity for the diagnosis of varicoceles when compared to selective venogrophy. One study developed ultrasound criteria for a significant varicocele that included three or more veins with a diameter of 3 mm at rest and which increased in size during the valsalva maneuver (42). In a more recent review of clinical ultrasound in the diagnosis of varicoceles (43), maximum vein diameter, sum of the diameters (plexus size) and changes in flow velocity during a valsalva maneuver were used to evaluate clinical varicoceles. Others used a simple pencil Doppler as part of the examination (5). The patients were examined in the standing position, with and without the valsalva maneuver. The probe was placed over the spermatic cord, and only continuous reflux was considered clinically meaningful. Grade 3 was visible, palpable and audible, Grade 2 was palpable and audible and Grade 1 was only audible. Regardless of grade, continuous reflux was needed to classify a clinical varicocele. These types of ultrasound protocols are now applicable for use in the office as part of the varicocele work up, and may be included in future varicocelectomy studies.

## 3.2 Consistent Varicocele Effects

Regardless of the clinical diversity, certain varicocele effects may be quite consistent because these lesions develop from retrograde blood flow down the internal spermatic veins and the cremasteric veins into the pampiniform plexus. The reversal of venous flow occurs because of absent or incomplete valves. Some anatomical dissections on men with varicoceles have demonstrated absence of the valve at the junction of the left renal vein and the internal spermatic vein (44). Other retrograde venography studies on men with varicoceles have demonstrated either absent or incompetent valves along the entire internal spermatic vein (45–47). The retrograde flow may produce varying increases in testicular temperature, hydrostatic pressure, stasis and release of substances from the endothelium from the inner walls of these veins.

These factors influence spermatogenesis in a variety of ways, but these conditions may be qualitatively and quantitatively different among individuals and represent another manifestation of clinical diversity. Human data related to intra testicular temperatures, increased hydrostatic pressures and stasis resulting from varicoceles overlap considerably among men with varicoceles and controls and may be too difficult to measure on a regular basis. However, the impact of these effects can be demonstrated consistently in animal models with varicoceles, because after the experimental surgery, the factors are always present and unrelenting. Therefore, data from these models are worthy of specific mention.

### 3.3 The Influence of Consistent Varicocele Effects in Animal Models

In humans, varicocele effects may vary under changing conditions, such as the time spent in a horizontal position during sleep, or with different clothing. Furthermore, these effects may trigger certain molecular and genetic changes that collectively produce the pathophysiology of varicoceles. In animal models, the varicocele effects are constant and unrelenting all the time, and the varicocele effects have been well documented.

Varicocele models have been created in at least four species of laboratory animals: rats (48), dogs (49), rabbits (50, 51), and monkeys (52–54). The "varicocele" was created by partial constriction of the left renal vein and/or left testicular vein leading to sustained partial obstruction with congestion and dilatation of the pampiniform plexus and testis vasculature. In the models that achieved visible evidence of venous distention, there was a reproducible increase in intra-testicular temperature and interstitial pressures in all species. Although these animals were fertile prior to the creation of the "varicocele effect," over time, 25–50% of the seminiferous tubules demonstrated a predictable pattern of hypospermatogenesis with premature sloughing of spermatocytes and spermatids. In the monkey model, sperm density dropped from a mean of 440 million sperm/ml to 227 million sperm/ml after 90 days, while in the rabbits it dropped from 300–450 million sperm/ml to 17–100 million sperm/ml.

These effects were reversible in the rat model following removal of the obstructing suture, so long as it was removed within 30 days after the creation of the varicocele (55). These results demonstrate that unrelenting varicocele effects influence spermatogenesis negatively, and lead to a progressive decline in the semen parameters, but that these processes are reversible.

Several studies have suggested that apoptosis may play an important role in the development of oligozoospermia among animal models and infertile men. In a rat model (56), there was increased germ cell apoptosis using the TUNEL assay. After 28 days, the model demonstrated 0.27 apoptotic cells per seminiferous tubule compared to 0.14 cells for controls ($p < 0.002$). In humans (57), there was increased apoptosis among varicocele patients. The mean percent apoptotic cells per total germ cells counted per high powered field was 14.7% for men with varicoceles compared to 2% for controls. In a report on ejaculated sperm (58), the investigators demonstrated that up to 10% of sperm cells in the ejaculate of men with varicoceles were apoptotic compared to 0.1% among fertile controls. Most recently, studies on testis tissue reported a bilateral increase in apoptosis even in cases of a unilateral varicocele (59). Thus, there seems to be a link between varicoceles and apoptosis, and the pathways leading to apoptosis, including oxidative stress, heat stress, androgen deprivation, and accumulation of toxic stimuli are discussed below.

## 4 Molecular/Genetic Responses Among Men with Varicoceles

### 4.1 NO, ROS and Oxidative Stress

Nitric oxide production is upregulated in the veins and testis of men with varicoceles because of pressure and stasis (60–63). This phenomenon is consistent with effects in other varicose veins within the body. The increase in NO concentration leads to increased expression of both endothelial nitric oxide synthase (eNOS) (64) and inducible NOS (iNOS) (64), and the

NO can lead to the production of reactive oxygen species (ROS) (hydrogen peroxide and free radicals such as OH and $O_2^-$) which are elevated in blood plasma, seminal plasma and testicular tissue of infertile men with varicoceles (57, 65, 66).

Low levels of reactive oxygen species may be involved in capacitation and induction of sperm motility, but elevated concentrations of ROS are associated with detrimental effects on the sperm (67). The oxidative stress associated with varicoceles produces are: 1) greater sperm DNA fragmentation (68), 2) greater testicular lipid peroxidation (69, 70), 3) increased numbers of immature sperm with cytoplasmic droplets in the ejaculate (71), 4) higher levels of proinflammatory cytokines in semen (72), and increased percentages of apoptotic (TUNEL-positive) sperm in the ejaculate (68).

Of patients attending an infertility clinic, 40% had detectable levels of reaction oxygen species (ROS) in their semen (73), whereas, reaction oxygen species were not detectable in the semen of normal volunteers (74). Recent studies suggest that varicocelectomy may reduce generation of NO and ROS, increase the antioxidant activities of seminal plasma, reduce lipid peroxidation, reduce retention of the cytoplasmic droplet during spermiation (71, 75, 76) and reduce the level of DNA damage. Some investigators have suggested that studies of oxidative stress should be included in the infertility workup (77), and future varicocelectomy studies may include indicators of oxidative stress as an entry criteria. A recent example of this study design reported a possible apoptosis-related phenotype of ejaculated sperm in patients with varicoceles (78). This protocol included four laboratory studies: the plasma membrane translocation of phosphatidylserine, evidence of mitochondrial dysfunction, nuclear DNA damage and single cell gel electrophoresis (Comet assay). These tests represent a coordinated laboratory protocol and they along with other markers may be used to stratify patients when evaluating outcomes of future varicocelectomy and/or ICSI studies.

## 4.2 Heat Stress and Apoptosis

Although the average scrotal temperature increases 2.5°C among men with varicoceles, it is unclear whether this increase is sufficient to initiate apoptosis (79). Experimentally, (80) the scrota of rats were exposed to 43°C for 15 min. The results of the heat stress lead to apoptosis, which was cell specific and stage specific. A separate report noted an early and increased expression of the proapoptotic Bax gene in susceptible germ cells after 30 min of scrotal heating (81).

Other markers of heat effect have been studied and well documented. Specific heat shock proteins (HSP70-2) are distributed over sperm cells and seem to be up regulated in heat stress (82). In the absence of heat shock proteins in a "knock out" mouse model there was a dramatic increase in apoptosis (83). Recently, the expression of HSP 70-1 was studied in the testis tissue as a defense mechanism of men with varicoceles (84). The men that demonstrated an HSP 70-1 response had less apoptosis and higher sperm densities vs. those with no response. Although the direct measurement of heat changes in men with varicoceles is difficult to carry out, identification of the markers of heat effect may be more practical and informative. Thus, identification of these markers may define the heat related conditions among men with varicoceles leading to apoptosis. These markers may be used to stratify patients for future varicocelectomy studies.

## 4.3 Androgen Deprivation and Apoptosis

Androgen deprivation may represent another apoptotic pathway in men with varicoceles. Specific studies of apoptosis and androgen deprivation have been carried out on rat models after a hypophysectomy (85), and with a gonadotropin-releasing hormone antagonist (86). These models demonstrated reduced sperm densities, but these effects were overcome with testosterone supplement (87). In other experimental studies, there was a sharp decline in intra-testicular testosterone in the varicocele rat model, without an effect on serum testosterone (88), and a failure of testicular tissue homogenates to convert $^3$H-pregnenolone to 3H-T in animal models and humans with varicoceles (89).

In the past, supplemental hCG, clomid and tamoxifen were used empirically following varicocelectomy (90, 91). In other studies, Leydig cells were quantified in biopsies from men with varicoceles and the findings were used to predict varicocelectomy outcomes (92), and semi-thin sections of testis biopsy material were evaluated for the function of Leydig cells based upon their histological appearance (93). In some of these cases, the Leydig cells appeared "burned out" which implied that this group would not benefit from varicocelectomy. Recently, the size and number of Leydig cells were quantified in testis tissue of men with varicoceles (94). These cells were reduced in number, but they appeared hypertrophied. In addition, the testis appeared to be mounting a protective response to reactive oxygen species by increased expression of inducible heme oxygenase-1 in Leydig cells, because the products of heme oxygenase-1 have antioxidant activities (94).

The use of hormonal supplements for men with varicoceles has been empiric, but in the future selective hormonal stimulation may be used on specific patients with evidence of intra testicular androgen deprivation. The diagnosis may require percutaneous aspiration biopsies of limited testis tissue, but this approach has proven safe with ultrasonic control (95). This type of testing for local androgen deficiency may lead to protocols for hormonal therapy, and entry criteria for future varicocelectomy studies.

### 4.4 *Toxic Agents and Apoptosis*

Toxic agents, such as 2-methoxyethanol, an ethylene glycol ether and its byproduct 2-methoxyacetic acid, have been shown to cause apoptosis in rats and mice leading to spermatocyte death (96–98). Some investigators have suggested that toxic adrenal byproducts could reflux down the internal spermatic vein to the testicle in men with varicoceles (99, 100). However, the toxic effects of cortisol and catacholamines were never proven. Others demonstrated higher levels of prostaglandin and serotonin in the spermatic veins of varicocele patients, but these compounds did not produce an antispermatogenesis affect (101, 102).

Perhaps, the most widely studied toxic agent related to infertility has been cigarette smoke. In smokers, the semen quality may shift into an infertile range (103) and oligozoospermia is ten times more common among men with varicoceles who smoke compared to men with varicoceles who did not smoke (104). In a separate study, cadmium has been suggested as a toxic agent that affected spermatogenesis because the serum levels of cadmium in smokers is more than double the values of nonsmokers (105). Recently, cadmium levels were studied in testicular tissue of infertile men with varicoceles who were undergoing a varicocelectomy, and 53% had elevated levels of tissue Cd (59, 95). The men with increased levels of testis Cd had increased levels of apoptosis and less improvement following varicocelectomy.

In a rat model, administration of cadmium (Cd) chloride induced the characteristic apoptosis ladder-like patterns of DNA on the agarose gel (106). Wister rats demonstrated oligozoospermia following varying doses of Cd in their drinking water (107). Furthermore, altered gene expressions were noted on microarray analysis and microdeletions were noted in the L-type voltage dependent calcium channels. A similar alteration of the calcium channel had been demonstrated in infertile humans with varicoceles, and the men with microdeletions had a poor response to varicocelectomy (59, 95).

In summary, the molecular and genetic effects contribute to the overall pathophysiology of varicoceles, and identification of molecular/genetic markers in semen or testis tissue may be used to stratify men with varicoceles, and increase the selectivity for surgery. Identification of some specific markers may be included with the entry criteria for candidates in future varicocelectomy studies, but the panel of markers needs greater clarification. These markers may be present as part of the intrinsic genetic make-up of the individuals, or they may develop from extrinsic causes related to the effects. In either case, these markers have led some investigators to introduce the concept of the "second hit hypothesis" (35, 108, 109).

These authors suggest that the varicocele was the "second hit" on top of underlying molecular/genetic defects. If there were no defects, then the men would remain fertile, despite the varicocele. If these defects were limited, then correction of the varicoceles would lead to improvement in the semen parameters and pregnancy rates. However, if the defects were advanced, then the varicocelectomy would probably fail. To illustrate these concepts, the genetic influences on varicocelectomies may be demonstrated in men with azoospermia and varicoceles.

## 5 Molecular/Genetic Differences Among Men with Azoospermia and Varicoceles

In a classic paper, Tulloch performed a varicocelectomy on an azoospermic male (110). After surgery, the semen parameters improved leading to pregnancy. This report has been the stimulus for varicocele surgery over the years, but until recently, most azoospermic men were excluded as candidates for varicocelectomy. With the development of IVF/ICSI, there has been renewed interest in varicocelectomy for azoospermic men (111), but the data suggest that the outcome of varicocelectomy may depend upon the preexisting genetic status. For example, sperm returned to the ejaculate following varicocelectomy in 55% of azoospermic men and pregnancy rate was 3 of 22 (13.6%) (112). In 28 men with varicoceles with nonobstructive azoospermia, 12 (43%) demonstrated sperm in the ejaculate after 24 months of follow up (113). However, the improvement occurred only in men who had testis histology with hypospermatogenesis or spermatogenic arrest at the spermatid level, but recent reports suggest that varicocelectomies may produce sperm in the ejaculate of some men with Sertoli Cell Only (114, 115). In contrast to these results, others considered the endpoint of varicocelectomy in men with azoospermia as the appearance of sperm in the ejaculate that were sufficient for ICSI. In these cases, varicocelectomy produced sufficient sperms for ICSI in only 9.6% of these cases (116). Although some azoospermic men improve after varicocelectomy, it may be reasonable to evaluate the histology of testicular biopsies to determine the underlying histology. Presently, limited percutaneous testis biopsies may be performed in an office setting with local anesthesia (95).

In addition to testicular histology, azoospermic men with varicoceles have been studied for other genetic factors. The Y chromosome microdeletion analysis was performed in 200 consecutive infertile men, and 2 of 70 men with varicoceles tested positive for Y chromosome micro deletions (117). This finding illustrates that genetic problems may coexist in patients with varicoceles. In a separate study on a group of azoospermic and oligozoospermic men, those with Y chromosome microdeletions or aneuploidy failed to improve following varicocelectomy (118). These data suggests that Y chromosome mapping and karyotype studies may be important in the workup of men with varicoceles and azoospermia or severe oligozoospermia, because the genetic findings may predict varicocelectomy outcome. Another 138 patients with nonobstructive azoospermia and varicoceles were evaluated, and 82 had Y chromosome studies (116). From among this group, seven had micro microdeletions. No sperm were retrieved with TESE from the men with deletions in the AZF b region, but some sperm were recovered with TESE in 2 of 3 men with micro deletions in the AZFc regions with or without varicocelectomies. An additional 14 patients had a varicocele and Kleinfelters Syndrome (47,XXY), and 11 (79%) had sperm at TESE regardless of a varicocelectomy,

Although the molecular/genetic aspects of an individual may contribute to the pathophysiology of infertile men with varicoceles, another variable should be considered when comparing the outcomes of varicocelectomy studies. There maybe significant differences in the success and failure rates based on the procedures themselves. The following section will examine some of these differences.

## 6 Variable Outcomes with Different Varicocelectomy Procedures

Evers et al. presented an updated systemic review for the Cochrane Collaboritave study entitled, "Surgery or embolization for varicoceles in subfertile men" (119). Based on data from nine PRTs they concluded that, "there is no evidence that treatment of varicoceles in men from couples with otherwise unexplained subfertility improves the couple's chance for conception." Their review included data from PRTs that utilized open surgery, percutaneous retrograde embolization with coils and antegrade sclerosis. None of the varicocelectomies were done with microsurgical procedures. The basic assumption in the article was that these procedures had similar outcomes. However, this assumption requires further analysis.

Surgical varicocelectomies were done for the treatment of pain early in the twentieth century (120). The original surgical procedures included exploration of the inguinal canal with ligation of the dilated internal spermatic veins (121), and a retroperitoneal approach with ligation of the entire spermatic cord at a level above the internal ring (122). Varicocele surgery was not used for the treatment of infertility until Tulloch in 1955 performed retroperitoneal surgery on a man with azoospermia (110). Subsequently, others popularized the inguinal approach for the treatment of infertile men with varicoceles (123), and now it is estimated that approximately 20,000–40,000 varicocelectomies are performed in the United States each year.

Although these techniques have been widely accepted in clinical practice, some reports described significant complications as a result of these surgeries including azoospermia after bilateral varicocelectomies and testicular atrophy after ipsilateral surgery (124, 125). To overcome these specific clinical problems associated with open surgery, the subinguinal microsurgical varicocelectomy was developed (9, 126). With these microsurgical techniques, the lymphatics and testicular arteries were preserved, hydroceles were eliminated and there was no testicular atrophy. More recently, laparoscopic varicocelectomies were introduced, but they are usually limited to the treatment of adolescents (127). Percutaneous retrograde sclerosis procedures (128, 129) and embolizations (130) were introduced as an alternative to surgery. More recently, a technique for antigrade sclerosis of varicoceles was introduced (131). These various procedures may have different outcomes, and unless these differences are accounted for in the varicocelectomy studies, they may affect the final statistical analysis.

With the clinical utilization of diagnostic venography, it became apparent that the recurrence rates following open surgical varicocelectomies were higher than previously reported or a frequency of recurrence of 5–20% (132). Often these failures were due to refluxive vessels that were overlooked during the surgical procedure, including refluxive cremasteric veins in 40% of these cases (133). With retrograde phlebography and embolization for therapy, some interventional radiologists reported technical problems during access to the venous drainage systems, and 5–18% of the cases were aborted (134). In some cases the balloons or coils migrated (135). Overall, when the reflexive veins were not obliterated, the failure rate was about 4.4% (136). In the case of antegrade sclerotherapy, the recurrence rates were higher at 9% (137).

The studies in the meta-analysis of Evers et al. utilized a variety of procedures for treatment, and several lacked information regarding the post treatment examinations and true failure rates (19, 119). Furthermore, none of the studies were microsurgical procedures. The Guidelines Committees on Infertility from the AUA and ASRM indicated that most specialists utilize microsurgery for the correction of varicoceles (1, 2), and in a recent "head to head" PRT (138) the authors demonstrated that the recurrence rate and postoperative pain was less with the microsurgical approach. The original recurrence rate for microsurgical repairs was 2.9%/patient, but with experience the recurrence rates dropped to 2.1%/patient or 1.6%/unit (5, 9). Since the recurrence rates may differ among procedures, each varicocelectomy study should include a statement of recurrences, because these rates may influence outcomes. Ideally, future systemic reviews of the effect of varicocelectomy on reproductive outcome should be limited to a single procedure.

Another aspect for consideration regarding future varicocelectomy studies will be the study design for the control group. The use of a "no treatment" arm may be not appropriate for control patients because it is contrary to the intent of the couple that is seeking help for infertility and a "no treatment" delay adds age to the female during the time of no treatment. One reviewer suggested that future varicocelectomy studies should offer a recognized treatment option such as IVF/ICSI in the control arm (21). Therefore, the next section will explore the relationship of varicocelectomy with assisted reproductive technologies (ART).

## 7 Varicocelectomy and Art

The statements at the beginning of this chapter suggest that some clinical decisions regarding varicocelectomies are partisan. For infertile men with palpable varicoceles and an abnormal semen parameter, urologists will often recommend surgery, whereas REs favor IVF/ICSI. However, recent literature on varicocelectomy and ART has taken this debate in a new direction. Some clinicians have combined these therapies with improved pregnancy outcomes and cost savings, and coined the term "progressive stacking therapy" (139). If the improvement after varicocelectomy was limited, they recommended ART in addition to surgery to maximize the benefits from both the procedures. Initially, some investigators were concerned that the sequence of varicocelectomy and ART would delay the inevitable and add age to the female partner (140). They warned that the average interval between varicocele repair and pregnancy may exceed 6 months, and that this natural delay may add at least 6 months to the female age who may become candidates for ART.

This concern is consistent with data from several investigators who have called attention to the importance of female age and the outcome with ART (13). The 2005 ART report of The Centers of Disease Control and Prevention supported these concern based on data based on 143,260 IVF cycles from 422 clinics (141). The women were classified by age: <35 years., 35–37, 38–40 and >41. The live birth rates per cycle were 37.3, 29.5, 19.7 and 10.6%, respectively. However, when other studies on women over 35 used a combination of surgery and ART, the age factor seemed to be minimized. The pregnancy outcomes for women over 35 years after combined varicocelectomy and ART was 35% and an additional 2 and 4% achieved pregnancy with IUI and IVF/ICSI respectively for an overall success rate of 41%. In a group with ART alone, 25% achieved a spontaneous pregnancy with management of the female partner, and an additional 7 and 9% achieved pregnancy with IUI and IVF/ICSI alone. Although the female age should be considered in all cases, other factors may influence the outcomes such as improved semen parameters after varicocelectomy.

## 7.1 Varicocelectomy and Postoperative Sperm Density and Financial Considerations

In a recent comprehensive review of the outcomes of varicocelectomy, the authors cited data from seven controlled and 19 uncontrolled studies since 1994 and suggested that the sperm density improved significantly after the surgery (142). Even an open critic of varicocelectomy reported statistically significant improvement of sperm density following surgery (13, 25). In a separate randomized clinical trial for IUI and superovulation, the authors established the threshold for fertility based on sperm density as a single variable at 13.5 million sperm/ml (143). The men with values below this threshold had an odds ratio for infertility of 5.3 (95% CI 3.3–8.3). Specific to a varicocelectomy, a 50% improvement of sperm density after surgery was a strong predictor of pregnancy (144). Therefore, if varicocelectomy procedures can significantly raise the sperm density, then why withhold these procedures from selected patients?

In some studies involving varicocelectomy and ART, the total motile sperm count was used as predictor of pregnancy outcome because a threshold value of greater than or equal to 5 million motile sperm was associated with elevated spontaneous pregnancy rates (145). In one study, the investigators classified 110 infertile men with clinical varicoceles by their total motile sperm count (TMC) (146). Overall, 66% of these men shifted to an improved category after surgery. The authors created three categories: Grade A, >20 million motile sperm, Grade B, 5-20 TMC and Grade C, <5 TMC. Following varicocelectomy, the mean TMC increased significantly for the group from 21.7 to 54.6 ($p = 0.015$), and the number of Grade A patients increased from 18 to 35. Among the group of Grade A patients, 12 achieved natural pregnancies, and 12 required the least number of ART procedures to achieve pregnancies: three IUI and nine IVF/ICSI.

In another study, investigators evaluated 540 infertile men with varicoceles (147) and the patients were classified into four categories based on their TMCs and each group received a clinical designation: Preoperatively, 154 were classified as ICSI candidates (TMC 0–1.5 million), 79 as IVF candidates (TMC 1.5–5.0 million), 151 as IUI candidates (TMC 5–20 million) and 156 as spontaneous pregnancy candidates (>20 million). After surgery, many candidates shifted their clinical classification: 31% of the ICSI group and 53% of IVF candidates achieved IUI or spontaneous pregnancy status, and 42% of the IUI group achieved spontaneous pregnancy status. The overall spontaneous pregnancy was 36.6% and the mean time to conception was 7 months (range 1–19 months). The authors concluded that varicocelectomy demonstrated a significant potential to shift the clinical category and reduce the need for IVF/ICSI.

In a separate study from Canada, pregnancy data were recorded for 610 infertile men with varicoceles who were counseled and given options for treatment (148). The options included surgery, IUI and IVF/ICSI. The patient decisions may be in part due to economic influences, because in Canada varicocelectomy is covered by the National Health Plan but ART is not. The authors estimated costs in US dollars, and figured the costs of three to six IUIs in the range of $1,000–2,000, and the cost of one IVF/ICSI cycle about $5,000–10,000. A total of 363 patients opted for a varicocelectomy and the spontaneous pregnancy rate after surgery alone was 39%. When IUI and ICSI were used in addition, the overall postoperative pregnancy rate for this group was 53%. The remaining 40% of the study group or 257 original patients rejected surgery and was considered the "observational" group. From among this group, 77 couples attempted ART for with an overall pregnancy rate of 56%. However, it is important to note that the remainder of the "observational" group opted for no treatment, and these results may have been skewed by economic decisions, and because the surgical population had significantly greater numbers of couples with primary infertility. These studies support the notion that varicocelectomies done on properly selected infertile men may lead to improved semen parameters, but the reality remains that many clinical decisions regarding the combination of surgery and ART may be based on other factors, such as cost.

The estimated costs per delivery were examined after a single cycle of IVF/ICSI vs varicocelectomy (149). The study utilized 1994 figures and the average delivery rates for ICSI were 28% single cycle, and 30% for varicocelectomy. The cost per delivery with ICSI was $89,091 whereas the cost per delivery after varicocelectomy was only $26,268. Another study evaluated the cost benefit analysis by applying a decision modeling technique, and by stratifying patients according to the total motile sperm count (150). The initial branch of the decision model included two choices, varicocelectomy or ART, and the second branch for the ART group split the patients into two groups, those with >10 million TMC and those with <10 million TMC. The cost per pregnancy was calculated using the cumulative costs in each branch divided by the number of pregnancies. In the varicocelectomy group, the pregnancy rate was 16.5% for men with <10 million sperm at a cost of $28,286/pregnancy, whereas in a similar ART group, the cost was $33,333. Following varicocelectomy for men with >10 million TMC the average pregnancy rate was 36.6% at an average cost of $10,694. In a similar group with ART, the cost per pregnancy was $18,733. When the TMCs were low, the ART patients required more IVF/ICI procedures at a cost of $10,000/cycle, whereas patients with higher scores used more IUI attempts which were less expensive at $500/attempt. So long as the pregnancy rate was >14% after surgery, the varicocelectomy was more cost effective than ART. For couples to make an informed decision, these types of cost analyses should be essential in any counseling session related varicocelectomy and ART.

## 8 Conclusions

The intent of this chapter was to examine the differences between two recent meta-analyses on the subject of varicocelectomy and fertility (1, 2) and to present general information related to the clinical diversity among men with varicoceles and some aspects of the pathophysiology of varicoceles in the light of current molecular and genetic studies. The chapter also presented potential differences among specific varicocelectomy procedures, and examined the outcomes of varicocele surgery combined with IUI and IVF/ICSI, including the costs. With this comprehensive information, it is hoped that the matter of varicocelectomies and pregnancies may be considered with greater understanding on both sides of the debate.

When Evers et al. stated, "there is no evidence that treatment of varicoceles in men from couples with otherwise unexplained subfertility improves the couple's chance for conception," perhaps their statement was too broad and not selective enough for application in clinical practice. Perhaps the position of the AUA and ASRM Guidelines, which stated, "correction of varicoceles is indicated for infertile men with palpable lesions and one or more abnormal semen parameters or an abnormal sperm function test" is now more understandable regarding the essential conditions for surgery. In the future, molecular/genetic markers may be used to better identify patients for surgery. Microsurgical corrections may have advantages over other procedures. Presently, it should be apparent to all clinicians that surgery and ART may be used together in protocols to improve outcomes. In the end, it is hoped that this publication presented some new ideas about varicoceles that may prove to be useful to all clinicians.

## References


1. Jarow JP, Sharlip ID, Belker AM, et al. Best practice policies for male infertility. The Journal of Urology 2002;167(5):2138–44.
2. Sharlip ID, Jarow JP, Belker AM, et al. Best practice policies for male infertility. Fertility and Sterility 2002;77(5):873–82.
3. Madgar I, Weissenberg R, Lunenfeld B, Karasik A, Goldwasser B. Controlled trial of high spermatic vein ligation for varicocele in infertile men. Fertility and Sterility 1995;63(1):120–4.
4. Okuyama A, Fujisue H, Matsui T, et al. Surgical repair of varicocele: effective treatment for subfertile men in a controlled study. European Urology 1988;14(4):298–300.
5. Schlesinger MH, Wilets IF, Nagler HM. Treatment outcome after varicocelectomy. A critical analysis. The Urologic Clinics of North America 1994;21(3):517–29.

6. Marmar JL, Kim Y. Subinguinal microsurgical varicocelectomy: a technical critique and statistical analysis of semen and pregnancy data. The Journal of Urology 1994;152(4): 1127–32.
7. Onozawa M, Endo F, Suetomi T, Takeshima H, Akaza H. Clinical study of varicocele: statistical analysis and the results of long-term follow-up. International Journal of Urology 2002;9(8):455–61.
8. Cayan S, Kadioglu TC, Tefekli A, Kadioglu A, Tellaloglu S. Comparison of results and complications of high ligation surgery and microsurgical high inguinal varicocelectomy in the treatment of varicocele. Urology 2000;55(5):750–4.
9. Goldstein M, Gilbert BR, Dicker AP, Dwosh J, Gnecco C. Microsurgical inguinal varicocelectomy with delivery of the testis: an artery and lymphatic sparing technique. The Journal of Urology 1992;148(6):1808–11.
10. Sayfan J, Soffer Y, Orda R. Varicocele treatment: prospective randomized trial of 3 methods. The Journal of Urology 1992;148(5):1447–9.
11. Segenreich E, Israilov SR, Shmueli J, Niv E, Servadio C. Correlation between semen parameters and retrograde flow into the pampiniform plexus before and after varicocelectomy. European Urology 1997;32(3):310–4.
12. Clinical guidelines: Fertility: assessment and treatment for people with fertility problems. National Collaborating Centre for Women's and Children's Health 2004:54–5.
13. Kamischke A, Nieschlag E. Varicocele treatment in the light of evidence-based andrology. Human Reproduction Update 2001;7(1):65–9.
14. Nilsson S, Edvinsson A, Nilsson B. Improvement of semen and pregnancy rate after ligation and division of the internal spermatic vein: fact or fiction? British Journal of Urology 1979;51(6):591–6.
15. Grasso M, Lania C, Castelli M, Galli L, Franzoso F, Rigatti P. Low-grade left varicocele in patients over 30 years old:the effect of spermatic vein ligation on fertility. BJU International 2000;85(3):305–7.
16. Breznik R, Vlaisavljevic V, Borko E. Treatment of varicocele and male fertility. Archives of andrology 1993;30(3):157–60.
17. Rageth JC, Unger C, DaRugna D, et al. Long-term results of varicocelectomy. Urologia Internationalis 1992;48(3): 327–31.
18. Krause W, Muller HH, Schafer H, Weidner W. Does treatment of varicocele improve male fertility? results of the 'Deutsche Varikozelenstudie', a multicentre study of 14 collaborating centres. Andrologia 2002;34(3):164–71.
19. Evers JL, Collins JA. Assessment of efficacy of varicocele repair for male subfertility: a systematic review. Lancet 2003;361(9372):1849–52.
20. Marmar JL, Agarwal A, Prabakaran S, et al. Reassessing the value of varicocelectomy as a treatment for male subfertility with a new meta-analysis. Fertility and Sterility 2007;88(3):639–48.
21. Templeton A. Varicocele and infertility. Lancet 2003; 361(9372):1838–9.
22. Marmar JL, Benoff S. Varicoceles. The Journal of Urology 2006;175(3 Pt 1):818–9.
23. Ficarra V, Cerruto MA, Liguori G, et al. Treatment of varicocele in subfertile men: The Cochrane Review–a contrary opinion. European Urology 2006;49(2):258–63.
24. Agarwal A, Deepinder F, Cocuzza M, et al. Efficacy of varicocelectomy in improving semen parameters: new meta-analytical approach. Urology 2007;70(3):532–8.
25. Nieschlag E, Hertle L, Fischedick A, Abshagen K, Behre HM. Update on treatment of varicocele: counselling as effective as occlusion of the vena spermatica. Human Reproduction (Oxford, England) 1998;13(8):2147–50.
26. Williams JK. Understanding evidence-based medicine: a primer. American Journal of Obstetrics and Gynecology 2001;185(2):275–8.
27. Peipert JF, Phipps MG. Observational studies. Clinical Obstetrics and Gynecology 1998;41(2):235–44.
28. Norris SL, Atkins D. Challenges in using nonrandomized studies in systematic reviews of treatment interventions. Annals of Internal Medicine 2005;142(12 Pt 2):1112–9.
29. Comhaire F. Clinical andrology: from evidence-base to ethics. The 'E' quintet in clinical andrology. Human Reproduction (Oxford, England) 2000;15(10):2067–71.
30. Cook DJ, Sackett DL, Spitzer WO. Methodologic guidelines for systematic reviews of randomized control trials in health care from the Potsdam Consultation on Meta-Analysis. Journal of Clinical Epidemiology 1995;48(1):167–71.
31. Stroup DF, Berlin JA, Morton SC, et al. Meta-analysis of observational studies in epidemiology: a proposal for reporting. Meta-analysis of observational studies in epidemiology (MOOSE) group. JAMA 2000;283(15):2008–12.
32. Yavetz H, Levy R, Papo J, et al. Efficacy of varicocele embolization versus ligation of the left internal spermatic vein for improvement of sperm quality. International Journal of Andrology 1992;15(4):338–44.
33. Shlansky-Goldberg RD, VanArsdalen KN, Rutter CM, et al. Percutaneous varicocele embolization versus surgical ligation for the treatment of infertility: changes in seminal parameters and pregnancy outcomes. Journal of Vascular and Interventional Radiology 1997;8(5):759–67.
34. Horwitz RI, Viscoli CM, Clemens JD, Sadock RT. Developing improved observational methods for evaluating therapeutic effectiveness. The American Journal of Medicine 1990;89(5):630–8.
35. Marmar JL. The pathophysiology of varicoceles in the light of current molecular and genetic information. Human Reproduction Update 2001;7(5):461–72.
36. Uehling DT. Fertility in men with varicocele. International journal of fertility 1968;13(1):58–60.
37. Kursh ED. What is the incidence of varicocele in a fertile population? Fertility and Sterility 1987;48(3):510–1.
38. Libman J, Jarvi K, Lo K, Zini A. Beneficial effect of microsurgical varicocelectomy is superior for men with bilateral versus unilateral repair. The Journal of Urology 2006;176(6 Pt 1):2602–5; discussion 5.
39. Steckel J, Dicker AP, Goldstein M. Relationship between varicocele size and response to varicocelectomy. The Journal of Urology 1993;149(4):769–71.
40. Tinga DJ, Jager S, Bruijnen CL, Kremer J, Mensink HJ. Factors related to semen improvement and fertility after varicocele operation. Fertility and Sterility 1984;41(3):404–10.
41. Dhabuwala CB, Hamid S, Moghissi KS. Clinical versus subclinical varicocele: improvement in fertility after varicocelectomy. Fertility and Sterility 1992;57(4):854–7.
42. McClure RD, Khoo D, Jarvi K, Hricak H. Subclinical varicocele: the effectiveness of varicocelectomy. The Journal of Urology 1991;145(4):789–91.
43. Yarborough MA, Burns JR, Keller FS. Incidence and clinical significance of subclinical scrotal varicoceles. The Journal of Urology 1989;141(6):1372–4.

44. Kohler FP. On the etiology of varicocele. The Journal of Urology 1967;97(4):741–2.
45. Ahlberg NE, Bartley O, Chidekel N, Fritjofsson A. Phlebography in varicocele scroti. Acta Radiologica: Diagnosis 1966;4(5):517–28.
46. Coolsaet BL. The varicocele syndrome: venography determining the optimal level for surgical management. The Journal of Urology 1980;124(6):833–9.
47. Comhaire F, Kunnen M. Selective retrograde venography of the internal spermatic vein: a conclusive approach to the diagnosis of varicocele. Andrologia 1976;8(1):11–24.
48. Turner TT, Jones CE, Roddy MS. Experimental varicocele does not affect the blood-testis barrier, epididymal electrolyte concentrations, or testicular blood gas concentrations. Biology of Reproduction 1987;36(4):926–32.
49. Saypol DC, Howards SS, Turner TT, Miller ED Jr. Influence of surgically induced varicocele on testicular blood flow, temperature, and histology in adult rats and dogs. The Journal of Clinical Investigation 1981;68(1):39–45.
50. Snydle FE, Cameron DF. Surgical induction of varicocele in the rabbit. The Journal of Urology 1983;130(5):1005–9.
51. Sofikitis N, Miyagawa I. Bilateral effect of unilateral varicocele on testicular metabolism in the rabbit. International Journal of Fertility and Menopausal Studies 1994;39(4):239–47.
52. Fussell E, Lewis R, Roberts JA, Harrison RM. Early ultrastructural findings in experimentally produced varicocele in the monkey testis. Journal of Andrology 1981;2:111–9.
53. Harrison RM, Lewis RW, Roberts JA. Pathophysiology of varicocele in nonhuman primates: long-term seminal and testicular changes. Fertility and Sterility 1986;46(3):500–10.
54. Kay R, Alexander NJ, Baugham WL. Induced varicoceles in rhesus monkeys. Fertility and Sterility 1979;31(2):195–9.
55. Green KF, Turner TT, Howards SS. Varicocele: reversal of the testicular blood flow and temperature effects by varicocele repair. The Journal of Urology 1984;131(6):1208–11.
56. Caruso A, Walsh R, Ross L, Trummer H, Meacham R. Experimental varicocele induces testicular germ cell apoptosis in the rat. The Journal of Urology 1999;161:280.
57. Sharma RK, Agarwal A. Role of reactive oxygen species in male infertility. Urology 1996;48(6):835–50.
58. Baccetti B, Collodel G, Piomboni P. Apoptosis in human ejaculated sperm cells (notulae seminologicae 9). Journal of Submicroscopic Cytology and Pathology 1996;28(4):587–96.
59. Benoff SH, Millan C, Hurley IR, Napolitano B, Marmar JL. Bilateral increased apoptosis and bilateral accumulation of cadmium in infertile men with left varicocele. Human Reproduction (Oxford, England) 2004;19(3):616–27.
60. Mitropoulos D, Deliconstantinos G, Zervas A, Villiotou V, Dimopoulos C, Stavrides J. Nitric oxide synthase and xanthine oxidase activities in the spermatic vein of patients with varicocele: a potential role for nitric oxide and peroxynitrite in sperm dysfunction. The Journal of Urology 1996;156(6):1952–8.
61. Middendorff R, Mueller D, Wichers S, Holstein A, Davidoff M. Evidence for production and functional activity of Nitric oxide in seminiferous tubules and blood vessels of the human testes. The Journal of Clinical Endocrinology and Metabolism 1997;82:4154–61.
62. Romeo C, Ientile R, Santoro G, et al. Nitric oxide production is increased in the spermatic veins of adolescents with left idiophatic varicocele. Journal of Pediatric Surgery 2001;36(2):389–93.
63. Santoro G, Romeo C, Impellizzeri P, et al. Nitric oxide synthase patterns in normal and varicocele testis in adolescents. BJU International 2001;88(9):967–73.
64. Benoff S, Hurley IR, Yuan L, Marmar JL. Endothelial nitric oxide synthase (eNOS) and inducible nitric oxide synthase (iNOS) are separately induced and have separable effects in varicocele infertility. Journal of Andrology 2006;27:57.
65. Weese DL, Peaster ML, Himsl KK, Leach GE, Lad PM, Zimmern PE. Stimulated reactive oxygen species generation in the spermatozoa of infertile men. The Journal of Urology 1993;149(1):64–7.
66. Hendin B, Kolettis P, Sharma RK, Thomas AJ, Agarwal A. Stimulated reactive oxygen species generation in spermatozoa of infertile men. The Journal of Urology 1999;161:1831–4.
67. de Lamirande E, Gagnon C. Reactive oxygen species and human spermatozoa. I. Effects on the motility of intact spermatozoa and on sperm axonemes. Journal of Andrology 1992;13(5):368–78.
68. Smith R, Kaune H, Parodi D, et al. Increased sperm DNA damage in patients with varicocele: relationship with seminal oxidative stress. Human Reproduction (Oxford, England) 2006;21(4):986–93.
69. Koksal IT, Usta M, Orhan I, Abbasoglu S, Kadioglu A. Potential role of reactive oxygen species on testicular pathology associated with infertility. Asian Journal of Andrology 2003;5(2):95–9.
70. Chen LP, Wang SQ, Zhao YZ, Liu L, Wang SX, Lu YZ. [The changes of IL-1 and NO levels in the testes of rats with experimental varicocele]. Zhonghua nan ke xue = National Journal of Andrology 2002;8(2):125–6.
71. Zini A, Buckspan M, Jamal M, Jarvi K. Effect of varicocelectomy on the abnormal retention of residual cytoplasm by human spermatozoa. Human Reproduction (Oxford, England) 1999;14(7):1791–3.
72. Nallella KP, Allamaneni SS, Pasqualotto FF, Sharma RK, Thomas AJ Jr, Agarwal A. Relationship of interleukin-6 with semen characteristics and oxidative stress in patients with varicocele. Urology 2004;64(5):1010–3.
73. Aitken RJ, Clarkson JS. Cellular basis of defective sperm function and its association with the genesis of reactive oxygen species by human spermatozoa. Journal of Reproduction and Fertility 1987;81(2):459–69.
74. Iwasaki A, Gagnon C. Formation of reactive oxygen species in spermatozoa of infertile patients. Fertility and Sterility 1992;57(2):409–16.
75. Mostafa T, Anis TH, El-Nashar A, Imam H, Othman IA. Varicocelectomy reduces reactive oxygen species levels and increases antioxidant activity of seminal plasma from infertile men with varicocele. International Journal of Andrology 2001;24(5):261–5.
76. Mancini A, Milardi D, Conte G, Festa R, De Marinis L, Littarru GP. Seminal antioxidants in humans: preoperative and postoperative evaluation of coenzyme Q10 in varicocele patients. Hormone and Metabolic Research Hormon- und Stoffwechselforschung 2005;37(7):428–32.
77. Deepinder F, Cocuzza M, Agarwal A. Should seminal oxidative stress measurement be offered routinely to men presenting for infertility evaluation? Endocrine Practice 2008;14(4):484–91.
78. Wu GJ, Chang FW, Lee SS, Cheng YY, Chen CH, Chen IC. Apoptosis-related phenotype of ejaculated spermatozoa in patients with varicocele. Fertility and Sterility 2008.

79. Goldstein M, Eid JF. Elevation of intratesticular and scrotal skin surface temperature in men with varicocele. The Journal of Urology 1989;142(3):743–5.
80. Lue YH, Lasley BL, Laughlin LS, et al. Mild testicular hyperthermia induces profound transitional spermatogenic suppression through increased germ cell apoptosis in adult cynomolgus monkeys (*Macaca fascicularis*). Journal of Andrology 2002;23(6):799–805.
81. Sinha Hikim AP, Lue Y, Diaz-Romero M, Yen PH, Wang C, Swerdloff RS. Deciphering the pathways of germ cell apoptosis in the testis. The Journal of Steroid Biochemistry and Molecular Biology 2003;85(2–5):175–82.
82. Miller D, Brough S, al-Harbi O. Characterization and cellular distribution of human spermatozoal heat shock proteins. Human Reproduction (Oxford, England) 1992;7(5):637–45.
83. Dix DJ, Allen JW, Collins BW, et al. Targeted gene disruption of Hsp70-2 results in failed meiosis, germ cell apoptosis, and male infertility. Proceedings of the National Academy of Sciences of the United States of America 1996;93(8):3264–8.
84. Brackin P, Marmar JL, Millan C, Benoff S. Identification of heat shock protein 70-1 (HSP 70-1) in testis tissue of men with varicocele. The Journal of Urology 2003;169:415.
85. Tapanainen JS, Tilly JL, Vihko KK, Hsueh AJ. Hormonal control of apoptotic cell death in the testis: gonadotropins and androgens as testicular cell survival factors. Molecular Endocrinology (Baltimore, MD) 1993;7(5):643–50.
86. Hikim AP, Swerdloff RS. Temporal and stage-specific effects of recombinant human follicle-stimulating hormone on the maintenance of spermatogenesis in gonadotropin-releasing hormone antagonist-treated rat. Endocrinology 1995;136(1):253–61.
87. Erkkila K, Henriksen K, Hirvonen V, et al. Testosterone regulates apoptosis in adult human seminiferous tubules in vitro. The Journal of Clinical Endocrinology and Metabolism 1997;82(7):2314–21.
88. Rajfer J, Turner TFR. Inhibition of testicular testosterone biosynthesis following experimental varicocele in rats. Biology of Reproduction 1997;36:933–7.
89. Weiss DB, Rodriguez-Rigau L, Smith KD, Chowdhury A, Steinberger E. Quantitation of Leydig cells in testicular biopsies of oligospermic men with varicocele. Fertility and Sterility 1978;30(3):305–12.
90. Amelar RD, Dubin L. Human chorionic gonadotrophin therapy in male infertility. JAMA 1977;237(22):2423.
91. Check JH. Improved semen quality in subfertile males with varicocele-associated oligospermia following treatment with clomiphene citrate. Fertility and Sterility 1980;33(4):423–6.
92. Rodriguez-Rigau LJ, Weiss DB, Zukerman Z, Grotjan HE, Smith KD, Steinberger E. A possible mechanism for the detrimental effect of varicocele on testicular function in man. Fertility and Sterility 1978;30(5):577–85.
93. Hadziselimovic F, Leibundgut B, Da Runga D. The value of testicular biopsy in patients with varicoceles. The Journal of Urology 1986;135:707–710.
94. Benoff S, Hurley IR, Xu H, Marmar JL. Alteration in Leydig cell nuymber and morphology among infertile men with varicoceles. Fertility and Sterility 2006;86(Supl 2):S48–9.
95. Marmar JL, Benoff S. The safety of ultrasonically guided testis aspiration biopsies and efficacy of use to predict varicocelectomy outcome. Human Reproduction (Oxford, England) 2005;20(8):2279–88.
96. Li L, Wine RN, Chapin RE. 2-Methoxyacetic acid (MAA) – induced spermatocyte apoptosis in human and rat testis: an in vitro comparison. Journal of Andrology 1996;17: 538–49.
97. Ku WW, Wine RN, Chae BY, Ghanayem BI, Chapin RE. Spermatocyte toxicity of 2-methoxyethanol (ME) in rats and guinea pigs: evidence for the induction of apoptosis. Toxicology and Applied Pharmacology 1995;134(1):100–10.
98. Brinkworth MH, Weinbauer GF, Bergmann M, Nieschlag E. Apoptosis as a mechanism of germ cell loss in elderly men. International Journal of Andrology 1997;20(4):222–8.
99. Cohen MS, Plaine L, Brown JS. The role of internal spermatic vein plasma catecholamine determinations in subfertile men with varicoceles. Fertility and Sterility 1975;26(12): 1243–9.
100. Comhaire F, Vermeulen A. Varicocele sterility: cortisol and catecholamines. Fertility and Sterility 1974;25(1):88–95.
101. Cockett AT, Takihara H, Cosentino MJ. The varicocele. Fertility and Sterility 1984;41(1):5–11.
102. Ito H, Fuse H, Minagawa H, Kawamura K, Murakami M, Shimazaki J. Internal spermatic vein prostaglandins in varicocele patients. Fertility and Sterility 1982;37(2):218–22.
103. Vine MF, Tse CK, Hu P, Truong KY. Cigarette smoking and semen quality. Fertility and Sterility 1996;65(4):835–42.
104. Klaiber EL, Broverman DM, Pokoly TB, Albert AJ, Howard PJ Jr, Sherer JF Jr. Interrelationships of cigarette smoking, testicular varicoceles, and seminal fluid indexes. Fertility and Sterility 1987;47(3):481–6.
105. Chia SE, Ong CN, Tsakok FM. Effects of cigarette smoking on human semen quality. Archives of Andrology 1994;33(3):163–8.
106. Jones MM, Xu C, Ladd PA. Selenite suppression of cadmium-induced testicular apoptosis. Toxicology 1997;116(1–3): 169–75.
107. Benoff S, Auborn K, Marmar JL, Hurley IR. Link between low-dose environmentally relevant cadmium exposures and asthenozoospermia in a rat model. Fertility and Sterility 2008;89(2 Suppl):e73–9.
108. Peng BC, Tomashefsky P, Nagler HM. The cofactor effect: varicocele and infertility. Fertility and Sterility 1990;54(1): 143–8.
109. Benoff S, Gilbert BR. Varicocele and male infertility: Part I. Preface. Human Reproduction Update 2001;7(1):47–54.
110. Tulloch WS. Varicocele in subfertility; results of treatment. British Medical Journal 1955;2(4935):356–8.
111. Czaplicki M, Bablock L, Janczewski Z. Varicocelectomy in patients with azoospermia. Archives of Andrology 1979;3:51–5.
112. Matthews GJ, Matthews ED, Goldstein M. Induction of spermatogenesis and achievement of pregnancy after microsurgical varicocelectomy in men with azoospermia and severe oligoasthenospermia. Fertility and Sterility 1998;70(1):71–5.
113. Kim ED, Leibman BB, Grinblat DM, Lipshultz LI. Varicocele repair improves semen parameters in azoospermic men with spermatogenic failure. The Journal of Urology 1999;162(3 Pt 1):737–40.
114. Lee JS, Park HJ, Seo JT. What is the indication of varicocelectomy in men with nonobstructive azoospermia? Urology 2007;69(2):352–5.
115. Pasqualotto FF, Sobreiro BP, Hallak J, Pasqualotto EB, Lucon AM. Induction of spermatogenesis in azoospermic

men after varicocelectomy repair: an update. Fertility and Sterility 2006;85(3):635–9.
116. Schlegel PN, Kaufmann J. Role of varicocelectomy in men with nonobstructive azoospermia. Fertility and Sterility 2004;81(6):1585–8.
117. Pryor JL, Kent-First M, Muallem A, et al. Microdeletions in the Y chromosome of infertile men. The New England Journal of Medicine 1997;336(8):534–9.
118. Turek PJ, Cayan S, Black L. The response to varicocelectomy in oligospermic men with and without genetic infertility. Fertility and Sterility 2000;74:528.
119. Evers JL, Collins JA, Clark J. Surgery or embolisation for varicocele in subfertile men. The Cochrane Library 2008; (3):CD000479.
120. Ivanissevich O, Gregorini H. A new operation for the care of varicocele. Semana Medica 1978;25:575.
121. Ivanissevich O. Left varicocele due to reflux; experience with 4,470 operative cases in forty-two years. The Journal of the International College of Surgeons 1960;34:742–55.
122. Palomo A. Radical cure of varicocele by a new technique: Preliminary report. The Journal of Urology 1948; 61:604–7.
123. Dubin L, Amelar RD. Etiologic factors in 1294 consecutive cases of male infertility. Fertility and Sterility 1971; 22(8):469–74.
124. Silber SJ. Microsurgical aspects of varicocele. Fertility and Sterility 1979;31(2):230–2.
125. Wosnitzer M, Roth JA. Optical magnification and Doppler ultrasound probe for varicocelectomy. Urology 1983;22(1):24–6.
126. Marmar JL, DeBenedictis TJ, Praiss D. The management of varicoceles by microdissection of the spermatic cord at the external inguinal ring. Fertility and Sterility 1985;43(4):583–8.
127. Zampieri N, Zuin V, Corroppolo M, Chironi C, Cervellione RM, Camoglio FS. Varicocele and adolescents: semen quality after 2 different laparoscopic procedures. Journal of Andrology 2007;28(5):727–33.
128. Iaccarino V. A nonsurgical treatment of varicocele: transcatheter sclerotherapy of gonadal veins. Annales de Radiologie 1980;23(4):369–70.
129. Lima SS, Castro MP, Costa OF. A new method for the treatment of varicocele. Andrologia 1978;10(2):103–6.
130. Walsh PC, White RI Jr. Balloon occlusion of the internal spermatic vein for the treatment of varicoceles. JAMA 1981;246(15):1701–2.
131. Tauber R, Johnsen N. Antegrade scrotal sclerotherapy for the treatment of varicocele: technique and late results. The Journal of Urology 1994;151(2):386–90.
132. Comhaire F, Kunnen M, Nahoum C. Radiological anatomy of the internal spermatic vein(s) in 200 retrograde venograms. International Journal of Andrology 1981;4(3):379–87.
133. Sayfan J, Adam YG, Soffer Y. A new entity in varicocele subfertility: the "cremasteric reflux". Fertility and Sterility 1980;33(1):88–90.
134. Feneley MR, Pal MK, Nockler IB, Hendry WF. Retrograde embolization and causes of failure in the primary treatment of varicocele. British Journal of Urology 1997;80(4):642–6.
135. Kaufman SL, Kadir S, Barth KH, Smyth JW, Walsh PC, White RI Jr. Mechanisms of recurrent varicocele after balloon occlusion or surgical ligation of the internal spermatic vein. Radiology 1983;147(2):435–40.
136. Zuckerman AM, Mitchell SE, Venbrux AC, et al. Percutaneous varicocele occlusion: long-term follow-up. Journal of Vascular and Interventional Radiology 1994;5(2):315–9.
137. Zucchi A, Mearini L, Mearini E, Costantini E, Bini V, Porena M. Treatment of varicocele: randomized prospective study on open surgery versus Tauber antegrade sclerotherapy. Journal of Andrology 2005;26(3):328–32.
138. Al-Said S, Al-Naimi A, Al-Ansari A, et al. Varicocelectomy for male infertility: a comparative study of open, laparoscopic and microsurgical approaches. The Journal of Urology 2008;180(1):266–70.
139. Galarneau G, Nagler HM. Cost effective infertility therapies in the 90s: to treat or to cure? Contemporary Urology 1999;11:32–45.
140. Cocuzza M, Cocuzza MA, Bragais FM, Agarwal A. The role of varicocele repair in the new era of assisted reproductive technology. Clinics (Sao Paulo, Brazil) 2008;63(3):395–404.
141. www.cdc.gov/reproductivehealth/index/htm.
142. Richardson I, Grotas AB, Nagler HM. Outcomes of varicocelectomy treatment: an updated critical analysis. The Urologic Clinics of North America 2008;35(2):191–209; viii.
143. Guzick DS, Overstreet JW, Factor-Litvak P, et al. Sperm morphology, motility, and concentration in fertile and infertile men. The New England Journal of Medicine 2001;345(19):1388–93.
144. Benoff S, Goodwin LO, Millan C, Hurley IR, Pergolizzi RG, Marmar JL. Deletions in L-type calcium channel alpha1 subunit testicular transcripts correlate with testicular cadmium and apoptosis in infertile men with varicoceles. Fertility and Sterility 2005;83(3):622–34.
145. O'Brien J, Bowles B, Kamal KM, Jarvi K, Zini A. Does the gonadotropin-releasing hormone stimulation test predict clinical outcomes after microsurgical varicocelectomy? Urology 2004;63(6):1143–7.
146. Matkov TG, Zenni M, Sandlow J, Levine LA. Preoperative semen analysis as a predictor of seminal improvement following varicocelectomy. Fertility and Sterility 2001;75(1):63–8.
147. Cayan S, Erdemir F, Ozbey I, Turek PJ, Kadioglu A, Tellaloglu S. Can varicocelectomy significantly change the way couples use assisted reproductive technologies? The Journal of Urology 2002;167(4):1749–52.
148. Zini A, Boman J, Baazeem A, Jarvi K, Libman J. Natural history of varicocele management in the era of intracytoplasmic sperm injection. Fertility and Sterility 2008.
149. Schlegel PN. Is assisted reproduction the optimal treatment for varicocele-associated male infertility? A cost-effectiveness analysis. Urology 1997;49(1):83–90.
150. Meng MV, Greene KL, Turek PJ. Surgery or assisted reproduction? A decision analysis of treatment costs in male infertility. The Journal of Urology 2005;174(5):1926–31; discussion 31.

# Does Preimplantation Genetic Screening (PGS) Improve IVF Outcome?

# The Role of Aneuploidy Screening in Human Preimplantation Embryos

Alan R. Thornhill and Alan H. Handyside

**Abstract** Aneuploidy screening in human preimplantation embryos or preimplantation genetic screening (PGS) has been clinically applied to different groups of IVF patients for over a decade but is generally considered too invasive and inaccurate for routine embryo selection following IVF. Nevertheless, for some women (e.g. those of advanced maternal age), high incidence of aneuploidy arising in female meiosis is clearly a major factor contributing to pregnancy failure, and PGS could still have a role in their clinical management. PGS should be considered a diagnostic procedure incorporating confirmatory molecular cytogenetic analysis of any screened embryos remaining after transfer. Consequently, patients benefit from detailed assessment of aneuploidy risk and avoid transfer of aneuploid embryos. To become a successful routine adjunct for all IVF patients, PGS must tip the cost-benefit ratio towards benefit by providing: (a) safer biopsy or non-invasive methods, (b) rapid testing at low cost (c) high accuracy, (d) comprehensive analysis of all chromosomes and (e) information to distinguish between chromosomal abnormalities of meiotic and mitotic origin.

**Keywords** Preimplantation genetic screening • Chromosomal aneuploidy • Chromosomal mosaicism • Fluore-scence in-situ hybridisation • Aneuploidy risk • Embryo biopsy • Blastomere • Polar body

A.R. Thornhill (✉) and A.H. Handyside
The London Bridge Fertility, Gynaecology and Genetics Centre, 1 St. Thomas Street, London, SE1 9RY, UK
e-mail: athornhill@thebridgecentre.co.uk

## 1 Introduction

Abnormalities of chromosome number (aneuploidy) are relatively common in human gametes and preimplantation embryos and are a major cause of developmental failure and abnormality. The genetic imbalance caused by trisomy (three copies of a chromosome) or monosomy (only a single copy) can result in developmental arrest before implantation, miscarriage, stillbirths or, rarely, viable but developmentally abnormal pregnancies depending on the chromosome(s) involved. Half of all miscarriages that can be karyotyped are associated with chromosomal aneuploidy. Sex chromosome aneuploidies and trisomies of some of the smaller autosomes – most commonly trisomy 21 (Down syndrome) – can be viable with abnormalities of varying degrees – although more than 80% of trisomy 21 concepti are lost through miscarriage (1).

Aneuploidy in gametes is typically caused by abnormal segregation or pre-division of chromosomes in one or both meiotic divisions, which should normally result in a haploid set of single chromosomes, one of each pair. Aneuploidy in embryos can arise via (a) meiotic error – through fertilisation with an aneuploid gamete, or (b) mitotic error – abnormal cell division of the embryo resulting in a chromosomally mosaic embryo with both euploid and aneuploid cells. The overall incidence of aneuploidy in sperm from a fertile male is estimated to be 1–2% (2). In some cases of severe male infertility, however, there can be a significantly increased incidence of aneuploidy of some or all chromosomes with an increase in sex chromosome aneusomy, specifically observed in oligozoospermic men with Klinefelter's syndrome (3). The incidence of aneuploidy in oocytes is estimated to be approximately 20% but increases dramatically with

D.T. Carrell et al. (eds.), *Biennial Review of Infertility,* DOI: 10.1007/978-1-60327-392-3_19

advancing maternal age from the mid 30s to menopause (2, 4, 5).

In cleavage stage human embryos analysed by sequential multicolour fluorescence in situ hybridisation (FISH) with probes specific for five autosome pairs (22, 21, 18, 16, and 13) plus X and Y, the incidence of abnormal chromosomal number, affecting all cells of the embryo (uniform aneuploidy) and assumed to arise from fertilisation with an aneuploid gamete, increases with maternal age (6, 7).

Embryo selection following cleavage stage embryo biopsy and chromosome analysis to identify aneuploid embryos has been performed worldwide for over a decade and has overtaken more conventional PGD for single gene disorders as the most common indication for preimplantation testing (8). However, PGS, in its current form, is considered by most clinics to be too invasive and potentially damaging for routine use in every couple having IVF/ICSI, or all women of advanced maternal age (9). The largest randomized multi-center clinical PGS trial to date (10) confirms this expectation and is valuable in quantifying the negative effect on pregnancy and live birth rates of using preimplantation genetic screening (PGS) for aneuploidy routinely for all women over 35. Nevertheless, for some women in their late 30s and early 40s, high incidence of aneuploidy arising in female meiosis is clearly a major factor contributing to pregnancy failure suggesting that the level of aneuploidy risk varies between patients. This chapter explores the premise underpinning the use of PGS in human cleavage stage embryos, current and future methodologies and its clinical applications (including possible harms, benefits, indications and strategies for use).

## 2 The Rise of PGS

Preimplantation genetic screening for aneuploidy is now in widespread practice for women of advanced maternal age, recurrent miscarriage, recurrent implantation failure and some severe male factor infertility indications across the world (8, 11). In the UK, clinical application has been slower than in the US as a result of the requirement for licensing to perform PGS. Despite this regulatory hurdle, PGS is currently licensed by the Human Fertilisation and Embryology Authority (HFEA) in eight clinics across the UK and looks set to increase as clinics try to find ways to help specific subgroups of patients in a regulatory environment moving towards single embryo transfer. Conventional cytogenetic analysis in the 1970s demonstrated that half of all spontaneous miscarriages are associated with aneuploidy and other structural chromosomal abnormalities, the incidence of which was higher in the first trimester suggesting a process of natural selection through pregnancy loss. By extrapolation, an average incidence of aneuploidy at conception of 25% was suggested which has been consistently and extensively confirmed by direct analysis of human IVF embryos using fluorescence in situ hybridisation (FISH) to identify specific chromosomes in interphase nuclei (7, 12, 13). For this reason, few disagree that the premise underpinning a screening test for chromosomal aneuploidy in human embryos is scientifically and clinically sound.

## 3 What Can We Learn from Clinical Trials?

Contradictory results have been noted on the benefits of aneuploidy screening among the various clinical indications, with a recent meta-analysis concluding that insufficient data was available to determine whether PGS is an effective intervention in IVF/ICSI for improving live birth rates (14).

However, in many other studies not included in the meta-analysis, outcome measures were improved but not significantly so – suggesting insufficient power (i.e. too few cases), or reflecting variability between patients (a feature which is clearly seen among our patients). It seems evident that any future trials, however large, involving heterogeneous target groups will likely show no beneficial effect of PGS (particularly as measured by increased pregnancy rates) since we observe heterogeneity in the incidence of aneuploidy in different treatment groups. Essentially, there are two main reasons for the poorer results in the PGS treatment group in the large clinical trial investigating the value of PGS for advanced maternal age (10): (a) embryo biopsy and (b) false positive results due to chromosomal mosaicism. Clearly embryo biopsy is invasive and can compromise embryo development (15) particularly when applied to embryos with already compromised development. There are also questions surrounding the efficacy of embryo biopsy in the hands of the centres involved in the trial, since biopsied embryos with no result that were transferred showed a much reduced implantation rate compared with non-biopsied embryos (11). Embryo biopsy is therefore only justifiable when the benefit of testing outweighs the cost to the embryo. With respect to chromosomal mosaicism, our experience shows that the incidence of false positive results decreases as the embryos are more at risk of aneuploidy. It follows that routine application of PGS, irrespective of *a priori* aneuploidy risk, will result in more unwanted false positive results and is clearly inappropriate. Since no follow-up analysis of embryos was reported in the large clinical trial (10), it is impossible to establish the actual aneuploidy risk for patients and accuracy of the PGS test used in the trial (both of which are critical when considering the efficacy of PGS).

Leaving these criticisms aside, there is a clear message from this trial about the futility of indiscriminate application of PGS for advanced maternal age. Ironically, although the conclusions from recent clinical trials are that PGS has no clinical benefit, a lot of data does actually point to some benefit to selecting against abnormality (10, 16–18). It is hard to otherwise explain maintenance of implantation rates following PGS vs. no-PGS controls having eliminated the majority of the cohort of embryos for transfer.

## 4 Current Methodologies

The majority of centres performing clinical PGS to date have investigated aneuploidy in cleavage stage embryos (8); but it is possible to perform aneuploidy screening on polar bodies (4, 5) and later at the blastocyst stage (19) with each stage having different diagnostic limitations (see Table 1). PGS at the cleavage stage typically involves the following steps: (1) removing single cells from each cleavage stage embryo, with five or more cells, early on day three post-insemination; (2) spreading of interphase nuclei on a microscope slide; (3) sequential Fluorescence in-situ hybridisation (FISH) analysis using between 5 and 12 different chromosome-specific probes, and (4) on day 4 or 5, transfer of embryos with the normal number of chromosomes for those tested. An additional step that can be incorporated for confirmation of single cell diagnosis and accurate assessment of aneuploidy risk is to perform whole embryo follow-up analysis of all nuclei from untransferred, non-cryopreserved embryos with or without prior single cell diagnosis. The choice of which chromosomes to analyse for PGS to be effective depends, to some extent, on the reason for applying PGS. Nevertheless, selection of the first eight or nine chromosomes to evaluate is relatively straightforward (namely 13, 14, 15, 16, 18, 21, 22, X, and Y) based on data from first trimester miscarriages (20) which has been largely confirmed following FISH analysis of human embryos (21). However, beyond nine chromosomes, it is less clear which chromosomes should next be tested in order of clinical significance. The obvious next step is to test for all 23 pairs of chromosomes in conjunction with the sex chromosomes. Although it is possible to perform multiple sequential rounds of FISH on the same single cell, FISH efficiency and hence accuracy decreases with each successive round and markedly so beyond the third round (22). The use of FISH on single blastomeres to deliver a PGS service to patients carries with it a degree of technical error and the inherent problem of chromosomal mosaicism in the embryo. However, both limitations are measurable and, as such, can be discussed with patients to allow fully informed consent. We are one of the few private

**Table 1** Detection of aneuploidy with respect to biopsy strategy

| | Method of biopsy | | | |
|---|---|---|---|---|
| Origin of aneuploidy | First polar body | First and second polar body | Cleavage stage blastomere(s) | Trophectoderm cells from blastocysts |
| | **Errors resulting in uniform aneuploidy** | | | |
| Maternal meiosis I | ✓ | ✓ | ✓ | ✓ |
| Maternal meiosis II | × | ✓ | ✓ | ✓ |
| Paternal meiosis I and II | × | × | ✓ | ✓ |
| Chromosome loss prior to 1st mitosis | × | × | ✓ | ✓ |
| | **Errors resulting in chromosomal mosaicism** | | | |
| Postzygotic malsegregation | × | × | ×✓ | ×✓ |

diagnostic laboratories worldwide to provide follow-up confirmation of diagnosis of any embryos remaining after transfer and/or cryopreservation. Thus we can provide quality assurance (in the form of accurate false negative and false positive rates) as well as useful diagnostic information that may lead to clinical closure for some patients. Indeed, for some patients, information gained from whole embryo chromosome analysis is more useful than the single cell result. With patient consent, follow-up of whole embryos allows us to categorise embryos as chromosomally chaotic (negligible viability), uniformly aneuploid (resulting in miscarriage or affected children as a result of meiotic errors in sperm or eggs), or to evaluate the degree of chromosomal mosaicism (see Fig. 1). Such follow-up analysis may be a key piece of diagnostic information in assessing the likelihood of a live birth or the time needed to achieve a live birth healthy with the patients' own gametes and embryos. We speculate that a small degree of mosaicism in an otherwise chromosomally normal embryo - in the absence of any other pathology - would likely result in a "normal" pregnancy.

## 5 Accuracy and Efficiency

Patients and providers alike are rightly focussed on the accuracy and efficiency of the FISH technique on single blastomeres. Follow-up analysis of embryos after PGS confirms the single cell result represents a uniform aneuploidy in approximately 85–90% of embryos. Of the remaining 10–15% in which the single cell result is not confirmed to be a uniform abnormality, most are false-positives i.e. an aneuploid test result is not confirmed in all cells of the biopsied embryo (most of which can be interpreted as caused by chromosomal mosaicism) and very few (approximately 1–2%) are false-negatives i.e. a normal test result in an otherwise uniformly aneuploid embryo. In addition, false-positives are less likely in patients at higher risk of aneuploidy. Figure 1 illustrates the mechanism by which false-positives and negatives can arise when testing embryos using a single blastomere. The efficiency of the sequential multicolour FISH technique on fixed blastomere nuclei is approximately 95%, but efficiency of the process from biopsy to result of the single cell analysis

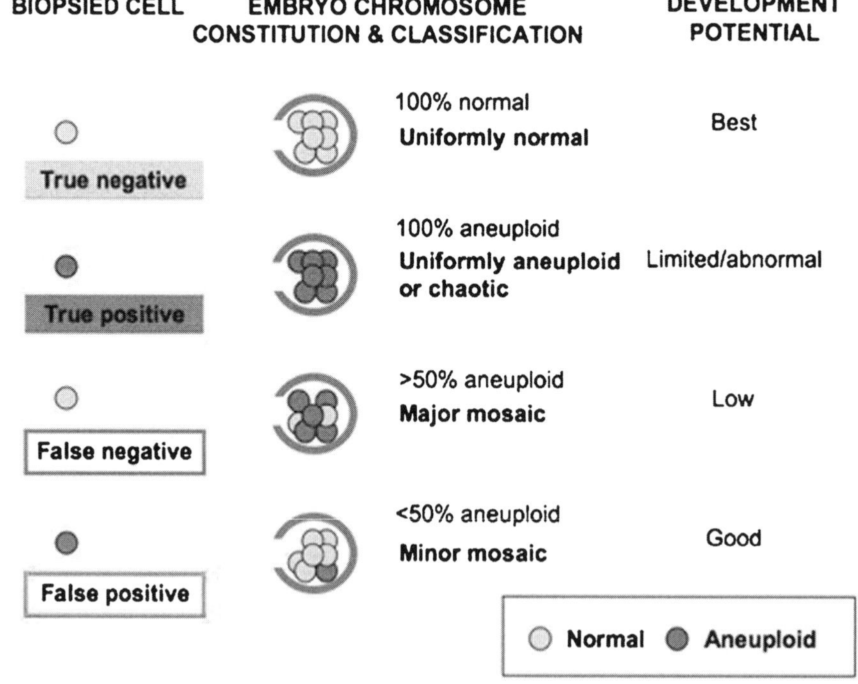


**Fig. 1** Embryo chromosome constitution and classification after single cell and whole embryo follow-up analysis. Schematic demonstration of the proportion of normal and abnormal cells to qualify as uniformly normal, minor mosaic, major mosaic, uniformly abnormal or chaotic in our classification system. Following single cell biopsy and FISH testing, both false-positives (FP) and false-negatives (FN) lead to adverse outcomes. FP results lead to a reduced chance of success (owing to a reduced pool of embryos for transfer) and FN results lead to increased chances of implantation failure, miscarriage or birth of an affected child

is slightly lower at 85%. In the remaining 15% either no nucleus is found or there is an inconclusive result – both of which observations support the view that nucleus spreading and fixation is critical to the success of the test. Patients therefore need to be aware that like any other prenatal tests, PGS is a screening test only and a conclusive result is not 100% guaranteed. For this reason, patients should consider carefully non-invasive and/or invasive testing (chorionic villus sampling or amniocentesis) of any pregnancy following PGS. Since (a) there is no universally agreed system for classifying chromosomal mosaicism in embryos; (b) embryos may be analysed by FISH at different developmental stages; (c) embryos from patients with different indications have been reported in the literature, estimates of embryo mosaicism vary widely, making comparisons between groups performing PGS difficult. However, chromosomal mosaicism certainly presents a problem for accurate assessment of chromosome constitution in embryos as illustrated in data we have collected from two different target groups where the embryos were analysed by seven chromosome FISH following single cell biopsy (see Table 2). Note that, in the better prognosis group (Group 1), despite an extremely low incidence of uniform aneuploidy, the incidence of mosaicism is still relatively high with potential for false-positives and subsequent discard of essentially chromosomally normal embryos.

In clinical scenarios in which there is a high prevalence of disease (for PGS this equates to chromosome abnormality within an embryo), an effective test can have relatively low specificity. In contrast, where the prevalence of chromosome abnormality (or specifically uniform abnormality) is lower, then both sensitivity and specificity need to be very high for the test to be considered effective. In clinical PGS, when using a clinical test of limited sensitivity and specificity, one would predict that the positive predictive value - PPV (the ability of the test to detect an abnormality when one exists) would be lower in a population with low incidence of uniform aneuploidy than that in the advanced maternal age group (in which prevalence of aneuploidy is higher). This is supported by our data comparing embryos from women whose ages were on average 30 vs. 40 completed years (see Table 2). It is not surprising therefore that in clinical trials of PGS for women in whom the rate of uniform chromosome abnormality may not be high (10), the risk of false positive results, largely as a result of chromosomal mosaicism in the cleavage stage embryo, is too high to justify the procedure and results in selection against and ultimately the discard of essentially normal embryos. As with any embryo selection method, the quality of embryos *per se* is not improved following selection of euploid embryos. Indeed embryo quality is slightly compromised since any invasive test, especially biopsy,

**Table 2** Incidence of aneuploidy in different target groups

| | Group 1 | Group 2 |
|---|---|---|
| Patients (*n*) | 29 | 52 |
| Cycles (*n*) | 29 | 64 |
| Maternal age in years (range) | 30.6 ± 3.9 (22–39) | 40.6 ± 2.4 (36–47) |
| % Embryo transfer/cycle | N/A | 66 |
| % Live birth/cycle | 83 | 10 |
| Embryos with single cell and whole embryo data[a] (*n*) | 122 | 161 |
| Patients with ≥1 uniform aneuploidy (%) | 1 (3) | 40 (77) |
| Uniform aneuploidy (%) | 0.8[b] | 53.4 |
| Major mosaic (%) | 23 | 13.7 |
| Abnormal (uniform aneuploid + major mosaic + chaotic + other) | 37.6 | 76.4 |
| Normal | 8.2 | 9.9 |
| Minor mosaic | 54.1[c] | 13.7 |
| Normal + minor mosaic | 62.4 | 23.6 |
| Positive predictive value | 0.63 | 0.82 |

*Group 1* Simulated aneuploidy screening using only surplus frozen embryos from successful clinical IVF cycles; *Group 2* Clinical aneuploidy screening in women of advanced maternal age

*Minor mosaic* when >50% nuclei are normal

*Major mosaic* when >50% nuclei are abnormal

*Normal* when >85% nuclei are normal

[a]Mean number nuclei scored/whole embryo is 30 vs. 12 (Group 1 vs. Group 2)

[b]One embryo with monosomy 21

[c]Majority with ≥75% nuclei of normal genotype

has a cost to the embryo (15). Moreover, embryos from some women of advanced maternal age may already be developmentally compromised even without biopsy and irrespective of their chromosomal status.

## 6 How Well Do We Select Genetically Healthy Embryos Based on Morphology Alone?

Most laboratories worldwide use a simple morphologic grading scheme for selecting embryos for transfer to the uterus. With an increasing focus on single embryo transfer, a battery of embryo selection tools (including morphology) is vital. PGS is one such tool. At present, in the context of a PGS treatment cycle, even limited chromosomal information is weighted above embryo morphology such that a morphologically high quality embryo testing positive for trisomy 18 (Edwards syndrome) will not be selected above a poorer quality embryo testing chromosomally normal. However, embryo morphology may take precedence if the abnormality detected is monosomy, as this could be a false positive. Even if the monosomy is a true positive result, transfer in most cases would not result in the birth of an affected child. Depending on the particular patient history, PGS may be more or less important than simple morphologic selection. The potential conflict in choosing between chromosomal and morphological information for specific embryos is illustrated in Fig. 2. Selection by morphology alone can

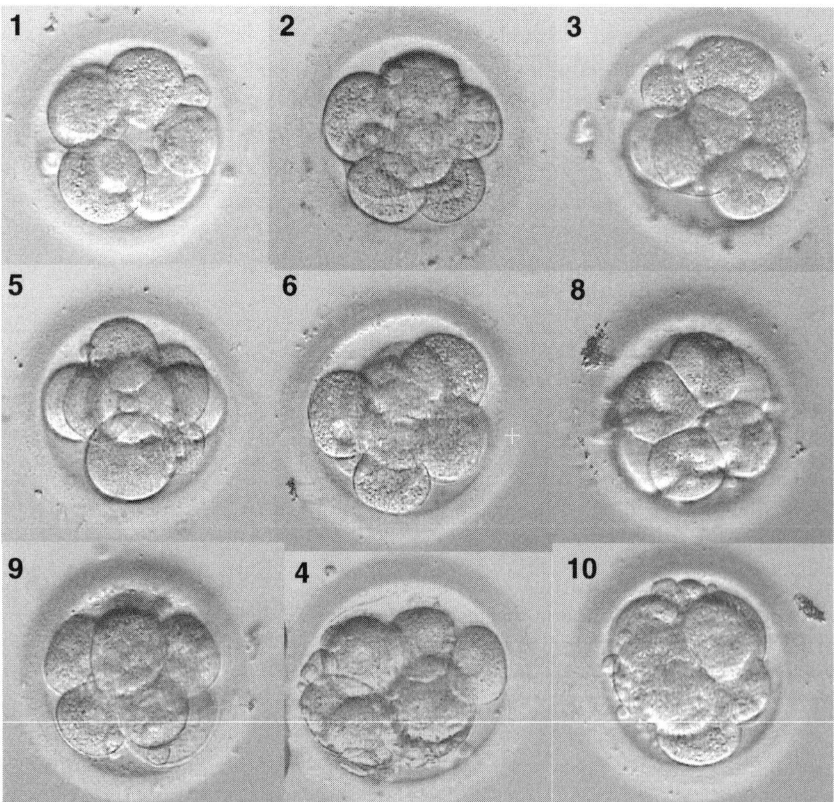


**Fig. 2** Assessment of day 3 human preimplantation embryos by a combination of morphologic and chromosomal assessment by 7-chromosome FISH. A cohort of day 3 embryos from a 38-year old women having PGS for chromosomes 13, 16, 18, 21, 22, X, and Y. All embryos had PGS performed on day 3 on a single biopsied cell. Embryos testing abnormal based on the single cell result were followed-up (confirmation of diagnosis from all remaining cells after whole embryo fixation). Embryo genotypes were confirmed as follows: (E1 – monosomy 21; E2 – monosomy 22; E3 – trisomy 21; E6 – trisomy 16 and 22; E9 – monosomy 16; E10 – chaotic). Two of the three embryos testing "normal" from the single cell result (E4, 5, and 8) were transferred to the uterus resulting in a healthy singleton live birth

eliminate embryos with gross chaotic chromosomal abnormalities but not the uniform abnormalities couples most wish to avoid (7, 23).

## 7 Future Methodologies

Despite the push to identify ever more chromosomes in PGS testing, for women over 40, a relatively small sample of chromosomes screened may be sufficient to avoid viable abnormalities and identify abnormalities incompatible with pregnancy and live birth. In contrast, for younger women with higher quality eggs having concomitantly fewer chromosomal abnormalities, a comprehensive 24-chromosome screen may be more effective at identifying chromosomal errors governing the embryo's ability to implant. Comprehensive chromosome screening has been performed clinically in human embryos (24, 25) and oocyte polar bodies (26) using comparative genomic hybridisation, but the technique is not in widespread use because it is labour-intensive and, in the case of embryos, cannot generally be performed in time following cleavage-stage biopsy. To this end, we, and others, are investigating the use of microarray technology to allow us to screen multiple regions of each chromosome simultaneously in single embryonic cells (27). Moreover, limited aneuploidy screening, using a DNA based approach with polymorphic markers is already incorporated into tests for specific single gene disorders (28, 29) and may be the most effective way of identifying clinically significant chromosome abnormalities such as viable trisomies. Once again, each of the methodologies has limitations with respect to diagnostic performance (see Table 3).

## 8 Clinical Applications

Few disagree that the premise underpinning a screening test for chromosomal aneuploidy in human embryos is scientifically and clinically sound. For women of advanced maternal age, this is particularly relevant since high levels of uniform aneuploidy have been confirmed in their embryos (7, 12, 13) (see Table 2). While chromosomal aneuploidy in embryos increases with increasing maternal age (7), the relationship between chromosomal mosaicism and maternal age in embryos is less clear (6, 21) and, it is difficult to accurately cite an average estimate of mosaicism from published data. Nevertheless, reports estimate chromosomal mosaicism in cleavage stage embryos at between 30 and 50% (7, 30), while elevated levels of mosaicism are strongly associated with poor morphology and development (7, 23). In our centre, after testing all cells from untransferred embryos, 80% of women aged 37–45 completed years having PGS were confirmed to have at least one uniformly aneuploid embryo among those tested and the incidence of aneuploidy per embryo in each cycle ranged from 20 to 75%. The incidence of double (16%) and triple (9%) aneusomies was also surprisingly high. With any indication for PGS the benefits of reducing the risk of aneuploid pregnancy are balanced by the costs of invasive testing and limitations of single cell analysis on clinical pregnancy rates (see Table 4). Indeed, while considering any improvements to aneuploidy screening, both costs and benefits need to be carefully assessed (see Table 5). Three aspects of PGS, as it is currently performed, remain contentious: (a) the exact method needed to accurately, reliably and comprehensively diagnose

**Table 3** Limitations of different aneuploidy detection methods on cleavage stage blastomeres

| | Multicolour sequential FISH | Haplotyping using DNA markers | Array CGH |
|---|---|---|---|
| *Aneuploidy detection method* | | | |
| Number of chromosomes identified | 7–12 | Limited | 24 |
| *Type of aneuploidy detected* | | | |
| Trisomy | ✓ | ✓ | ✓ |
| Monosomy | ✓ | ✓ | ✓ |
| Haploid | ✓ | ✓ | ×✓ |
| Tetraploid | ✓ | × | × |
| Structural imbalance | ✓ | Limited | Limited |
| Uniparental disomy | × | ×✓ | ×✓ |
| *Uniform vs. mosaic aneuploidy* | | | |
| | × | Trisomy | × |

**Table 4** Costs and benefits associated with aneuploidy screening using FISH

| Costs | Benefits |
|---|---|
| Damage to embryo from non-invasive/invasive selection/ biopsy methods, particularly low quality embryos in poor prognosis patients | Lower risk of aneuploid pregnancy and live birth |
| Elimination of chromosomally normal embryos for transfer because of chromosomal mosaicism/technical errors, resulting in lower live birth rate | Assessment of aneuploidy risk by follow-up analysis of embryos identified as aneuploid |
| Test specificity normal embryos << aneuploid embryos<br>Low positive predictive value in low aneuploidy risk<br>Unforeseen long-term effects of invasive biopsy methods | Improved pregnancy and miscarriage rates *only* if moderate incidence of aneuploidy *and* other chromosomally normal, good quality embryos available for transfer |

**Table 5** Possible approaches for improving the efficiency of aneuploidy screening at cleavage stages

| Measure | Limitations | Benefits |
|---|---|---|
| *Improve clinical management* | | |
| More stringent patient selection | Procedure offered to fewer patients | Procedure focussed on eligible patients only |
| Algorithm to incorporate cumulative patient PGS experience | Requires large body of comparable data to make accurate assumptions | Identify patients most likely to benefit |
| Transfer selected monosomic embryos | Small chance of viable abnormal pregnancy | Fewer embryos discarded as false-positives/ mosaics |
| *Safer biopsy* | | |
| Demonstrated competency | Reduced access to patients initially | Standardised, high quality service |
| "Safer" methods (e.g. mechanical biopsy) | Additional training required | Improved viability post-biopsy and post-freezing |
| *High quality single cell testing* | | |
| Chromosomes appropriate to indication | Not yet clear which are most important for specific patient target groups | Eliminate use of redundant chromosomes from diagnostic test, improve accuracy and reduce false-positives |
| 24 chromosome test (successive rounds of FISH) | Increased chance of false-positives | More comprehensive test |
| External quality assessment | Additional staff resource | More accurate and reproducible test and reporting |
| Pre-test Validation to identify possible polymorphic regions on parental chromosomes | Test development required at extra cost and time delay | More accurate test |
| Rescue probes | Additional cost and procedure time | More accurate test; fewer embryos discarded as false positives |
| Optimised cell spreading/fixing techniques | Additional training required | More accurate, reproducible test |
| Pre-cycle aneuploidy risk assessment | Discarded embryos may be unrepresentative of therapeutic cohort | Uses only discarded embryos from therapeutic cycle |
| *Incorporate routine follow-up analysis of embryos* | | |
| Confirm single cell diagnosis | Additional cost and procedure time | Establish ongoing accurate false positive/ negative rates |
| Estimate aneuploidy risk for individual patients | Relatively small embryo cohort | Determine for individual patients:<br>Utility of aneuploidy screening<br>Likelihood of IVF success using own eggs |

aneuploidy in single embryonic cells (whether it be the precise chromosomes to identify or the number of cells to biopsy), (b) the appropriate patients to target to obtain maximum benefit from the technique and (c) the strategy required to overcome the reduced test specificity due to high incidence of chromosomal mosaicism in human preimplantation embryos. Whatever the precise method to be used, PGS test results need to be relatively simple and easy to comprehend for clinicians, embryologists and patients since most centres providing PGS do not incorporate genetic counselling into the process and have not yet been recommended to do so (31).

## 9 Indications

Clearly, there are a number of indications for which PGS may be of benefit (since they are each associated with an increased risk of chromosomal aneuploidy). These include advanced maternal age, recurrent miscarriage, recurrent implantation failure and severe male factor infertility (11) – The situation becomes more complex when several indications co-exist in a single patient or couple (for example, advanced maternal age and recurrent miscarriage). Moreover, within each indication there is likely to be a degree of biological variance such that there is heterogeneity within each group with some patients more at risk of chromosomal aneuploidy than others. Other indications in which patients may benefit from aneuploidy screening include (a) risk of chromosomally unbalanced embryos as a result of a structural chromosomal aberration and (b) single gene disorders with an additional aneuploidy risk factor, such as age. A high proportion of embryos screening normal for specific chromosomes involved in the translocation have been found to be chromosomally abnormal when a five-chromosome screen for common aneuploidies was applied (32). Contraindications include (a) women with low egg and embryo numbers (if using PGS primarily for positive embryo selection) and (b) poor embryo quality in which case the cost-benefit ratio for PGS is shifted towards cost to the embryo.

Even with current test limitations, detailed follow-up of developmental and chromosomal abnormalities in embryos is an extremely powerful way of assessing risk for some patients. PGS should be considered a diagnostic procedure effective for aneuploidy detection (but not necessarily for embryo selection) incorporating confirmatory molecular cytogenetic analysis of any screened embryos remaining after transfer. Confirmatory analysis provides quality assurance, an assessment of true aneuploidy risk for individual patients and a detailed assessment of a patient's future prospects including clinical closure in some cases.

In view of equivocal and, in some case, poorer outcomes following PGS in clinical trials (10, 16, 19) and the professional recommendations which followed (33, 34), it is easy to forget that chromosomal aneuploidy may be the main cause of morbidity in the human preimplantation embryo. If one accepts the biological significance of chromosomal aneuploidy in the human embryo, then the question is not whether to test for chromosomally abnormal embryos, but how to test and in which target groups. Indeed, a significant proportion of women would prefer PGS to spontaneous pregnancy with prenatal diagnosis if the risk of Down syndrome was reduced by 80% and pregnancy rate was unaffected (35). Current PGS tests should be targeted only to "at-risk" patients and include follow-up of untransferred embryos to provide accurate quality assurance and risk estimates for patients. However, the "ideal test" to screen for chromosomally abnormal embryos could be used more liberally if it was inexpensive, rapid, and comprehensive for all 24 chromosomes, high resolution, accurate, non-invasive or minimally invasive and could distinguish meiotic from mitotic errors. Such a test would tip the cost/benefit ratio in favour of benefit, even in lower risk patients and regardless of the indication.

## 10 The Changing Role of Aneuploidy Screening: Focus on Follow-Up Analysis

Of the tens of thousands of embryos undergoing PGS, only a small proportion have been analysed in their entirety following single blastomere analysis and many of the published data are inadequately reported or report embryos as "normal" when up to 37% of the constituent cells are abnormal (7). Thus, limited, accurate data exists regarding the incidence of false-positives and false-negatives – both of which determine the strength of a diagnostic test. At our center, PGS is targeted to women with previous failed IVF cycles, miscarriage or termination of an abnormal pregnancy and, importantly, we strongly recommend that following PGS, particularly in the first cycle, the single cell test is followed up by analysis of every cell from the abnormal embryos. This follow-up analysis serves as a confirmatory diagnosis and helps to accurately assess the level of risk of chromosomal aneuploidy (both uniform and mosaic) for individual patients. This ensures that couples who are not at risk of uniform aneuploidy do not have repeated cycles of PGS and for women in their forties it helps to determine the likelihood of a live birth when using their own oocytes.

We propose a broader perspective of PGS following analysis of embryos identified as aneuploid from single cell biopsies, to incorporate not only (a) embryo selection (to improve pregnancy rates), but also (b) screening (to reduce miscarriage) and (c) comprehensive diagnostic information from untransferred embryos to provide patients with a realistic roadmap towards future treatments as follows:

(a) *Selection*

When more than two or three embryos (depending on age) have developed to an appropriate stage on day 3 post-insemination, PGS can be used to enhance embryo selection. Although 1 in 10, predominantly mosaic embryos, may be excluded from transfer because of false positive results, avoiding uniformly aneuploid embryos must *de facto* reduce the chance of implantation failure, miscarriage or aneuploid live birth and this is apparent on closer analysis of data from clinical trials (10, 16). Following PGS for selection, if all embryos have an aneuploid or no result, the patient may decide that one or more embryos should be transferred because of the possibility of false positive results. In such cases, the preference would be to transfer monosomic embryos, rather than trisomic embryos, based on the latter group's reduced developmental potential if uniformly aneuploid.

(b) *Screening*

The main application is to reduce chance of miscarriage or viable aneuploid birth in women at increased risk because of advanced maternal age and/or previous aneuploid pregnancy. In this scenario, PGS is performed even if there is only a single embryo that has reached the appropriate stage for biopsy on day 3 post-insemination and only screened "normal" embryos are selected for transfer.

(c) *Diagnostic*

Detailed follow-up of untransferred embryos following IVF cycles with or without PGS will reveal uniform aneuploidies or major mosaic patterns of chromosome abnormalities incompatible with a healthy live birth.

In evaluating respective goals of patients and providers, clearly, for patients, a healthy live birth within a reasonable time frame should be the primary focus. As providers, we must also take great care to help couples achieve pregnancy without the disappointment of miscarriage and resulting delay to future treatments. Indeed, we have a moral obligation to avoid the transfer of embryos that are chromosomally abnormal and also have a responsibility for the health of children born following assisted reproduction. Even current PGS, with its limitations, has been shown to improve pregnancy rates (17) and reduce common miscarriages (18) and for these reasons, may be of value to at-risk couples.

Clearly PGS has been overused as a solution to declining IVF results in women in their late 30s and early 40s and many clinics, particularly in the US, were quick to make it available to all patients. We now know that when applied to all women of advanced maternal age (10) and women under 35 with no other indication (16) the average pregnancy and live birth rates are not significantly increased and can even be reduced. Clearly, in older women the removal of a blastomere, the obligatory extended culture period and additional stress of procedures, such as biopsy (15) could further weaken an already developmentally compromised embryo. In young women, prevalence of uniformly aneuploid embryos is lower than in their older counterparts and discard of essentially normal embryos occurs owing to false positive PGS results as a result of chromosomal mosaicism. However, we believe strongly that when combined with detailed follow-up of embryos screened as abnormal from the single cell test to confirm risk, PGS is an effective method for identifying embryos with abnormal numbers of the chromosomes tested. If there is now a moral obligation to prevent multiple pregnancies and resulting increased perinatal morbidity, because it is possible to limit the numbers of embryos transferred, there must surely be an equal obligation to avoid the transfer of genetically abnormal embryos, which are either not viable, cause miscarriage or rarely can result in severely abnormal babies.

## 11 What of Clinical Relevance Have We Learned from PGS?

Chromosomal mosaicism is a fact of life when dealing with IVF embryos generated after superovulation and may be linked to the high levels of gonadotropin (36) or the *in vitro* culture system used (37). In this respect, any test - however powerful and accurate - may be limited in its ability to identify uniformly abnormal embryos unless it can identify mosaicism (through discrimination of mitotic and meiotic errors). Of more fundamental interest is the preponderance of monosomies among early human embryos. Based on a non-disjunction model for aneuploidy origin, one would predict approximately equal numbers of monosomic and trisomic embryos. Instead we have observed a distortion in the monosomy: trisomy ratio of approximately 0.63:0.37 in follow-up analysis of whole preimplantation stage embryos in agreement with previous reports (21) – presumably as the result of chromosome loss prior to the first mitotic division.

## 12 Conclusion

PGS for aneuploidy is an effective method for identifying uniformly aneuploid embryos that if transferred, would have limited or no viability or may cause miscarriage or developmental abnormality. Follow-up analysis confirms high incidence of uniformly aneuploid embryos in some, but not all, patients. The challenge for the future of PGS is to identify patients who will benefit using the safest, most cost-effective and accurate test available. In a regulatory environment moving inexorably towards single embryo transfer, we have a duty to avoid the transfer of chromosomally abnormal embryos, not necessarily to improve pregnancy rates but to avoid miscarriage and children with abnormalities. Identification of a group of embryos with uniform chromosome abnormalities may not only provide closure to the patient in terms of using her own eggs but also prevent future fruitless IVF cycles at additional expense to the couple – an expense that vastly outweighs the additional expense of PGS. Chromosomal mosaicism combined with inherent limitations of the current FISH-based test makes PGS a test of limited value if applied routinely and without targeting at-risk patients. Indeed, it is tempting to speculate that if the main embryo morbidity factor derives from maternal meiotic errors, the focus should be on diagnosing polar bodies and not blastomeres. With our current technology, however, appropriate application of PGS can provide immense benefit to a sub-group of at-risk patients. With improved microarray technology, the use of algorithms to determine eligibility and robust information to fully inform patients, aneuploidy screening could become a mainstream tool for embryo selection for many more patients and would likely complement rather than replace other selection methods.

## References

1. Gardner RJM, Sutherland GR. Chromosome Abnormalities and Genetic Counselling. 3rd Edition, Oxford University Press, Oxford, 2004.
2. Martin, RH. Meiotic errors in human oogenesis and spermato-genesis. Reprod Biomed Online 2007;16(4):523–31.
3. Griffin DK, Finch KA. The genetic and cytogenetic basis of male infertility. Hum Fertil (Camb) 2005;8(1):19–26.
4. Munné S, Dailey T, Sultan KM, et al. The use of first polar bodies for preimplantation diagnosis of aneuploidy. Hum Reprod 1995;10(4):1014–20.
5. Verlinsky Y, Cieslak J, Freidine M, et al. Pregnancies following pre-conception diagnosis of common aneuploidies by fluorescent in-situ hybridization. Hum Reprod 1995;10(7):1923–7.
6. Munné S, Sandalinas M, Escudero T, et al. Chromosome mosaicism in cleavage-stage human embryos: evidence of a maternal age effect. Reprod Biomed Online 2002;4(3): 223–32.
7. Munné S, Bahçe M, Sandalinas M, et al. Differences in chromosome susceptibility to aneuploidy and survival to first trimester. Reprod Biomed Online 2004;8(1):81–90.
8. Harper JC, de Die-Smulders C, Goossens V, et al. ESHRE PGD consortium data collection VII: cycles from January to December 2004 with pregnancy follow-up to October 2005. Hum Reprod 2008; 23(4):741–55. Epub 31 Jan 2008.
9. Handyside AH, Thornhill AR. In vitro fertilization with preimplantation genetic screening. N Engl J Med 2007;357: 1769–71.
10. Mastenbroek S, Twisk M, van Echten-Arends J, et al. In vitro fertilization with preimplantation genetic screening. N Engl J Med 2007;357:9–17.

11. Harper JC, Sermon KD, Geraedts JP, et al. What next for preimplantation genetic screening (PGS)? Hum Reprod 2008;23(3):478–80.
12. Gianaroli L, Magli MC, Ferraretti AP, et al. Preimplantation genetic diagnosis increases the implantation rate in human in vitro fertilization by avoiding the transfer of chromosomally abnormal embryos. Fertil Steril 1997;68(6): 1128–31.
13. Mantzaratou A., et al. Variable aneuploidy mechanisms in embryos from couples with poor reproductive histories undergoing preimplantation genetic screening. Hum Reprod 2007;22(7):1844–53.
14. Twisk M, Mastenbroek S, van Wely M, et al. Preimplantation genetic screening for abnormal number of chromosomes (aneuploidies) in in vitro fertilisation or intracytoplasmic sperm injection. Cochrane Database Syst Rev Jan 2006;25(1):CD005291.
15. Cohen J., Wells D, Munné S. Removal of 2 cells from cleavage stage embryos is likely to reduce the efficacy of chromosomal tests that are used to enhance implantation rates. Fertil Steril 2007;87(3):496–503.
16. Staessen C, Platteau P, Van Assche E, et al. Comparison of blastocyst transfer with or without preimplantation genetic diagnosis for aneuploidy screening in couples with advanced maternal age: a prospective randomized controlled trial. Hum Reprod 2004;19:2849–58.
17. Mersereau JE, Pergament E, Zhang X, et al. Preim-plantation genetic screening to improve in vitro fertilization pregnancy rates: a prospective randomized controlled trial. Fertil Steril 2008;90:1287–89.
18. Schoolcraft WB, Katz-Jaffe MG, Stevens J, et al. Preimplantation aneuploidy testing for infertile patients of advanced maternal age: a randomized prospective trial. Fertil Steril 2008; Aug 8 [Epub ahead of print].
19. Jansen RP, Bowman, MC, de Boer, KA, et al. What next for preimplantation genetic screening (PGS)? Experience with blastocyst biopsy and testing for aneuploidy. Hum Reprod 2008;23:1476–8.
20. Jalal SM, Adeyinka A, Thornhill AR. Chromosome analysis in prenatal diagnosis. In: Handbook of Clinical Laboratory Testing During Pregnancy. Current Clinical Pathology. Ann M Gronowski, Editor: Humana, NJ, 2004: 139–58.
21. Munné S, Chen S, Colls P, et al. Maternal age, morphology, development and chromosome abnormalities in over 6000 cleavage-stage embryos. Reprod Biomed Online 2007;14(5):628–34.
22. Harrison RH, Kuo HC, Scriven PN, et al Lack of cell cycle checkpoints in human cleavage stage embryos revealed by a clonal pattern of chromosomal mosaicism analysed by sequential multicolour FISH. Zygote 2008;(3):217–24.
23. Magli MC, Gianaroli L, Ferraretti AP, Ruberti A, Farfalli V, et al. Embryo morphology and development are dependent on the chromosomal complement. Fertil Steril 2007;87(3):534–41.
24. Wells D, Sherlock JK, Handyside AH, et al. Detailed chromosomal and molecular genetic analysis of single cells by whole genome amplification and comparative genomic hybridisation. Nucleic Acids Res 1999; 27(4):1214–18.
25. Voullaire L, Slater H, Williamson R, et al. L. Chromosome analysis of blastomeres from human embryos by using comparative genomic hybridisation. Hum Genet 2000;106: 210–17.
26. Wells D, Escudero T, Levy B, et al. First clinical application of comparative genomic hybridization and polar body testing for preimplantation genetic diagnosis of aneuploidy. Fertil Steril 2002;78(3):543–9.
27. Le Caignec C, Spits C, Sermon K, et al. Single-cell chromosomal imbalances detection by array CGH. Nucleic Acids Res 2006;34(9):e68.
28. Fiorentino F, Biricik A, Nuccitelli A, et al. Strategies and clinical outcome of 250 cycles of preimplantation genetic diagnosis for single gene disorders. Hum Reprod 2006; 21(3):670–84.
29. Rechitsky S, Kuliev A, Sharapova T, et al. Preimplantation HLA typing with aneuploidy testing. Reprod Biomed Online 2006;12(1):89–100.
30. Delhanty JD, Harper JC, Ao A, et al. Multicolour FISH detects frequent chromosomal mosaicism and chaotic division in normal preimplantation embryos from fertile patients. Hum Genet 1997;99:755–60.
31. Thornhill AR, deDie-Smulders CE, Geraedts JP, et al. ESHRE PGD Consortium "Best practice guidelines for clinical preimplantation genetic diagnosis (PGD) and preimplantation genetic screening (PGS)." Hum Reprod 2005;20 (1):35–48.
32. Pujol A, Benet J, Staessen C, et al. The importance of aneuploidy screening in reciprocal translocation carriers. Reproduction 2006;131(6):1025–35.
33. Practice Committee of the Society for Assisted Reproductive Technology; Practice Committee of the American Society for Reproductive Medicine. Preimplantation genetic testing: a practice committee opinion. Fertil Steril 2007;88(6):1497–504.
34. Anderson RA, Pickering S. The current status of preimplantation genetic screening: British fertility society policy and practice guidelines. Hum Fertil (Camb) 2008;11(2):71–5.
35. Twisk M, Haadsma ML, van der Veen F, et al. Preimplantation genetic screening as an alternative to prenatal testing for Down syndrome: preferences of women undergoing in vitro fertilization/intracytoplasmic sperm injection treatment. Fertil Steril 2007;88:804–10.
36. Baart EB, Martini E, Eijkemans MJ, et al. Milder ovarian stimulation for in-vitro fertilization reduces aneuploidy in the human preimplantation embryo: a randomized controlled trial. Hum Reprod 2007;22(4):980–8.
37. Bean CJ, Hassold TJ, Judis L, et al. Fertilization in vitro increases non-disjunction during early cleavage divisions in a mouse model system. Hum Reprod 2002;17(9):2362–7.

# Lack of Benefit of Pre-Implantation Genetic Screening

Glenn L. Schattman

**Abstract** While there have been more than 3 million babies born from the assisted reproductive technologies (ART) worldwide, success in a cycle is not guaranteed. In an effort to overcome inefficiencies in human reproduction, additional embryos are often transferred into the uterus, increasing the risk of multiple pregnancies. Despite the transfer of supra-numerary embryos, the probability of achieving pregnancy is less than 50%. Pre-implantation genetic screening (PGS) has been utilized by some programs in addition to standard IVF procedure in an effort to increase delivery rates in patients with poor prognosis for conception (advanced maternal age or prior failed IVF cycles) or to reduce the chance of subsequent miscarriage in patients with a history of recurrent pregnancy loss. Additionally, PGS has been used in an attempt to select the "perfect" embryo to reduce risk of multifetal gestation. Due to difficulties with the technique of fluorescence in-situ hybridization (FISH) used to detect aneuploidy in embryos, as well as biologic limitations of embryonic development, the goal of increasing live birth rates with ART does not appear to have been reached. In fact, in two randomized controlled trials, PGS might actually have had the opposite effect and reduced a woman's chance of having a child.

**Keywords** Assisted reproductive technology • Preimplantation genetic screening • Aneuploidy • Live birth

G.L. Schattman
Reproductive Medicine, Weill Medical College of Cornell University, 1305 York Avenue, 7th Floor, New York, NY 10021, USA
e-mail: glschatt@med.cornell.edu

## 1 Introduction

Assisted reproductive technology (ART) has helped more than 3 million couples conceive and deliver children. Pre-implantation genetic testing (PGT) is a technique that can be used in conjunction with ART where removal of one or more nuclei from oocytes (polar bodies) or embryos (blastomeres or trophoectoderm cells) allows for detection of mutations in gene sequence or aneuploidy before embryo transfer (1). PGT includes both pre-implantation genetic diagnosis (PGD) where one or both potential parents are known to carry a genetic defect and pre-implantation genetic screening (PGS) where both genetic parents are presumed to be karyotypically normal and screening is performed for the possibility of a de-novo aneuploidy in each embryo.

Pre-implantation genetic screening (PGS) has been utilized by some programs in addition to the standard IVF procedure in an effort to increase delivery rates in patients with poor prognosis for conception (advanced maternal age or prior failed IVF cycles) or to reduce the chance of subsequent miscarriage in patients with a history of recurrent pregnancy loss. Additionally, PGS has been used in an attempt to select the "perfect" embryo to transfer in an effort to reduce the risk of multi-fetal gestation. PGS has even been championed as a technique that should be utilized in every ART cycle.

In patients with previous IVF failures, recurrent miscarriages and advanced maternal age where a higher than normal rate of aneuploidy is expected to be the primary etiology for reproductive failure, PGS in theory should improve the probability of transferring chromosomally normal embryos. However, PGS has technical limitations including the possibility of misdiagnosis due to overlapping or split signals and failed

D.T. Carrell et al. (eds.), *Biennial Review of Infertility,* DOI: 10.1007/978-1-60327-327-3_20

hybridization, as well as biologic limitations including embryo mosaicism and self-correction that reduces the clinical significance of an abnormal result from a single cell in a multi-cell embryo. Additionally, when there is a limited number of embryos to test or transfer, as is often the case in the population of patients at risk of aneuploidy, increasing the probability of live birth seems unlikely, and misdiagnosis can only further reduce the possibility of success. Is the failure of implantation always due to embryo aneuploidy? Is it possible that screening for aneuploidy analyzing less than the entire complement of chromosomes in each embryo can eliminate the chance for miscarriage or are there other potential causes of miscarriage and ART failure that make this goal impossible to achieve? A critical review of the literature regarding outcomes following PGS appears to cast doubt on the clinical benefit of PGS as it is currently performed.

## 2 PGS Techniques

### 2.1 *Biopsy of Cells for Analysis*

Genetic analysis is usually performed on one or two nucleated blastomeres removed from the embryo, 3 days after fertilization. Genetic analysis can also be performed on the oocyte by removing the first and sometimes, the second polar body and by inferring the genetic composition of the oocyte from the result (2, 3). Alternatively, mural trophectoderm cells can be removed from the embryo for analysis at the blastocyst stage. To remove cells from an oocyte or embryo, an opening in the zona pellucida is created using a laser, a sharpened glass needle or acid Tyrode's solution. The polar body or blastomere(s) then may be removed through the opening using a small suction pipette or by gently compressing the embryo to extrude cells through the opening.

The decision to remove one or two blastomeres from a day 3 embryo depends on the quality of the embryo although it has been suggested that removal of two blastomeres can potentially compromise embryonic developmental competence (4). Unfortunately, this argument comes from extrapolation of data looking at cell survival after cryopreservation and thawing and may not be applicable to the biopsy procedure in normally developing embryos. Loss of one or more blastomeres from cryopreservation and thawing together with the negative impact of the cellular debris remaining in the embryo is not equivalent to the removal of one or two cells from a 7–8-cell embryo. Biologic differences between an embryo that doesn't fully survive the cryopreservation process and one that does are also not considered in this model used to refute the negative findings of a randomized controlled trial from an experienced center. Polar body biopsy avoids the possible detrimental effect of removal of biomass from the embryo; however it still subjects the embryo to possible negative impact of the biopsy procedure itself and does not account for post-meiotic events.

### 2.2 *Genetic Analysis for PGS*

Fluorescence in-situ hybridization (FISH) employs DNA probes labeled with distinctly colored fluorochromes that bind to specific DNA sequences unique to each chromosome. FISH is used to detect missing or excess chromosomal material in the oocytes or embryos. After removal of the blastomere, the nucleus of each cell removed is fixed on a glass slide and fluorescent DNA probes are added. The DNA is heat denatured and the probes allowed to hybridize to the matching chromosome. The number of fluorescent signals of a particular color reflects the number of copies of each of the corresponding chromosomal segments.

The specific chromosomes evaluated are those involved in the most common aneuploidies identified in spontaneous miscarriages, or are chosen according to the patient's prior history. The number of chromosome pairs from each nucleus that can be evaluated by FISH at present is incomplete (usually 9–11) due to technical limitations. Alternatively, the entire genome (all 23 chromosome pairs) can be amplified using random primers for analysis by comparative genomic hybridization (CGH) (5). CGH is a technique in which test and reference samples are amplified simultaneously using red (test sample) and green (reference sample) fluorochromes. The amplified products are allowed to hybridize with a normal male metaphase chromosome spread for 2–3 days. Image-processing software is used to analyze relative amounts of red and green signal to determine chromosome numbers and identify any structural chromosomal abnormalities. Newer methods of detecting aneuploidy in all 23 chromosome pairs which do not require the arduous and technically difficult task of fixing each blastomere and spreading the nucleus in a time frame that would be consistent with current limitations are in development.

## 3 Limitations in Single Cell Testing

### 3.1 Technical Limitations of Single Cell Testing

Because of the limited number of chromosome pairs that can currently be evaluated by FISH, the possibility of missing aneuploidies and transferring what appear to be normal embryos exists. Studies comparing results obtained with FISH and CGH have revealed that up to 25% of aneuploid embryos would be judged normal by FISH because the abnormal chromosome pair(s) were not among those included in the analysis. (6)

Approximately 10% of cells removed for screening yield no results, or results not confirmed by analysis of the remaining cells in embryos not transferred. The likelihood of obtaining no result or an incorrect result with FISH depends on the number of blastomeres and the number of chromosomes that are analyzed (7–9). No result may be obtained if the labeled probes fail to hybridize with the denatured chromosomes. Erroneous results may be obtained from polymorphisms or cross-hybridization or when the orientation or overlapping of chromosomes yields split or diffused signals that are misinterpreted (10). Despite best efforts to reduce this error, technical challenges remain. Even in one of the most experienced labs, the probability of not getting interpretable results from each cell was 11.6 and 15.4% using 5 and 9 probes respectively (10). Using an additional round of hybridization with probes binding to a different locus than the original probe used or subtelomeric probes, the authors were able to obtain information on 87.4% of blastomeres where they had either obtained no results or results were inconclusive. Blastomeres from embryos that had "no result" were not re-analyzed and were discarded when additional embryos with results were available for transfer. While this reduced the probability of technical errors with interpreting signals to 3.1% from 7.5% of blastomeres analyzed, some potentially normal embryos were discarded due to technical limitations of the fixation and FISH. Re-analysis also does not eliminate the possibility of other diagnostic errors.

### 3.2 Biologic Limitations of Single Cell Testing

Aneuploidy may arise in several ways. When non-disjunction occurs during meiosis, all of the cells in the embryo should be aneuploid. In contrast, mitotic non-disjunction yields two or more distinct cell lines and results in an embryo that contains both normal and abnormal cells; the actual proportions of normal and abnormal cells will vary, depending on the point at which the abnormal segregation occurred. These mosaic embryos can only be potentially identified if at least two cells are removed and analyzed. Even then, the true proportions of normal and abnormal cells cannot be determined unless all the cells are analyzed, thus destroying the embryo. In one study (11), removal of two cells resulted in discordant results (one normal and one abnormal, or both abnormal for different chromosomes) in 50% of cases. Almost 50% of these "mosaic" embryos were euploid after all cells were analyzed. Potentially, up to half of all embryos identified as aneuploid at the cleavage stage will "self correct" by the blastocyst stage (12–14). Theories proposed to explain the discordant results include embryonic mosaicism in which abnormal cell lines fail to proliferate, self-correction of the embryo weeding out the abnormal cell line, correction of the mosaicism through biopsy procedure or the possibility that the initial diagnosis was incorrect (13, 14). However, because the actual proportion of euploid cells required for normal development is unknown, abnormal results-even when discordant- must be considered potentially abnormal and therefore be reanalyzed at the blastocyst stage or the embryo discarded. Therefore, an abnormal result from FISH analysis of a single blastomere removed from a day 3 embryo is not proof-positive that the embryo is abnormal and non-viable.

## 4 Appropriate Outcome Measures

The only outcome truly relevant to a discussion on the merits of PGS is live birth rate per cycle started. Most non-controlled trials evaluating the merits of PGS use inappropriate outcome measures such as implantation rate, pregnancy rate per transfer, pregnancy loss rate or chromosomal abnormalities detected in miscarriages. Since the denominator in implantation rate (No. of embryos transferred) depends on strategy and not on the design, it cannot be used. Additionally, if approximately 20% of patients undergoing PGS have no embryo transfer performed, and these patients discard potentially viable embryos due to falsely categorizing an embryo as abnormal when in fact it was not, pregnancy rate per transfer procedure will be falsely elevated at the expense of patients who were not given a chance to conceive.

## 5 PGS for Advanced Maternal Age

The risk of miscarriage increases with advancing maternal age in both naturally conceived and IVF pregnancies and the percentage of abnormal karyotypes identified increases as women get older. (15–17). The reason for this can be traced back to the preimplantation embryo since the majority of day 3 embryos that are analyzed by FISH are aneuploid. (18, 14). Using a panel of nine chromosome pairs (X, Y, 13, 15, 16, 18, 21, 22) only 40% of embryos from women <35 years of age and 20% of embryos from women >40 were found to be normal (19). As the detection of aneuploidy among embryos increases using an expanded panel of probes, it is quite surprising that anyone ever conceives a pregnancy following ART procedures. However, with the addition of each new chromosome screened for, the risk of mis-diagnosis also increases. Despite this pessimistic outlook, PGS in theory should increase the likelihood that embryos selected for transfer will be euploid and thus result in improved implantation, pregnancy and live birth rates. However, the results achieved with PGS so far for advanced maternal age have not lived-up to that expectation.

One prospective study observed a significantly higher implantation rate (26%) in a group of 73 women who had PGS, compared to a group of 84 "controls" (14%) who chose not to have PGS but underwent assisted hatching (20). As stated previously, this study used both an inappropriate control group -since patients selected their treatment -as well as an inappropriate outcome measure- implantation rate. In a prospective, randomized, controlled trial, 400 women age 37 years or older agreed prior to oocyte retrieval to be randomized to blastocyst transfer with or without PGS performed on their day 3 embryos (21). In the PGS group, 148/200 women (74%) and 141/200 (71%) of controls went to oocyte retrieval. In the PGS group, 130/148 (88%) had embryos suitable for biopsy; one blastomere was removed from embryos having five cells and two were removed from those containing six or more cells on day 3 after fertilization. Among 685 embryo biopsies analyzed by FISH (7 chromosomes; X, Y, 13, 16, 18, 21, 22), 653 (95%) yielded results. Only 240/653 embryos (37%) were normally diploid; 353/653 (54%) exhibited a variety of abnormalities, and the remaining 60 embryos (9%) contained one normal and one abnormal cell. In the PGS group, 81/148 (55% of retrievals) received an embryo transfer, compared with 121/141 (86% of retrievals) in the control group. In the control group, 15/141 women (11%) had no blastocysts available for transfer. In the PGS group, 11/130 women with analyzed embryos (8%) had no morula or blastocysts derived from genetically normal embryos and 38/130 (29%) had no genetically normal embryos. FISH was successfully performed on the rest of the cells in 43/67 (64%) embryos considered normal on day 3 but morphologically not suitable for transfer. All contained a majority of normal cells (0% false-negative). Among 285/413 (69%) abnormal embryos reanalyzed successfully, 18% were mosaic and 8% were normal (false-positive). Among the 49/130 women in the PGS group having only genetically abnormal embryos (38/49; 78%) or no morula or blastocyst derived from normal embryos (11/49; 22%), reanalysis identified normal embryos in 2/38 (5.2%) and 1/11 (0.9%), respectively. In 6% of PGS cycles patients unfortunately did not have an embryo transfer due to false positive results. This is probably the most compelling argument against doing PGS in this study. There were 22 ongoing pregnancies in the PGS group (15% per retrieval, 27% per transfer), compared with 29 among controls (21% per retrieval, 24% per transfer) (NS). Overall, the pregnancy loss rates (including preclinical and clinical abortions) in the PGS (7/29, 24%) and control (10/39, 26%) groups were also not different.

In the only other double-blind controlled trial undertaken to evaluate the effects of PGS in older women, 408 women ages 35–41 having no previous IVF failures were randomized to undergo up to three cycles of IVF with or without PGS (22). Neither the patients nor the physicians were aware of group assignment or the number or quality of embryos transferred on day 4 after fertilization. A maximum of two embryos were transferred. Extra embryos of sufficient quality were cryopreserved, and if pregnancy did not result, cryopreserved embryos were thawed and transferred before a new cycle was initiated. In the PGS group, a single blastomere was removed from all embryos containing at least four cells. FISH was performed for eight chromosomes (X, Y, 1, 13, 16, 17, 18, and 21). If no chromosomally normal embryos with good morphologic features were available for transfer to women assigned to PGS, embryos of undetermined chromosomal composition (failed biopsy, absent or incomplete nucleus after fixation, failed FISH) were transferred. In the control group, selection of embryos for transfer was based solely on morphologic features. There were 434 completed cycles in patients randomized to PGS and 402 cycles in patients whose embryos were not biopsied. While the implantation rate for genetically "undetermined" embryos transferred into women who had no normal embryos was only 6% (6/100), there were still pregnancies from this cohort of embryos. Overall, the cumulative ongoing pregnancy and live birth rates for the group of women assigned to PGS (25% and 24%, respectively) were significantly lower than those observed among controls (37% and 35%, respectively). Since PGS in this prospective RCT actually decreased the probability of pregnancy, another way to look at these results is to identify the number needed to harm. In other words, for every nine women aged 35–41 who plan to undergo up to three cycles of IVF, there will be one MORE live birth if PGS is NOT performed (23).

## 6 PGS for Recurrent Pregnancy Loss

Recurrent pregnancy loss (RPL) is defined as three or more pregnancy losses under 500 g (before 20 weeks' gestation). If no specific cause or predisposing factor can be identified, the probability for a subsequent successful pregnancy in patients with RPL is approximately 70%, depending on the number of previous miscarriages and the karyotype of prior abortuses (24–26). Women with RPL have a high likelihood of having chromosomally abnormal miscarriages (46%) and embryos (>70%) independent of the age of the female partner (27–29). Some patients with RPL have karyotypically normal abortuses. These patients have worse prognosis for subsequent live births compared to women whose abortus was karytypically abnormal and screening of their embryos for aneuploidy is not likely to be informative or beneficial (24). PGS for aneuploidy has been proposed in an attempt to decrease the risk of implanting an aneuploid conceptus and improve live-birth rates in women with RPL.

No randomized controlled trials have been conducted to evaluate if indeed PGS improves outcome in patients with RPL. In one prospective study, 71 patients with RPL undergoing PGS for aneuploidy were compared to 28 patients having PGD performed for a sex-linked disease (controls) (28). Twenty two percent (19/86) of cycles in patients with RPL did not proceed to embryo transfer as no "normal" embryos were identified. The ongoing/delivered pregnancy rate was 26% per cycle and 33% per transfer in the RPL group, compared with 29% per cycle and 32% per transfer among controls. In the RPL group, three miscarriages (12%) occurred despite PGS while there were none in the control group. Interestingly, 71% of embryos were aneuploid in both younger (<37) and older (≥37) patient groups compared with 45% in the controls. It was also observed in this study that 62% of euploid embryos reached the blastocyst stage, while only 25% of aneuploid embryos made blastocysts- an observation suggesting that extended culture itself might help in selection of euploid embryos for transfer.

Platteau (30) prospectively compared outcomes in both younger (age <37; 35 cycles) and older (age ≥37; 34 cycles) women with a history of RPL undergoing a cycle of IVF with PGS. A large proportion of embryos were aneuploid in both younger (44%) and older patients (67%). The ongoing pregnancy rates/cycle in both the younger women (26%, mean age 32.5 ± 2.7 years) and the older patients (2.9%, mean age 40.2 ± 2.5 years) did not differ significantly from those achieved in the general IVF population. No embryo transfer was performed in 11.4% of younger patients and 47% of cycles from women ≥37 because they had no normal embryos. The conclusion of this study was that RPL patients did not derive any benefit from PGS, but the finding of no normal embryos with PGS will help with the decision to utilize donor oocytes. However, because the prevalence of aneuploidy in the embryos of women with RPL is already so high, and the possibility of misdiagnosis with PGS persists, the threshold level that would justify such a recommendation is difficult to determine.

## 7 PGS for Repeated Implantation Failure

Patients would like to know the reasons for IVF failure. This is especially true after more than one failed IVF attempt. Most PGS studies point to the embryo and aneuploidy as a possible reason for embryonic demise. PGS has therefore been suggested as a means to improve outcome with IVF in future cycles in these patients. Unfortunately, no randomized controlled trials are available to evaluate critically if PGS is of benefit to this population. One retrospective study showed that the rate of aneuploidy in patients with recurrent implantation failure is quite high; in patients <37 years of age with an average of 8.9 embryos per patient, 65.4% were chromosomally abnormal. In patients ≥37 years of age who had an average of 7.5 embryos biopsied, 70.7% were chromosomally abnormal. They observed a 31% ongoing pregnancy rate/retrieval in patients <37 years of age and a 16% ongoing pregnancy rate in patients ≥37 years of age after IVF/ICSI with PGS in a group of patients with an average of 4.2 previous failed IVF cycles. This result compared favorably with a pregnancy rate of 33% in a group of women who received IVF with PGS for sex-linked diseases (mean age of 31.6 ± 2.5 y) (31). Even with PGS, miscarriage rate was 12.5%. If we compare these findings to a group of young egg donors with a mean age of 25.4, only 43% of their embryos were considered normal after PGS with an experienced program performing the biopsy and FISH. If embryos from 25-year-old women are abnormal more than 50% of the time, the argument that aneuploidy is the main reason for repeated failed implantation is hard to justify. Additionally, PGS to screen embryos from young egg donors did not increase the chance for pregnancy in the recipients which was only 50% (mean of 2.1 embryos transferred), as the LIVE birth rate with egg donation nationally is 54% with a mean of 2.2 embryos transferred on day 3 or 5 (32).

Two other retrospective studies did not identify a difference, even in implantation rates between patients with >2 prior failed cycles and a "control" group. Patients who elected PGS were matched to a control group whose embryos underwent assisted hatching on day 3 (20). In the 27 patients with recurrent implantation failure, 54% of the embryos analyzed by PGS were aneuploid. While implantation rate appeared higher due to the use of an inappropriate denominator in the PGS group compared to the control group (17.3 vs. 9.5%), no difference in the clinical pregnancy rate or miscarriage rate was observed (22 and 20% respectively in both groups). Yet another study observed a 14.3% implantation rate in 54 cycles in patients aged 35 or older with recurrent implantation failure (2 or more failed IVF cycles), compared to 11.5% in a group of controls matched retrospectively (NS) (33). Nineteen patients (14%) had no embryo transfer due to all their embryos testing abnormal. Unfortunately the error rate for a false positive result was at least 12% in re-analyzed embryos- meaning that two patients in this group would have had a transfer of potentially genetically normal embryos and might have been pregnant had they not done PGS.

## 8 PGS for Selection of Best Embryo for Elective Single Embryo Transfer

Multiple pregnancies (twins or greater) account for 28.8% of all ART pregnancies. While the overwhelming majority of these pregnancies are twins, ideally the ability to select the single best embryo most likely to implant would improve the efficiency of the ART process and reduce the need to transfer supra-numerary embryos with its associated risks. While elective single embryo transfer has met with success in a limited population of patients (younger patients, first attempt, good quality embryos), most patients undergoing ART in the U.S. do not fall into this category and transfer of a single embryo will significantly limit their chance for success. Freezing success rates in most programs however, are not as good as success rates with fresh embryos (32), and for this reason, transferring a single embryo will decrease the chance of having a child.

One recent prospective controlled trial (34) randomized young women (age <38 years) with at least two blastocysts to either trophectoderm biopsy and PGS with analysis of 5 chromosome pairs or no biopsy with transfer of the single best blastocyst. The trial had to be terminated early as patients randomized to the no biopsy group had a statistically significantly higher live birth rate than patients who had PGS performed (58.7% vs. 35.7%, $p = 0.03$). The no biopsy control group was similar to patients who did not participate in the study and all underwent elective single blastocyst transfer. Additionally, patients who did not have PGS performed had more embryos cryopreserved for future attempts.

Are there non-invasive measures of aneuploidy in pre-implantation embryos? Morphology has traditionally been the basis for embryo selection and there are numerous classification schemes that have been developed; however the value of morphologic parameters up to day 3 of culture to predict a normal chromosomal complement or implantation potential is limited. (35–38) Extended culture however appears to be one way that aneuploid embryos will differentiate themselves. As mentioned previously, it was observed that 62% of euploid embryos reached the blastocyst stage, while only 25% of aneuploid embryos reached this developmental milestone, indicating that extended culture itself, not PGS might be helpful in selecting euploid embryos for transfer.

## 9 Conclusions

Women subjecting themselves to ovarian stimulation, oocyte retrieval and all the associated risks of ART usually do not step foot into the doctor's office and ask "what is my implantation rate?" The clinical outcome they are most interested in is the chance of having a live-birth if they start gonadotropin stimulation and proceed to oocyte retrieval. It is imperative that appropriate outcome measures are used when comparing treatments; the only appropriate measure for these patients being live birth rate per started cycle.

It has been stated that there are four potential benefits of screening for numerical chromosomal abnormalities (33). The first and second goal is to "prevent trisomic offspring" and "reduce spontaneous abortions". Nature already does this quite well as most trisomic and all monosomic (with the exception of 45XO) conceptions do not survive up to the stage of viability. Most conceptions that make it up to 13 weeks gestation will be picked-up on routine screening during pregnancy or at amniocentesis or CVS. Miscarriage rates in the Mastenbroek study were identical between the PGS arm (18%) and the control arm (18%). Likewise, there was no significant difference in either preclinical or clinical losses in the only other RCT (21). Additionally, even in the most experienced lab, patients undergoing IVF with PGS still had a miscarriage rate of 14.3% (8).

The third goal is to "minimize the number of embryos necessary for replacement and successful pregnancy". Clearly, based on the above discussions and data, PGS falls far short of this goal. If all the embryos of the patient were subjected to extended culture, embryo self-selection will help identify the best suited embryo for transfer. As PGS only "works" for patients with $\geq 8$ embryos of good enough quality to biopsy (33), these are the same patients who would be candidates for extended culture. Since the embryo biopsy itself and the removal of 12.5–25% of the embryo biomass cannot be advantageous to the development of the embryo, embryo biopsy will possibly reduce the potential for each embryo to survive.

The last goal is to "improve implantation". While PGS may be able to achieve this false goal, it does so at the expense of discarding potentially viable embryos and actually reducing the number of women who will have a child as a result of the ART procedure. By artificially controlling the denominator, total number of embryos transferred, patients are misled by an apparent improvement in a false outcome measure. As already mentioned, in doing PGS, the number needed to harm is only nine (23). For every nine patients undergoing IVF with PGS, there will be one fewer baby born. It is essential that patients considering PGS be made aware of the available evidence that no benefit is derived from PGS to improve live birth rate as it is currently performed and it may potentially lower their chance of having a child. Until data from well-designed studies is presented that unequivocally demonstrates the benefit of PGS for improving live-birth rate per started cycle, PGS should be considered experimental and should not be done outside of appropriately designed, IRB approved research protocols.

## References

1. Handyside A, Kontogianni EH, Hardy K, Winston RM. Pregnancies from biopsied human preimplantation embryos sexed by Y-specific DNA amplification. Nature 1990; 344(6268):768–70.
2. Verlinsky Y, Rechitsky S, Verlinsky O, Ivanchnenko V, Lifchez A, Kaplan B, et al. Prepregnancy testing for single-gene disorders by polar body analysis. Genet Test 1999; 3:185–90.

3. Verlinsky Y, Cieslak J, Ivanchnenko V, Evsikov S, Wolf G, White M, et al. Prepregnancy genetic testing for age-related aneuploidies by polar body analysis. Genet Test 1997–1998; 1:231–5.
4. Cohen J, Wells D, Munne S. Removal of 2 cells from cleavage stage embryos is likely to reduce the efficacy of chromosomal tests that are used to enhance implantation rates. Fertil Steril 2007; 87:496–503.
5. Wilton L, Williamson R, McBain J, Edgar D, Voullaire L. Birth of a healthy infant after preimplantation confirmation of euploidy by comparative genomic hybridization. N Eng J Med 2001; 345:1537–41.
6. Wilton L, Voullaire L, Sargeant P, Williamson R, McBain J. Preimplantation aneuploidy screening using comparative genomic hybridization or fluorescence in situ hybridization of embryos from patients with recurrent implantation failure. Fertil Steril 2003; 80:860–8.
7. Munne S, Magli C, Bahce M, Fung J, Legator M, Morrison L, et al. Preimplantation diagnosis of the aneuploidies most commonly found in spontaneous abortions and live births:XY,13,14,15,16,18,21,22. Prenatal Diag 1998; 18: 1459–66.
8. Munne S, Magli C, Cohen J, Morton P, Sadowy S, Gianaroli L, et al. Positive outcome after preimplantation genetic diagnosis of aneuploidy in human embryos. Hum Reprod 1999; 14:2191–99.
9. Michiels A, Van Assche E, Liebars I, Van Steirteghem A, Staessen C. The analysis of one or two blastomeres for PGD using fluorescence in-situ hybridization. Hum Reprod 2006; 21(9):2396–2402.
10. Colls P, Escudero T, Cekleniak N, Sadowy S, Cohen J, Munne S. Increased efficiency of Preimplantation genetic diagnosis for infertility using "no result rescue." Fertil Steril 2007; 88:53–61.
11. Baart EB, Martini E, van den Berg I, Macklon NS, Galjaard R-J H, Fauser BCJM, Van Opstal D. Preimplantation genetic screening reveals a high incidence of aneuploidy and mosaicism in embryos from young women undergoing IVF. Hum Reprod 2006; 2:223–33.
12. Magli MC, Jones GM, Gras L, Gianaroli L, Korman I, Trounson AO. Chromosome mosaicism in day 3 aneuploid embryos that developed to morphologically normal blastocysts in vitro. Hum Reprod 2000; 15:1781–86.
13. Li M, DeUgarte C, Surrey M, Danzer H, DeCherney A, Hill D. Flourescence in situ hybridization reanalysis of day 6 human blastocysts diagnosed with aneuploidy on day 3. Fertil Steril 2005; 84:1395–1400.
14. Munne S, Chen S, Fischer J, Colls P, Zheng X, Stevens J, Escudero T, Oter M, Schoolcraft B, Simpson J, Cohen J. Preimplantation genetic diagnosis reduces pregnancy loss in women aged 35 years and older with a history of recurrent miscarriages. Fertil Steril 2005; 84:331–5.
15. Simpson JL. Genes, chromosomes and reproductive failure. Fertil Steril 1980; 33:107–16.
16. Warburton D, Stein Z, Kilne J, Susser M. Chromosome abnormalities in spontaneous abortions: data from the New York City study. In: Porter LH, Hook EB, eds. Human embryonic and fetal death. New York, Academic, 1980: 261–67.
17. Eiben B, Bartels I, Bahr-Porch S, Borgmann S, Gatz G, Geller G. Cytogenetic analysis of 750 spontaneous abortions with the direct preparation method of chorionic villi and it's implications for studying genetic causes of pregnancy wastage. Am J Human Genet 1990; 47:656–63.
18. Platteau P, Staessen C, An M, Van Steirteghem A, Liebaers I, Devroey P. Preimplantation genetic diagnosis for aneuploidy screening in women older than 37 years. Fertil Steril 2005; 84:319–24.
19. Munne S, Chen S, Colls P, Garrisi J, Zheng X, Cekleniak N, Lenzi M, Hughes P, Fischer J, Garrisi M, Tomkin G, Cohen J. Maternal age, morphology, development and chromosome abnormalities in over 6,000 cleavage stage embryos. Reprod Biomed Online 2007; 14:628–34.
20. Gianaroli L, Magli MC, Ferraretti AP. Preimplantation genetic diagnosis for aneuploidies in patients undergoing IVF with a poor prognosis: identification of the categories in which it should be proposed. Fertil Steril 1999; 72:837–44.
21. Staessen C, Platteau P, Van Assche E, An M, Tournaye H, Camus M, et al. Comparison of blastocyst transfer with or without preimplantation genetic diagnosis for aneuploidy screening in couples with advanced maternal age: a prospective randomized controlled trial. Hum Reprod 2004; 19:2849–58.
22. Mastenbroek S, Twisk M, Echten-Arends J, Sikkema-Raddatz B, Korevaar JC, Verhoeve HR, et al. In vitro fertilization with preimplantation genetic screening. NEJM 2007; 357(1):9–17.
23. Collins JA. Preimplantation genetic screening in older mothers. N Eng J Med, 2007; 357:61–3.
24. Ogasawara M, Aoki K, Okada S, Suzumori K. Embryonic karyotype of abortuses in relation to the number of previous miscarriages. Fertil Steril 2000; 73:300–4.
25. Balasch J, Creus M, Fabregues F, Civico S, Carmona F, Martorell J, et al. In vitro fertilization treatment for unexplained recurrent abortion: a pilot study. Hum Reprod 1996; 11:1579–82.
26. Clifford K, Rai R, Regan L. Future pregnancy outcome in unexplained recurrent first trimester miscarriage. Hum Reprod 1997; 12:387–89.
27. Stephenson MD, Awartani KA, Robinson WP. Cytogenetic analysis of miscarriages from couples with recurrent miscarriage: a case-control study. Hum Reprod 2002; 17:446–51.
28. Rubio C, Simon C, Vidal F, Rodrigo L, Pehlivan T, Remohi J, et al. Chromosomal abnormalities and embryo development in recurrent miscarriage couples. Hum Reprod 2003; 18: 182–8.
29. Kahraman S, Benkhalifa M, Donmez E, Biricik A, Sertyel S, Findikili N, et al. The results of aneuploidy screening in 276 couples undergoing assisted reproductive techniques. Prenat Diag 2004; 24:307–11.
30. Platteau P, Staessen C, Michiels A, Van Steirteghem A, Liebaers I, Devroey P. Preimplantation genetic diagnosis for aneuploidy screening in patients with unexplained recurrent miscarriages. Fertil Steril 2005; 83:393–7.
31. Pehlivan T, Rubio C, Rodrigo L, Romero J, Remohi J, Simon C, et al. Impact of preimplantation genetic diagnosis on IVF outcome in implantation failure patients. Reprod Biomed Online 2002; 6:232–7.
32. Society for Assisted Reproductive Technology. 2006 (https://www.sartcorsonline.com/rptCSR_PublicMultYear.aspx?ClinicPKID=0).
33. Munne S, Sandalinas M, Escudero T, Velilla E, Walmsley R, Sadowy S, et al. Improved implantation after preimplantation

genetic diagnosis of aneuploidy. Reprod Biomed Online 2003; 7:91–7.
34. Jansen RPS, Bowman MC, de Boer KA, Leigh DA, Lieberman DB, McArthur SJ. What next for preimplantation genetic screening (PGS)? Experience with blastocyst biopsy and testing for aneuploidy. Hum Reprod 2008; 23:1476–78.
35. Pellestor F, Giradet A, Andreo B, Arnal F, Humeau C. Relationship between morphology and chromosomal constitution in human Preimplantation embryo. Mol Reprod Dev 1994; 39:141–46.
36. Munne S, Alikani M Tomkin G, Grifo J, Cohen J. Embryo morphology, developmental rates and maternal age are correlated with chromosomal abnormalities. Fertil Steril 1995; 64:382–91.
37. Munne S. Chromosome abnormalities and their relationship to morphology and development of human embryos. Reprod Biomed Online 2006; 12:234–53.
38. Moayeri SE, Allen RB, Brewster WR, Kim MH, Porto M, Werlin LB. Day 3 embryo morphology predicts euploidy among older subjects. Fertil Steril 2008; 89:118–23.

# The Benefits of Preimplantation Genetic Diagnosis for Chromosomal Aneuploidy

Anver Kuliev and Yury Verlinsky

**Abstract** Despite recent controversy, preimplantation genetic diagnosis (PGD) for aneuploidies is becoming a practical means in assisted reproduction technology (ART) to select embryos with higher developmental potential for improving in vitro fertilization (IVF) effectiveness. Available PGD experience for chromosomal disorders shows that at least half of the oocytes and embryos obtained from poor prognosis IVF patients are aneuploid and clearly should not be transfered, which makes PGD of direct clinical relevance to IVF. The current selection of embryos for transfer, based on morphologic criteria, cannot guarantee avoiding the transfer of aneuploid embryos destined to be lost in pre and post-implantation developments. This may explain the fact that thousands of PGD cycles have been performed for poor prognosis IVF patients, including those of advanced reproductive age, with repeated IVF failure, and recurrent spontaneous abortions, with the majority demonstrating a positive impact of preselection of aneuploid-free embryos on IVF outcome. The present review demonstrates that because of the potential benefit of PGD for chromosomal disorders, it may soon become a valuable addition to the required standards of IVF.

**Keywords** Preimplantation genetic diagnosis (PGD) • PGS • Aneuploidy • Chromosomal disorders • Oocytes • Embryos • IVF outcome

A. Kuliev (✉) and Y. Verlinsky
Reproductive Genetics Institute, 2825 North Halsted Street, Chicago, IL, USA
e-mail: anverkuliev@hotmail.com

## 1 Introduction

Preimplantation genetic diagnosis (PGD) was introduced almost two decades ago with the initial purpose of providing at-risk couples with an option to avoid the birth of affected offspring with inherited disorders, without facing pregnancy termination. It has since become obvious that the detection and avoidance of transfer of embryos with chromosomal abnormalities may allow preselection of embryos with higher developmental potential as an alternative to traditional selection of embryos, based on morphologic criteria during in vitro fertilization (IVF) because, despite possible correlation between normal morphology and euploidy, many morphologically normal embryos still have chromosome abnormalities (1–3).

Because of the potential of improved implantation rates, decreased spontaneous abortion rates, and lowered multiple pregnancy rates, PGD has now been applied in several thousand IVF cycles (4–6). It is presently performed by either the first and second polar body (PB1 and PB2) removal, or by embryo biopsy at the cleavage or blastocyst stage, and the biopsied material is tested for chromosomal abnormalities using fluorescent in-situ hybridization (FISH) analysis (2, 7) to select and transfer embryos free from numerical and structural chromosome anomalies. Although each of the biopsy methods may be used separately depending on the circumstances, the most accurate and reliable diagnosis may be achieved by a combination of two or even three different methods. For example, paternally derived chromosomal abnormalities will be missed by PB analysis, while mosaicism derived from trisomy rescue following female meiotic errors will be missed in embryo biopsy. Although more data has to be collected to exclude completely short and/or long-term side effects of multiple

D.T. Carrell et al. (eds.), *Biennial Review of Inferility,* DOI: 10.1007/978-1-60327-392-3_21 biopsy procedures, presently available data provides no evidence for a detrimental effect of PB, single blastomere, or blastocyst biopsy (8, 9).

This chapter reviews the available data on preimplantation aneuploidy testing and suggests that it is potentially beneficial for improving IVF outcome.

## 2 The Basis for Potential Benefit of Preimplantation Aneuploidy Testing

The potential benefit of pre-selecting euploid embryos for transfer is in agreement with the fact that approximately half of the oocytes and embryos tested in poor prognosis IVF patients contain chromosomal abnormalities (1, 10–14). It is established that 95% of these abnormalities originate from female meiosis, with only 5% deriving from paternal meiosis or mitotic nondisjunction (15). This is in agreement with the sperm karyotyping data, showing 1.8% aneuploidy rate on the average, with a certain increase of disomy frequency for chromosome 21 and sex chromosomes (16). On the other hand, direct testing of oocytes from IVF patients of advanced reproductive age by PB1 and PB2 analysis with fluorescent probes specific for chromosomes 13, 16, 18, 21, and 22, revealed 52% aneuploidies, of which 41% had errors in meiosis I, 31% in meiosis II, and 28% in both meiosis I and II (10, 11). It is understood that the tested oocytes were obtained from stimulated IVF patients of advanced reproductive age, which may explain the higher aneuploidy rate than described previously (17). Also the aneuploidy rates strongly depend on the overall maternal age, and may almost double in oocytes obtained from patients of 40 years and older (1, 2, 10–13).

Results of direct testing of female meiotic errors show two times higher frequency for nullisomies compared to disomies in meiosis I, in contrast to a comparable distribution of nullisomines and disomies in meiosis II (10–11). Also, the meiosis I errors of chromatid nature were observed ten times more frequently than chromosome type anomalies, with the majority of the chromatid and chromosome errors resulting in disomies in MII oocytes, which is in agreement with a higher frequency of trisomies over monosomies, described in spontaneous abortions and affected children.

It is also of note that approximately one quarter of abnormalities resulting from female meiosis I and II are of complex types, represented by different types of errors, or errors of different chromosomes. As expected, the most frequent chromosomes involved in meiotic error were the smaller chromosomes 21 and 22, although chromosome 22 errors were mainly originated from meiosis II, while chromosome 21 errors originated comparably from meiosis I and II. The other chromosome errors, originating predominantly in meiosis II, were chromosome 16 errors, while chromosome 18 errors originated predominantly in meiosis I. Involvement in meiotic error of chromosomes 13, 16, and 18 was less frequent with a specific error pattern for each of them (10, 11).

Data show that the genotype of the resulting zygote cannot be predicted without testing the outcomes of both meiotic divisions, which can be inferred from PB1 and PB2 analyses. It is of clinical significance that the testing of meiosis I errors alone reduce aneuploidy rate in the resulting embryos by at least two-thirds. Although one-third of these oocytes will still be aneuploid following the second meiotic division, PB1 testing alone may in practice improve the implantation and pregnancy rates in poor prognosis IVF patients, just by applying ICSI selectively to the oocytes with aneuploidy-free PB1. This has recently been applied in a setting in which only a few oocytes are allowed to be fertilized (12), allowing generation of only zygotes free from meiosis I errors. Although the results of testing of only the first 527 oocytes were reported, significant improvement in clinical pregnancy rate was observed, with reduction in fetal loss rate. The overall high aneuploidy rate of 59% in this series may be due to the inclusion in testing of immature oocytes, matured in vitro, in which the aneuploidy rate was 70%.

However, only half of meiosis II errors are detected by PB1 analysis; so to avoid the transfer of the embryos with all types of meiotic errors, testing of both PB1 and PB2 is still required. In contrast to other micromanipulation procedures involving embryo biopsy which may potentially affect viability of the embryo, PB1 and PB2 are extruded in a normal process of oocyte maturation and fertilization, having no biological significance in pre- and post-implantation development. Therefore, PB removal and testing may become a useful tool in assisted reproduction practices to identify aneuploidy-free oocytes, which should help in the preselection of embryos with the highest potential for establishing a viable pregnancy.

In agreement with the above PB data, 60–80% cleavage stage embryos are aneuploid (1–3, 13). Although the reported prevalence and types of aneuploidies may differ depending on the average reproductive age of patients, up to 50% of these abnormalities may be represented by mosaicism. The proportion of mosaicisms may differ depending on the morphology of the embryos and their rate of cleavage (3, 13, 17), and it cannot be excluded that the observed mosaicism, especially those with chaotic errors, may actually be the direct consequence rather than the cause of developmental anomalies or arrest of the embryos. In the majority of these cases, it is not known if the mosaic embryos were aneuploid from the onset, or became chromosomally abnormal following mitotic errors during cleavage. It may therefore be suggested, that a significant proportion of mosaic embryos originate from aneuploid oocytes, through a process of trisomy rescue (8). A possible high rate of further mitotic errors in cleaving embryos, deriving from the oocytes with complex aneuploidies, may also explain the phenomenon of chaotic embryos. A comparable prevalence of aneuploidies in oocytes and embryos, with differences in the types of chromosomal anomalies, may also support a prezygotic origin of the majority of embryo chromosome abnormalities (8).

The exact rate of mosaicism in preimplantation development is not known, because only a limited number of preimplantation embryos have been fully studied. The majority of data available from PGD for aneuploidies was obtained through a single biopsied blastomere, which may not be representative of the whole embryo. Although some fraction of postzygotic mitotic errors may derive from the cleavage stage embryos euploid from the onset, the proportion of aneuploidy and mosaicism stemming from these errors, as well as the impact of these postzygotic errors on the pre and post-implantation embryo development, is not known. Despite the high rate of mosaicism, most of them are chaotic or diploid/polyploid mosaics, associated with developmental abnormalities, and rarely reach the blastocyst stage (8). Also, only a small proportion of mosaicism, represented by aneuploid mosaics, is thought to affect the accuracy of PGD, mainly due to false negative diagnoses, evaluated to occur in 4.3%, while the false positive rate is estimated to happen in 1.3%, not actually affecting the accuracy as these embryos are not transferred anyway (13). On the other hand, for clinical purposes, such results might still not be acceptable, because the probability of mistake cannot be excluded, which may result in transferring an aneuploid embryo, or not transferring an otherwise perfectly normal embryo, because of the false positive result, unless the corresponding oocyte information is available.

A possible overestimate of aneuploidy rate, detected by blastomere analysis, may also be suggested by the significantly higher prevalence of autosomal monosomies over trisomies reported in cleaving embryos (13), which is in conflict with the above oocyte data, predicting a 3:1 disomy/nullisomy ratio (11). However, as mentioned, data on the predominance of trisomies over monosomies is in agreement with spontaneous abortions data, and may suggest that the higher prevalence of autosomal monosomies over trisomies detected in cleaving embryos, may originate from the postzygotic errors in the early cleavage, which might not have biological significance and will actually form euploid embryos with appropriate developmental potential (8, 18).

On the basis of this data, it may be suggested that the most accurate preselection of embryos for transfer in PGD for aneuploidies may be performed by a sequential testing of meiosis I, meiosis II and mitotic errors, through sequential PB1 and PB2, followed by blastomere sampling. This may allow the avoidance of transfer of embryos with prezygotic chromosomal errors, which seem to be the major source of chromosomal abnormalities in the embryo, and also the detection of possible mitotic errors in embryos resulting from the euploid zygotes, some of which may not be of clinical significance.

According to the presented information, aneuploidy testing should potentially exclude from transfer almost half the cohort of embryos, which might be aneuploid and would clearly contribute to the low pregnancy outcome of the poor prognosis IVF patients. If undetected, the majority of these chromosomally abnormal embryos will be eliminated before implantation, because only one in ten of them are expected to survive through recognized pregnancies, thereby being responsible for implantation and pregnancy failures in poor prognosis IVF patients.

## 3 PGD Experience on Aneuploidy Testing in Relation to IVF Outcome

The above data provides the background for the clinical application of aneuploidy testing, making it obvious that recent controversy about PGD application in IVF is not about its benefit, as the transfer of chromosomally abnormal embryos should clearly be avoided, but solely concerns the safety, accuracy and reliability of the testing. The high aneuploidy prevalence in oocytes and embryos makes it obvious that without the detection and avoidance of chromosomally abnormal embryos, there is a 50% chance of transferring abnormal embryos, destined to be lost during implantation or post-implantation development. So, in addition to the clear benefit of avoiding aneuploid embryos from transfer, which contributes to the improvement of the pregnancy outcome of poor prognosis IVF patients, this should improve the overall standard of medical practice, upgrading the current selection of embryos by morphological criteria to include testing for aneuploidy.

The expected obvious benefit of avoiding aneuploid embryos from transfer may explain the widespread application of aneuploidy testing, which has been performed in thousands of IVF cycles in the effort to preselect the embryos with highest developmental potential. It is not surprising that most of the large studies have demonstrated the clinical benefit of aneuploidy testing, in terms of improved IVF outcome through improved implantation and pregnancy rates, reduction of spontaneous abortions and improved take-home baby rate in poor prognosis IVF patients, including those of advanced reproductive age, repeated IVF failures and recurrent spontaneous abortions (1, 4, 5, 19, 20).

On the other hand, PGD is still a highly sophisticated procedure, involving oocyte and/or embryo biopsy, which may have a detrimental effect on embryo development if not performed up to standards (21), as well as the FISH technique applied on single cells, also requiring sufficient training and experience due to its present limitations. So the failure of observing the positive effect of aneuploidy testing on reproductive outcome in a few smaller studies may be due to possible methodological problems (22–24). In two of these reports, two (instead of one) blastomeres were removed from day 3 embryos (22, 23), which definitely reduced the implantation potential of the biopsied embryos to an extent that could not be compensated, even by preselection of aneuploidy-free embryos (25). Instead, the data were misinterpreted as the lack of PGD impact on pregnancy outcome (22, 23, 26–28), although even the absence of differences between PGD and non-PGD groups in the above study may suggest the possible beneficial effect of preselection of aneuploidy-free embryos, compensating for the detrimental effect of the two-cell biopsy on day 3 (25). In the other study also, there was a clearly detrimental effect of embryo biopsy even after single blastomere biopsy, in addition to the lack of a sufficient success rate of aneuploidy testing that could have affected the appropriate preselection of embryos for transfer (24).

Although randomized controlled studies may still be designed to further quantify the clinical impact of pre-selection of aneuploidy-free zygotes for embryo transfer, the positive impact of PGD is also obvious from the comparison of reproductive outcome in the same patients with and without PGD, as previous reproductive experience of the patients may be an adequate control for PGD impact. In the two large studies devoted to this issue, the reproductive outcome of >500 couples was investigated before and after PGD, including implantation rate, spontaneous abortions and take-home baby rates, demonstrating significant improvement after PGD (29, 30). This included an almost fivefold improvement in implantation rate, and a threefold reduction of spontaneous abortion rate, which contributed to a more than twofold increase of take-home baby rate after PGD, suggesting the obvious clinical usefulness of aneuploidy testing for IVF patients with poor reproductive performance. These results have recently been further reproduced by a number of reports presented during the eighth PGDIS 2008 Barcelona Conference, covering overall the total reproductive outcomes from thousand of patients (31). The impact of PGD is even higher in translocation patients, with a considerable reduction of spontaneous abortion rate after PGD, resulting in a corresponding increase in the take-home baby rate (30).

In the light of the data presented above, the current IVF practice of selection of embryos for transfer on the basis of morphologic criteria may hardly be an acceptable procedure for poor prognosis IVF patients at present. Without PGD there is an extremely high risk of establishing an effected pregnancy from the onset and there will be a significant compromise in the very poor chances of the IVF patients to become pregnant, especially with the current tendency of limiting the number of transferred embryos to only two, thus leaving only a single embryo on the average with a potential chance of reaching full term.

Although culturing embryos to day 5 (blastocyst) before transfer may allow, to some extent, the preselection of more developmentally competent embryos compared to day 3, at least some aneuploid embryos will still be capable of developing to blastocyst (32–33). So, these abnormal embryos will not be eliminated in the current shift to blastocyst transfer, and may implant and lead to spontaneous abortions, compromising the outcome of pregnancies resulting from the implanted normal embryos in multiple pregnancies. In fact, multiple pregnancies represent a severe complication of IVF, which may in the future be avoided by preselection and transfer of a single euploid blastocyst with the greatest developmental potential to result in healthy pregnancy.

While it may be predicted that PGD will soon become an important addition to the practice in poor prognosis IVF patients, it cannot be excluded that preselection of aneuploid-free embryos may appear of value for any IVF patient, and in future contribute to improving the overall standards of assisted reproduction practices.

## 4 Conclusions

Preimplantation genetic diagnosis is a realistic option in assisted reproduction technology (ART), to allow detection and avoid transfer of embryos with chromosomal abnormalities, with the purpose of improving pregnancy outcome. Because more than half of in vitro fertilization (IVF) patients are of advanced reproductive age, and therefore at risk of producing offspring with age-related aneuploidies, PGD may appear an important tool in improving IVF efficiency. In this context, exclusion of aneuploid embryos from transfer may clearly be considered a useful tool in any future effort in improving the effectiveness of IVF, because otherwise these embryos are destined to be lost during implantation or post-implantation development. In other words, PGD for chromosomal aneuploidies may in the future be a more valuable component in identifying embryos with higher implantation potential and in the avoidance of the transfer of aneuploid embryos, than present strategies, which mainly concentrate on morphological criteria, can guarantee. Despite the present controversy about the use of PGD for aneuploidies,the majority of available experiences, presently involving as much as dozens of thousands of PGD cycles, suggest that there is a definite positive effect of PGD on IVF outcome, if performed accurately, avoiding embryo damage. So, with the future improvement of reliability of aneuploidy testing, PGD may soon become a useful addition in the pre-selection of a single embryo with the best potential of implantation and produce a healthy pregnancy.

## References


1. Gianaroli L, Magli MC, Ferraretti AP. The in vivo and in vitro efficiency and efficacy of PGD for aneuploidy. Mol Cell Endocrin 2001; 183:S13–S18.
2. Verlinsky Y, Kuliev A. Atlas of Preimplantation Genetic Diagnosis. Taylor & Francis, London, 2005; pp. 288.
3. Munne S. Chromosome abnormalities and their relationship to morphology and development of human embryos. Reprod Biomed Online 2006; 12:234–253.
4. Verlinsky Y, Cohen J, Munne S, Gianaroli L, Simpson JL, Ferraretti AP, Kuliev A. Over a decade of preimplantation genetic diagnosis experience – a multicenter report. Fertil Steril 2004; 82:292–294.
5. Munne S. Chromosomal status of human embryo. In: Human Preimplantation Embryo Selection. Edited by Elder K, Cohen J. Informa Healthcare, London, UK, 2007; 209–234.
6. Harper JC, de Die-Smulders C, Goosens V, et al. ESHRE preimplantation genetic diagnosis consortium data collection VII: cycles from January to December 2004 with pregnancy follow-up to October 2005. Hum Reprod 2008; 23:741–755.
7. McArthur SJ, Leigh D, Marshall JT, de Boer KA, Jansen RPS. Pregnancies and live births after trophectoderm biopsy and preimplantation genetic testing of human blastocysts. Fertil Steril 2005; 84:1628–1636.
8. Verlinsky Y, Kuliev A. Practical Preimplantation Genetic Diagnosis. Springer, Berlin, 2006; XII, 204 pp.
9. Cieslak J, Tur-Kaspa I, Ilkevitch Y, Bernal A, Morris R, Verlinsky Y. Multiple micromanipulations for preimplantation genetic diagnosis do not affect embryo development to the blastocyst stage. Fertil Steril 2006; 85:1826–1829.
10. Kuliev A, Cieslak J, Illkewitch Y, Verlinsky Y. Chromosomal abnormalities in a series of 6733 human oocytes in preimplantation diagnosis of age-related aneuploidies. Reprod BioMed Online 2003; 6:54–59.
11. Kuliev A, Cieslak J, Verlinsky Y. Frequency and distribution of chromosomal abnormalities in human oocytes. Cytogenet Genome Res 2005; 111:193–198.
12. Magli C, Ferraretti A, Crippa A, Lappi M, Feliciani E, Gianaroli L. First meiosis errors in immature oocytes generated by stimulated cycles. Fertil Steril 2006; 86:629–635.
13. Munné S, Serena C, Colls P, et al. Maternal age, morphology, development and chromosome abnormalities in over 6000 cleavage-stage embryos. Reprod Biomed Online 2007;14:628–634.
14. Hassord T and Hunt P. To err in human: the genesis of human aneuploidy. Nat Rev Genet 2001; 2:280–291.

15. Templado C, Bosch M, Benet J. Frequency and distribution of chromosome abnormalities in human spermatozoa. Cytogenet Genome Res 2005; 111:199–205.
16. Pellestor F. Andreo B, Armal F, Humeau C, Demaille J. Mechanisms of non-disjunction in human female meiosis: the co-existence of two modes of malsegregation evidenced by the karyotyping of 1397 in-vitro unfertilized oocytes. Hum Reprod 2002; 17:2134–2145.
17. Munné S, Sandalinas M, Escudero T, Marquuez C, Cohen J. Chromosome mosaicism in cleavage stage human embryos: evidence of a maternal age effect. Reprod Biomed Online, 2002; 4:223–232.
18. Munne S, Velilla E, Colls P, Bermudes MG, Vemuri MC, Steuerwald N, Garrisis J, Cohen J. Self-correction of chromosomally abnormal embryos in culture and implications for stem cell production. Ferlil Steril 2005; 84:1328–1334.
19. Munné S, Sandalinas M, Escudero T, Velilla E, Walmsley R, Sadowy S, Cohen J, Sable D. Improved implantation after preimplantation genetic diagnosis of aneuploidy. Reprod Biomed Online 2003; 7:91–97.
20. Munne S, Fisher J, Warner A, Chen S, Zouves C, Cohen J, and referring centers PGD group. Preimplantation genetic diagnosis significantly reduces pregnancy loss in infertile couples: A Multi-Center Study. Fertil Steril 2006; 85:326–332.
21. PGDIS. Guidelines for good practice in PGD: program requirements and laboratory quality assurance. Reprod Biomed Online 2008; 16:134–147.
22. Staessen C, Platteau P, Van Assche E, Michels A, Tournaye H, Camus M, Devroey P, Liebaers I, Van Steirteghem A. Comparison of blastocyst transfer with or without preimplantation genetic diagnosis for aneuploidy in couples with advanced maternal age: a prospective randomized controlled trial. Hum Reprod 2004; 19:2849–2858.
23. Platteau P, Staessen C, Michiels A, Van Steirteghem A, Liebaers I, Devroey P. Preimplantation genetic diagnosis for aneuploidy in patients with unexplained recurrent miscarriages. Fertil Steril 2005; 83:393–397.
24. Mastenbroek S, Twisk M, Van Echten-Arends J, et al. In vitro fertilization with preimplantation genetic screening. NEJM 2007; 357:9–17.
25. Cohen J, Wells D, Munné S. Removal of two cells from cleavage stage embryos is likely to reduce the efficacy of chromosomal tests employed to enhance implantation rates. Fertil Steril 2007; 87:496–503.
26. Shahine LK, Cedar MI. Preimplantation genetic diagnosis does not increase pregnancy rates in patients at risk for aneuploidy. Fertil Steril 2006; 85:51–56.
27. Twisk M, Mastenbroek S, Van Wely, Neineman M, Van Der Veen F, Repping S. Preimplantation genetic screening for abnormal number of chromosomes (aneuploidies) in in vitro fertilization or introcytoplasmic spem injection. Coehrane Database Syst Rev 2006; 25:CD005291.
28. Denoso P, Staessen C, Fauser BCJM, Devroey P. Current value of preimplantation genetic aneuploidy screening in IVF. Hum Reprod Update 2007; 13:15–25.
29. Gianaroli L, Magli MC, Ferraretti A, Tabanelli C, Trengia V, Fargalli V, CavalliniG. The beneficial effects of PGD for aneuploidy support extensive clinical application. Reprod Biomed Online 2004; 10:633–640.
30. Verlinsky Y, Tur-Kaspa I, Cieslak J, Bernal A, Morris R, Taranissi M, Kaplan B, Kuliev A. Preimplantation testing for chromosomal disorders improves reproductive outcome of poor-prognosis IVF patients. Reprod Biomed Online 2005; 11:219–225.
31. PGDIS. Eighth international symposium on preimplantation genetic diagnosis. Reprod Biomed Online 2008; 16 (Suppl 3): 60 pp.
32. Magli MC, Jones GM, Gras L, Gianaroli L, Korman I, Trounson AO. Chromosome mosaicism in day 3 aneuploid embryos that develop to morphologically normal blastocysts in vitro. Hum Reprod 2000; 15:1781–1786.
33. Sandalinas M, Sadowy S, Alikani M, Calderon, G, Cohen J, Munne S. Developmental ability of chromosomally abnormal human embryos to develop to the blastocyst stage. Hum Reprod 2001; 16:1954–1958.

# The Inefficacy of Preimplantation Genetic Screening

Sebastiaan Mastenbroek, Fulco van der Veen, and Sjoerd Repping

**Abstract** Preimplantation genetic screening (PGS) was introduced into clinical practice to improve the disappointingly low ongoing pregnancy rates in subfertile couples in assisted reproduction, based on the assumption that the high rates of chromosomal aneuploidy in the cleavage stage embryos of these couples were the underlying cause. However, despite its wide availability and usage during the past 10 years, PGS has never been shown to actually increase ongoing pregnancy rates after assisted reproduction. In fact, meta-analysis of all properly designed studies conducted for the indication advanced maternal age shows a significant reduction in ongoing pregnancy rates. This lack of evidence for the efficacy of PGS and the accumulating evidence for its harm for the indication advanced maternal age, means that PGS should not be offered as a routine treatment in clinical practice.

**Keywords** Preimplantation genetic screening • Advanced maternal age • IVF outcome • Aneuploidy • FISH • Embryo quality • Mosaicism

PGS has evolved from preimplantation genetic diagnosis (PGD). In PGD a blastomere is aspirated from an *in vitro* embryo and selection of embryos for transfer is based on the subsequent genetic analysis of these cells. PGD was developed to prevent the transmission of genetic disorders from a fertile couple in which one or both partners carries a genetic abnormality (1). In 1992, 2 years after the first reported pregnancies after PGD, blastomere gender determination by fluorescence in situ hybridisation (FISH) analysis was introduced for PGD of X-linked diseases (2). Further development of this FISH analysis made it possible to determine the ploidy status of multiple chromosomes in a single blastomere and soon aneuploidy screening became a tool in itself and as such is nowadays referred to as PGS (3, 4). It was introduced into clinical practice to improve pregnancy rates of subfertile couples, based on the assumption that high rates of chromosomal aneuploidy, frequently found in the cleavage stage embryos of these couples, were responsible for the disappointingly low pregnancy rates using ART (5).

Since the first reported pregnancies after PGS in 1995 (4), there has been a steady increase in the use of this technique. The most extensive registry available to date is that of the European Society for Human Reproduction and Embryology (ESHRE) PGD Consortium, which reported on 116 cycles of PGS performed worldwide in 1997–1998 and 2,087 cycles in 2004 (6). The preliminary analysis of data from 2005 follows this trend with 2,316 PGS cycles (Fig. 1) (7). The total number of cycles performed worldwide each year is much higher, since only a limited number of PGS centers report their data to the consortium. A survey in 2005 among all US-based infertility centers showed that 127 out of 186 centres (68%) performed PGS, with a total of 2,197 cycles (8).

During this decade of increasing use of PGS, many papers have been published on this topic, but PGS has never been shown to do what it promised, which is to increase ongoing pregnancy rates after ART. Non-randomised studies comparing the outcomes of ART cycles with and without PGS did show an increase in implantation rate (the proportion of transferred embryos that successfully implant in the uterus), but no effect on clinical pregnancy rate (the proportion of

S. Mastenbroek(✉), F. van der Veen, and S. Repping
Center for Reproductive Medicine, Academic Medical Center, University of Amsterdam, Meibergdreef 9, 1105 AZ Amsterdam, The Netherlands
e-mail: S.Mastenbroek@amc.uva.nl

D.T. Carrell et al. (eds.), *Biennial Review of Infertility*, DOI: 10.1007/978-1-60327-392-3_22

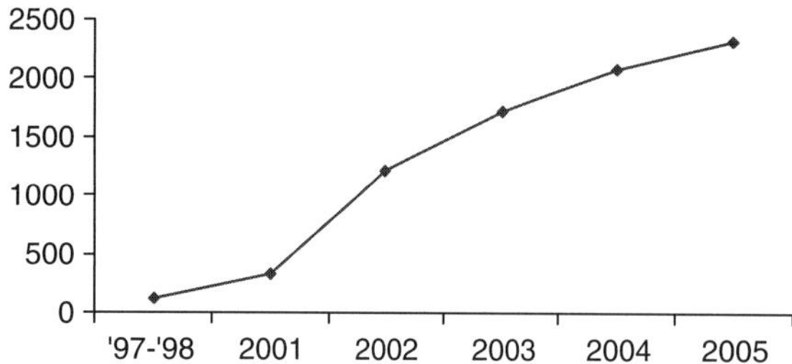


**Fig. 1** An increasing use of PGS as shown by the data collection of the European Society for Human Reproduction and Embryology (ESHRE) PGD Consortium (7)

women with a gestational sac). Surprisingly, no data on ongoing pregnancy and live birth was provided in these studies. From 2004 onwards five randomised controlled trials in women of advanced maternal age, i.e. women aged 35 years and up, were published (9–13). Combining the available data from these trials shows a ongoing pregnancy rate per cycle of 13% (92 out of 696) after PGS, vs. 21% (132 out of 638) in the control group (odds ratio 0.56 (95% CI 0.42–0.76) (Fig. 2). In other words, PGS causes a significant reduction in ongoing pregnancies in women of advanced maternal age.

Although advanced maternal age is the most common indication for PGS, PGS has also been applied for other indications like recurrent implantation failure, recurrent early pregnancy loss, severe male factor infertility and more recently good prognosis patients (6). Only one trial, presented as a poster at the ESHRE meeting in Barcelona (Blockeel, P-522), is available for patients with repeated implantation failure. This trial included 140 cycles and showed that the relative risk of clinical pregnancy per cycle after PGS is 0.60 (95% CI 0.35–1.03). For the indications recurrent early pregnancy loss and severe male factor infertility no trials have been performed. Four trials have been performed with multiple good quality embryos (14–17). for good prognosis patients, i.e. younger infertile women (<38 years of age) with multiple good quality embryos, four trials have been performed. No benefit of PGS was found in any of these trials.

PGS advocates are disputing the outcomes of the randomised controlled trials, especially the trials on PGS for advanced maternal age, on grounds of insufficient expertise of the investigators and inappropriate methods such as (1) the aspiration of two blastomeres instead of one, (2) the use of incomplete panels of probes, and (3) the low success rates of biopsy-, fixation- and FISH-procedures resulting in high rates of embryos without a diagnosis (18–22). Ad 1: Although the aspiration of two blastomeres instead of one has been shown to negatively influence embryo development, it does not seem to affect live birth rates (23). Ad 2: The selection of probes to be used in PGS is in fact quite arbitrary since there are no large detailed studies on the frequency of numerical abnormalities of all 23 chromosome pairs in cleavage stage embryos. In addition, prospective studies comparing different probe sets in relation to live birth rates after PGS have not been conducted. Ad 3: The success rates of the technical steps in PGS, i.e. biopsy, fixation and FISH-analysis, seem to be similar between the two centers that performed the largest randomised controlled trials on PGS: 97.2 and 94.2% successfully biopsied embryos, 89.1 and 93.6% successfully fixated blastomeres, and 92.3 and 92.9% blastomeres with successful FISH analysis for the centers in Amsterdam and Brussels, respectively (11, 24). No other center has ever reported their success rates per technical step making any

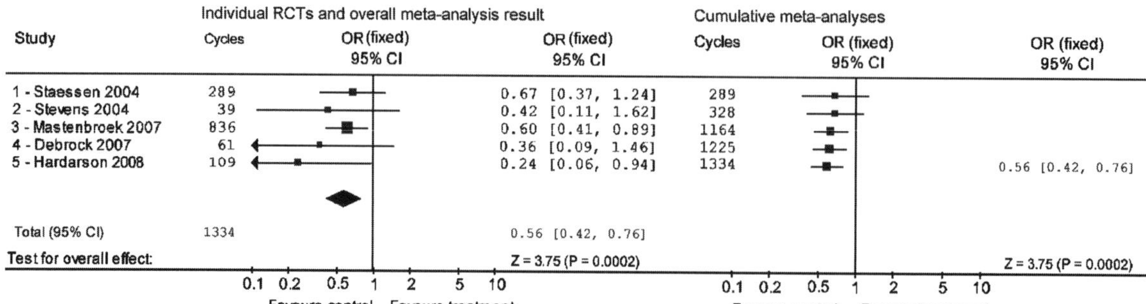


**Fig. 2** Meta-analysis of the available randomised controlled trials on PGS for the indication advanced maternal age shows a significant reduction in ongoing pregnancies per cycle after PGS. On the left is the traditional meta-analysis and on the right the same data are presented as cumulative meta-analyses (adapted from (34))

comparison unfair. Combined data of the ESHRE PGD consortium data collection on PGS shows a somewhat higher success rates (98.7% successful biopsied embryos and 89.3% blastomeres with successful fixation and FISH). This could be due to the fact that this data collection was not a prospective study with an intention to treat analysis, but a voluntary retrospective data collection (6). Thus, there are no scientific data that substantiate the claim of PGS advocates that the RCTs were of inferior technical quality.

Another commentary on the PGS RCTs for advanced maternal age was that these trials included women from 35 years onwards whereas PGS would only have a beneficial effect in older patients. Although no specific trial for patients above 40 years of age has thus far been performed, subgroup analysis from the largest trial available to date shows that also in even older patients there is no beneficial effect of PGS (25). More precisely, the rate ratio for women between 35 and 38 years of age was 0.83 and for women 38 years and older the rate ratio was 0.47 (25). Thus, although not significantly different, the effect of PGS was even worse in the subgroup of older patients. This also seems apparent from two RCTs performed by the group from Brussels (12, 17). When studying the effect of PGS on ongoing pregnancy rates in young patients (under 36 years of age) they found a relative risk of 0.90 and when they studied the effect of PGS on ongoing pregnancy rates in older patients (over 37 years of age) they found a relative risk of 0.72 (12, 17). Of note, additional subgroup analysis also indicated no benefit of PGS in subgroups of women with increased risk of embryonic aneuploidy, i.e. women with a male partner with low semen quality, women receiving high dose FSH during ovarian hyperstimulation and women with a history of recurrent miscarriage (25).

What are the possible causes for the inefficacy of PGS? First, the biopsy procedure per se may be more harmful for the potential of an embryo to successfully implant than previously thought (26). Data regarding the effect of biopsy alone on pregnancy rates are not available.

Second, the techniques used for PGS have -as do all other laboratory techniques- a certain failure rate as discussed above. Third, FISH analysis is not 100% accurate. The estimated accuracy of FISH probes used for PGS is 92–98% per probe. An accuracy of 98% per probe will result in an estimated 15% error rate for an eight-probe panel ($0.98^8$), while an accuracy of 92% per probe will result in an estimated 49% error rate ($0.92^8$). The low positive predicative accuracy of the test results in the exclusion of embryos for consideration for transfer which have the potential to be successful. Fourth, many preimplantation embryos are mosaic, which may well be the most important contributor to the inefficacy of PGS. A recent review of the literature reported that 58% of 260 cleavage stage embryos that were analysed with five or more chromosomes were diploid-aneuploid mosaic, with a mean of 61% diploid blastomeres in these embryos (van Echten et al., submitted). This means that in 35% of all embryos (0.58 × 0.61) a diploid blastomere is aspirated during the PGS procedure, which will reduce the proportion of diploid blastomeres in these embryos and lead to transfer or cryopreservation of embryos with an increased proportion of abnormal cells. Conversely, in 23% of all embryos (0.58 × 0.39) an aneuploid blastomere will be aspirated during the PGS procedure, which will lead to discarding of these embryos, despite the fact that the proportion of normal blastomeres is increased and the fact that they have potential to be viable.

Several observations support the idea that these discarded diploid-aneuploid embryos are viable. First, frozen-thawed embryos that have lost nearly half of their blastomeres due to the cryopreservation procedure are still able to result in live births, implying that not all blastomeres of human preimplantation embryos are necessary for proper development into a child (28). Second, mosaic embryos are suggested to contain rescue mechanisms that lead to the disappearance of aneuploid blastomeres once the embryonic genome has been activated (29). Interestingly, in humans the embryonic genome is not activated until the 8-cell stage which is exactly the time when PGS is generally performed (30). Third, experiments using tetraploid embryo complementation, a technique in which mice originate from ES cells that are injected in tetraploid blastocysts, have shown that even the injection of donor ES cells of which only a small percentage are diploid (20% diploid cells combined with 80% cells with chromosomal abnormalities) results in a fully diploid normal adult mice (31).

It can of course not be excluded that eventually an improved form of PGS (technically or conceptually) will help (some) couples to improve their chance to achieve an ongoing pregnancy. Such new forms of PGS however, should not be introduced into routine clinical practice before pilot studies have shown promising results which should then be confirmed in well-designed randomised clinical trials. One example is the emerging technology that provides the ability to analyse all 23 chromosome pairs in a single blastomere and not just the 5–9 chromosomes typically analysed with current techniques (32). Although these new techniques can detect aneuploidy for more chromosomes than analysed at present (and possibly with increased accuracy), they will never be able to circumvent the biological phenomenon of chromosomal mosaicism. In the light of current evidence it should be assumed that the patient will not benefit from having their embryos tested with PGS until proven otherwise.

The primary principle in medicine is to do no harm (primum non nocere). Given the currently available tools in clinical research, this ideally translates into proof of safety and effectiveness of a treatment through clinical trials first, and introduction into routine clinical practice thereafter. The days should now be behind us where a technique is routinely applied just because it is widely promoted and accepted by some professionals, such as for instance voluminous bloodletting, that persisted from antiquity well into the nineteenth century (33). The lack of evidence for the effectiveness of PGS after all these years, combined with the accumulating evidence for its harm in women of advanced maternal age, means that PGS should not be offered as routine clinical practice and to do so in fact violates the primary principle in medicine.

## References

1. Handyside AH, Kontogianni EH, Hardy K, Winston RM. Pregnancies from biopsied human preimplantation embryos sexed by Y-specific DNA amplification. Nature 1990; 344:768–770.
2. Griffin DK, Wilton LJ, Handyside AH, Winston RM, Delhanty JD. Dual fluorescent in situ hybridisation for simultaneous detection of X and Y chromosome-specific probes for the sexing of human preimplantation embryonic nuclei. Hum Genet 1992; 89:18–22.
3. Munne S, Lee A, Rosenwaks Z, Grifo J, Cohen J. Diagnosis of major chromosome aneuploidies in human preimplantation embryos. Hum Reprod 1993; 8:2185–2191.
4. Verlinsky Y, Cieslak J, Freidine M, et al. Pregnancies following pre-conception diagnosis of common aneuploidies by fluorescent in-situ hybridization. Hum Reprod 1995; 10:1923–1927.
5. Wilton L. Preimplantation genetic diagnosis for aneuploidy screening in early human embryos: a review. Prenat Diagn 2002; 22:512–518.
6. Harper JC, Die-Smulders C, Goossens V, et al. ESHRE PGD consortium data collection VII: cycles from January to December 2004 with pregnancy follow-up to October 2005. Hum Reprod 2008; 23:741–755.
7. Harper J, Sermon K, Geraedts J, et al. What next for preimplantation genetic screening? Hum Reprod 2008; 23:478–480.
8. Baruch S, Kaufman D, Hudson KL. Genetic testing of embryos: practices and perspectives of US in vitro fertilization clinics. Fertil Steril 2008; 89:1053–1058.
9. Debrock S, Melotte C, Vermeesch J, Spiessens C, Vanneste E, D'Hooghe TM. Preimplantation genetic screening (PGS) for aneuploidy in embryos after in vitro fertilization (IVF) does not improve reproductive outcome in women over 35: a prospective controlled randomized study. Fertil Steril 2007; 88:S237.
10. Hardarson T, Hanson C, Lundin K, et al. Preimplantation genetic screening in women of advanced maternal age caused a decrease in clinical pregnancy rate: a randomized controlled trial. Hum Reprod 2008.
11. Mastenbroek S, Twisk M, van Echten-Arends J, et al. In vitro fertilization with preimplantation genetic screening. N Engl J Med 2007; 357:9–17.
12. Staessen C, Platteau P, Van Assche E, et al. Comparison of blastocyst transfer with or without preimplantation genetic diagnosis for aneuploidy screening in couples with advanced maternal age: a prospective randomized controlled trial. Hum Reprod 2004; 19:2849–2858.
13. Stevens J, Wale P, Surrey ES, Schoolcraft WB, Gardner DK. Is aneuploidy screening for patients aged 35 or over beneficial? A prospective randomized trial. Fertil Steril 2004; 82:S249.
14. Jansen RP, Bowman MC, de Boer KA, Leigh DA, Lieberman DB, McArthur SJ. What next for preimplantation genetic screening (PGS)? Experience with blastocyst biopsy and testing for aneuploidy. Hum Reprod 2008; 23:1476–1478.
15. Mersereau JE, Pergament E, Zhang X, Milad MP. Preimplantation genetic screening to improve in vitro fertilization pregnancy rates: a prospective randomized controlled trial. Fertil Steril 2007; 90:1287–1289.
16. Meyer LR, Hazlett D, Nasta T, Mangan P, Klipstein S, Karande V. Does pre-implantation genetic diagnosis (PGD) improve cycle outcome in the "good-prognosis" patient? Fertil Steril 2006; 86:S72.
17. Staessen C, Michiels A, Verpoest W, Van der Elst J, Liebaers I, Devroey P. Does PGS improve pregnancy rates in young patients with single-embryo transfer? Hum Reprod 2007; 22:i31–i33.
18. Cohen J, Wells D, Munne S. Removal of 2 cells from cleavage stage embryos is likely to reduce the efficacy of chromosomal tests that are used to enhance implantation rates. Fertil Steril 2007; 87:496–503.
19. Cohen J, Munne S. Staessen et al. (2004). Two-cell biopsy and PGD pregnancy outcome. Hum Reprod 2005; 20:2363–2364.
20. Cohen J, Grifo JA. Multicentre trial of preimplantation genetic screening reported in the New England Journal of Medicine: an in-depth look at the findings. Reprod Biomed Online 2007; 15:365–366.
21. Kuliev A, Verlinsky Y. Impact of preimplantation genetic diagnosis for chromosomal disorders on reproductive outcome. Reprod Biomed Online 2008; 16:9–10.

22. Munne S, Gianaroli L, Tur-Kaspa I et al. Substandard application of preimplantation genetic screening may interfere with its clinical success. Fertil Steril 2007; 88:781–784.
23. Goossens V, De Rycke M, De Vos A, et al. Diagnostic efficiency, embryonic development and clinical outcome after the biopsy of one or two blastomeres for preimplantation genetic diagnosis. Hum Reprod 2008; 23:481–492.
24. Michiels A, Van Assche E, Liebaers I, Van Steirteghem A, Staessen C. The analysis of one or two blastomeres for PGD using fluorescence in-situ hybridization. Hum Reprod 2006; 21:2396–2402.
25. Twisk M, Mastenbroek S, Hoek A, et al. No beneficial effect of preimplantation genetic screening in women of advanced maternal age with a high risk for embryonic aneuploidy. Hum Reprod 2008; 23:2813–2817.
26. De Vos A, Van Steirteghem A. Aspects of biopsy procedures prior to preimplantation genetic diagnosis. Prenat Diagn 2001; 21:767–780.
27. Deugarte CM, Li M, Surrey M, Danzer H, Hill D, Decherney AH. Accuracy of FISH analysis in predicting chromosomal status in patients undergoing preimplantation genetic diagnosis. Fertil Steril 2008; 90:1049–1054.
28. Munne S, Sultan KM, Weier HU, Grifo JA, Cohen J, Rosenwaks Z. Assessment of numeric abnormalities of X, Y, 18, and 16 chromosomes in preimplantation human embryos before transfer. Am J Obstet Gynecol 1995; 172:1191–1199.
29. Los FJ, Van Opstal D, van den BC, et al. Uniparental disomy with and without confined placental mosaicism: a model for trisomic zygote rescue. Prenat Diagn 1998; 18:659–668.
30. Braude P, Bolton V, Moore S. Human gene expression first occurs between the four- and eight-cell stages of preimplantation development. Nature 1988; 332:459–461.
31. Eggan K, Rode A, Jentsch I, et al. Male and female mice derived from the same embryonic stem cell clone by tetraploid embryo complementation. Nat Biotechnol 2002; 20:455–459.
32. Le Caignec C, Spits C, Sermon K, et al. Single-cell chromosomal imbalances detection by array CGH. Nucleic Acids Res 2006; 34:e68.
33. Niebyl PH. The English bloodletting revolution, or modern medicine before 1850. Bull Hist Med 1977; 51:464–483.
34. Antman EM, Lau J, Kupelnick B, Mosteller F, Chalmers TC. A comparison of results of meta-analyses of randomized control trials and recommendations of clinical experts. Treatments for myocardial infarction. JAMA 1992; 268:240–248.

# Index